Brain Metastases

Mikhail Dolgushin • Valery Kornienko
Igor Pronin

Brain Metastases

Advanced Neuroimaging

Springer

Mikhail Dolgushin
N.N. Blockhin Russian Cancer Research Center
Moscow
Russia

Igor Pronin
N.N. Burdenko National Scientific and
Practical Center for Neurosurgery
Moscow
Russia

Valery Kornienko
N.N. Burdenko National Scientific and
Practical Center for Neurosurgery
Moscow
Russia

ISBN 978-3-319-86240-8 ISBN 978-3-319-57760-9 (eBook)
DOI 10.1007/978-3-319-57760-9

Softcover reprint of the hardcover 1st edition 2017

Printed on acid-free paper

This Springer imprint is published by Springer Nature
The registered company is Springer International Publishing AG
The registered company address is: Gewerbestrasse 11, 6330 Cham, Switzerland

Foreword

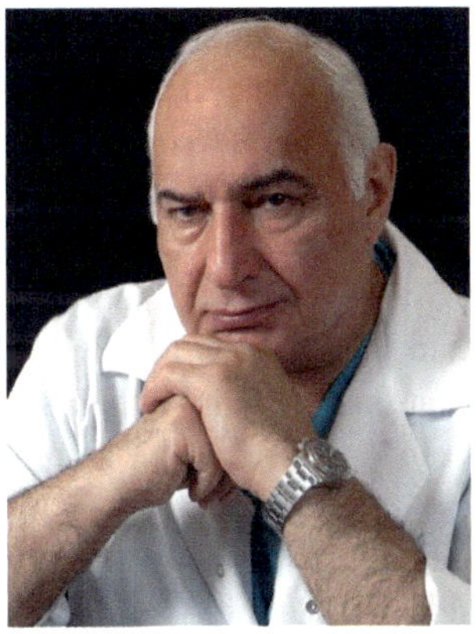

Dear colleagues,

With great pleasure, I present in this monograph the result of many years of scientific and practical collaboration between the two largest clinical research institutions of the Ministry of Health of the Russian Federation, the N. N. Blokhin Russian Cancer Research Center and N. N. Burdenko National Scientific and Practical Center for Neurosurgery, in investigation and improvement of the methods of differential diagnosis and treatment of focal cerebral lesions.

This fundamental scientific work is based on the results of the diagnosis and treatment of more than 3000 patients with brain metastases from malignancies with various natures and different sites. The authors performed a comparative analysis of the comparable number of cases of primary tumors and other focal brain lesions in order to develop effective approaches for differential diagnosis, prognosis, and treatment for conditions that differ by their nature but have similar clinical and neuroimaging manifestations.

Neuroimaging is one of the most rapidly developing areas in radiology. Until recently by historical standards, we were able to look inside the skull only during surgery, and only a very limited area of a surgical wound was available for such an inspection. In order to extend these boundaries, to make visible the entire brain and its surrounding structures, CT and MRI technologies were developed in the late 1980s, and the first patients, who underwent these studies, were patients with focal brain lesions.

Until now, neuro-oncology traditionally has been a separate branch of clinical oncology. Today the key fundamentals of cancer therapy are based on the consensus regarding manifestations of oncological diseases in the organism, including the brain, from the point of view of development, prognosis, and modern treatment options (surgery, radiation, and drug therapy).

Primary brain tumors have their patterns of growth and development; they rarely metastasize and often are the object of professional interest of neuro-oncologists and neurosurgeons. At the same time, the secondary tumors in the brain—tumor metastases—represent a common issue for oncologists with any specialization.

The reality confirmed by statistics is that the number of patients with metastatic brain lesions is growing, due to improved quality of treatment of cancer patients—patients live longer and, as expected, this increases the long-term risk of distant metastases.

Brain metastases are indicative of advanced cancer. Until recently, therapeutic measures for patients with brain metastases were limited only to providing symptomatic relief to the patient. It would be wrong to assert that a bias toward the symptomatic treatment for patients with advanced tumors is completely eliminated, but nevertheless the success of modern oncology reduces the level of hopelessness and despair: a breakthrough in drug treatment and radiation therapy technology allows for a full response therapy even for patients with multiple metastases.

At the same time, a successful treatment cannot be imagined without a preceding qualitative investigation aimed at assessing the state of all organs and systems, including the brain. This is also applicable to interim investigations to assess the effectiveness of the therapy.

The comprehensive approach used by the authors to study this issue appears to be particularly valuable. Biological characteristics of metastasis and invasion of secondary tumors into the brain substance are presented in detail. A number of specific manifestations of brain metastases are described based on the morphology of the primary tumor. Some technical capabilities of neuroimaging are presented that are to be used in the diagnostician's everyday practice. The authors provide excellent illustrations for the variants of manifestations of brain metastases from various primary tumors using radiation diagnostic technologies: from direct angiography to CT, MRI, and PET.

Differential diagnosis of focal lesions and ways of solving differential diagnostic difficulties in the context of secondary brain tumors are also presented in this monograph. The authors pay particular attention to identification, verification, and differential diagnosis of treatment-induced changes in the brain tissue at the tumor lesion, caused by different treatments. The issue of identifying post-radiation changes (necrosis) after various radiotherapy regimens concerns almost half of cases of patients who received this treatment, and this area (evaluation of antitumor treatment) is reflected in this monograph.

The professional authority of the authors is beyond argument. Valery Nikolaevich Kornienko (academician, professor, corresponding member of the Russian Academy of Sciences), Igor Nikolaevich Pronin (professor), and Mikhail Borisovich Dolgushin (professor) are known Russian neuroradiologists. It is significant that this treatise by highly respected authors is a logical continuation of a series of monographs previously published by the team.

The represented monograph will be very useful not only for entry-level specialists in diagnostic radiology but also for experienced and wordly wise colleagues, as well as neurosurgeons, surgeons, oncologists, neurologists, chemotherapists, and radiation therapists.

Mikhail Davydov
Academician of the Russian Academy
of Sciences, Chief Oncologist
of the Russian Ministry of Health,
Director of the N. N. Blokhin
Russian Cancer Research Center,
Honored Scientist, Doctor
of Medicine Sciences,
Moscow, Russia

Preface

The monograph presented to the professional audience is the result of many years of study of one of the most complex issues in oncology—the diagnosis of metastatic brain lesions. Clinical and research work that allowed to accumulate our unique clinical material was carried out in close cooperation with the personnel of the N. N. Blokhin Russian Cancer Research Center and N. N. Burdenko National Scientific and Practical Center for Neurosurgery and is based on the analysis of over 3000 clinical cases.

The first part of the monograph is devoted to the epidemiology and etiopathogenesis of tumor lesions in the brain, biological bases and pathophysiological mechanisms of primary and metastatic tumors, factors and conditions that contribute to "unauthorized" crossing of the blood-brain barrier, clinical manifestations, and treatment of patients with metastatic brain lesions.

The second part presents a comprehensive range of modern diagnostic methods and techniques in the service of a neuroradiologist. We describe the physical and mathematical foundations of a qualitative and quantitative analysis of findings obtained using high-tech applications and characterize radiological semiology and basic parametric properties of metastases in the brain from various primary tumors, obtained using both standard CT and MR sequences, as well as the entire arsenal of supplemental CT and MR applications. The PET method is also adequately presented: in particular, its possibilities in the diagnosis of intra- and extracranial diseases.

The third part is devoted to the analysis of characteristics of pathophysiological processes occurring in the brain substance when it is affected by metastases from primary tumors of various origins and morphogenesis. We provided the information related to the methods of use of parametric data obtained by means of modern diagnostic technologies: a "map" for establishing a justified differential diagnosis aimed at the indication of intracerebral metastases and identification of their organ and tissue of origin. This section is illustrated by many typical clinical examples.

The fourth part is devoted to neoplastic and non-neoplastic diseases characterized by focal changes in the brain substance. In a basis — the analysis of the diagnostic data obtained by means of routine and modern diagnostic technologies. Approaches to the recognition of specifics of focal lesions among possible biological varieties, as well as the principles of differential diagnosis, are described. Specifics of the diagnostic information that should be considered for the justified construction of a differential diagnostic series are also discussed.

The book is intended for radiologists, oncologists, neuroradiologists, neurosurgeons, neurologists, scientists, and, of course, young medical specialists starting their professional career in the field of clinical medicine such as postgraduate students, residents, and medical students.

Moscow, Russia Mikhail Dolgushin

Contents

About the Authors

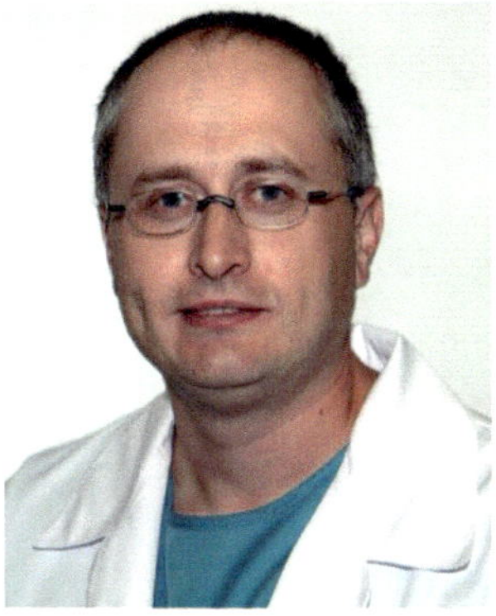

Mikhail Dolgushin M.D., Ph.D. is a professor of the Russian Academy of Sciences and head of PET Department of the N. N. Blokhin Russian Cancer Research Center in Moscow. He is the author of more than 100 scientific publications.

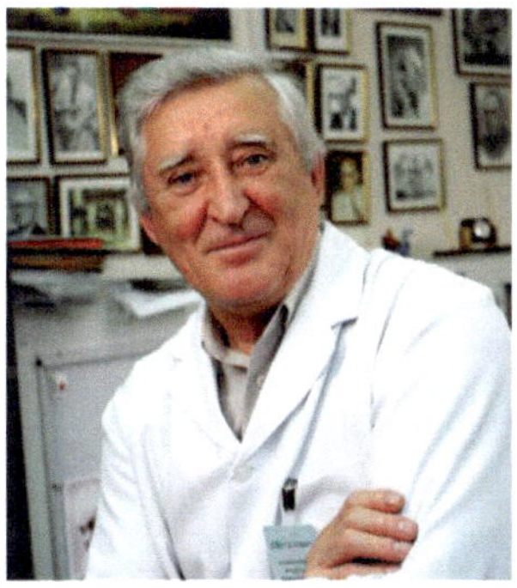

Valery Kornienko M.D., Ph.D. is an academician of the Russian Academy of Sciences, a famous Russian neuroradiologist in the former Russian School of Neuroradiology, and a full member of the Russian and American Society of Neuroradiology. He is the author of 21 monographs (two of them in Springer) as well as more than 500 scientific publications in the field of neuroradiology.

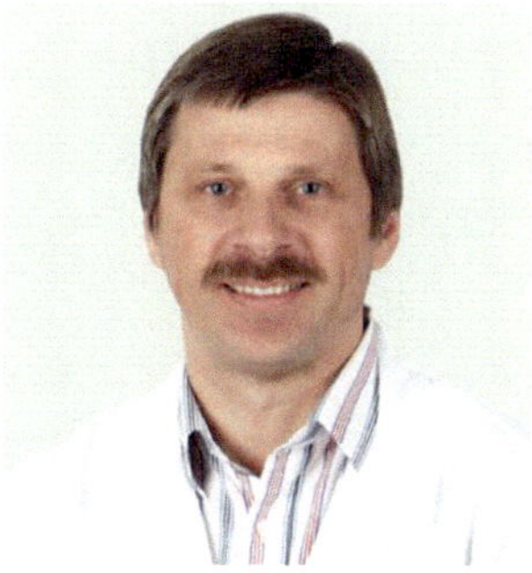

Igor Pronin M.D., Ph.D. is the head of the Neuroimaging Department of the N. N. Burdenko National Scientific and Practical Center for Neurosurgery by the Russian Ministry of Health. He is an academician of the Russian Academy of Sciences, a professor, and a neuroradiologist and the author of 14 monographs (two of them in Springer) and more than 350 scientific publications in the field of neuroradiology.

Part I

Etiology, Pathogenesis, Symptoms and Treatment of Brain Metastates

Prevalence of Brain Metastases

1

From the standpoint of radiology, the brain is a unique organ, whose substance enclosed in a rather thin bone "shell" could be differentiated as gray and white matter due to its relative homogeneity and immobility as early as on images obtained using the first models of CT scanners. Subsequently, imaging techniques, particularly MRI, allowed for a more accurate visualization of cerebral structural features and better identification of pathological changes in the brain structure than with CT. Requirements of clinicians for quantitative and most importantly qualitative content of the obtained diagnostic findings are constantly growing. In terms of diagnostic requests of modern medicine, a mere statement of the fact of visualization of a focal brain lesion is definitely not enough in most cases. The actual clinical situation is such that a formal description of syntopical features of focal brain lesions is the distant past of continuously developing neuroimaging methods. Today, there is a demand for technology allowing to obtain information that brings findings of noninvasive radiation diagnostic methods as close as possible to the exact interpretation of the histologic nature of lesions, an objective assessment of the characteristics of their blood supply, etc., without any techniques with traumatic access to abnormal sites.

In neuroimaging, a differential diagnostic series in focal brain lesions includes primary tumors, metastases of tumors from other sites, and ischemia. It is important to remember that an X-ray pattern in metastatic brain lesions is characterized by a variety of manifestations and dynamic development of secondary tumors, which is essential for the interpretation of diagnostic evidence in patients without history of tumors. The right selection of treatment tactics for such patients directly depends on the reliability of neuroradiological findings that should indicate the secondary nature of intracranial neoplasms as accurately as possible.

This monograph is based on the analysis of clinical cases of more than 3000 patients with metastatic brain lesions, including the steps of the primary and differential diagnosis, as well as various stages of treatment at the N.N. Blokhin Russian Cancer Research Center and N.N. Burdenko Research Institute of Neurosurgery. We did our best to highlight the ways of solving the main problems related to both the issues of primary and differential diagnosis (including modern methods of determining a true site of primary tumor and the disease extent in general), as well as some aspects of diagnosis of treatment-induced changes in the brain tissue, developing after surgery, radiotherapy, and antitumor drug treatment, involving capabilities of the entire range of modern diagnostic methods (computed, magnetic resonance, and positron emission tomography).

A *metastasis* (from the Greek μετάστασις, "transference, removal, change") is a distant secondary focus of a pathological process caused by the transfer of its origin (tumor cells, microorganisms) from the primary site through the body tissues. In the modern sense, a metastasis usually characterizes local spread of cancer cells (Encyclopedia).

The fact that malignant tumors can metastasize into the brain has long been known; however, such metastases used to be identified very rarely; therefore, the treatment of such patients was associated with considerable difficulties. In 1888, Cowers divided intracranial lesions by their frequency into six categories, with metastatic carcinoma being on the third place by its frequency. Also in 1888, Bramwell noted that brain metastases could originate from any organ system but in particular from the lungs and that the latter, in turn, were a certain "filter" for metastases of tumors from other sites. In 1889, Paget proposed the theory of metastasizing, according to which the brain substance was presented as a great culture medium for foreign organisms. He suggested that metastasizing was not a spontaneous process but occurred only in cases where there was a specific interaction between the migrating tumor cells and a recipient organ—the seed and soil hypothesis.

Further study of the issue did not result in any significant advances, and many tumors described as carcinoma actually had a metastatic nature. Only in 1927, Globus and Selinsky published their paper that described clinical and pathological

M. Dolgushin et al., *Brain Metastases*, DOI 10.1007/978-3-319-57760-9_1

manifestations of the disease in 12 patients with brain metastases, and already in 1933, a symptomatic classification was developed based on clinical manifestations of brain metastases that may differ from other manifestations of intracranial tumors. This classification became the first differential diagnostic algorithm for brain neoplasms. From that moment on, approaches to the treatment of secondary tumors in the brain began to differ from those generally accepted.

The quantitative criterion gives particular relevance to the issue of metastatic brain lesions: it is a fair assumption to say that patients with metastatic brain tumors already make up more than half of the entire cohort of neuro-oncological patients. The majority of patients receive a complex therapy with an emphasis on radiosurgical treatment. As such, surgical removal of metastatic brain tumors becomes a more and more rare treatment strategy and is performed either for solitary lesions or after failure of other methods of cancer treatment. The key point in deciding on the tactics of treatment becomes criteria of patient's objective status, the presence and extent of metastatic involvement of other organs. For this reason, patients with metastatic brain lesions cannot be regarded solely as neuro-oncological patients: the extent of neoplastic lesions in the body and foci of metastatic lesions, whose manifestations are dominant in the clinical picture of the disease, should be taken into account.

According to Langer and Mehta (2005), the number of new cases of metastatic brain lesions in malignant tumors identified in the USA each year is more than 170,000, and, according to Smedby et al. (2009), it tends to increase. Analyzing the statistics of the incidence of malignant tumors in Russia and taking into account average results of cooperative studies on the incidence of cerebral metastases, it can be assumed that it is actually 70,000 persons a year. A number of factors may contribute to an increased incidence of cerebral metastases, including introduction of high-tech neuroimaging techniques and increased life expectancy of cancer patients. Based on WHO prognoses, the number of cancer cases will continue to grow from 14 million in 2012 to 22 million in the next decade.

According to the international project GLOBOCAN 2012 of the WHO International Agency for Research on Cancer (*IARC*), including statistics from 184 countries around the world, the most frequent carcinomas in the male population are as follows: lung cancer (16.7% of all cancers), prostate cancer (15.0%), colorectal cancer (10.0%), gastric cancer (8.5%), and liver cancer (7.5%). At the same time, mortality among men is 23.6% from lung cancer, 11.2% from liver cancer, and 10.1% from stomach cancer. Lung cancer in the male population has the highest incidence rate—34.2 per 100,000—and the highest mortality rate, 30.0 per 100,000 persons. The incidence rate of prostate cancer that occupies the second place among all cancers is 31.1 per 100,000 persons, but its mortality is significantly lower—7.8 per 100,000 compared to lung cancer. In the women's population, breast cancer has the highest incidence (25.2%). It is followed by colorectal cancer (9.2%), lung cancer (8.7%), cervical cancer (7.9%), and stomach cancer (4.8%). Note that the mortality from breast cancer has decreased to 14.7% as compared to 2011 and mortality from lung cancer in women accounts for 13.8%.

Taking into account both sexes, according to GLOBOCAN 2012, the most prevalent are lung cancer (13.0%), breast cancer (11.9%), colorectal cancer (9.7%), prostate cancer (7.9%), and gastric cancer (6.8%). The incidence of cancer increases dramatically with age. Thus, the incidence of cancer in the pediatric population (0–14 years of age) is 10 per 100,000; it becomes 150 per 100,000 by 40–44 years of age and more than 500 per 100,000 by 60–64 years of age (GLOBOCAN 2012).

The highest cancer rates are reported in industrialized countries of North America, Western Europe, as well as in Japan, the Republic of Korea, Australia, and New Zealand. Medium incidence is observed in Central and South America, East European countries, and Southeast Asian countries, including China. The lowest rate is reported in Africa and in western and southern parts of Asia, including India. In the industrialized countries of Europe, in the USA, and in Canada, the prevalent cancers are prostate cancer, breast cancer, lung cancer, and colorectal cancer. In Eastern and Central Asia with the most densely populated regions (57% of the global population, including 19% for China, 18% for India), lung cancer and gastrointestinal carcinoma are most commonly identified in the male population. In female population from these regions, breast cancer, lung cancer, cervical cancer, colorectal cancer, and gastric cancer prevail. Table 1.1 shows the statistical data on cancer incidence in the world population and in Russia, according to the WHO for 2012 (GLOBOCAN 2012).

The risk of malignant tumor metastasizing increases with the age of patients. Thus, according to Walker et al. (1985), one case of metastasizing per 100,000 is detected in individuals younger than 35 years of age, and 30 cases per 100,000 are detected in persons over 60 years of age. Brain metastases are often identified in elderly patients. Thus, according to Raizer et al. (2007), up to 60% of metastatic brain lesions are detected in patients aged 50–70 years of age, which correlates with the highest incidence of malignant neoplasms; 70% of deaths from cancer in the USA are reported in patients older than 65 years of age (Yancik and Ries 2004). However, several authors point out that there is a higher risk of brain metastases in young patients with carcinoma with any site than in older patients, which indicates a more aggressive course of the disease (Graus et al. 1986; Tasdemiroglu and Patchell 1997; Schouten et al. 2002; Pronin et al. 2005).

Table 1.1 Cancer statistics in Russia and worldwide (WHO 2012)

Primary site	RF/total	Incidence Abs.	(%)	ASR(W)	Morbidity Abs.	%
Lungs	RF	55,805	12.2	24.0	5,450,888	17.2
	Total	1,824,701	13.0	23.1	1,589,925	19.4
Breast	RF	57,502	12.5	45.6	24,544	8.3
	Total	1,671,149	11.9	43.1	521,907	6.4
Melanoma	RF	8717	1.9	4.1	3632	1.2
	Total	232,130	1.7	3.0	55,488	0.7
Colorectal	RF	59,928	13.1	24.5	39,907	13.5
	Total	1,360,602	9.7	17.2	693,933	8.5
Kidneys	RF	19,313	4.2	8.9	9025	3.1
	Total	337,860	2.4	4.4	143,406	1.7
Stomach	RF	38,417	8.4	16.0	32,854	11.1
	Total	951,594	6.8	12.1	723,073	8.8
Esophagus	RF	7263	1.6	3.1	6499	2.2
	Total	455,784	3.2	5.9	400,169	4.9
Pancreas	RF	14,512	3.2	6.0	16,371	5.5
	Total	337,872	2.4	4.2	330,391	4.0
Cervix	RF	15,342	3.3	15.3	7371	2.5
	Total	527,624	3.8	14.0	265,672	3.2
Uterine body	RF	20,972	4.6	16.1	5477	1.9
	Total	319,605	2.3	8.3	76,160	0.9
Ovaries	RF	13,373	2.9	11.3	7971	2.7
	Total	238,719	1.7	6.1	151,917	1.9
Prostate	RF	26,885	5.9	30.1	11,480	3.9
	Total	1,094,916	7.8	30.7	307,481	3.7
Testicles	RF	1330	0.3	1.8	399	0.1
	Total	55,266	0.4	1.5	10,351	0.1
Thyroid	RF	10,174	2.2	5.2	2020	0.7
	Total	298,102	2.1	4.0	39,771	0.5
Liver	RF	6812	1.5	2.9	8521	2.9
	Total	782,451	5.6	10.1	745,533	9.1
Gallbladder	RF	3411	0.7	1.3	2834	1.0
	Total	178,101	1.3	2.2	142,823	1.7
Larynx	RF	6421	1.4	2.9	4309	1.5
	Total	156,877	1.1	2.1	83,376	1.0
Bladder	RF	13,853	3.0	5.7	6843	2.3
	Total	429,793	3.1	5.3	165,084	2.0
Other	RF	78,352	17.1	–	54,352	18.4
	Total	2,814,748	19.7	–	1,755,115	21.5
All cancers	RF	458,382	100.0	204.3	295,357	100.0
	Total	14,067,894	100.0	182.0	8,201,575	100.0

Note. ASR (W)—Standardized incidence of cancers in the world (% per 100,000)

Brain metastases in children occur in 4–13% (Vannucci and Baten 1974; Graus et al. 1983; Posner 1995; Tasdemiroglu and Patchell 1997; Paulino et al. 2003; Kebudi et al. 2005; Yoshida 2007; Salvati et al. 2010). The average time of MTS development after the identification of the primary tumor is 327 days. The most common tumors in children under 15 years of age are lymphoma, osteosarcoma, rhabdomyosarcoma, and Ewing's sarcoma (Graus et al. 1983). Embryonal tumors typically metastasize in patients aged 15–22 years. Rhabdomyosarcoma metastasizes more frequently than Ewing's sarcoma. According to Rodriguez-Galindo et al. (1997), melanoma metastases in the brain developed in 18% of cases (analysis of 44 pediatric cases).

Brain metastases are the most common tumor-related abnormality in the central nervous system and the most common intracranial tumor lesion that surpasses the number of primary brain tumors by several times. An autopsy identifies brain metastases in 20–40% of patients with metastatic cancers.

Walker et al. (1985) reported that the risk of brain metastases from malignant tumors is higher in males than in females (9.7 and 7.1 per 100,000, respectively). Lung cancer most often metastasizes in men (6.1 and 2.2 per 100,000, respectively), while in women, breast cancer metastasizes most often. However, one recent study by Nieder et al. (2010) that analyzed the changes in the epidemiology of brain metastases within the last two decades revealed the prevalence of the female population. The authors attribute this fact to an increase in the lung cancer incidence among women lately.

Based on the results of numerous studies on the diagnosis and treatment of brain metastases, we can confidently say that lung cancer is the most common cause of secondary tumor brain lesions (Baker et al. 1951; Nugent et al. 1979; Emami and Graham 1997; Andre et al. 2004; Smedby et al. 2009; Nieder et al. 2010).

Frequency of brain metastases by primary tumor site is provided in Table 1.2.

The greatest increase in the number of patients with brain metastases over the past two decades may be associated not only with an increased epidemiological factor of specific histological forms of cancers (Barnholtz-Sloan et al. 2004; Pestalozzi et al. 2006; Pelletier et al. 2010) but also with a broader introduction of high-tech diagnostic equipment.

Findings of numerous authors indicate a decrease in the detection rate of solitary metastases from 63% to 29% (Delattre et al. 1988; Gaspar et al. 1997; Sperduto et al. 2008; Eichler et al. 2008; Nieder et al. 2010) and a significant increase in multiple (three or more) metastases from 17% to 36% (Villà et al. 2011; Nieder et al. 2010; Fabi et al. 2011) over the past two decades. In general, about 10–20% of brain metastases represent a single lesion, and more than 80% represent multifocal brain lesions.

Recent studies show that simultaneous diagnosis of intracranial metastases and identification of the primary tumor is a more common diagnostic tactics, especially if MRI is used (Heon et al. 2010; Villà et al. 2011; Vuong et al. 2011; Zakaria et al. 2014). Whole-body studies based on new MRI technologies in patients with newly diagnosed metastatic brain lesions allow to suggest the site of the primary tumor and assess the disease extent in general as part of one investigation.

Metastases with an unknown primary origin (UPO) make up 5–10% of cases. In these cases, the primary origin may be cancer of unknown primary origin or rare metastatic tumors. Thus, Brehar et al. (2013) identified multifocal brain metastases with UPO; immunohistochemistry diagnosed endocrine cancer that rarely metastasizes to the brain. Araujo (2013) identified several sub- and cortical space-occupying lesions in both cerebral hemispheres. The investigations conducted, including chest CT, showed no abnormalities. Due to the impossibility of performing spectroscopic and perfusion studies, a stereotactic biopsy was performed that verified by the diagnosis of primary papillary lung adenocarcinoma. In general, cancer from UPO is a complex still unresolved issue in clinical oncology.

Table 1.2 Frequency of brain metastases of malignant tumors with various sites (according to Nussbaum et al. 1996)

Primary tumor site	Frequency of metastasizing (%)	Single metastases (%)	Multiple metastases (%)
Lung	40	48	52
Breast	17	49	51
Melanoma	11	49	51
Kidney	6	56	44
GIT	6	67	33
Uterus/vagina	5	53	47
Unknown origin	5	70	30
Ovary	2	57	43
Bladder	2	64	36
Prostate	2	82	18
Testicles	2	55	45
Other	4	65	47
TOTAL	100	53	47

1.1 Lung Cancer Metastases

Lung cancer (LC) is one of the most common human malignancies. Worldwide, about one million of people develop lung cancer each year; the tumor occupies the first place in the structure of cancer among men in Russia. According to numerous authors, lung cancer metastasizes in 18 to 65% of cases (Baker 1942; Abrams et al. 1950; Baker et al. 1951; Nugent et al. 1979; Takakura et al. 1982; Graf et al. 1988; Burt et al. 1992; Ceresoli et al. 2004), with 40% of the total number of lung metastases constituting metastases of small cell cancer (SCLC) and adenocarcinoma: these tumors are two times more likely to metastasize than other lung cancers (Cox et al. 1986; Sen et al. 1998).

According to Alexander et al. (1996), brain metastases are identified in 10% of SCLC patients at their initial presentation to a healthcare provider and are identified during treatment in more than 20% of patients. Autopsy findings indicate that 40 to 60% of SCLC patients have brain metastases at time of death. High risk of cerebral metastases was the main reason for the inclusion of prophylactic cranial irradiation (PCI) in the treatment program for patients with SCLC and a mandatory MRI or CT with contrast enhancement (Babchin et al. 1974a, b; Idrisov 1980; Halimova 1982; Ragayshene

1985; Kristijansen 1989; Lester et al. 2005; Slotman et al. 2007; Gustavo et al. 2009).

Several authors noted that supratentorial intracerebral metastases with multiple characters (60–70%) are most often (80–93%) observed in SCLC and they are combined with distant metastases in other organs and tissues, most often in bones, liver, and lungs, in 50–93% of cases (Posner 1977; Oneschuk and Bruera 1998; Vecht 1998, Tomiak 2001; Nieder et al. 2010; de Groot and Munden 2012).

1.2 Breast Cancer Metastases

Breast cancer (BC) is the most common malignancy in women. While studying the epidemiology of MTS in breast cancer and assessing the economic costs, Pelletier et al. (2008) noted an increase in the proportion of cases with brain metastases from 6.61% in 2002 to 11.78% in 2004. Brain metastases of breast cancer usually develop between the second and third years from the time of the diagnosis (van Eck et al. 1965; Nussbaum et al. 1996; Yawn et al. 2003; Sperduto et al. 2012a, b). In metastatic breast cancer, chemotherapy is effective in 70–80%, while patients with treatment failure die from distant metastases. Autopsy identifies brain metastases of breast cancer in 30% of cases (Chissov and Davydov 2008). The average life expectancy of patients with stage IV breast cancer is 18–24 months, but the real figure depends on the site of metastatic lesions. The 5-year survival rate of patients with breast cancer with distant metastases is 19%, with the disease having the worst prognosis in cases of visceral metastases (Zimm et al. 1981).

1.3 Melanoma Metastases

Melanoma is the third by the frequency of metastasizing into the brain. Melanoma metastases constitute 5–21% of the total cases of secondary brain malignancies, in spite of the fact that the proportion of melanoma in the structure of the latter is only about 4% (Greenlee et al. 2001). According to Douglas and Margolin (2002), melanoma is characterized by the maximum metastasizing rate: up to 20% of patients with stage IV disease have brain metastases (Amer et al. 1978; Douglas and Margolin 2002). Melanoma metastasizes more often in men than in women. In recent years, the number of melanoma cases has been increasing, and the tumor is more common at a young age (Durnov et al. 2000).

Typically, the primary tumor is located in the skin (97%); 2–3% of cases are melanomas of vaginal mucosa, anorectal skin and mucosa, and choroid. In 1% of cases, primary melanoma is located in the CNS and usually develops in the choroidal plexus or the pial membrane of the fourth ventricle or around the brainstem (especially in the ventral regions), as well as in the upper sections of the spinal cord, since these areas contain the greatest concentration of melanocytes (Gebarski and Blaivas 1996; Arbelaez et al. 1999; Saparadin et al. 2012).

1.4 Renal Cancer Metastases

Renal cancer quite often metastasizes to the brain: a series of autopsies in patients with kidney adenocarcinoma showed brain involvement in 11% of cases (Saitoh 1981). According to Harada et al. (1999), among 325 patients treated for kidney cancer at the Osaka University Hospital from 1957 to 1993, 5.5% of cases were with brain metastases. Metastatic lesions in the meninges and cranial bones in renal cancer occur more frequently than with other histological types of tumors; their growth is quite active, since secondary tumors often mimic meningioma. It should be noted that "aggressive" relapses with involvement of the meninges and cranial bones, even on a complex treatment, are more often observed with renal cancer metastases than with other metastatic tumors. Multiple brain metastases of renal cancer are more typical for a young age ($p < 0.001$) (Bianchi et al. 2012).

1.5 Gastrointestinal Cancer Metastases

There has been an increase in the colorectal cancer (CRC) rate within the last decades in many countries around the world, including Russia. According to Vogel et al. (2000), due to active screening programs, 80% of patients have tumors that can be surgically removed. Metastases of colorectal cancer account for 1.8 to 4.8% of all metastatic brain lesions (Vogel et al. 2000). According to Temple et al. (1982), the incidence of secondary brain metastases reaches 10% in patients with colorectal cancer. The main risk factor for colorectal cancer is elderly age: the likelihood of CRC increases significantly after the age of 55 and becomes maximum after 70–75 years of age (Boyle and Leon 2002; Faivre et al. 2002; Papapolychroniadis 2004).

Gastric cancer patients with brain metastases amount to not more than 1% of all cases of brain metastases, both according to autopsy findings and clinical manifestations (Zimm et al. 1981; Graf et al. 1988). Brain metastases develop 1–23 months after the diagnosis of gastric cancer, with the overall survival of patients with metastatic brain lesions of about 9 weeks (York et al. 1999).

In most cases, brain metastases develop in patients with large primary esophageal tumors and metastatic involvement of distant lymph nodes. Metastases of esophageal cancer amount to less than 1% of all malignant tumor MTS in the brain (Zimm et al. 1981; Graf et al. 1988).

1.6 Metastatic Tumors of the Reproductive System

Prostate cancer metastasizes to the brain in 0.6–4.4% of cases (Catane et al. 1976; Castaldo et al. 1983). On average, prostate cancer metastasizes to the brain 28 months after the initial diagnosis. Small cell carcinoma of the prostate and transitional cell carcinoma of the prostate are associated with development of brain metastases more often than adenocarcinoma (Zimm et al. 1981; McCutcheon et al. 1999; Hatzoglou et al. 2014).

The incidence of brain metastases from *testicular* cancer is not more than 2% (Guenot et al. 1994). Brain metastases of endometrial cancer are identified very rarely (0.3%). Low-grade endometrial carcinoma with signs of vascular invasion can metastasize to the brain even before clinical manifestations of the primary tumor develop (Martinez-Manas et al. 1998). Henriksen (1975), based on findings of autopsies performed on patients who died from endometrial cancer, discovered cranial metastases in 5% of cases, including brain metastases in 3%.

Independent studies by Behney (1933) and Brunschwig and Pierce (1948) in the analysis of 181 patients with *cervical cancer* did not found any brain metastases, while Holzaepfel and Ezell (1955) revealed metastatic brain lesions in 1.5–2.3% of cases. The time interval from the detection of primary cervical tumor to the detection of metastatic brain lesions may reach 8 years (30 months on average).

Findings by Hardy et al. (1990), related to a small number of *ovarian carcinoma* cases, showed brain MTS in 11.6% of cases. Mayer et al. (1978) found brain metastases in 0.9% of 567 autopsies of patients who died from ovarian cancer.

1.7 Metastases of Thyroid Cancer

The frequency of metastatic brain lesions in thyroid cancer (TC) is 0.1–5.0% (Jyothirmayi et al. 1995; Altimari-Romero et al. 1997), while the average time to the development of secondary brain lesions varies from 1 to 12 years. According to Salvati et al. (1995), the time from detection of the primary tumor to detection of brain metastases of thyroid cancer is 2.8 years for papillary cancer and 1.2 years for anaplastic cancer.

2 The Mechanism of Development of Brain Metastases

Before primary tumor cells are transferred to the brain, they grow into the surrounding lymph and blood vessels. Once in the lymph vessels and, rarely, blood vessels, single tumor cells or groups of cells migrate with the current of blood or lymph. A tumor embolus must preserve its viability after it overcomes the action of the immune system or another humoral body defense system, turbulence, and circulation, and only then it "settles" in the capillary bed of the recipient organ, penetrates its parenchyma, proliferates, and forms micrometastases. Not all tumor cells that get into the lymph or blood flow will eventually provide the basis for the growth of a metastatic tumor. Thus, according to Liotta and Kohn (2003), the number of tumor microemboli that eventually form metastases is about 0.01%. The potential to metastasize depends on the number of tumor cell emboli and the specifics of interaction between the latter and homeostatic mechanisms of the host (Fidler 1997; Langley and Fidler 2013).

The development of most cancers is associated with the need for a blood supply sufficient to meet the needs of increased tumor metabolism. This, in turn, leads to the formation of additional, abnormally shaped and branched vasculature, so-called abnormal tumor vasculature (Shweiki et al. 1992; McDonald and Choyke 2003; Pronin et al. 2005; Bulakbasi et al. 2005). According to Li et al. (2000), as early as 24 h after an injection of 20–50 tumor cells to animals, healthy vessels surrounded by the tumor begin to deform and take a convoluted shape. All the above conditions result in the formation of a relatively independent vascular structure of a metastasis, different from the normal intracranial vasculature. Thus, vascular proliferation and tumor angiogenesis are the most important factors in the biology of secondary brain malignancies (Chaudhry et al. 2001; Fitzgerald et al. 2008).

Leenders et al. (2003) pointed out that the process of metastasizing is highly specific and involves some successive transformations. After implantation of the embolus cell and primary cell growth, the tumor tissue should become vascularized (it is usually noticeable when the tumor mass reaches 1 mm^3 in diameter). Vascular endothelial growth factor (VEGF) that primarily affects the activity of tumor vasculature formation also affects the surrounding tissue, which results in the formation of anastomoses between the vasculature, the tumor, and the body. This factor can promote initial tumor growth even without "own" tumor angiogenesis (Kusters et al. 2003).

A metastatic tumor growing in the brain parenchyma certainly interacts with various protective mechanisms and structures, particularly, with the structures of the blood-brain barrier (BBB). In contrast to primary lesions, metastatic tumor cells should reach brain microvessels, "attach" to their endothelium, and then penetrate into the brain parenchyma, start active proliferation, and produce a number of factors to promote angiogenesis. Formation of a local metastasis starts with the interaction of tumor cells and BBB endothelial cells, which occurs with active contribution of growth factors (Nicolson et al. 1996; Kim et al. 2004). Inhibition of VEGF and activation of anti-angiogenic factors greatly reduce the chance for a metastatic tumor to "catch" in the brain tissues. It should be noted that certain of these endogenous factors, on the contrary, "help" metastatic cells to grow into the brain matter. Analysis of cases with patients treated with adjuvant chemotherapy showed that administered drugs may affect the BBB, so that the probability of metastasizing into the brain increases (Bouffet et al. 1997; Kolomainen et al. 2002; Bendell et al. 2003).

The main elements of the BBB structure are endothelial cells. Intercellular gaps between endothelial cells, astrocytes, pericytes, and BBB are smaller than the gaps between the cells in other tissues. These three cell types represent the structural basis of the BBB (Fig. 2.1). Cerebral vessels are characterized by the presence of tight junctions between endothelial cells and the absence of both fenestrations and intercellular gaps between them. Tight junctions between endothelial cells inhibit intercellular (paracellular) passive transport. Thus, the endothelial lining of the brain capillaries is continuous. Another difference between the cerebral capil-

M. Dolgushin et al., *Brain Metastases*, DOI 10.1007/978-3-319-57760-9_2

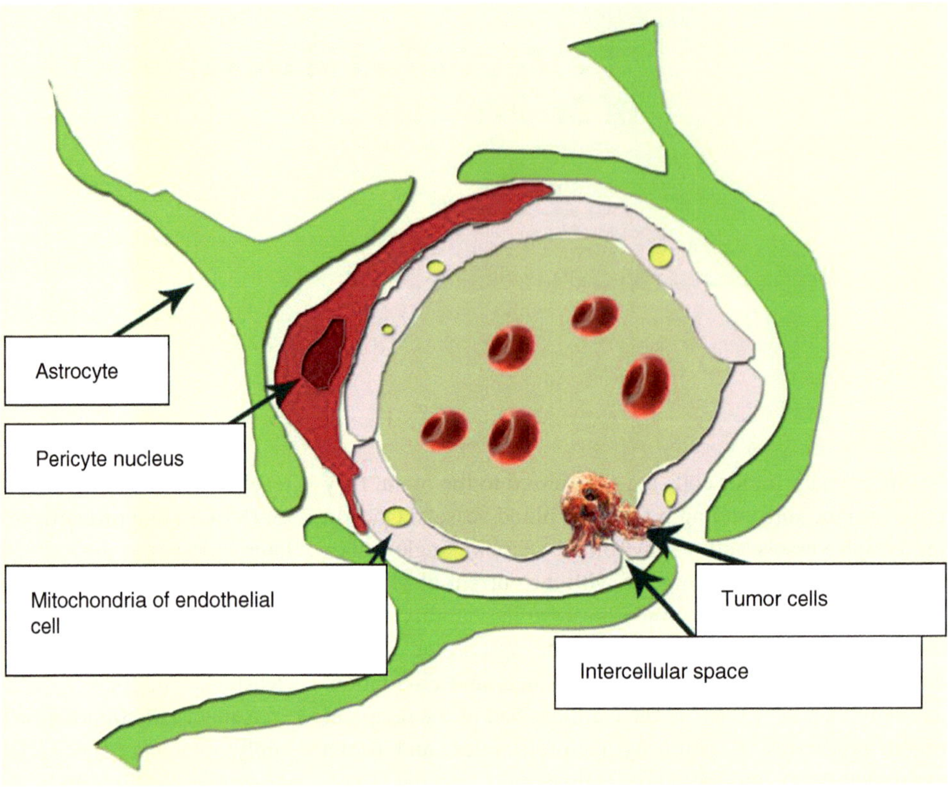

Fig. 2.1 The structural BBB unit. A distinctive characteristics of the relationship between a capillary and the brain substance is a close contact of endothelial cells, as well as presence of pericytes with a contractile function, which prevents large blood elements from penetration outside the capillary

lary endothelium and the peripheral capillary endothelium is a low content of pinocytosis vesicles. All of this is aimed at preventing the penetration of various unwanted substances from the bloodstream into the brain tissue.

Every second to fourth endothelial cell has a contact with a pericyte. Pericytes are mainly located at the points of contact of endothelial cells. Pericytes are present in almost all arterioles, venules, and capillaries of the body. The level of their coverage of the endothelial capillary layer correlates with the permeability of the vascular wall. Pericytes are tightly bound to endothelial cells. This binding occurs through three types of contacts: gap junctions, focal adhesions, and membrane invagination from one cell to the cavity of another. Gap junctions directly connect cytoplasm of two cells, while being permeable to ions and small molecules. This is typical only for cerebral pericytes. They perform the macrophage function in the cerebral capillary network. Accordingly, the cytoplasm of cerebral pericytes contains a large number of lysosomes. The ability of pericytes to perform phagocytosis and antigen presentation was confirmed in tissue culture (Peppiatt et al. 2006).

Pericytes also synthesize a number of vasoactive substances and play an important role in angiogenesis. Macrophage properties of pericytes constitute a "second line of defense of the brain" from neurotoxic molecules that have overcome the barrier of endothelial cells. Thus, they are an important part of the cerebra immune system, which, along with other factors, significantly hinders penetration of metastatic cells into the brain substance.

In particular, the above properties of neoplastic growth of colorectal cancer are controlled by the genes responsible for angiogenesis, invasion, and metastasizing that promote production of so-called matrix metalloproteinases (MMPs) by tumor cells (Delektorskaya et al. 2007; Ganusevich 2010; Said et al. 2014). The MMP1, MMP2, and MMP9 expression was demonstrated to represent an unfavorable prognostic factor for colon cancer. Similar associations were found for other protease family—uPA (urokinase-type plasminogen activator). Glycoprotein CD44 performing the adhesive function and apparently promoting the attachment of tumor cells in anatomically distant tissues and organs is one of the best known markers of metastasizing (Pasche et al. 2002; Kahlenberg et al. 2003).

In case of invasion of melanoma cells, for example, neurotrophins—proteins that support the viability of neurons and stimulate their growth and activity—facilitate local destruction of the basement membrane of the BBB cells and promote the release of angiogenic factors by increasing the production of extracellular matrix (ECM) degradation enzymes, such as heparanase. Heparanase produces an effect on the growth of melanoma and other malignant tumors and promotes their invasion into distant organs. There is an increased number of neurotrophins on the tumor-brain interface (Nakajima et al. 1988; Yano et al. 2000; Vlodavsky and Friedmann 2001; Denkins et al. 2004).

Findings of Wikman et al. (2012), who studied the profiles of chromosomal aberrations (whole genome) in primary breast cancer and brain metastases using comparative genomic hybridization (CGH) to microarrays, showed that brain metastases in general contain the same chromosomal aberrations as the primary tumor, but their occurrence is a few times higher. A statistically significant difference was obtained for nine different loci with an increased EGFR (7p11,2) content and amplification—epidermal growth factor receptor from the tyrosine kinase group—and a decrease in 10q22,3-qter as the most relevant and significant aberrations in the metastasis ($p < 0.01$, false positives <0.04). An allelic mismatch in 10q was confirmed in 77 primary tumors and 21 metastases. A mismatch in the PTEN locus (phosphatase and tensin homolog), an enzyme that suppresses the tumor cell activity, was greater in metastases (52%) and in primary tumors with a brain relapse (59%) as compared to primary tumors (18%, $p = 0.003$) or a non-brain relapse (12%, $p = 0.006$). A decrease in PTEN expression is most common in HER-2 negative metastases (64%). Furthermore, expression of a micro-PHK PTEN was decreased in brain metastases as compared to the primary tumor. PTEN mutation was often detected in metastases. These findings demonstrate that brain metastases contain a very complex set of genomic aberrations, suggestive of a possible role of PTEN and EGFR in their formation.

The ability of invasive growth and metastasis growth rate are associated with its original nature. This theory is based, according to Radinsky et al. (1998), on the following three principles. First, tumors are biologically heterogeneous and contain subpopulations of cells with a variety of angiogenic, invasive, and metastatic properties. Second, metastatic process depends on the activity of invasion, embolization, survival of the tumor embolus cell in the circulation, and its entrapment in distant capillaries and spread with cell division in the parenchyma of the target organ. Third, a great deal depends on the multiplicity of invading cells, their ability to oppose the homeostatic mechanisms of the host. The tumor can "attract" inflammatory cells that provide more favorable conditions for a further growth of metastases and "affect" the BBB (Egeblad and Werb 2002). During the development of a metastatic tumor in the brain, its volume increases, and it invades into the brain tissue underdriven by growth factors produced by astrocytes (provided the tumor cell has specific receptors) (Gavrilovic and Posner 2005).

Not all metastatic cells actively develop after their invasion. Some of them die, while another become "silent" for years. This phenomenon of "silence" is the most characteristic of metastatic melanoma and breast cancer (Chambers et al. 2002).

Close interaction of metastatic tumors with the surrounding brain tissue almost always results in edema. Cerebral edema in metastases is caused by morphologic vascular disorders (increased permeability) followed by fluid egress into the brain substance and modification in the BBB structure, resulting in the penetration of plasma proteins, large molecules, and water-soluble substances into the extracellular space of the brain parenchyma (Bradbury 1983; Weissman 1988; Zedeler et al. 1992; Broadwell and Sofroniew 1993; Sierra et al. 1997; Zhang and Olsson 1997; Bliznyukov et al. 2001).

There are several papers studying the effect of K+, Na+, and Cl- channel inhibitors on migration of tumor cells in publications. According to Sontheimer (2011), ion channels, in particular K+, affect the degree of activity of abnormal growth, while inhibitors of these channels cause a tumor growth delay. The coordinated activity of K+ and Cl channels activates the growth of tumors. After an increase in intracellular Ca^{+2} levels, these channels activate the release of K+ and Cl-ions with bound water, which results in the inhibition of tumor grows (Cuddapah and Sontheimer 2011).

A microscopic picture of cells and tissue structure of metastases can be very similar to that of the primary tumor (renal cancer, pigmented melanoma, follicular thyroid carcinoma). At the same time, it may be somewhat different, for example, amelanotic metastases of primary pigmented melanoma (Bishop 1991; Sawaya et al. 2004). This process increases the autonomy of tumor cells and results in the heterogeneity of the cell population in general. In addition, each subset has its own growth characteristics and ability to invade. Over time, tumor cells evolutionarily become more resistant to the immune system and may transform based on the changing conditions (Maxwell et al. 1999). A variety of histological forms is, respectively, reflected on diagnostic images.

3 Clinical Symptoms

Before the advent of instrumental methods, including radiation ones, diagnosis of metastases, as well as of other intracranial tumors, was based on clinical symptoms. Neurological symptoms in metastatic brain lesions, as in case of primary tumors, are diverse and, above all, are determined by the lesion site, their number, size, and presence of perifocal edema, indicating a vascular barrier breach in the tumor tissue. Majority of cerebral metastases are located in the cerebral hemispheres (80%), cerebellar hemispheres (up to 17%), and brainstem (3%) (Tikhtman and Patchell 1995). According to Delattre et al. (1988), among the various areas of the cerebral hemispheres, the largest part of the metastatic lesions is accounted for the frontal (21%), parietal (19%), and temporoparietal-occipital (19%) lobes rather than for the temporal and occipital lobes. Typical focal symptoms (paresis, hemianopsia, aphasia, impaired hearing, vision, etc.) accompany the developing overall clinical picture with intense headache, often with nausea, vomiting, and impaired consciousness and later with increased intracranial pressure (Table 3.1).

An acute or subacute onset with progressive cerebral symptoms is characteristic of the presence of metastatic brain lesions. Thus, according to Hochberg and Pruitt (1980), metastatic tumors at the area of a transition of gray matter into the white matter—the area most frequently affected by metastases—are mostly characterized by occurrence of acute symptoms that manifest for a few days or weeks, as compared with primary tumors with the same location.

Table 3.1 The main clinical symptoms of metastatic brain lesions (Posner 1995)

General symptoms	%	Focal	%
Headache	49	Hemiparesis	59
Mental disorders	32	Cognitive disorders	58
Weakness	30	Sensory disturbances	21
Ataxia	21	Congested optic disk	20
Seizures	18	Ataxia	19
Speech disorders	12	Movement disorders	18

Focal symptoms primarily caused by compression of the adjacent brain regions by the metastatic lesion become pronounced and increase with the tumor growth, development of edema/swelling of the brain tissue, and displacement of nearby structures. Often, the clinical picture is aggravated by the development of ischemia due to vascular occlusion with a metastatic embolus. However, the developing local symptoms are milder than those with primary malignant brain tumors.

The principal symptom of a brain tumor lesion is progressive headache. Early headache in brain metastases is usually acute and localized and is often accompanied by nausea and vomiting. As compared to primary tumors, headaches are more intense, which may result from the development of early toxicity effects on the brain tissue and its membranes (Romodanov et al. 1973).

Early symptoms of brain metastases also include pronounced mental disorders (impaired consciousness, cognitive decline), occurring in 64–95% of cases, which, according to some authors, is more characteristic of metastatic brain lesions (Babchin et al. 1974a, b; Abasheev-Konstantinovsky 1973; Levine et al. 1978; Passik and Ricketts 1998). Thus, according to Finegold (1977), headaches, vomiting, stagnant nipples optic nerves, slow heart rate, dizziness, and general seizures occur much more frequently in primary intracerebral tumors, while mental disorders are more common in metastatic tumors. According to Kalkun (1963), mental disorders manifest as asthenia, lethargy, apathy, sleepiness, slow associative processes, memory impairment in 82% of cases. Confusion is noted in 65% of cases (Mehta et al. 2003). The development of a delirious state in function of the duration and severity of the process, according to Lawlor et al. (2000), is observed in 10–70% of cases.

One of the main focal symptoms is motor insufficiency, rarely (34%) Jackson's seizures (Kalkun 1963). Thus, in

M. Dolgushin et al., *Brain Metastases*, DOI 10.1007/978-3-319-57760-9_3

subcortical metastases, focal manifestations occur as motor and sensory disorders and may have remitting intensity. Local and generalized seizures may occur in 40% of patients, while being the first manifestation of metastases in 10% of patients (Steblov and Mandelbeym 1962; Smirnov 1962; Ragayshene 1985; Kristijansen 1989; Flowers and Levin 1993; Emami and Graham 1997; Nakagawa et al. 1997; Helfre and Pierga 1999). It was noted that convulsive disorder is more common in metastatic renal cell carcinoma and melanoma that are radioresistant tumors. Gaidar et al. (2005) attribute this to their predisposition to hemorrhage.

Meningeal symptoms are more common with metastatic lesions in the occipital lobe and cerebellum (Christiaans et al. 2002; Kaal et al. 2005a, b). A symptom such as "stagnant nipples optic nerves" develops at later stages of the disease with progression of intracranial hypertension (Babchin et al. 1974a, b; Likhterman 1979; Kurennaya 1986; Soffietti et al. 2002; Davey 2002).

According to Steblov and Mandelbeym (1962), autopsies of patients who died of tumors with brain metastases always identified clear signs of increased intracranial pressure: meningeal tension. During the lifetime, this manifested as obvious meningeal symptoms resembling those in meningitis, smoothness of sulci, flattening of gyri, venous congestion, edema, and swelling of the brain substance, occasionally an expansion of the brain ventricles.

Cases with small lesions located in the cortical parts of the frontal and parietal regions are clinically less significant. However, the most expressed clinical picture is observed in brainstem lesions.

Lesions in the meninges may involve cranial nerves with corresponding symptoms. Secondary malignancies with the characteristic involvement of meninges include melanoma, lung adenocarcinoma, breast adenocarcinoma, and gastrointestinal tract adenocarcinoma. It should be noted that meningeal symptoms are detected more frequently in brain metastases than in primary tumors (42% and 19%, respectively). The clinical picture of a metastatic lesion in the dura mater and the skull bones is distinguished by basal (due to the presence of metastases in the dura mater of the basal parts of the brain) and convexital (due to the localization of metastases in the dura mater covering the convex surface of the cerebral hemispheres) syndromes (Krasovsky 1958).

Metastasizing into the sellar structures completely mimics the clinic picture of pituitary adenoma with signs of weight loss and hypopituitarism (Kovacs 1973). This has been noted to be much more common in breast cancer (Cairncross et al. 1980; Hirsch et al. 1982; Marin et al. 1992). Due to the blood supply specifics of the sellar structures, the neurohypophysis is initially affected.

Involvement of the temporal bone manifests by the damage to the branches of the facial nerve or impaired hearing.

Metastasizing into the pineal region rarely occurs, with the involvement of the pineal gland (1.5–3.8% of all metastases) and other deep structures, manifests as a severe intracranial hypertension syndrome, and is often accompanied by hydrocephalus (Ortega et al. 1951; Chason et al. 1963; Kashiwagi et al. 1989; Schuster et al. 1998). Local symptoms caused by the tumor compression of the midbrain structures can manifest as oculomotor disorders and other syndromes due to selective involvement of deep structures (Konovalov and Pitskhelauri 2004).

Small metastases are characterized by asymptomatic course, which is also possible if meninges are involved (Kalkun 1963; Laigle-Donadey et al. 2005; Gavrilovic and Posner 2005). It was noted that clinical manifestations of lung cancer metastases in the brain can be less pronounced. According to Snee and Rodger (1985), autopsies detected metastases in the brain in 44%, with the third of patients not being clinically diagnosed during their lifetime. Most often the frequency of MTS detection in the brain is underestimated due to asymptomatic course, with up to a third of all cases of metastatic brain lesions being diagnosed only at autopsy after patient's death (Posner 1977).

The clinical picture of multiple metastases first of all depends on the activity of growth of certain tumor lesions and their impact on the surrounding tissue. The clinical picture of multiple metastases is mostly characterized by depression, apathy, fatigue, drowsiness, lack of euphoria, subsequent confusion, and all kinds of hallucinations and delusions due to the toxic effects of cancer metabolites (Smirnov 1962; Alperovich 1975). According to Sheehan et al. (2005), multiple brain metastases do not clinically manifest in 26%.

It is not uncommon when the primary tumor located outside the central nervous system is asymptomatic in patients with metastatic brain lesions (Gavrilovic and Posner 2005), and intracranial symptoms prevail, especially, if the frontal lobes are affected (Abrakov 1955; Adamovich-Razumovskaya and Goryukova 1958; Kalkun 1963; Gavrilovic and Posner 2005). This is very typical for bronchogenic cancer that is clinically asymptomatic for a long time. Findings from studies by Ryabukha et al. (2010) in cases with brain metastases of lung cancer with various histological structures showed the following relationship: manifestations of cerebral metastases in undifferentiated cancer, squamous cell cancer, adenocarcinoma, and small cell carcinoma occurred before clinical manifestations of the primary tumor in 100%, 56.55%, and 44.4% of cases and in only one (1) case, respectively. In cases when metastases were diagnosed after the detection of the primary tumor and average time to their clinical manifestation slightly differed, the average duration was 10.2, 11, and 11.4 months in metastases of squamous cell carcinoma, adenocarcinoma, and small cell cancer, respectively. The authors noted that women had a more aggressive course of metastatic brain lesions—cerebral metastases manifested clinically before the primary tumor in 80% and were multiple in 50% of cases (while in men in 32.2% of cases). In cases when the primary tumor manifested earlier, the average time to clinical manifestations was 5 months.

The clinical picture can significantly deteriorate as a result of a hemorrhage (intratumoral, intracerebral) that occurs on average in 14% of total cases with metastatic brain lesions (Maiuri et al. 2000; Biswas et al. 2006). The risk of hemorrhage is primarily related to the histological structure of the tumor lesion. The greatest number of hemorrhages is characteristic of aggressive metastatic tumors—metastases of melanoma (50%), renal cell carcinoma (70%), lung cancer (adenocarcinoma), and rarely metastases of colorectal cancer and ovarian cancer (Navi et al. 2010; Heon et al. 2010).

Acute insult-like clinical course of the disease is characterized by the highest level of hemorrhages of up to 70% (Kondziolka et al. 1987). A cerebral hemorrhage is often the first clinically significant manifestation of cancer: according to Mandybur (1977), 2/3 of patients with cerebral metastases were diagnosed with cancer only after the detection of a hemorrhage.

When analyzing clinical manifestations of metastatic brain lesions from malignant tumors with various sites, a significant increase in treatment-induced neurological disorders should be noted, resulting from extensive use of modern methods of cancer treatment (chemotherapy, radiation therapy, etc.). Moreover, an increase in the life expectancy of cancer patients resulted in the growth of late toxic effects manifested by certain neurologic deficits, such as cognitive decline and memory impairment after radiotherapy.

4 Basic Principles of Treatment of Brain Metastases

The objective of treatment of brain metastases, in addition to a probable prolongation of life by monitoring the intracranial disease progression, is to reduce the severity of neurological symptoms or prevent their occurrence in order to preserve patient's quality of life as long as possible. Due to the treatment success in general, the duration of life of cancer patients increases and, therefore, increased the frequency of detection of tumor metastases in the brain. Effective therapy and local control of brain metastases are of paramount importance for prognosis and ensuring a satisfactory quality of life (Law et al. 2002; Chiang et al. 2004; Opstad et al. 2004).

The choice of treatment, whether surgical removal of metastases, radiation exposure (hypofractionated radiation therapy, radiosurgery, whole-brain radiotherapy), or drug therapy, is based on an assessment of three main parameters: patient's general status, morphological structure of malignant tumor, and the number and characteristics of sites of metastatic lesions. The key point for the clinician when selecting the treatment tactics is the expected extent of radical treatment; therefore, the possibility of surgical removal of the tumor(s) is estimated during the first phase.

4.1 Surgery

In 1926, Grant published his experience in resection of a metastatic tumor in the brain. In his opinion, a surgery for brain metastatic tumors is not only contraindicated but also "may harm patients." Pessimism regarding the surgical treatment of cerebral metastases began to decrease after the publication by Oldberg (1933), who described three cases of removal of brain metastases with long-term positive outcomes: one patient with breast cancer metastases lived for 2 years after the surgery. In 1951, Stortebecker, based on the analysis of 125 cases of patients who underwent surgery for brain metastases, concluded that the removal of metastases increased the life expectancy of patients. Randomized trials in 1990s of the last century showed a significant increase in the life expectancy of patients with solitary metastases, who underwent a surgical removal of secondary tumors and subsequent brain radiotherapy, as compared with patients who received only brain radiotherapy (Patchell et al. 1990a, b; Vecht et al. 1993; Mintz et al. 1996). The most favorable outcomes with a median survival of patients from 10 to 15 months after the surgical removal of intracranial metastases were achieved for breast cancer (Defesche 1982; Wronski et al. 1996; Cappuzzo et al. 2000; Iwadate et al. 2000). Good outcomes of complex treatment in patients with solitary brain metastases with additional implantation carmustine wafers into the resected tumor bed and subsequent radiotherapy were published in the paper by Ewend (2001).

Despite the occurrence of alternative methods within the last decade and changes in the treatment paradigm for intracranial metastases, the role of surgery for certain groups of patients with metastatic brain lesions is fundamental for creating optimal conditions for the further complex antitumor treatment (Kalkanis et al. 2010; Caroli et al. 2011; Patel et al. 2012; Mut 2012; Owonikoko et al. 2014).

A surgical resection followed by whole-brain radiotherapy (WBRT) is currently the standard treatment for resectable solitary cerebral metastases. The presence of brain metastases with an untreated or undetected primary tumor is not a contraindication for surgery (Kryuchkov and Yartsev 1974; Lang and Sawaya 1996; Nakagawa et al. 1997; Iwadate et al. 2000).

The key factors affecting the survival of patients include the histological tumor structure and the extent of administered (adjuvant) treatment for postoperative cerebral metastases, the disease extent and the duration of a disease-free period, and the patient's age and neurological status (Sundaresan and Galicich 1985; Pieper et al. 1997; Lagerwaard et al. 1999; Hatiboglu et al. 2011; Zaitsev et al. 2015). The best overall survival rates are achieved in patients with high performance status ($\geq$80 on the Karnofsky scale) and control of extracranial tumor process. It should be remembered that low performance status in some patients may be due to the

M. Dolgushin et al., *Brain Metastases*, DOI 10.1007/978-3-319-57760-9_4

mass effect and can be improved as a result of a surgical removal of the tumor.

In case of multiple brain metastases, the role of surgery is limited to obtaining a biopsy or eliminating mass effect symptoms caused by large lesions (Loshakov 2005; Paek et al. 2005; Stark et al. 2005). There are some retrospective findings showing the benefits of a surgical tumor resection (best overall survival) for certain patients with a good prognosis and limited (2–3 lesions) brain metastases (Mintz et al. 1996; Schackert et al. 2000).

Surgical treatment is indicated in the presence of metastatic lesions causing:

- Clinical manifestations of mass effect, accompanied by signs of intracranial hypertension
- A dislocation of midline brain structures
- An extensive perifocal swelling spreading to the nearby lobes and the opposite hemisphere
- A threat of blocking the cerebrospinal fluid pathways

Accordingly, a surgical intervention solves the following issues: the maximum extent of tumor removal, while observing the principles of anatomical justification and functional safety, exact determination of the histological tumor structure, reduction of the tumor impact on the unaffected brain structures, and restoration of impaired liquor circulation. The main factor determining a favorable outcome of the surgical treatment is complete removal of metastases. To this end, the best methods of postoperative assessment are CT (2–7 days) or MRI studies with contrast enhancement (1–2 days).

Removal of intracerebral metastases is indicated with a limited (≤3) number of focal lesions and the presence of a resectable lesion greater than 3 cm in diameter. In case of solitary metastases (one metastasis in the brain and absence of extracranial manifestations), surgical treatment is indicated if the latter are >3 cm. When metastases are <3 cm, located in functionally important areas, and symptomatic (neurological symptoms) and there is no response to the steroid test (administration of 8–24 mg of dexamethasone per day for 5 days), a surgical removal can be considered. However, when choosing between surgical and radiosurgical methods, one should consider a higher probability of persistent residual neurological deficit after the surgery.

In cases of radioresistant metastases (kidney cancer, melanoma) sized up to 3 cm, surgical treatment is preferable. In case of solitary metastases and extracranial manifestations of the disease, indications for surgical treatment are similar to the indications for treatment of solitary metastases. Surgical treatment is the most effective, provided control of extracranial metastases and presence of systemic treatment reserves.

Surgical treatment is also possible in multiple brain metastases and with at least one >3 cm lesion determining the severity of patient's condition. Favorable outcomes depend on the control of extracranial manifestations and/or existence of systemic treatment reserves.

Surgery of brain metastases is characterized by removal of a metastasis as a single unit with the surrounding perifocal and perivascular area. This removal method reduces the risk of local recurrence up to 5%, in contrast to piecemeal removal, where the risk of local recurrence is 40%.

Surgery is also indicated in case of local recurrence of a brain metastasis or active progression of post-radiation necrosis. Surgical removal of an abnormal lesion is also possible in active pseudotumor course of post-radiation necrosis with mass effect and development of persistent disabling neurological symptoms. In this case, the point of surgery is to remove (not radically) the major part of the necrotic tissue in order to eliminate the mass effect.

Thus, despite a broad discussion on the role of surgical treatment of brain metastases and selection of alternative methods, we believe that to date surgery has no alternatives in identification of the histological tumor structure, rapid elimination of the tumor mass effect, perifocal edema, management of clinical symptoms caused by the tumor, and improvement of patient's neurological status in general. As noted above, surgery helps create conditions for continued complex treatment of patients.

4.2 Radiosurgery

Radiosurgery (RS) in many cases is a direct alternative to surgical treatment. The choice in favor of radiosurgery is based mainly on the size of the locally irradiated area, which depends on the volume of the largest metastatic lesions or a total volume of the adjacent tumor foci forming a conglomerate.

According to RTOG 90-05 (Shaw et al. 2000), the maximum permissible doses of ionizing radiation during radiosurgical treatment of brain metastases (MTSs) are as follows:

- 15 Gy—for MTSs with the maximum diameter of 3–3.5 cm (recommended level 1)
- 18 Gy—for MTSs with the maximum diameter of 2–3 cm (recommended level 1)
- 24 Gy—for MTSs with the maximum diameter of 2 cm (recommended level 1)

Radiosurgical treatment is limited by the brain tissue volume irradiated with the dose 12 Gy, which should not exceed 15 cm^3. This rule approximately corresponds to the limitation of an irradiated lesion size (not more than 14 cm^3), which is a more useful parameter when considering the possibility of radiosurgery. When the volume is difficult to calculate, the maximum lesion diameter of ≤3 cm (14 cm^3) is an alternative to the volume calculation.

A direct indication for radiosurgery is the presence of a limited number of metastases (≤3 foci) (lesions with the maximum diameter ≤3 cm). Patients with multiple (3–10) MTSs can also be candidates for radiosurgery (Golan et al. 2015).

Radiosurgical treatment as a separate method of treatment requires careful monitoring of patients in order to early detect a possible relapse and subsequently repeat the radiosurgical treatment. The usual practice is to perform follow-up using thin-slice (1 mm) MRIs of the brain and intravenous administration of gadolinium-containing contrast agent at least once in 3 months.

Another treatment option is a combination of radiosurgery and whole-brain radiotherapy (WBRT) that is often used in case of multiple metastatic lesions (more than 10 MTSs). In this case, radiosurgery is performed on lesions with the diameter greater than 1 cm, followed by (in 1–2 weeks) WBRT. For this combination, the recommended radiation dose is reduced by 20–25% from the usual dose.

Hypofractionated stereotactic radiotherapy is recommended for the treatment of large, inoperable lesions or conglomerates (>3 cm in diameter).

An important feature of radiosurgical treatment is the possibility of repeated treatment, both for local relapses and for the treatment of "new" distant metastases.

4.3 Hypofractionated Stereotactic Radiotherapy

Stereotactic radiation therapy (SRT) of brain metastases can be considered an effective method to achieve a certain level of local control for large (>3 cm in diameter) MTSs. This level for large tumors can probably be improved using higher doses of radiation with a large number of factions in a hypofractionated mode. In phase II of a prospective study, Ammirati et al. (2010) confirmed the effectiveness of CPT regimen with total boost dose (TBD) = 30 Gy in 5 fractions. A biologically equivalent dose (BED) was calculated as 40 Gy (SBD = 2 Gy) for acute effects and as a 60 Gy (SBD = 2 Gy) for delayed effects, assuming the ratio of α/β = 10 Gy for acute effects and α/β = 2 Gy for delayed effects (Mehta et al. 2010). This study allowed to use equivalent (for BED) fractionation modes: 3 fractions of 8 Gy, TBD = 24 Gy; 5 fractions of 6 Gy, TBD = 30 Gy; and 7 fractions of 5 Gy, TBD = 35 Gy.

According to published studies and our own experience, adjuvant CPT on the resected tumor bed in certain clinical situations may replace preventive WBRT. Using high TBD on the minimum volume of surrounding normal brain tissue around the removed metastasis bed improves local control by 70% (for WBRT) to 85.5% (for stereotactic radiation therapy) and has low neurotoxicity (Golan et al. 2015).

Indications for hypofractionated stereotactic radiotherapy are as follows:

- Metastases larger than 2.5–3 cm in diameter
- Metastases located in critical brain structures
- The bed of a removed single metastasis in the postoperative period
- Metastatic lesions at the skull base, orbit, and posterior pole of the eye

A promising option is so-called staged radiosurgery when a 3 cm lesion is initially irradiated with a recommended dose of 10–12 Gy with a view to achieve a short-term reduction of the metastasis and to decrease the risk of local radiation necrosis. The effect of such treatment is unstable; therefore, within 1 month after the first treatment session, provided a reduction in the tumor volume, the second stage of treatment is performed with a higher recommended dose, to reinforce the desired effect. Preliminary results are encouraging but require a more detailed further study.

4.4 Whole-Brain Radiation Therapy

Whole-brain radiation therapy (WBRT) is used in cases of multiple metastatic lesions (≥10 MTSs) and presence of metastatic dissemination in the pia and dura mater or the cerebrospinal fluid pathways, regardless of the number of metastatic foci. In case of brain metastases from radiosensitive tumors (breast cancer, lung cancer), the use of WBRT is appropriate in the presence of >5 metastatic lesions in the brain. In patients with small cell lung cancer (SCLC), preventive WBRT reduces the development of metastases in the brain. An optimal radiation schedule in this case is considered SBD 2.5 Gy × 10 fractions. Increasing SBD to 36 Gy is accompanied by a significant increase in neurotoxicity (especially in patients older than 60 years of age). SBD in WBRT should not exceed 30 Gy in case it is used concomitantly with chemotherapy.

The available evidence suggests that changes in the radiation schedule and WBRT fractionation do not result in significant differences in median overall survival, local control, or frequency of neurocognitive changes after the treatment in comparison with the "standard" WBRT fractionation regimen: TBD 30 Gy, SBD 3 Gy (10 fractions), or TBD 37.5 Gy, SBD 2.5 Gy (15 fractions). Increasing the SBD above 3 Gy results in an increase in the frequency of neurocognitive impairment in patients.

WBRT is also used as a separate treatment (either as prevention or as therapy) or in combination with surgery or radiosurgery. In case surgical treatment is impossible, WBRT can be used as an independent treatment method or in combination with stereotactic radiotherapy (radiosurgery or hypofractionation, based on the clinical situation).

4.5 Drug Therapy

In view of low survival rates, it is urgent to study new drugs and treatment regimens for patients with metastatic brain tumors, in combination with radiation therapy and surgery.

At the first stage, patients with brain metastases undergo molecular genetic studies of the tumor, (1) MGMT methylation (melanoma patients); (2) EGFR mutation of exons 18–21; (3) ALK translocation and KRAS mutation (in patients with non-small cell lung cancer); (4) BRAF mutation (melanoma patients); and (5) KRAS, NRAS, and BRAF mutations (in patients with colorectal cancer), and immunohistochemical studies: (1) MGMT expression (melanoma patients) and (2) Her-2/neu expression (in breast cancer patients).

The immediate effectiveness and long-term results of drug treatment in patients with metastatic brain tumors can vary widely depending on the morphology and biological properties of the primary tumor and the drug therapy regimen.

Thus, in non-small cell lung cancer, the best results are achieved with EGFR inhibitors (erlotinib, gefitinib) in patients with EGFR mutations in exons 18–21 (75% of complete and partial responses in the brain, median survival of 18 months).

In patients with small cell lung cancer, chemotherapy regimens with irinotecan and cisplatin showed high efficacy in the treatment of brain metastases (87.5% of complete and partial responses), with the median survival of 11 months.

In patients with disseminated melanoma, best results are observed with a combination chemotherapy regimen (temozolomide and cisplatin): 34.4% of complete and partial responses in the brain, median survival of 8 months, with 12.5% of patients living for more than 3 years (this subgroup of patients lacks MGMT expression in the tumor). The use of targeted therapy (vemurafenib, dabrafenib, trametinib + dabrafenib) in melanoma patients with BRAF mutation allows to achieve complete and partial responses in the brain in 30–40% of patients, with a median survival of 8 months.

In the group of patients with breast cancer, the most significant progress is achieved in the subgroup of patients with Her-2/neu overexpression (up to 50% of complete and partial responses in the brain, with the median time to progression of 11 months and the median survival of 17.5 months).

In patients with renal cell carcinoma, the use of targeted therapy (sorafenib, pazopanib, sunitinib, etc.) can increase the median survival up to 10 months as compared to a median survival of 5 months in patients treated with cytokines. The majority of patients (54.5%) experienced stabilization of the disease in the brain.

First-line systemic antitumor therapy (chemotherapy and targeted therapy) is indicated in patients:

- With asymptomatic brain metastases
- Sensitive to systemic treatment (chemotherapy and targeted therapy):
  - With breast cancer (positive for Her-2 overexpression)
  - With small cell lung cancer (positive for EGFR mutation or ALK translocation)
  - With small cell lung cancer and ovarian cancer

Table 4.1 shows the regimens of current drug therapy options for brain metastases.

The effect of drug treatment is evaluated out every two to three cycles for chemotherapy or every 2–3 months for targeted therapy. Treatment is administered until the detection of disease progression. In case of targeted therapy for an isolated metastatic brain lesion or tumor progression in the brain, targeted therapy can be continued in combination with local tumor control (neurosurgical treatment, stereotactic radiotherapy/radiosurgery, whole-brain radiation therapy) in the brain.

In the case the first-line treatment consists of a surgical removal of a brain metastasis, it is recommended to investigate morphological and biological characteristics of the tumor removed for subsequent planning anticancer drug therapy.

Table 4.1 Regimen of anticancer drug therapy in patients with brain metastases depending on the site and biological characteristics of the primary tumor

Lung cancer	Small cell cancer (SCLC)	• Irinotecan + cisplatin • Irinotecan + carboplatin • Topotecan • Etoposide + carboplatin **EP regimen**: etoposide + cisplatin **VAC regimen**: vincristine + doxorubicin + cyclophosphamide
	Adenocarcinoma (negative for EGFR mutations, ALK translocations)	• Paclitaxel + carboplatin (in the absence of brain hemorrhages, chemotherapy in combination with bevacizumab) • Pemetrexed + cisplatin • Pemetrexed • Pembrolizumab (PD-L1 expression >50% – first-line treatment) • Pembrolizumab (PD—L1 expression 1–50% – second-line treatment) • Nivolumab (second-line treatment)
	Squamous cell cancer	• Gemcitabine + cisplatin • Gemcitabine + carboplatin
	Adenocarcinoma (EGFR mutation in exons 19 and 21)	• Gefitinib • Erlotinib • Afatinib
	Adenocarcinoma (translocation ALK)	• Crizotinib
Breast cancer	In the absence of Her-2 overexpression	• Capecitabine • Gemcitabine + cisplatin • Paclitaxel + carboplatin **FAC regimen**: cyclophosphamide + doxorubicin + 5-fluorouracil (for treatment-naive patients) **AC regimen**: doxorubicin + cyclophosphamide (for treatment-naive patients) **CMF regimen:** cyclophosphamide + methotrexate + 5-fluorouracil (for treatment-naive patients)
	Overexpressing Her-2 (Her-2+++ by immunohistochemistry or FISH+):	• Capecitabine + lapatinib • Capecitabine + lapatinib + trastuzumab • Trastuzumab + chemotherapy with taxanes (for treatment-naive) or change of chemotherapy regimen (for previously treated) + local tumor control in the brain (whole-brain radiation therapy or radiosurgical treatment) • Pertuzumab + trastuzumab + taxanes + local tumor control (whole-brain radiation therapy or radiosurgical treatment) • Trastuzumab emtansine (T-DM1) + local control of tumor (whole-brain radiation therapy or radiosurgical treatment)
Melanoma	Negative for BRAF mutations	• Temozolomide • Fotemustine • Lomustine • Temozolomide + cisplatin • Ipilimumab • Nivolumab • Pembrolizumab
	Positive for V600 BRAF mutations	• Vemurafenib • Dabrafenib • Dabrafenib + trametinib • Vemurafenib + cobimetinib

(continued)

Table 4.1 (continued)

Renal cancer	First-line treatment	• Sunitinib • Pazopanib • Sorafenib • Bevacizumab (+ interferons)
	Second and subsequent lines of treatment	• Sunitinib • Pazopanib • Sorafenib • Temsirolimus • Bevacizumab • Everolimus + lenvatinib • Axitinib • Nivolumab • Cabozantinib
Colorectal cancer		• Capecitabine • CapeOx regimen: capecitabine + oxaliplatin • FOLFIRI regimen: irinotecan + leucovorin + 5-fluorouracil • Raltitrexed • Bevacizumab (in combination with chemotherapy) Negative for KRAS, NRAS, BRAF mutations: • Cetuximab (in combination with chemotherapy) • Panitumumab (in combination with chemotherapy)

4.6 Treatment Algorithms for Patients with Brain Metastases

1. Patients with a single MTS

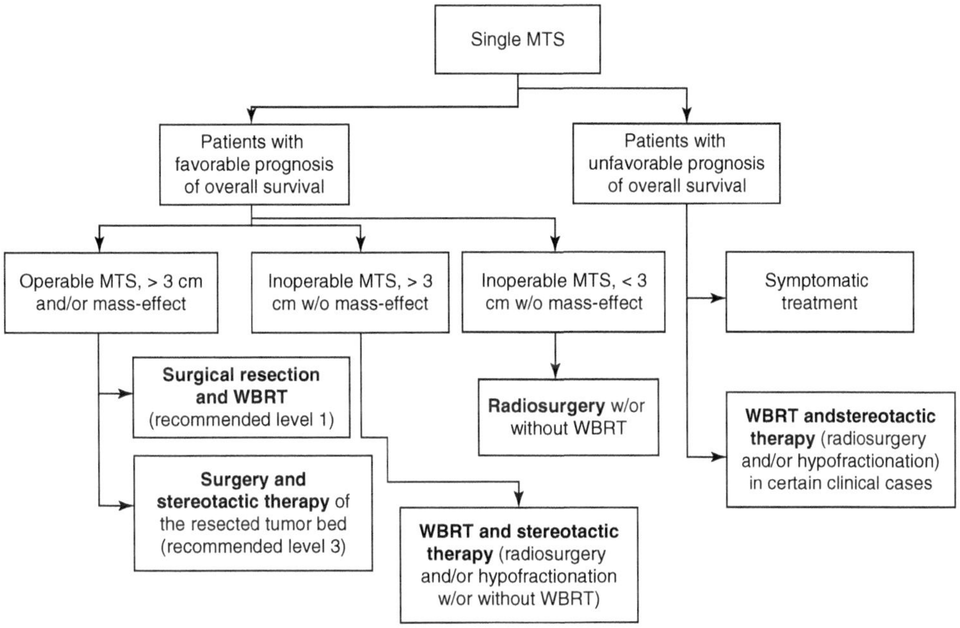

2. Patients with limited (two to three lesions)MTSs

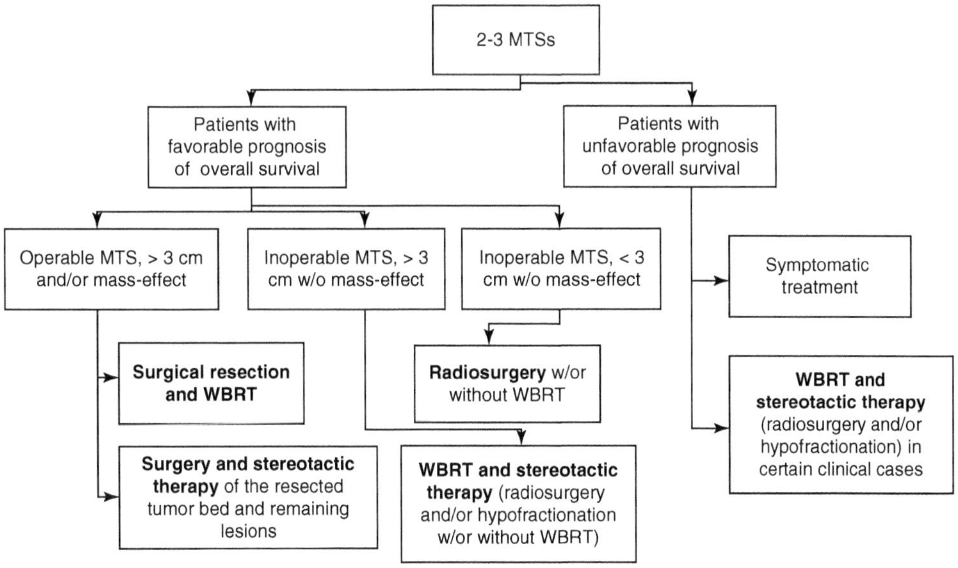

Part II

Neuroimaging Techniques in the Diagnosis of Brain Cancer Metastases

Introduction to Neuroimaging Techniques in the Diagnosis of Brain Cancer Metastases

5

Before the advent of X-ray imaging, cases of metastatic brain lesions were considered rare; furthermore, the direct application of this diagnostic method revolutionary for that time did not allow to identify brain tumors on radiographs, with exception of defects in the skull bones indirectly indicative of their tumor origin (Oppenheim 1901). In the early twentieth century, air encephalography (1919) was put into practice, followed by cerebral angiography (1931), allowing to detect changes in the brain vasculature and identify tumor vessels by their contrast enhancement (Dandy 1919 and Monitz 1927). In 1936, the method of electroencephalography (EEG) discovered as early as in 1875 was first applied to determine locations of brain tumors.

The advent of computed tomography (CT) in the late 1970s of twentieth century for the first time made possible direct X-ray imaging of brain tumors. However, only the introduction of CT contrast agents provided an opportunity for detection and identification of metastases among other brain tumors (Konovalov and Kornienko 1985a, b; Hardy et al. 1990; Khanjanasthiti et al. 1989). New opportunities in the diagnosis of brain metastases of malignant tumors with various locations occurred with the advent of magnetic resonance imaging (MRI) (Sze et al. 1990; Kuhn et al. 1994; Akeson et al. 1995; Schellinger et al. 1999). The development of radioisotope diagnosis, in particular single-photon emission computed tomography (SPECT) and positron emission tomography (PET), expanded the scope of the resulting visual information about tumors in various organs and tissues of the body and estimates of metabolic disorders in the brain substance and allowed to identify metastatic lesions, including those in the brain (Kitajima et al. 2009; Abdelmalik et al. 2013). It should be noted that X-ray imaging and cerebral angiography were the first imaging techniques used in neuro-oncology (Arutyunov and Kornienko 1971).

Among a variety of diagnostic techniques currently in use for investigation of internal human tissues and body fluids, it is impossible to single out one that best displays all the information necessary for clinicians, characterizing brain metastases. According to most neuroradiologists, a comprehensive diagnosis is required to assess brain metastases, including cerebral angiography, CT, MRI, single-photon emission computed tomography, and positron emission tomography (Kornienko and Pronin 2010; Abdelmalik et al. 2013). These techniques do not duplicate each other, since they differ in their "specialization"; therefore, each of them is used as part of the diagnostic system to solve only those problems where it has an advantage over the others: one is used to identify the primary foci; the other one for the detection of metastatic lesions, evaluation of their structure, and relationship with surrounding tissues; and the third one to clarify tumor growth and blood supply patterns. In addition, they allow to study changes in tumor growth, carry out a postoperative monitoring of patients, and evaluate the effectiveness of cancer treatment.

M. Dolgushin et al., *Brain Metastases*, DOI 10.1007/978-3-319-57760-9_5

6 Radiography

During the "pre-CT period," the diagnosis of brain lesions was based on the analysis of clinical symptoms, X-ray images, EEG data, radionuclide studies, cerebral angiography, air encephalography, ventriculography, and lumbar puncture (Moniz 1934; Engeset and Kristiansen 1940; Shlifer 1941; Lima 1950; Ecker and Riemenschneider 1955; Decker 1960; Robertson 1967). Despite such a large arsenal of diagnostic methods, diagnostic errors occurred quite a lot. Thus, according to Nisce et al. (1971), autopsies did not detect any brain tumors in 48 of 136 patients who underwent radiation therapy for brain metastases diagnosed based on the conclusions of radiological diagnostic methods. Of course, it is impossible to detect a tumor in the brain parenchyma and estimate its volume, structure, as well as the number of lesions based on X-ray findings. However, metastases in the bone structures of the skull can be diagnosed by X-ray imaging. Thus, metastases of malignant tumors of various origins in the cranial vault can be comparatively easily found on X-ray in frontal and lateral views. Figure 6.1 shows bone lesions of the cranial vault in breast cancer metastases. Metastatic changes in the cranial bones sometimes require X-ray images in special views in addition to the standard ones.

According to Kopylov (1968), the greatest difficulties in the differential diagnostic radiology of cranial tumors occurred in cases of destructive solitary metastatic lesions. The true nature of these lesions, according to the author, can be recognized based mainly on findings of general clinical examinations or repeated X-ray examinations. The presence of several destructive lesions with various sizes, often irregularly shaped without any noticeable reactive changes in the surrounding bone tissue, creates a sufficiently characteristic pattern of malignant metastases. Recently, in the era of CT and MRI, craniography and spondylography in the diagnosis of metastatic lesions are practically not used.

M. Dolgushin et al., *Brain Metastases*, DOI 10.1007/978-3-319-57760-9_6

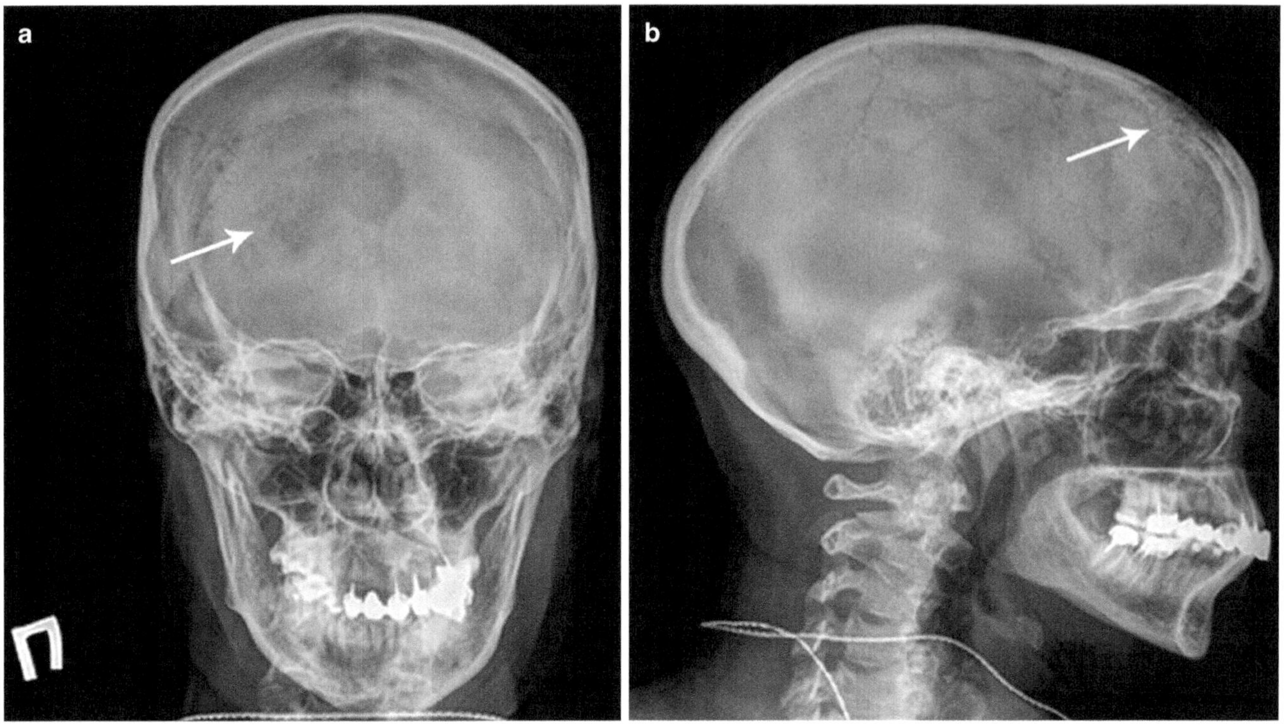

Fig. 6.1 Breast cancer metastases in the frontal lobe. Radiography. Images in frontal (**a**) and lateral (**b**) views in the squama of the frontal bone show an irregularly shaped area of bone destruction, which is an indirect evidence of a space-occupying lesion in the frontal lobe of the brain, growing into the frontal bone (*arrows*)

7 Cerebral Angiography

CAG is an X-ray technique of studying the vascular brain and spinal cord system, whose first stage is an artery puncture (usually the femoral artery) and its subsequent catheterization (Bryusova 1951; Galperin 1962; Arutyunov and Kornienko 1971; Krayenbuhl et al. 1979). Under fluoroscopic control, a catheter is inserted in the vascular pool of interest (selective angiography) or a separate vessel (superselective angiography) of the brain, followed by intra-arterial administration of a contrast agent with serial shots of the skull in the corresponding view (frontal, oblique, lateral). When studying the characteristics of the vascular structure of brain tumors based on cerebral angiography, Olivecrona and Tonnis (1954) noted that when metastases are located convexitally, their architectonics can have a picture similar to the architectonics of meningiomas. The authors failed to discover differences in metastases of different origins based on the characteristics of vasculature architectonics. Subsequently, some researchers reported that the vascular pattern of melanoma metastases in the brain was characterized by a "porous structure" with clear outlines; however, in cystic lesions, abnormal vasculature was sometimes not detected, but vessel dislocation might be observed (Rosner et al. 1986). According to CAG findings, solid metastases in the brain have a relatively homogeneous pattern of accumulation of a contrast medium, while the vasculature of glioblastomas is characterized by the presence of multiple arteriovenous shunts; therefore, the contrast agent accumulation pattern in these lesions is nonuniform (Kornienko and Pronin 2008a, b; Dolgushin 2012).

Figure 7.1 illustrates the results of an X-ray angiographic study of a melanoma metastasis in the brain: a marked tumor vasculature and a large draining vein running toward the superior sagittal sinus.

CT and MRI filled up the arsenal of high-tech diagnostic tools in the late 1970s and 1980s of the twentieth century and allowed to have a fresh look at current issues of neuro-oncology. Today, there is a possibility to investigate the location and structure of brain tumors and their relationship with the surrounding tissues.

M. Dolgushin et al., *Brain Metastases*, DOI 10.1007/978-3-319-57760-9_7

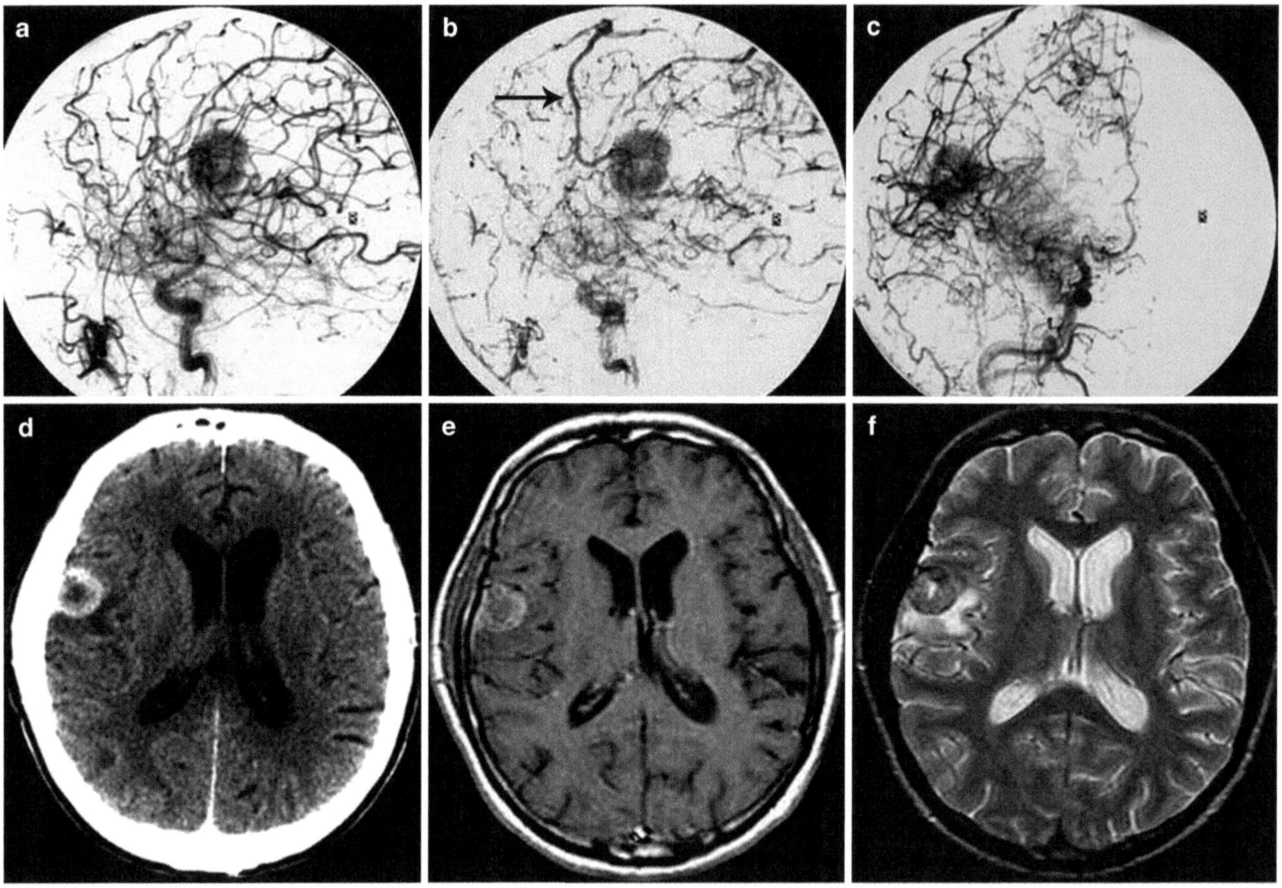

Fig. 7.1 Melanoma metastases in the right temporal region of the brain. An angiography (**a**–**c**) shows a marked tumor vasculature and a large draining vein (*arrow*). A CT scan (**d**) with contrast enhancement shows a rounded formation with annular contrast agent accumulation closely adjacent to the meninges. On T1 contrast-enhanced and T2-weighted MRI (**e**, **f**) images, the tumor is accompanied by a minimal peritumoral edema and has a moderately low T2 signal but a heterogeneously increased T1 signal

Computed Tomography (CT)

8

X-ray computed tomography (*CT*) has replaced X-ray projection techniques. CT provides images of brain cross sections in "digital" quality. In CT, an X-ray tube and detectors mounted on the opposite side in relation to the object move in a circle, with the object under study being in the center. During the movement of the tube, detectors sequentially record a plurality of projection data—ray sums—from different directions. Each ray sum includes the result of X-ray attenuation from each element of the object—a voxel—through which an X-ray beam passes from the tube to the detector.

The first layered sections of the object (phantom) were built based on repeated measurements of the total X-ray attenuation by Cormak in 1963, using an algorithm developed by him, which is now used in CT scanners. This is an algorithm to restore an object from its projections (filtered back projection).

The first device for X-ray examinations of the head was presented by Ambrose and Hounsfield (1973) at the annual congress of the British Institute of Radiology. The first CT scanner—an "EMI scanner" that produced a digital image of the head cross section—was built in England in 1972. Using it, Hounsfield and Ambrose clinically tested a new method. In 1973, Hounsfield published a detailed description of his "computer cross-scan system (axial scan)," as he called this method, as opposed to the so-called longitudinal scanning.

The first CT scanner used an algebraic method to calculate the X-ray attenuation coefficients μ (x, y) to find the X-ray attenuation in each cell layer—a voxel. Hounsfield proposed to display on the screen attenuation coefficients μ_T (x, y) in each volumetric pixel (voxel) of a layer in the form of so-called CT densities or X-ray attenuation values in the tissue, taken with respect to μ_{water} for water:

$$CT_{density} = \frac{\mu_T - \mu_{water}}{\mu_{water}} \times 1000\text{HU} \qquad (8.1)$$

Units of measurement of CT density, or a CT number, are called Hounsfield units (HU) in honor of the creator of the CT method. The CT density of water and any tissue with high water content, whose $\mu_T \approx \mu_{water}$ on the Hounsfield scale, corresponds to the value zero. The air has a negative CT density. The CT density of water and air in Hounsfield units is not dependent on the X-ray energy and takes specific, fixed values, 0 HU for water and 1000 HU for air, which are established when calibrating a CT scanner. Lung tissue and fat, due to their lower density relative to water and smaller attenuation ($\mu_{lung\ tissue} < \mu_{water}$), also have a negative CT density. Most tissues in the human body have a positive CT density. An element with the highest atomic number largest in the composition of bones and calcifications is calcium (CT density of 2000–3000 HU). The values of CT density of bone structures depend on the mineral composition of the bones.

Modern CT scanners use a range of CT densities from 1024 to 3071 HU. The greatest and the lowest values of μ on an image correspond to white and black areas, respectively, while intermediate values correspond to shades of gray. Images of transverse (axial) cross sections of an object are composed of individual elements—pixels—whose brightness in Hounsfield units is calculated by a computer based on the value of projection ray sums recorded when scanning an object.

Cormak and Hounsfield received the Nobel Prize in 1979 in Physiology or Medicine for the development of the method of computer tomography and creation of a CT scanner. CT has made breakthrough changes in neuroradiology, making possible the resolution between normal and abnormal tissues of the brain parenchyma with similar density (density resolution). This technique became known as the most important invention since the discovery of X-rays by Roentgen.

Currently neuro-oncology widely utilizes the so-called multislice scanners (MSCT) that use a multilayered matrix system of detectors and produce the data registration simultaneously for several spiral trajectories. The transition from a scanner with a single row of detectors and the period of tube rotation of 1 s to a scanner with a four-row detector system and the period of tube rotation of 0.5 s resulted in a potential

M. Dolgushin et al., *Brain Metastases*, DOI 10.1007/978-3-319-57760-9_8

eightfold increase in the efficiency of the X-ray use in scanning. The effectiveness of scanning of a 16-slice helical scanner increases 38 times. Currently, the number of detectors in scanners may be 256, 320, or more, i.e., scanners have become multidetector systems. Since during the scanning, a multislice scanner records the data for a certain area (volume) of the patient's body, these devices are sometimes referred to as three-dimensional CT scanners. The main advantage of multislice CT is high resolution (thin slices) and high speed of scanning. An important point is a reduced irradiation dose for the patient, which is achieved by decreasing the force of the anode current of the tube, reducing the exposure time, as well as using specialized image reconstruction algorithms to effectively reduce noise when recording the signals.

With a native (without contrast enhancement) CT study, metastases often look like isodense lesions or lesions with a low density relative to the density of the normal brain matter. In most cases, it is extremely difficult to determine a clear boundary between the tumor edge and gray matter, as the tumor "merges" with the deformed cortical brain substance. The boundaries between an edema and a tumor are better visible on CT slices, since the latter has a higher CT density relative to the edema area.

Today, the use of intravenous contrast enhancement is an integral part of CT examination protocols for patients with a suspected tumor in the brain. The current generation of diagnostic CT contrast agents consists of nonionic X-ray contrast agents containing 240–370 mg of iodine per 1 ml. The use of contrast enhancement significantly improves the sensitivity and specificity of CT examinations (Kornienko and Pronin 2006). According to Evert (2005), CT without contrast enhancement achieved positive results in only 3 of 38 patients with brain metastases and only due to the detection of perifocal edema in the brain substance.

Previously, it was thought that the use of CT with contrast enhancement allows detection of lesions in the brain in almost 100% of cases (Potts and Abbott 1980). However, as real practice shows, this is not the case; exceptions are lesions of less than 5 mm in diameter and lesions located convexitally (Fig. 8.1). According to our data, a large part of metastatic lesions almost always accumulates a contrast agent (~100%). However, even if a metastasis has a relatively large (up to 2 cm) size, especially if it is located in the convexital brain regions and

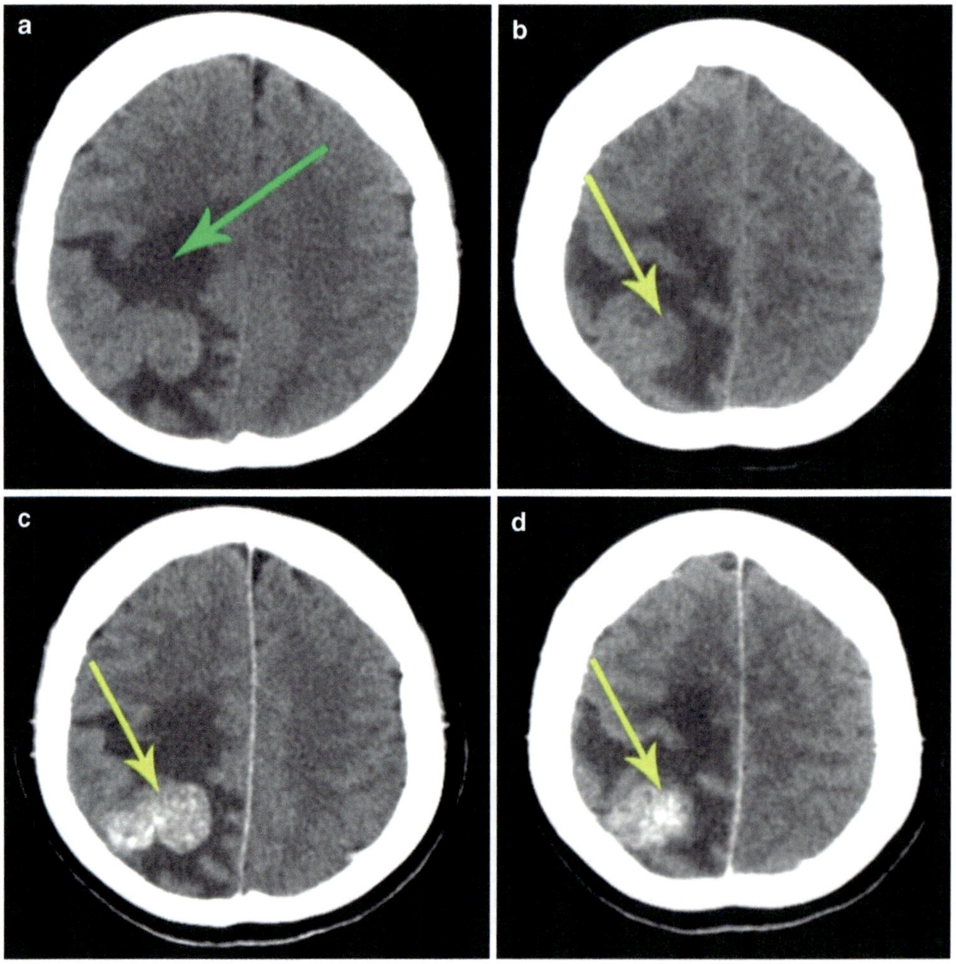

Fig. 8.1 A single breast cancer metastasis in the brain. Brain CT in the axial view before (**a**, **b**) and after (**c**, **d**) administration of the contrast agent. Along with an expressed perifocal edema (**a**), there is a large space-occupying lesion in the right parietal region. Prior to the introduction of the contrast agent, the lesion borders merge with the gray matter and are visualized only after an intravenous injection of the contrast agent

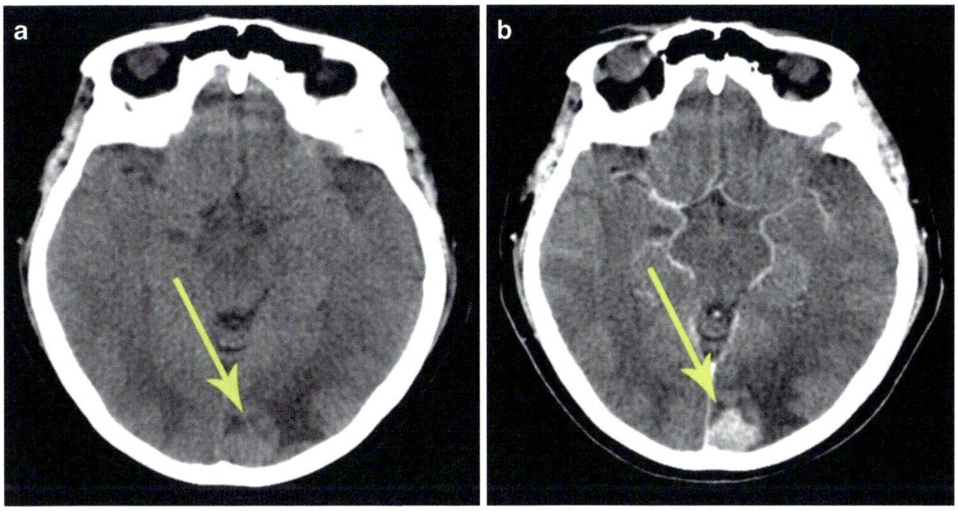

Fig. 8.2 A breast cancer metastasis in the brain. Brain CT before (**a**) and after (**b**) the administration of the contrast agent. In the projection of the left occipital region, there is a hypodense area (edema); a tumor lesion has a CT density similar to the CT density of the brain substance. After administration of the contrast agent, a parasagittal tumor lesion (*arrows*) is clearly visualized

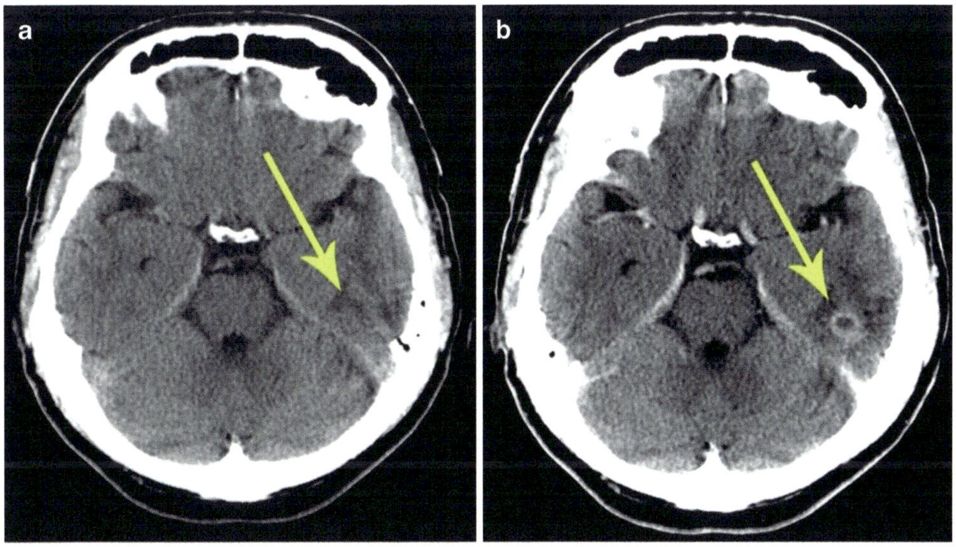

Fig. 8.3 A squamous cell lung cancer metastasis in the brain. Brain CT before (**a**) and after (**b**) the administration of the contrast agent. In the projection of the basal parts of the left temporal region, there is a hypodense lesion, while the tumor is not visualized. After administration of the contrast agent, the metastasis has a clear rounded shape and signs of central necrosis, which, on the background of an edema, gives a picture of ring enhancement (*arrows*)

with a minimum edema of the brain matter, it can be difficult to determine the tumor without contrast enhancement (Fig. 8.2).

Determination of the contrast enhancement border in cystic tumors (a thin solid component) is also difficult with small (less than 1 cm) sizes of metastases and in case of their proximity to the bone structures, in particular, with basal locations (Fig. 8.3).

With intravenous contrast enhancement, ring enhancement—a pathognomonic sign for most metastatic tumors—can be observed, which manifests as an increased density of the boundaries of a solid part of the tumor relative to the central necrotic areas on the background of the hypodense edematous brain substance. This sign is often not related to the size of metastatic lesions (Fig. 8.4).

In multiple brain metastases, lesions with central necrosis and hemorrhages (a high-density area on CT) can be observed along with homogeneous solid lesions (usually small). The cause of a hemorrhage is likely to be the damage to the blood vessel walls located in the tumor tissue (Fig. 8.5).

A perifocal edema of the brain substance in metastatic lesions can manifest in different ways, regardless of the structure and size of lesions, which may be associated with differences in the time of lesion occurrence, specifics of their blood supply, their proximity to the venous structures, and specifics of their own angiogenesis. The analysis of 958 CT observations showed that there was a severe, moderate, and insignificant (mild) perifocal edema, significantly larger than the tumor area in 76% of cases, with an equal size or smaller than the size of the metastasis in 23%, respectively, and only in 1% of cases, the edema was completely missing (Dolgushin 2012) (Table 8.1).

According to our data, in case of multiple metastases, a perifocal brain edema is not detected around some lesions and detected around other ones, even in the same patient (Fig. 8.6).

An interesting but inexplicable fact is that a perifocal edema can sometimes be absent altogether, despite the large size of a metastasis: most often, this is typical of a tumor located in the posterior fossa (Fig. 8.7).

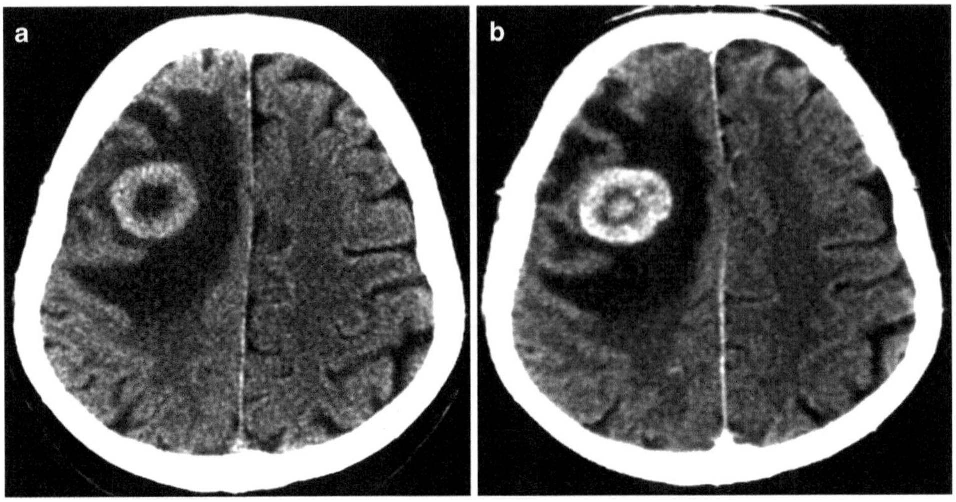

Fig. 8.4 A kidney cancer metastasis in the brain. In brain CT, the metastasis in the brain matter is well visualized both before (**a**) and after (**b**) intravenous administration of the contrast agent. The metastatic lesion has hyperdense characteristics before administration of the contrast agent (**a**). After contrast enhancement (**b**), there is a pronounced inhomogeneous accumulation of the contrast agent in the tumor

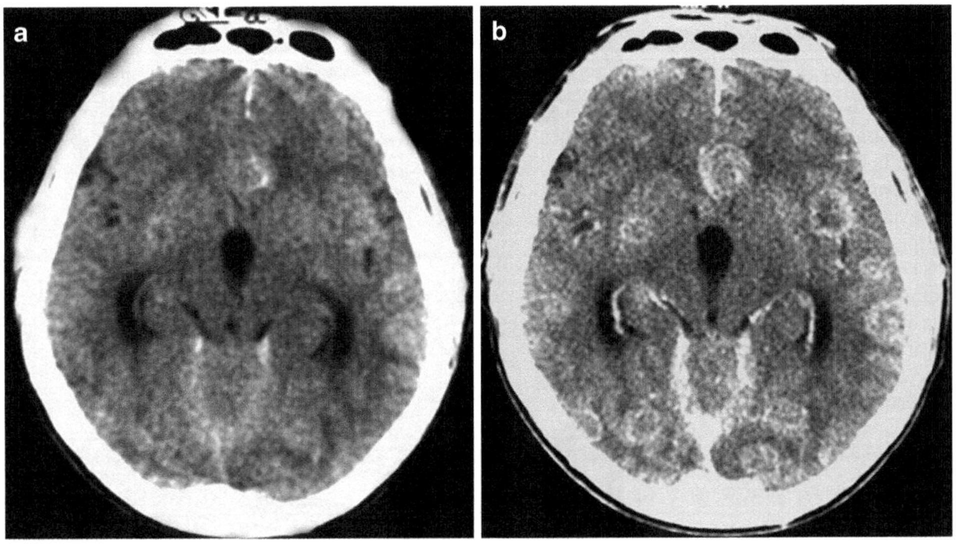

Fig. 8.5 Multiple lung cancer metastases in the brain. High-density areas can be seen on a CT scan before contrast enhancement (**a**) (due to hemorrhages in the tumor tissue). (**b**) After intravenous contrast enhancement, a large number of tumor lesions of various sizes can be observed

Table 8.1 Severity of perifocal edema on CT in patients with metastatic brain lesions ($n = 958$)

Perifocal edema (%)				
Severe	Moderate	Mild	Absence	Total (n)
728 (76)	172 (18)	46 (4.8)	12 (1.2)	958

Routine CT is not the method of choice for the diagnosis of metastatic brain lesions in general, since even studies with contrast enhancement do not fully visualize the true picture of the disease spread. Selection of CT imaging for primary diagnosis is a single option only in clinics where there is no MRI scanner. It should be remembered that the objectives of CT studies are not only to suggest (confirm, exclude) the secondary nature of brain lesions but also to search for a possible primary source of the tumor lesions in other organs and tissues. The assumption of the metastatic character of brain lesions requires an expansion of a CT imaging area, including studies of the chest, since, according to some authors, the lungs are a sort of a "transfer post" for metastases before they spread into the brain (Nersesyants et al. 1951, 1955).

In recent years, the method of brain CT has been significantly enriched by additional protocols and techniques that include 3D visualization, angiography, and perfusion studies.

8.1 3D Imaging Technology

3D imaging technology for constructing images improved the quality of neurosurgical diagnostics in general (Turkin and Belov 2000; Kornienko and Pronin 2009a, b, c, d, 2012). An important advantage of this technique is the possibility to assess bone changes (Fig. 8.8). CT allows to clearly visualize the extent of bone involvement and destruction of bone tissue. Three-dimensional processing allows to obtain additional information to clarify the location of an abnormal lesion in relation to the surrounding tissues and helps surgeons plan the extent of a surgical intervention and the subsequent bone reconstruction.

Most often, breast cancer (47–85%), prostate cancer (54–85%), and thyroid cancer (28–60%) metastasize to the cranial

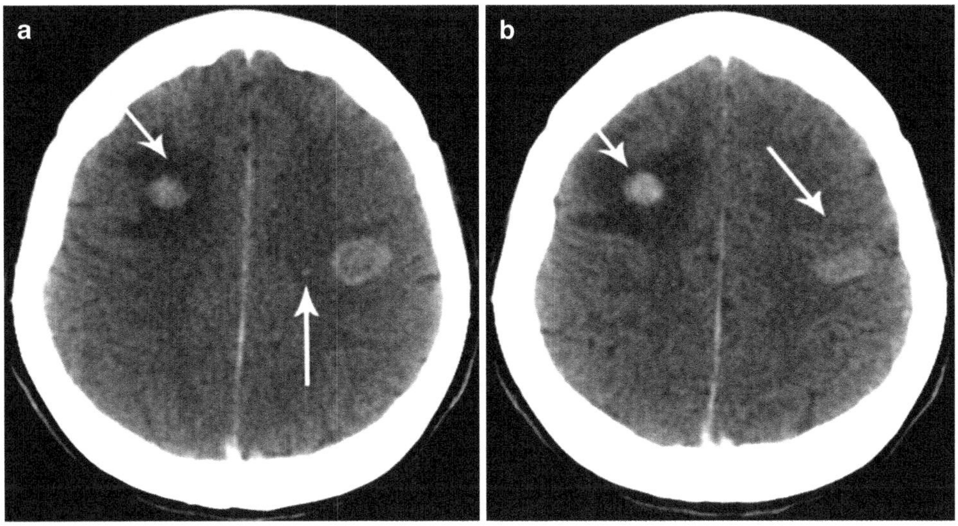

Fig. 8.6 Lung cancer metastases in the brain. Brain CT in the axial view before and after administration of the contrast agent. In the projections of the frontal areas, multiple metastatic tumors are observed in the right hemisphere of the brain with a pronounced perifocal edema, while there is no edema in the left one, in spite of the larger size of the lesion (**a**, **b**). Furthermore, contrast enhancement allows to identify micrometastases (**a**) (*arrows*)

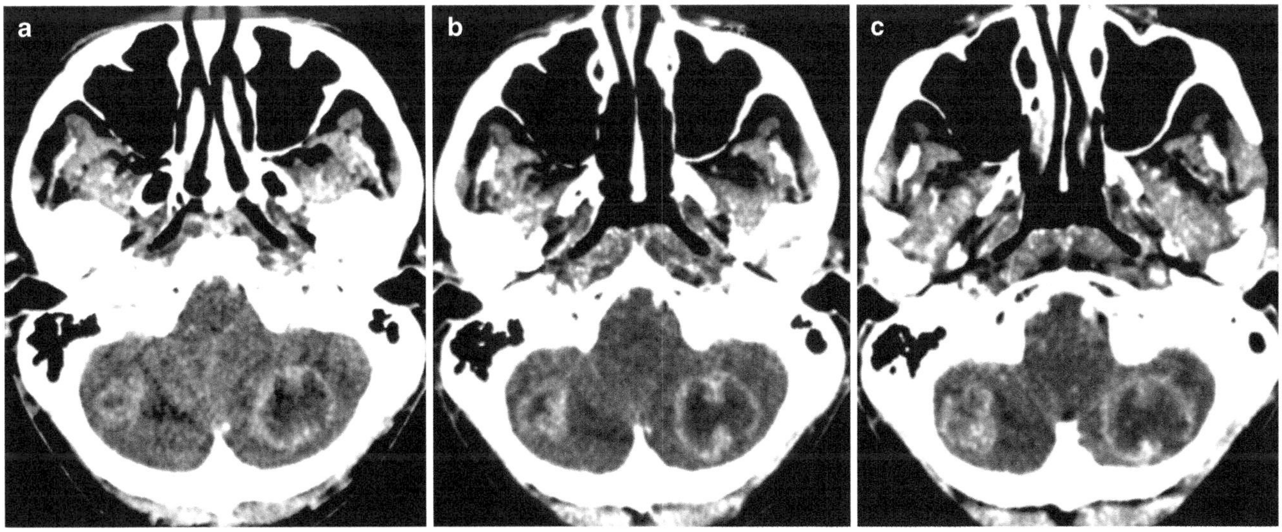

Fig. 8.7 Multiple breast cancer metastases in the brain. CT with contrast enhancement (**a**–**c**). In the projection of the basal parts of both cerebellar hemispheres, there are tumor lesions with necrosis in the center and a contrast-enhanced thin peripheral part. There is almost no perifocal edema

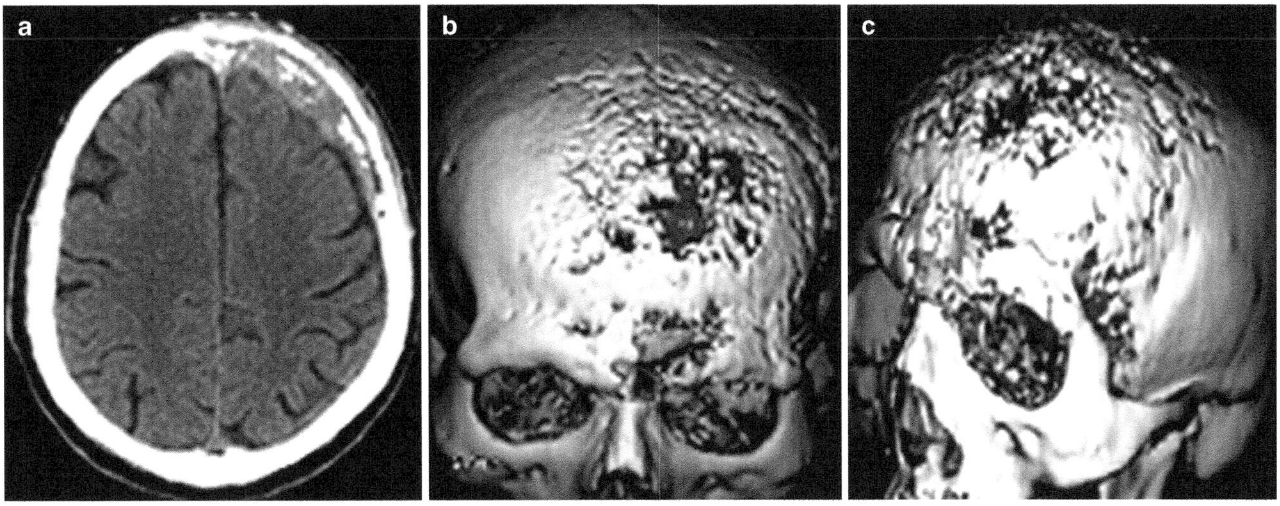

Fig. 8.8 A breast cancer metastasis in the cranial bones in a male patient. Brain CT in the axial projection (**a**) and a 3D reconstruction of the skull (**b**, **c**). There are significant destructive changes in the squama of the frontal bone, mostly on the left. 3D images well determine the lesion size and the involvement of the frontal, parietal and temporal bones. No changes in the brain substance (**a**) are identified

bones, followed by kidney cancer (33–40%), lung cancer (32–40%), melanoma (12%), ovarian cancer (9%), esophageal cancer (5–7%), and colorectal cancer (8–13%) (Dolgushin 2012). The cranial bones are affected in 20% of all cases of bone metastases. Hematogenous metastasizing into the vertebral bodies and cranial bones can occur not only through the systemic blood flow but also through the vertebral venous plexus, via a valveless system of venous anastomoses running along the spine from the brain to the lesser pelvis. Tumor cells are brought by bloodstream into the bone marrow. They secrete a variety of factors that start to affect osteoclasts, increasing their activity and accelerating the process of bone destruction (osteolytic metastases). Hence, bone thinning and vertebral fractures occur even at low physical activity. In some tumors (e.g., in prostate cancer), osteoblasts are activated, which leads to excessive growth of bone tissue (osteoplastic metastases). The type of a metastasis, osteolytic or osteoblastic, depends on the osteoclast to osteoblast activity ratio.

Multiplanar reconstructions based on SCT, along with 3D images, increase the informative value of diagnostic data on the relationship between a metastatic tumor with brain structures, vault bones, and bone structures of the skull base, the posterior cranial fossa.

8.2 SCT Angiography (CTA)

SCT angiography (*CTA*) is successfully competing with subtraction angiography in the detection of vascular abnormalities. Unlike direct cerebral angiography, in head and neck vascular CTA, a contrast agent flows through the venous system. High-density and spatial resolution of spiral CT allows to construct volumetric (3D) models of the vascular system. Modern helical CT scanners have a high spatial resolution of anatomical details (512 × 512 image matrix) and high temporal resolution—the duration of one data acquisition cycle takes less than 0.5 s. Administration of 60–80 ml of a contrast agent in CTA is performed using an automatic injector at 4–5 ml/s rate. Dynamic 4D SCT allows to simultaneously receive data for both angiography (arterial blood flow) and perfusion CT (capillary blood flow). The scanning in SCT angiography is carried out with a minimum slice thickness (0.5–1.25 mm). Isolation of sections corresponding to arterial or venous phases from a dynamic series allows to construct cerebral arterio- and venograms in different projections, independent of each other. CTA, similar to cerebral AG, provides information on the sources of tumor blood supply and their relationship with the major cerebral arteries, which allows to plan a surgical access and an extent of tumor resection.

A dynamic series of sections for the capillary phase of the contrast agent transit allows to evaluate the pathophysiological specifics of perfusion in metastatic lesions, obtaining quantitative estimates of hemodynamic perfusion parameters (cerebral blood flow (CBF), cerebral blood volume (CBV), mean transit time (MTT) of blood through the vascular network, and microvascular permeability PS), as well as to monitor the effectiveness of the cancer treatment and to carry out postoperative monitoring. A quantitative evaluation as part of diagnostic studies in brain tumors is relevant for modern neuroradiology and especially neuro-oncology.

8.3 Perfusion CT (PCT)

A new trend in using the possibilities of computed tomography is a quantitative assessment of changes in density characteristics of the tissue following intravenous bolus administration of a contrast agent—CT perfusion. An important factor in this regard is the possibility of obtaining multilateral quantitative characteristics related to the hemodynamics in the brain tissue, its tumors, and their adjacent areas. Perfusion methods estimate and quantify blood flow feeding the brain tissue through the capillary system. A theoretical rationale for evaluating the basic parameters of cerebral blood flow, such as velocity (CBF) and volume (CBV) of the latter using intravascular bolus administration of a contrast agent (CA), was developed in the 1950s of the twentieth century (Meier and Zierler 1954; Kety and Schmidt 1948). With the advent of CT, Axel (1983) proposed a method for measuring cerebral perfusion via dynamic scanning: registration of CT slice images $i =$ of the same location as the contrast agent bolus passes through the vasculature.

At present, for the data processing of dynamic CT series, specialized workstations or modern personal computers with the perfusion parameter-processing software are used; they perform the required calculations for each voxel with the possibility of constructing parametric CBV, CBF, MTT, and PS maps.

The first clinical use of CT perfusion was undertaken to assess the extent of ischemic brain damage in stroke by visualizing the brain hypoperfusion areas on parametric CBF and CBV maps within the first minutes after the onset of an acute ischemic attack (Lev and Nichols 2000; Konig 2003). Extension of the PCT scope allowed to obtain additional information (to detect areas of hyperperfusion) for the diagnosis of brain tumors and their differentiation from other focal lesions based on their hemodynamic features (Eastwood and Provenzale 2003; Pronin et al. 2005, 2007; Dolgushin et al. 2015).

The so-called principle of the central volume underlies study methods of tissue perfusion, which is the law of conservation of mass in relation to the cerebral circulation. According to this principle,

$$CBV = MTT \times CBF, \quad (8.2)$$

where CBV is cerebral blood volume passing through 100 g of a substance, measured in ml/100 g of the brain tissue; CBF is a cerebral blood flow in ml/100 g/min; and MTT is mean transit time in seconds.

The classic method of visual perfusion analysis is the construction of perfusion maps, where the brightness (and color) is proportional to the value of the selected quantitative perfusion parameter—MTT, CBF, and CBV.

Methods of CT evaluation of tissue perfusion use shape and temporal characteristics of the contrast enhancement profile in supplying arteries and draining veins in the brain tissue after intravenous bolus administration of a contrast agent (Fig. 8.9). To obtain similar time dependences, a series of sequential CT scans at predetermined levels is performed.

A PCT algorithm involves performing a standard plain CT to determine location of sections for a perfusion study. A contrast agent with a high iodine concentration (350–370 mg/ml) in an amount of 40 ml (plus 20 ml of saline after CA administration) is administered via a bolus injection in the cubital vein of a patient using an automatic syringe at 4 ml/s (administration rate of 4 ml/s is sufficient for most dynamic data processing programs). CA administration per protocol starts 5 s before the scanning. Data logging is performed for 40–50 s, at intervals of 1 s and with the X-ray tube voltage of 80 kV. If necessary, a "post-contrast" CT is performed; however, the appropriateness of the latter should be considered in each individual case, as an additional CT scanning increases the radiation dose for the patient (Wintermark et al. 2004; Konstas et al. 2009).

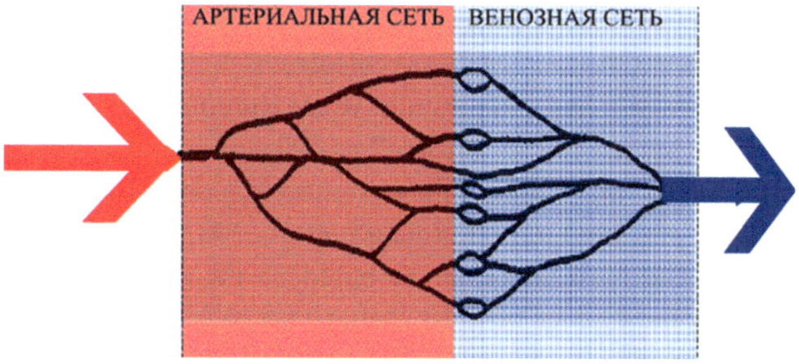

Fig. 8.9 The scheme of vasculature at the tissue level is represented by a system of randomly oriented arterioles, capillaries, and venules (from Meier and Zierler 1954)

CT density values recorded in a perfusion study depend on the amount of contrast agent contained in the tissue at the moment. The curve of CT density changes in each slice voxel as bolus of a contrast medium passes is characterized by the concentration-time dependence. The shape of this curve in the artery and vein determines an inlet (arterial) and outlet (venous) function, respectively (Fig. 8.10). According

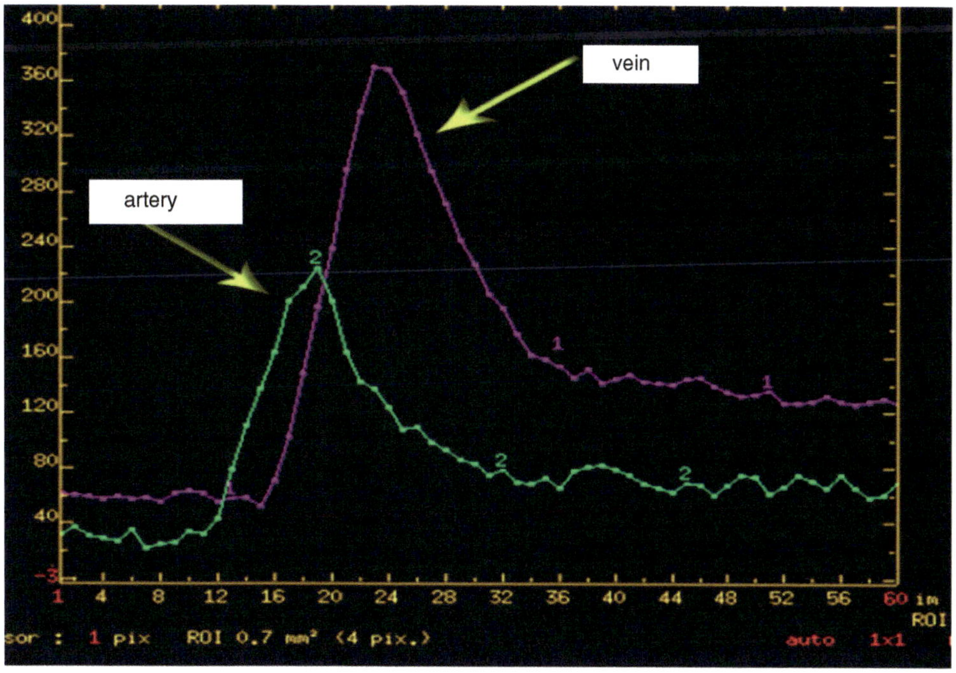

Fig. 8.10 The curve of CT density characteristics as bolus of a contrast medium passes. The "concentration-time" curves for arteries and veins are indicated by arrows

to the concentration-time curve, hemodynamic tissue parameters CBV, CBF, and MTT are calculated.

Perfusion maps and quantitative measurement of the data are constructed in the "off-line" mode on specialized workstations; the algorithm of their construction can be found in the relevant literature (Kornienko et al. 2007; Miles et al. 2007). The main algorithm is based on the deconvolution method, the essence of which is that if we look at some tissue volume at time t, the amount of CA in the volume *C*(*t*) will consist of the volume *V*(*t*) of the substance brought by arterial blood flow at this tissue site at the moment, plus a part of *W*(*t*) of the contrast agent that was brought earlier but had not yet "left" the investigated tissue volume. The volume *V*(*t*) brought in this short time interval Δt should be equal to the product of CA volume in the artery by F = CBV via this volume:

$$V(t) = F \times C_a(t) \times \Delta t \quad (8.3)$$

The volume *W*(*t*) can be represented by the sum of earlier "infusions" $F \times C_a(t-\Delta t) \times \Delta t$, multiplied by a factor $R(t-\Delta t)$ ("residual function") indicating the percentage of these earlier infusions that did not have time to leave the given volume (i.e., $0<R(t-\Delta t)<1$). As a result, the CA concentration in the tissue can be determined using the following equation:

$$C(t)=V(t)+W(t)=F_t \cdot \int C_a(u) \cdot R(t-u) \cdot du = C_a \otimes F_t \cdot R(t) \quad (8.4)$$

where the mathematical symbol ⊗ represents the convolution operation, or "convolution," and the function *R*(*t*) is considered monotonically decreasing, and $R(0) = 1$. The equation must be solved to find the flow F and "residual function" *R*(*t*), which has been called "deconvolution."

Duration of the flat portion in the graph *R*(*t*) (Fig. 8.11) is the minimum transit time of blood through the vascular system, and the area under the curve *R*(*t*) corresponds to the mean MTT value. Cerebral blood flow volume CBV is the product of *CBF* and *MTT*.

Of greatest interest in evaluating the specific features of metastatic tumors is their solid component that contains the greatest number of viable tumor tissue, having all the properties of the primary tumor to the maximum extent. This part of the neoplasm usually intensively accumulates contrast agent.

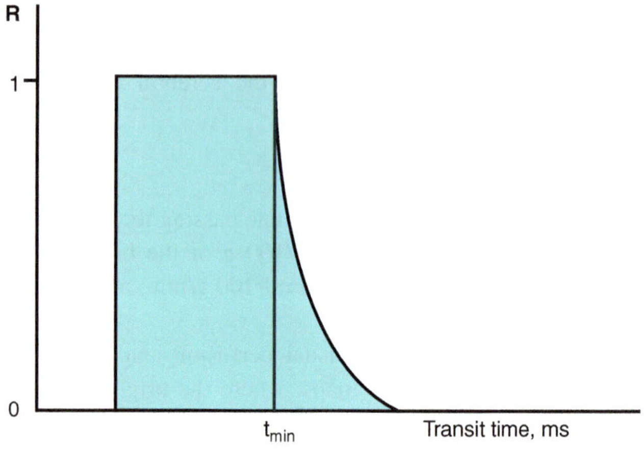

Fig. 8.11 *R*(*t*) is the "residual function," indicating which part of the earlier CA infusion has not yet left this volume. Duration of the flat portion in the graph *R*(*t*) is the minimum transit time of blood through the vascular system, and the area under the curve *R*(*t*) corresponds to the mean MTT value

The development of most cancers is associated with the need for a blood supply sufficient to meet the needs of increased tumor metabolism. This, in turn, results in the formation of additional abnormally formed or branched vasculature, which is reflected in increased perfusion parameters. Data received from perfusion CT (n = 126) allowed us to analyze the perfusion values in metastatic tumors in the brain based on the nature and location of the primary source (Dolgushin et al. 2015).

8.4 CBV (Cerebral Blood Volume)

Using perfusion maps, mean and maximum CBV values are measured in the solid portion of metastatic tumors depending on the location of their primary source (Fig. 8.12).

Comparative CBV values for brain metastases from various primary sources are listed in Table 8.2 (Dolgushin et al. 2007, 2015).

Maximum CBV values were obtained for brain metastases of kidney cancer (21.01 ± 6.21 ml/100 g), followed by, in a descending order, melanoma, breast cancer, and lung cancer (15.03 ± 9.75–11.27 ± 3.21 ml/100 g) and uterine and colorectal cancer (8.94 ± 3.33–8.14 ± 3.71 ml/100 g). The lowest CBV value was obtained for ovarian cancer metastases (5.34 ± 1.45 ml/100 g).

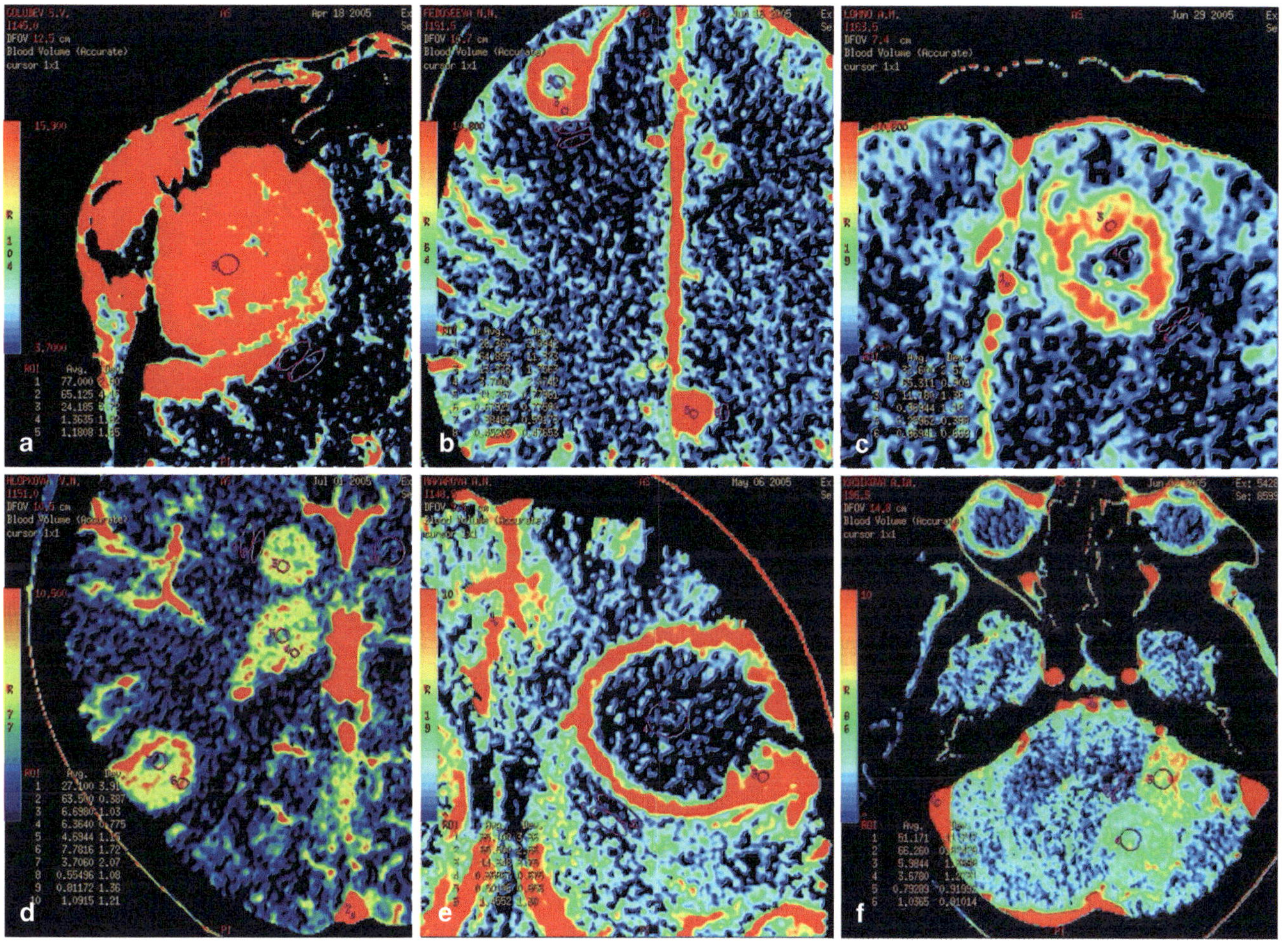

Fig. 8.12 CBV maps of brain CT perfusion in patients with metastases of kidney cancer in the right frontal region (**a**), melanoma in the right frontal region (**b**), lung cancer in the left frontal region (**c**), breast cancer in the right subcortical nuclei and in the parietal region (**d**), cervical cancer in the left frontal region (**e**), and ovarian cancer in the left hemisphere of the cerebellum (**f**). There is a marked increase in CBV values in tumor foci characterized by intense staining in *red* or *yellow-red* in all cases, except for the metastasis of ovarian cancer (**f**) *green color*, which reflects a relatively low CBV value

Table 8.2 CBV values in a solid structure of brain metastases from primary tumors with different locations (n = 126)

Location of the primary tumor	Average values (ml/100 g)	Standard deviations (ml/100 g)
Breast	11.57	5.79
Lung	11.27	3.21
Kidney	21.01	6.21
Colon	8.14	3.71
Melanoma	15.03	9.75
Ovary	5.34	1.45
Uterus	8.94	3.33

8.5 CBF (Cerebral Blood Flow)

This hemodynamic parameter represents the velocity of blood flow in the capillary network and is the next important factor quantifying tumor hemodynamics (Fig. 8.13).

Comparative CBF values of brain metastases from a variety of primary tumors are listed in Table 8.3.

The maximum CBF values were obtained for melanoma metastases (113.35 ± 24.25 ml/100 g/min), followed by, in a descending order, metastases of uterine, breast, lung, colorectal, and kidney cancer (102.59 ± 16.35–72.13 ± 35.35 ml/100 g/

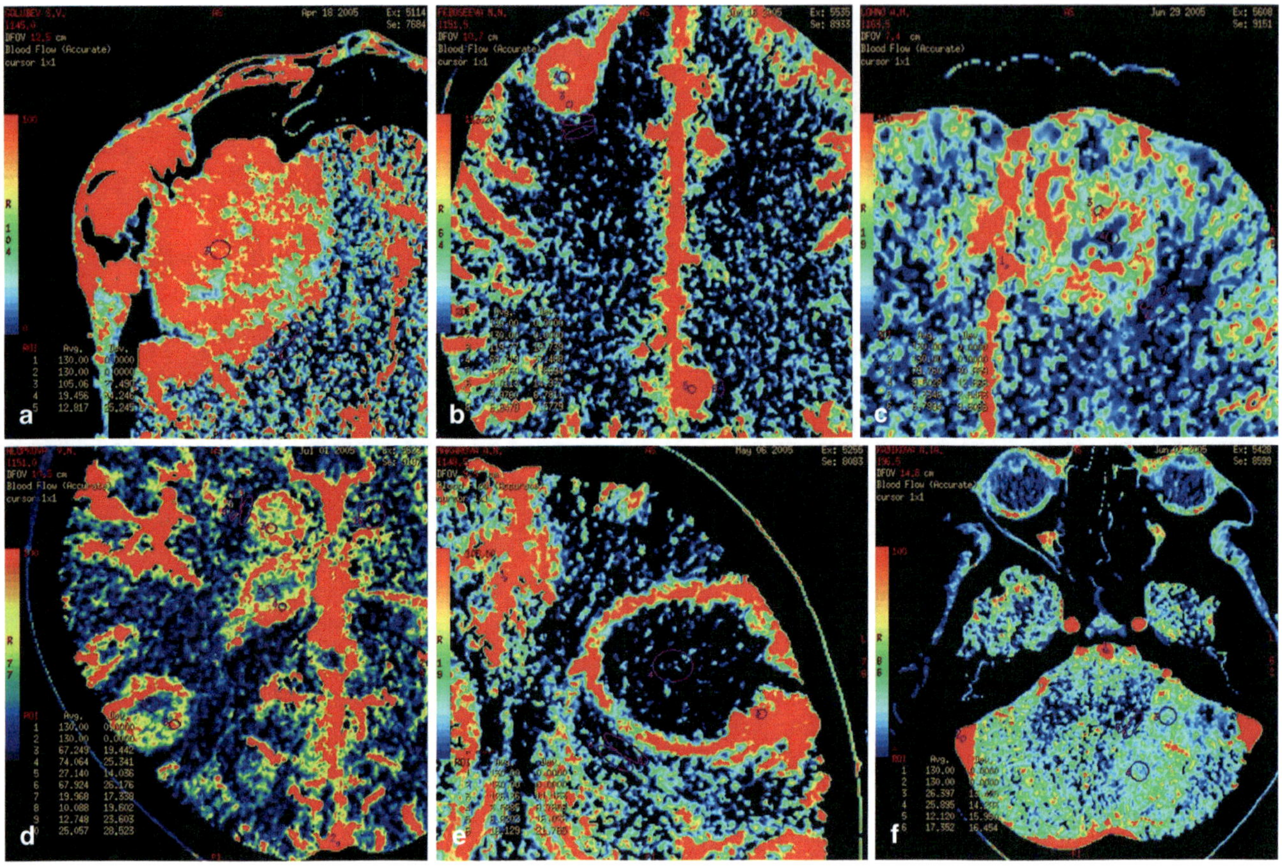

Fig. 8.13 CBF maps of brain CT perfusion in patients with metastases of kidney cancer in the right frontal region (**a**), melanoma in the right frontal region (**b**), lung cancer in the left frontal region (**c**), breast cancer in the right subcortical nuclei and in the parietal region (**d**), cervical cancer in the left frontal region (**e**), and ovarian cancer in the left hemisphere of the cerebellum (**f**). There is a marked increase in CBF values in tumor foci characterized by intense staining in *red*, except for the metastasis of ovarian cancer (**f**) *green color*, which reflects relatively low CBF values

Table 8.3 CBF values in the solid structure of brain metastases from primary tumors with different locations ($n = 126$)

Location of the primary tumor	Average values (ml/100 g/min)	Standard deviations (ml/100 g/min)
Breast	92.04	29.93
Lung	85.03	19.56
Kidney	73.93	27.59
Colon	72.13	35.35
Melanoma	113.35	24.25
Ovary	49.51	19.6
Uterus	102.59	16.35

min). The lowest CBF value was obtained for ovarian cancer metastases (49.51 ± 19.60 ml/100 g/min) (Dolgushin et al. 2007).

8.6 MTT (Mean Transit Time)

Another important perfusion indicator is MTT that characterizes the transit of CA through a capillary network of a unit of volume of the solid part of the metastasis (Fig. 8.14).

MTT shows not the duration of the contrast agent transit through a pixel but the CA delay time in the tumor tissue. Mean MTT values in the solid part of the brain metastases from primary tumors with different locations are listed in Table 8.4 (Dolgushin et al. 2007).

Table 8.4 shows that metastases of uterine cancer (5.36 ± 0.74 s) and melanoma (MTT = 7.22 ± 2.1 s) pass the blood the fastest (low MTT values). The slowest blood transit is through the tissue of kidney cancer metastases (18.38 ± 1.37 s), with these values being more than twofold higher than MTT values of melanoma metastases. It should be noted that the choice of an area for the measurement of MTS values for melanoma perfusion is complicated in cases where there are foci of hemorrhages in the tumor structure.

When measuring and analyzing the mean transit time of the blood through the unit volume of the tissue (MTT), take into account that the greater the numerical value, the slower the blood with contrast agent (CA) passes through the tissue per unit of time.

An important condition for obtaining the required image quality for further quantitative data is to select the largest artery on the affected side for reading the parametric data (Kornienko and Pronin 2009a, b, c, d). Often, when tumors

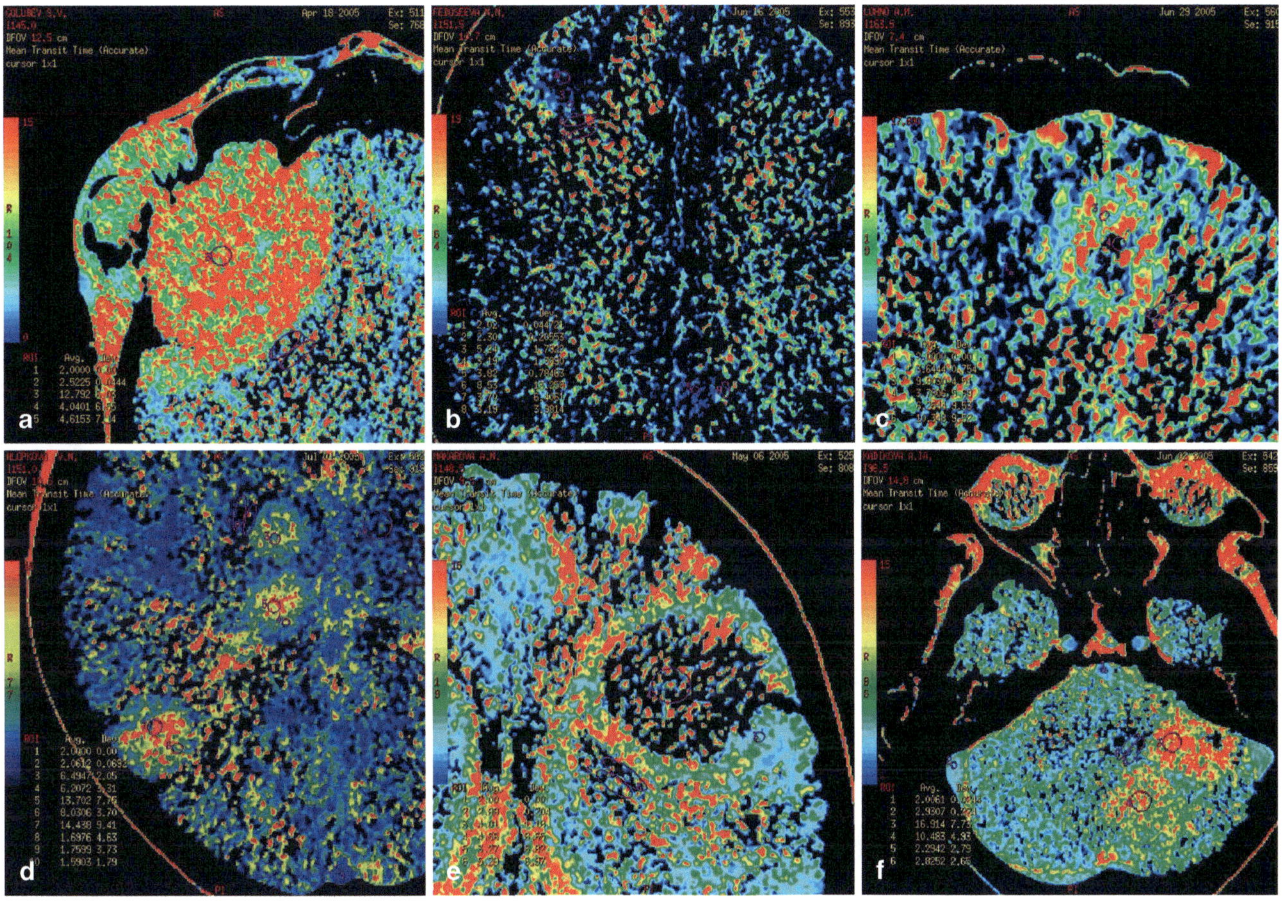

Fig. 8.14 MTT maps of brain CT perfusion in patients with metastases of kidney cancer in the right frontal region (**a**), melanoma in the right frontal region (**b**), lung cancer in the left frontal region (**c**), breast cancer in the right subcortical nuclei and in the parietal region (**d**), cervical cancer in the left frontal region (**e**), and ovarian cancer in the left hemisphere of the cerebellum (**f**). There is a decrease in MTT values in tumor foci, characterized by weak staining of melanoma tissue (**b**), which reflects the high level of blood flow. MTT values in other metastases are higher

Table 8.4 Mean transit time (MTT) of contrast agent via a solid portion of the capillary network in the brain metastases from primary tumors with different locations ($n = 126$)

Location of the primary tumor	Mean values (s)	Standard deviations (s)
Breast	7.60	3.11
Lung	8.83	2.85
Kidney	18.38	1.37
Colon	7.72	3.26
Melanoma	7.22	2.1
Ovary	10.58	6.27
Uterus	5.36	0.74

are located in the cortical areas of the frontal and parietal regions and the plane of sections is planned in parallel to the base of the anterior cranial fossa, or, if necessary, when studying several tumor sites located in different brain regions (upper sections of the parietal region and basal temporal area), a situation may arise in which the arteries in the section do not meet the necessary requirements (a small diameter, a tortuous course). In such cases, "oblique" slices are justified, being achieved by placing the patient's head at a certain angle relative to the axis of the passing beam and tilting the CT scanner gantry, which does not result in the loss of the study quality and distortion of the results of the quantitative data analysis. In turn, obtaining thin post-contrast enhancement sections allows to transform the images obtained in conventional axial sections if necessary. Typically, the choice of venous structures is not an issue, because large venous sinuses can be easily found at certain levels of tomographic sections.

The introduction into clinical practice of modern multiple row detector spiral CT scanners (64, 128, 256, 320, and more) allows to minimize these issues with the choice of arteries due to a large primary coverage of anatomical zones.

Figure 8.15 presents a case of the patient with lung cancer metastases in the brain, who underwent a CT perfusion study with his head turned to the right. Such patient's position gives a possibility to select an artery located in the depth to read the arterial parametric data. On a CT section, the lesion prior to the administration of

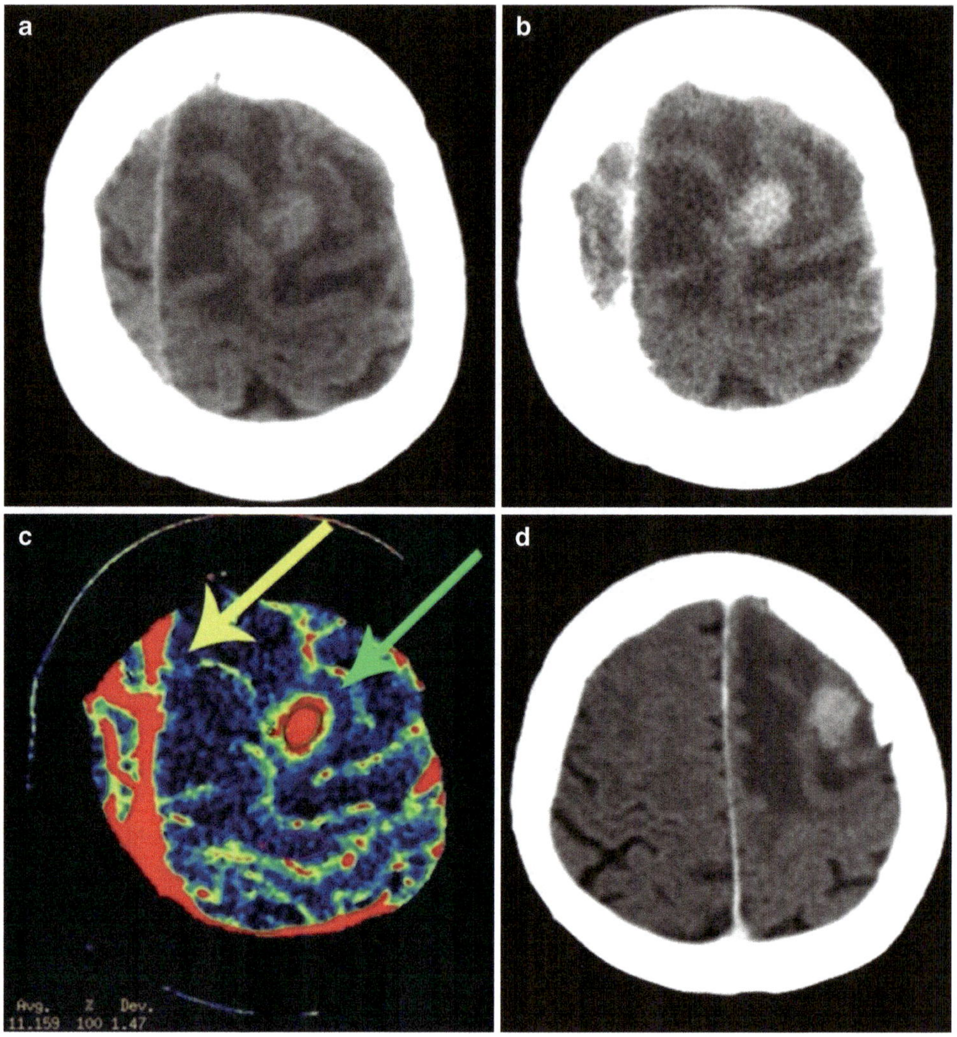

Fig. 8.15 A relapse of melanoma metastasis in the left frontal region. On a CT scan with the patient's head turned to the right, the lesion is indistinguishable from cerebral convolutions before the administration of the contrast medium (**a**); after an intravenous injection of the contrast agent (**b**), there is an intense accumulation of the latter in the tumor. On a CBV perfusion map (**c**), arrows indicate the superior sagittal sinus displaced right and a tumor. A strictly axial reformat of post-contrast enhancement series of images (**d**)

the contrast medium is isodense and is surrounded by a pronounced perifocal edema. The CT perfusion study performed with the head turn allowed to more accurately select the region of interest (ROI) (arrow) on the oblique section. The superior sagittal sinus on the section is displaced to the right (arrow), with the tumor site being displayed in the center of the image and sufficiently spaced from the bone structures, with which the metastatic lesion would merge in case of a conventional positioning of the patient's head (Fig. 8.15d).

A comparative assessment of perfusion parameters in multiple lesions showed the following relationship: CBV and CBF values in a larger lesion were usually higher than those in smaller lesions (Fig. 8.16). MTT values did not differ significantly.

8.7 CT Perfusion in Evaluating the Results of Treatment of Patients with Brain Metastases

The CT perfusion method is available, does not require extensive training, and is currently successfully used in the monitoring of radiosurgical (RS) treatment of patients with metastatic brain lesions.

In our clinical practice, the CT perfusion method was used not only for primary diagnosis of metastatic brain tumors but also for assessing post-radiation changes at any stage of patient treatment (n = 78). Thus, dynamic changes in the main perfusion parameters (CBV, CBF, and MTT) allowed us to monitor the effectiveness of radiation therapy already at an early stage (up to 2 months) after the

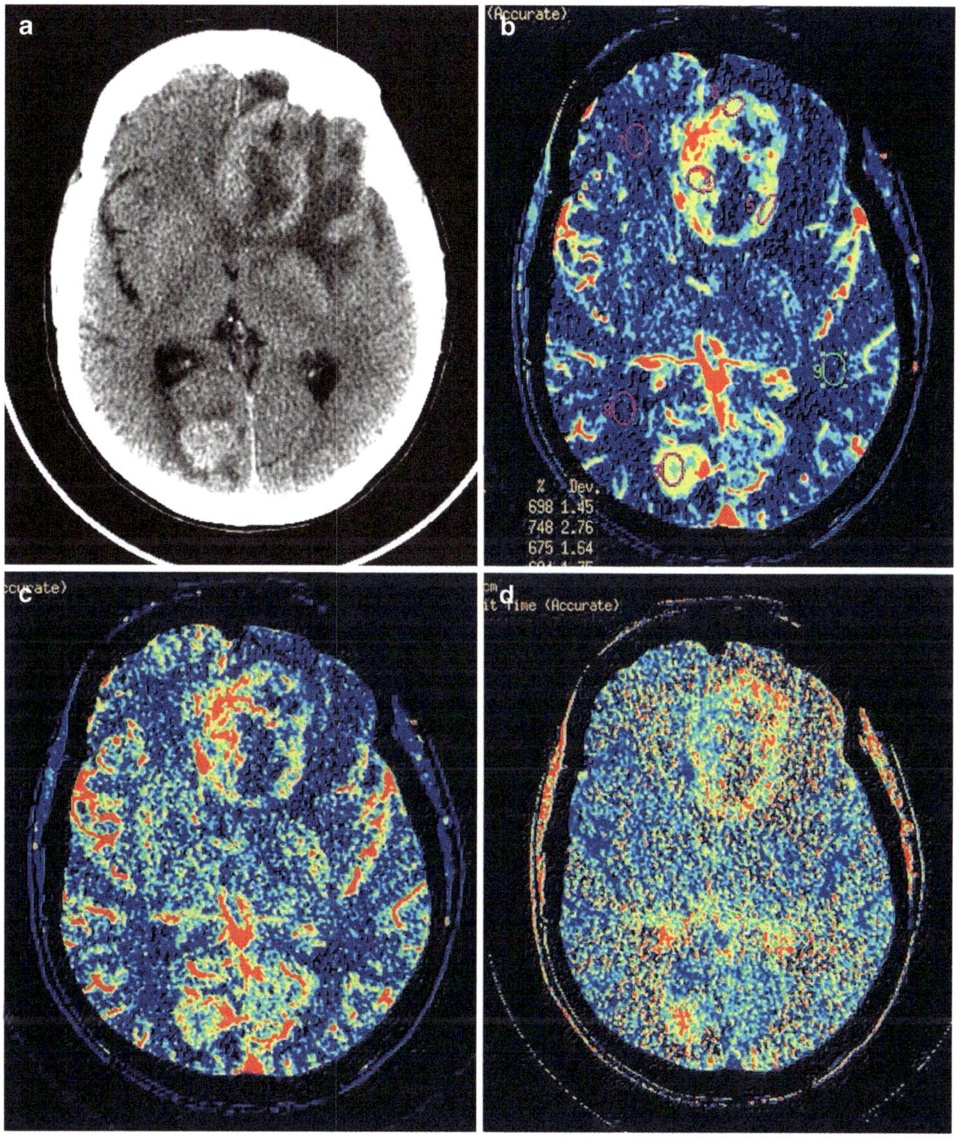

Fig. 8.16 Multiple melanoma metastases in the brain. CT with contrast enhancement (**a**) shows multiple, large lesions in the left frontal and right parietal regions, accompanied by a perifocal edema. On perfusion maps CBV (**b**), CBF (**c**), and MTT (**d**), unevenly increased CBF and CBV are observed in solid tumor fragments, while MTT values are heterogeneous

completion of radiation therapy, whereas other neuroimaging methods (CT and MRI with contrast enhancement) proved to be ineffective in assessing the dynamic changes occurring in the irradiated tumor in the early period after the treatment completion.

Changes in the main perfusion parameters within the first month after the radiosurgical treatment are shown in Fig. 8.17. Analysis of CBV, CBF, and MTT values in this group of patients ($n = 12$) showed that within 3 weeks after the treatment, a slight decrease in CBF and CBV values and an increase in MTT ($p \geq 0.05$) in the solid component of the tumor were noted.

The results of CT perfusion studies carried out 1, 4, and 6 months after the radiosurgery in patients ($n = 46$) with metastases in the brain are shown in Figs. 8.18, 8.19, and 8.20. The mean CBV values in the solid part of metastases were CBV = 7.03 ± 1.48 (ml/100 g). One month after, there was a decrease in CBV values down to 5.2 ± 1.4 (ml/100 g) and a further decrease down to 1.3 ± 0.7 ml/100 g over the next 3 months in CBV values. A control CT perfusion study 6 months after the treatment revealed a further decrease in CBV values down to 1.04 ± 0.12 ml/100 g.

Analysis of CBF values showed changes with time similar to those for CBV. Figure 8.19 shows a graph of changes in CBF values 1, 4, and 6 months after the radiosurgical treatment.

The vector of changes in MTT values differed from the above results of CBV and CBF data analysis and had a multidirectional nature. So, 1, 3, and 6 months after the radiosurgical

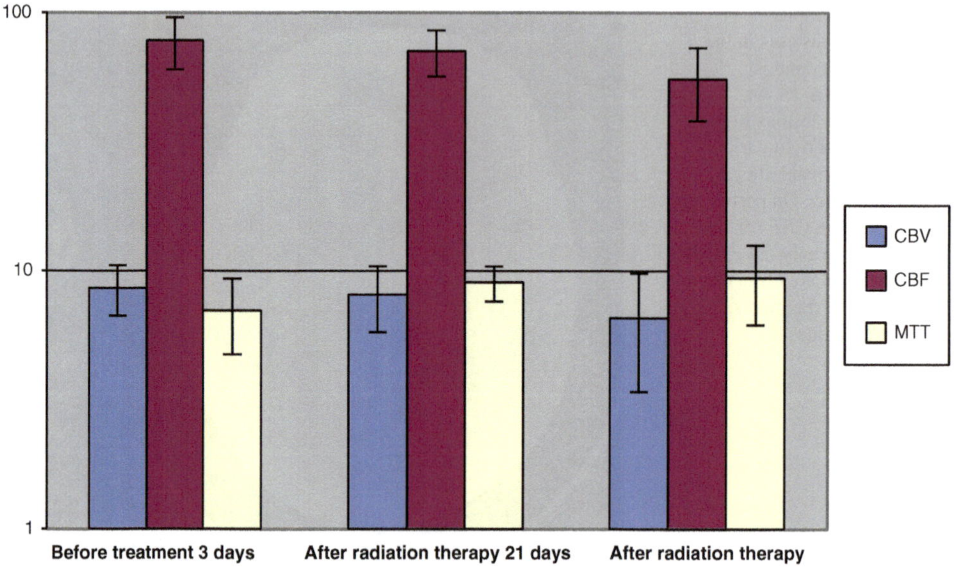

Fig. 8.17 Mean values of main CT perfusion parameters: before, 3 days after and 21 days after the completion of the radiation therapy. A moderate decrease in CBV and CBF was observed within the first 3 weeks after treatment, while MTT values increased

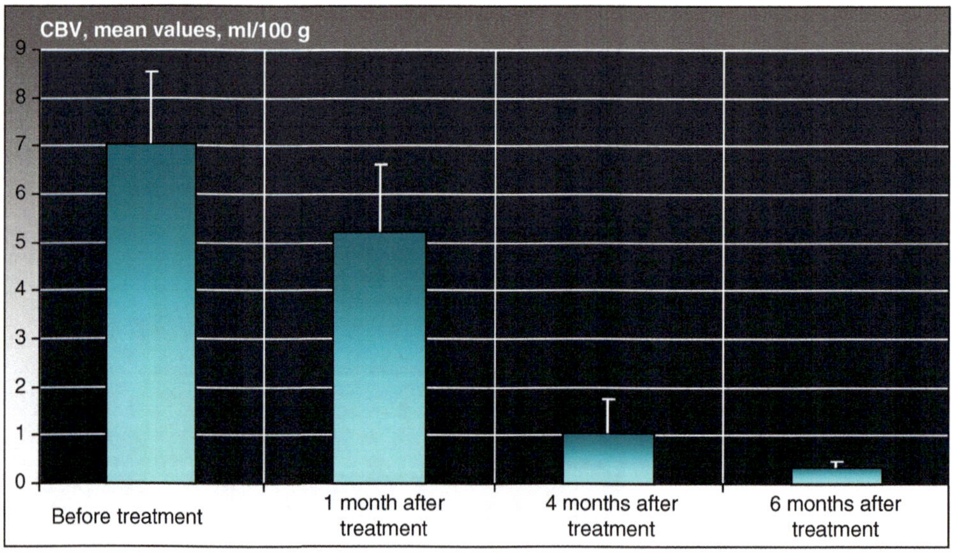

Fig. 8.18 The mean CBV values in the solid part of metastases within the first 6 months after the radiosurgical treatment. A significant decrease in the values

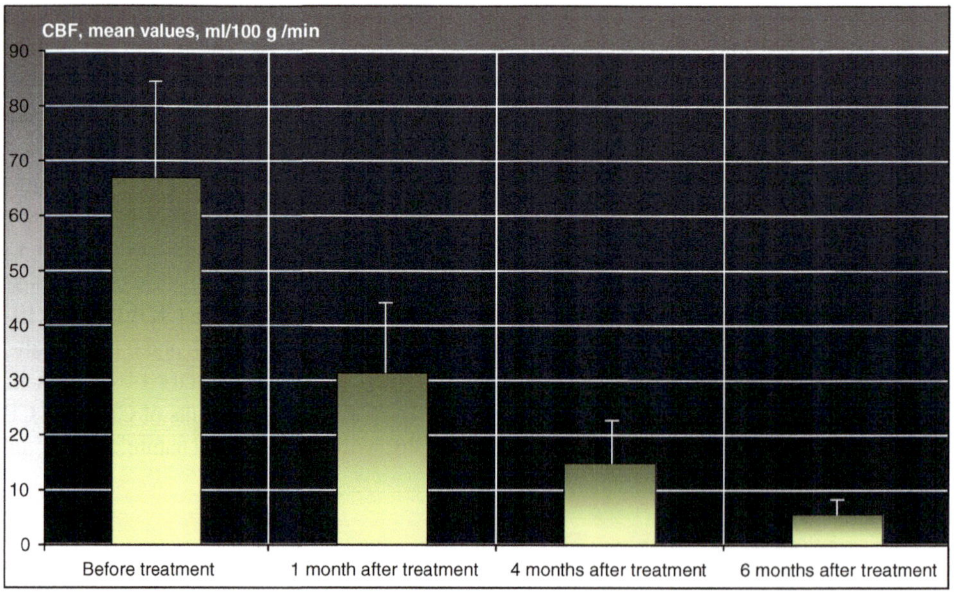

Fig. 8.19 The mean CBF values in the solid part of metastases within the first 6 months after the radiosurgical treatment. A significant decrease in the values

treatment, there was nearly a twofold increase in MTT values from 7.62 ± 2.42 (s) to 13.2 ± 3.08 (s), a decrease down to 3.6 ± 2.12 (s), and values were 5.4 ± 2.4 (s), respectively.

Abrupt changes in MTT values may be associated with the BBB state and development of associated post-radiation necrotic processes (Fig. 8.20). The initial increase in MTT values probably indicates a destruction of the tumor microvasculature and a slower blood flow through its tissue. Apoptosis and related post-radiation vascular changes are reflected in the decrease in CBV and CBF values and an increase in MTT values in the CT perfusion study. An increase in MTT values in the tumor structure is characteristic of the post-radiation changes (Fig. 8.21).

A dynamic decrease in CBV and CBF values and an increase in MTT were indicative of the post-radiation nature of changes in 100% of cases (Fig. 8.22). In this case, the mean CBV and CBF values in the solid part of metastases (more than 3 months) decrease by more than threefold ($p < 0.04$ and $p < 0.02$, respectively) in the later period after the radiosurgery, and the time of the contrast agent transit through tumor tissue (MTT) increased almost twice ($p < 0.06$).

The resulting perfusion characteristics shown in Fig. 8.22 reflect the positive ("expected") dynamics in post-radiation changes—a reduction in tumor size and a decrease in the edema surrounding the brain tissue (in MR study), while improving the patient's clinical condition. The data obtained were used for further comparative assessment of dynamic changes, while deviations of perfusion parameters from those specified above were considered as predictors of disease recurrence or treatment failure. It should be noted that, in routine follow-up CT and MRI with contrast enhancement, radiographic manifestations such as a reduction in the volume of the contrast-enhanced part and a decrease in edema around the metastases were observed 2–3 months later with respect to the changes in CT perfusion parameters.

Actively proliferating metastases tend to have increased CBV and CBF values and low MTT values, which characterizes a rapid blood flow in this lesion. Therefore, we considered that high CBV and CBF values or their increase with time, with an increasing size of a portion of abnormal contrast enhancement on MR scans, indicates extended tumor growth (Fig. 8.23).

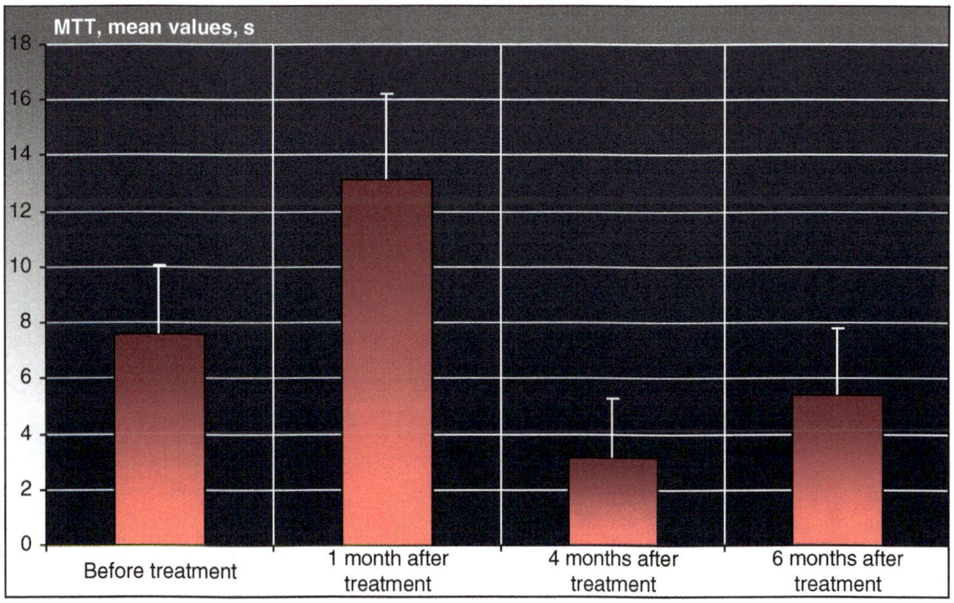

Fig. 8.20 The mean CBF values in the solid part of metastases within the first 6 months after the radiosurgical treatment. Multidirectional changes in parameters

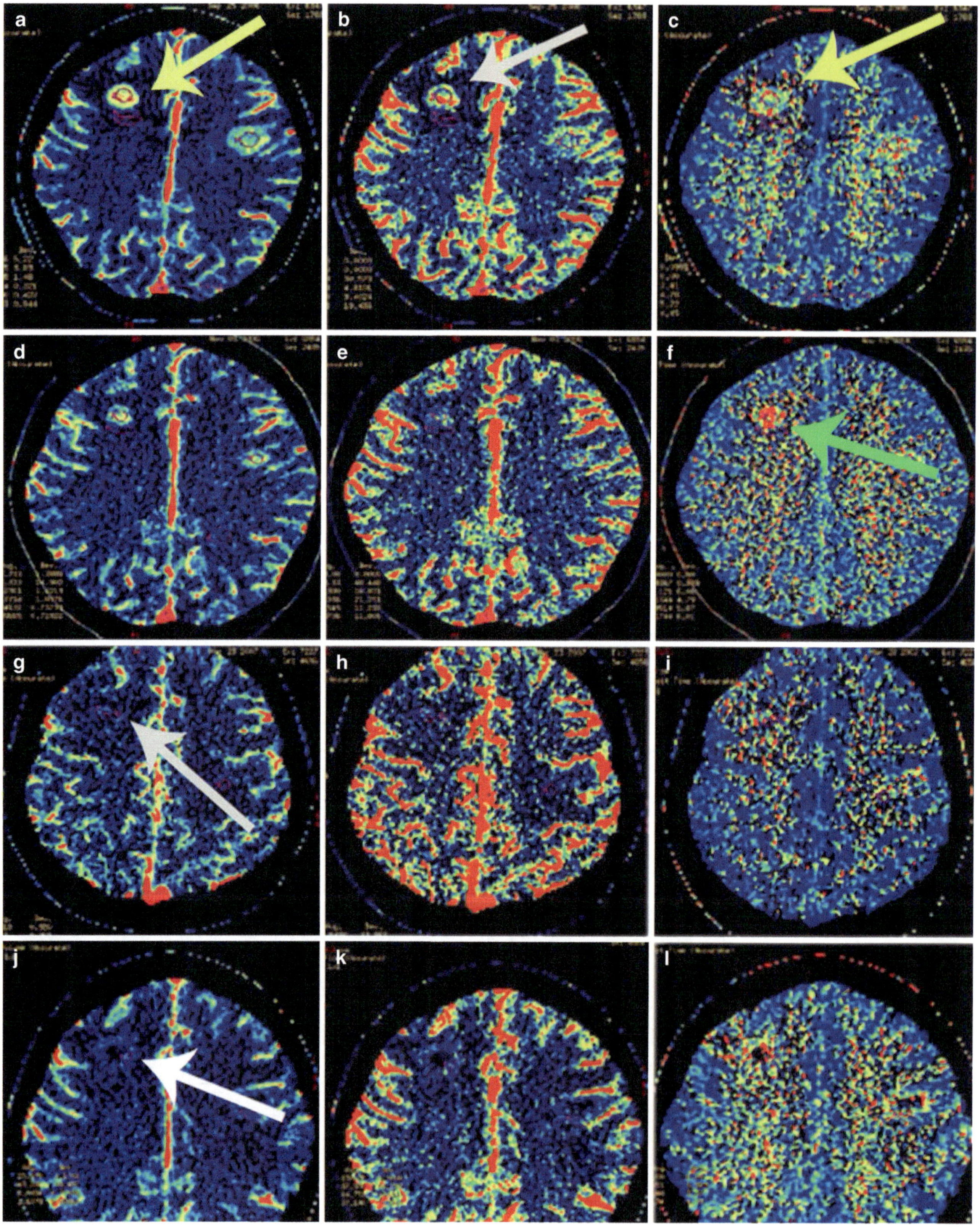

Fig. 8.21 Multiple lung cancer metastases in the brain. Perfusion maps of changes in CT perfusion parameters for 6 months after radiation therapy. Before treatment (**a–c**), there were high CBF and CBV values and mean MTT values in the solid component of the metastasis located in the right frontal area. These values indicate a significant blood supply to the tumor. On CT perfusion maps, the metastatic lesion is shown in *bright red* and *yellow* (*yellow arrows*). One month after the treatment (**d–f**), CBV and CBF values decreased, while MTT significantly increased (*bright red–green arrow*). The size of metastatic foci decreased. Four months after the treatment (**g–i**) lesions were not visualized, indicating the "alignment" of perfusion values between the tumor lesions and the surrounding brain substance. Six months after the treatment (**j–l**), there was a formation of a zone with low CBV and CBF values (*dark areas*) and increased MTT (**l**)

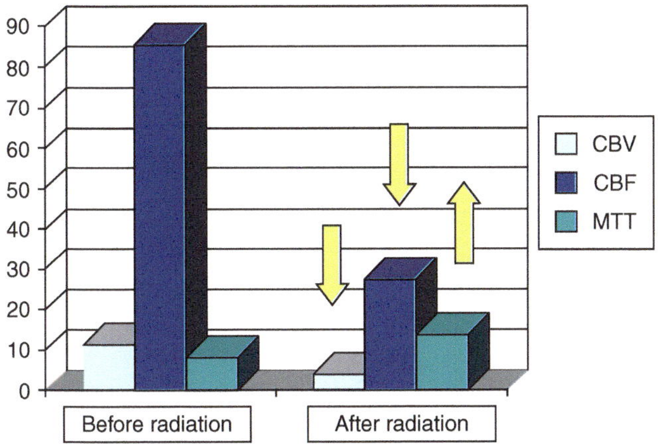

Fig. 8.22 The mean values of CT perfusion parameters before and 3 months after the radiosurgery. There is a marked decrease in CBF and CBV and an increase in MTT values

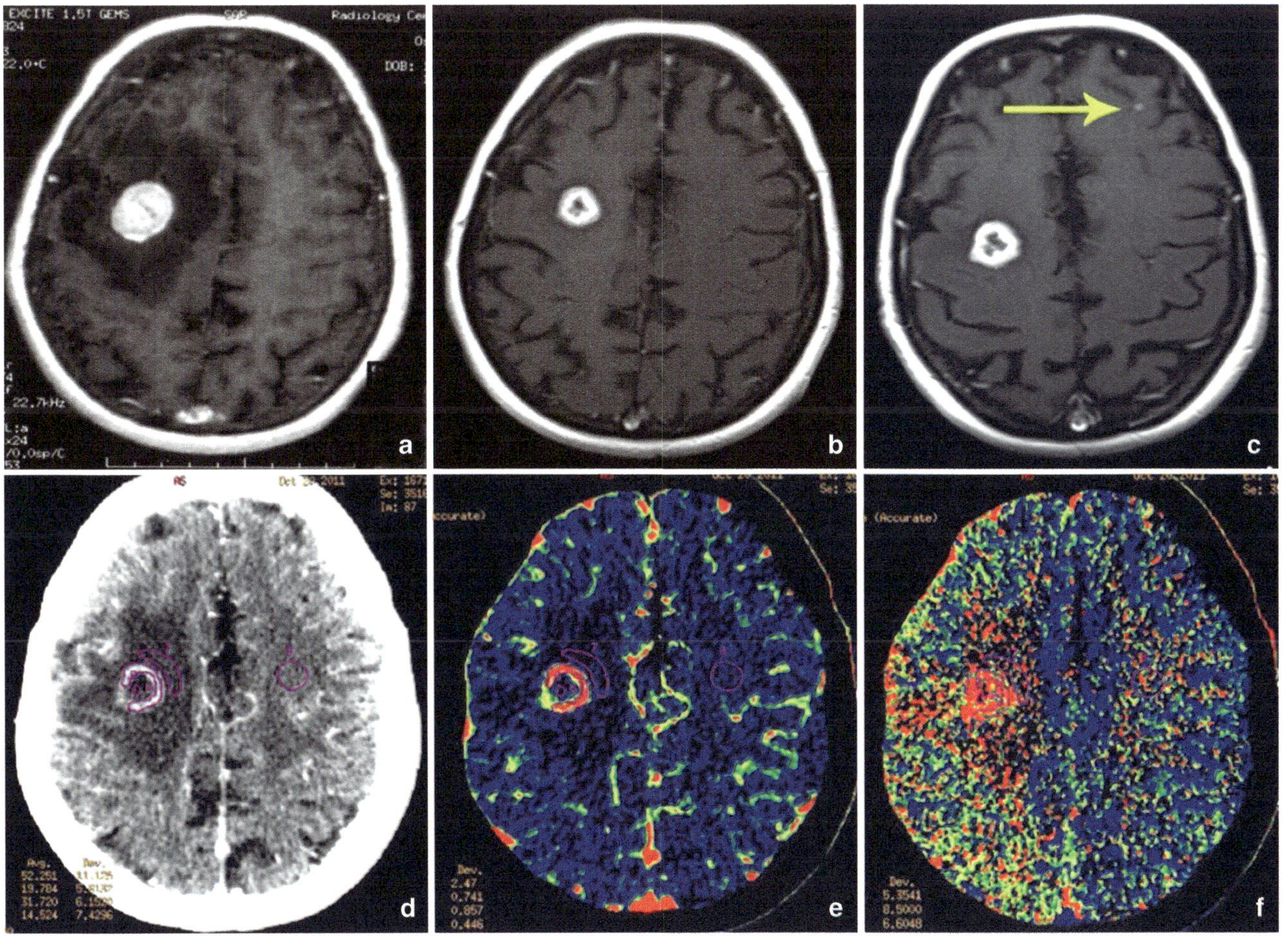

Fig. 8.23 Multiple breast cancer metastases in the brain. (**a**) MRI before the treatment (Gamma Knife), (**b**) 6 months after the treatment (tumor shrinkage), (**c**) 7 months after the treatment (a slight increase in the lesion size), as well as the occurrence of a "new" small area of abnormal contrast enhancement in the opposite brain hemisphere (the *arrow*). On CT scan after the treatment, there is an intense accumulation of contrast agent along the lesion contour (**d**); on CBV maps (**e**), there is an increase in perfusion values (7.89 ml/100 g), which indicates the presence of a residual tumor. On the periphery of the previously irradiated large metastatic lesion and in its projection, MTT values (**f**) are also unevenly increased (12.2 s)—post-radiation changes. Based on the obtained diagnostic findings, a decision was made to include all detected abnormal brain structures in the radiation treatment plan, including repeated radiosurgery of the "first" metastasis

9 Magnetic Resonance Imaging (MRI)

The phenomenon of nuclear magnetic resonance (NMR) was discovered and studied in the 1950s of the twentieth century. Two groups of British physicists under the leadership of Bloch and Pursell determined physical and chemical factors, such as proton density and the so-called relaxation parameters, times of longitudinal (T1) and transverse (T2) substance relaxation, on which the value of the detected MR signal depended. Hahn (1950) developed an in vitro method for measuring the substance relaxation parameters using a sequence of radio pulses, called a pulse sequence (PS) "spin echo" (SE) (Hahn 1950; Bloch et al. 1946; Pursell et al. 1946).

In 1973 Lauterbour proposed to separate the MR signal from a layer inside an object with an additional magnetic field G_z, changing linearly with distance in the direction of the main magnetic field of the magnet (gradient magnetic field). In the same year, Mansfield established a link between the frequency (phase) change of MR signals and the coordinates of voxels in the layer. He used two additional mutually perpendicular gradient magnetic fields G_x and G_y to set the coordinates of each element in the tomographic section and applied the Fourier analysis to extract MR signals from the registered data from each voxel in a given layer. This approach allowed to reduce the time obtaining tomographic cross sections down to a few minutes (Mansfield 1977). Lauterbour and Mansfield were awarded the Nobel Prize in Physiology or Medicine Prize in 2003 for the creation of MR imaging methods that were implemented in modern MRI scanners.

A detailed description of NMR physics and imaging principles intended for diagnosticians can be found in many monographs (Edelman et al. 1996; Konovalov et al. 1997a, b, c; Rink 2003).

A variety of tissue contrast ranges in MR images provide a wide set of pulse sequences, which represents greater possibilities for characterization of various CNS tissues than CT and is one of the advantages of MRI.

Standard or routine sequences used in the study of patients with brain metastases are T1, T2, and T2*. T1-weighted images are fundamental for detection of impairment and abnormalities of normal brain anatomy. Volumetric scanning 3DSPGR or VIBE allows to obtain T1-weighted high-resolution images with a 1.0 mm slice thickness and is currently used in routine diagnosis of metastatic brain lesions.

T2-weighted images are intended for visualization of edema and the presence of water in the tissues; SP T2-FLAIR suppresses the MR signal from free water (e.g., CSF) and better identifies hydration foci, demyelination, and hemorrhages in the brain tissue.

*T2-weighted images reflect the tissue magnetic susceptibility (Haacke et al. 2010, Kornienko and Pronin 2009a, b, c, d, 2010). The next step in the use of SP gradient echo became SWI (SWAN) sequences that are used to detect hemorrhages in metastatic brain lesions (Pronin et al. 2011; Dolgushin et al. 2012a, b; Haacke et al. 2010).

T1 MRI with intravenous contrast enhancement is often used in the diagnosis of neoplastic brain lesions, including metastases. MRI contrast agents (MRCA) are agents based on a paramagnetic material gadolinium (Gd), which shorten the T1 relaxation time. As a result, images of tissues that have accumulated MRCA will be bright in T1-weighted MRI. The concentration of gadolinium surrounded by a chelate providing stability of the product in the internal media of the human body may be from 0.5 mM/ml and 1.0 mM/ml in MRCA. During the standard procedure (neuro-oncology), a patient is administered 0.2 ml of the drug at the concentration 0.5 mm/ml/kg of body weight and 0.1 ml at the concentration 1.0 mM/ml. For a qualitative assessment of MRI signs of a tumor on tomograms, a subjective scale is generally utilized: the MR signal in the tumor can be isointense as compared to the brain matter on the contralateral side, hypointense or hyperintense. On T1-weighted images, MRI with contrast enhancement assesses only the degree of an increase in the MR signal intensity in the tumor (no enhancement, moderate and significant enhancement). A semiquantitative assessment of an increase in the relative tumor

M. Dolgushin et al., *Brain Metastases*, DOI 10.1007/978-3-319-57760-9_9

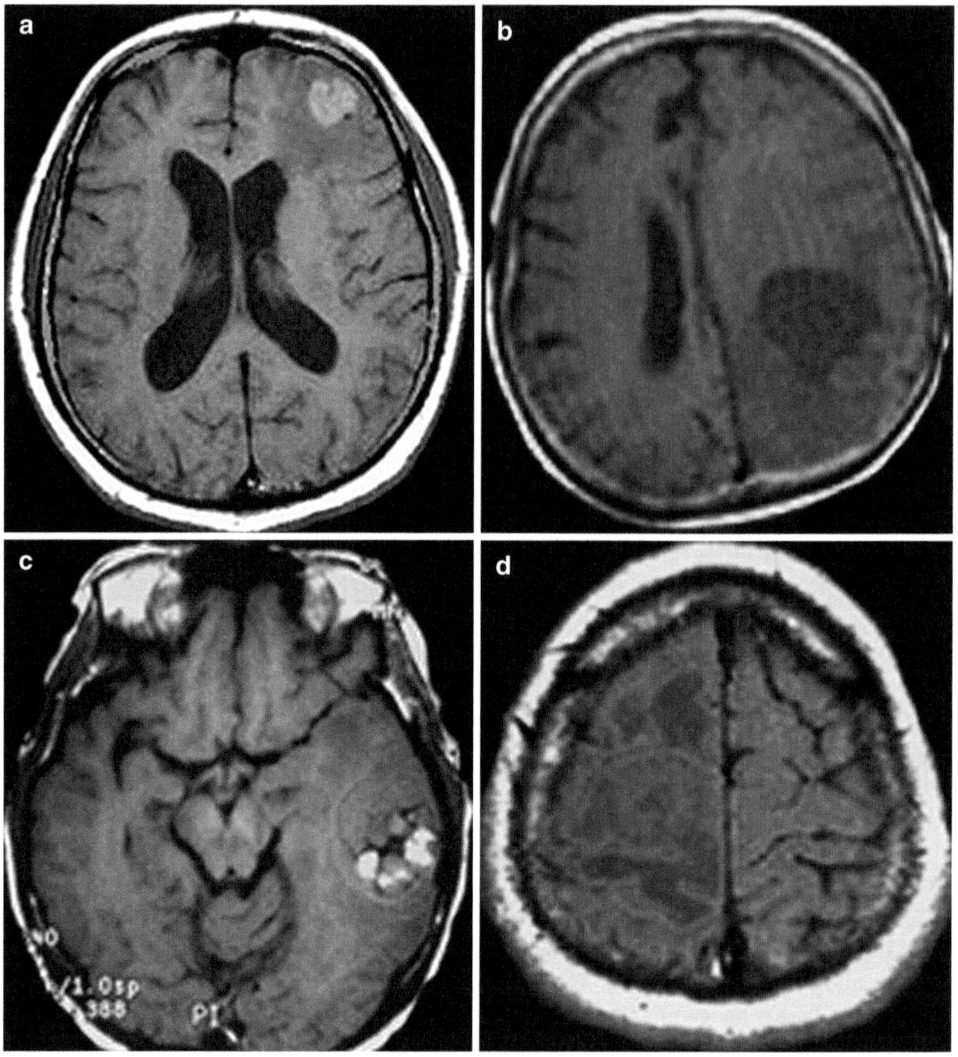

Fig. 9.1 Brain metastases from a variety of primary tumors. Variants of signal intensity on T1-weighted images in relation to the brain substance: (**a**) hyperintense, (**b**) hypointense, (**c**) heterogeneous, and (**d**) isointense

intensity on MRI with contrast enhancement (CE) is widely used in neuro-oncology, because of the simplicity of calculations and the information value of this parameter for neoplastic and nonneoplastic CNS lesions.

With contrast enhancement, even in the absence of clinical symptoms, metastases are detected in nearly 100% of cases (Kornienko et al. 2007). The use of intravenous bolus administration of MRCA allows to utilize the perfusion technique based on a decrease in the MR signal intensity on the T2 and T2* MRI in the diagnosis of brain metastases (Huisman and Sorensen et al. 2004).

Semiotics and differential diagnostic criteria for metastatic brain lesions, based on the results of the use of routine sequences (T1, T2, and T2-FLAIR) on the background of various doses of contrast agent, were discussed in sufficient detail in numerous publications (Konovalov et al. 1997a, b, c; Osborn 1994; Sze et al. 1998; Kornienko and Pronin 2008a, b, 2009a, b, c, d).

Standard MRI sequences can detect tumors and intratumoral changes (hemorrhage, necrosis) and assess the size of a peritumoral edema. In **T1**-weighted image, metastases may have various signal characteristics with respect to the brain substance. If the tumor lesion has a lower signal (Fig. 9.1) than the intact brain substance, edematous brain tissue that is hypointense in this sequence makes it difficult to clarify the size, shape, and boundaries of the tumor. In case of a mild edema and a small metastasis (less than 1 cm in diameter), the latter may not be detected in T1-weighted image. According to our data, in T1-weighted image, metastases mainly (90%) have a hypo- and isointense MR signal in relation to the brain substance. A hyperintense signal within an MTS is less common (up to 5.5% of the cases) and is generally encountered in case of a hemorrhage (metastatic melanoma, renal cell carcinoma).

Some metastatic tumors have a number of pathognomonic imaging manifestations that allow to assume the nature of the primary tumor with a high probability, even based on routine investigations. Thus, the characteristic feature of melanoma in an MRI study is an increased signal in T1-weighted image before contrast enhancement, since

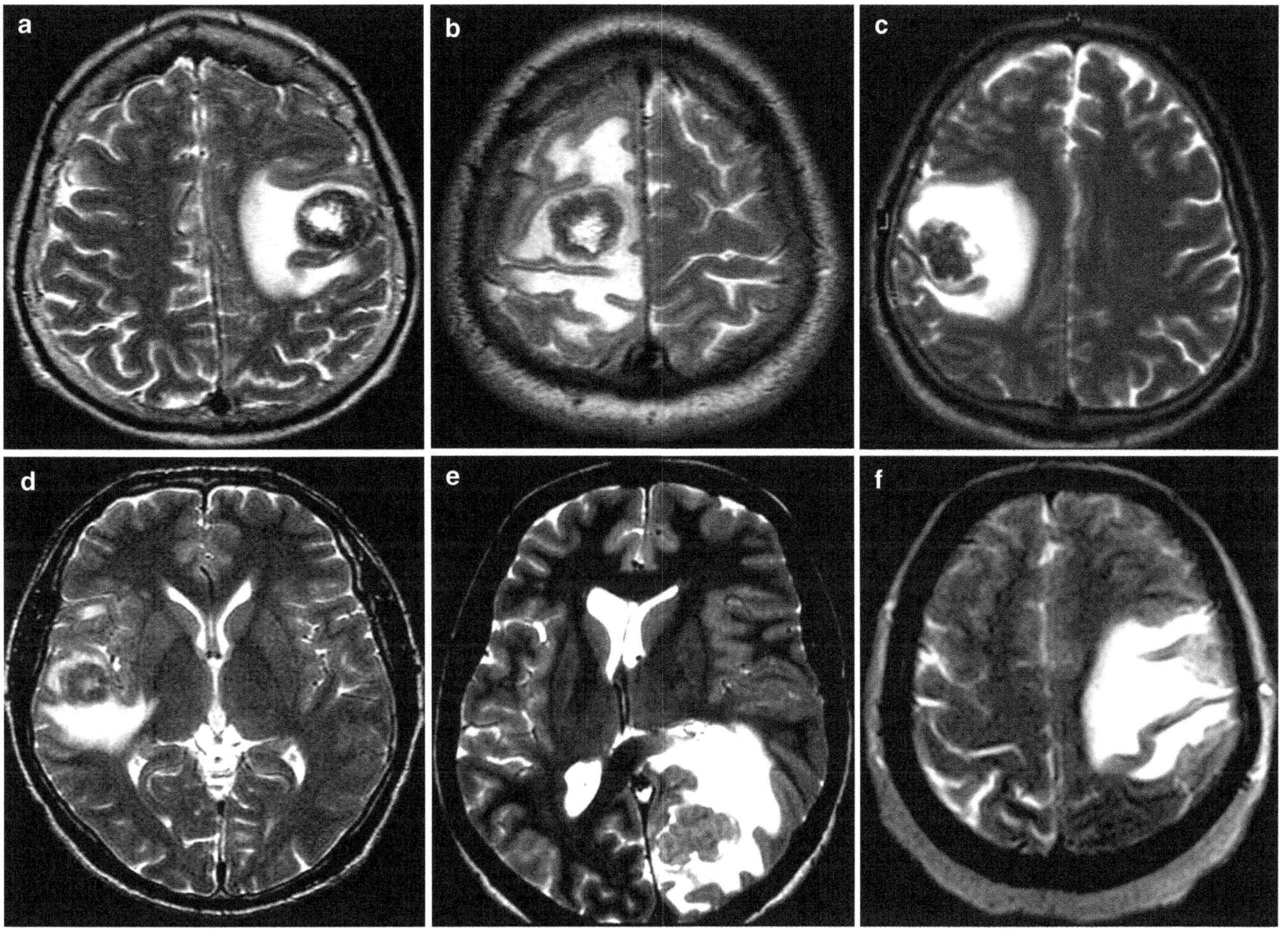

Fig. 9.2 Visualization of colorectal cancer metastases in the brain in T2-weighted image. A solid tumor component has a hypointense (**a**–**d**) or iso-hyperintense (**e**, **f**) signal in relation to the brain substance. In some cases, there are signs of central necrosis in metastatic lesions

melanin is characterized by paramagnetic properties. A heterogeneous and increased MR signal in many observations is usually associated with the presence of a hemorrhage in the tumor tissue.

On **T2**-weighted images, metastases are characterized by an iso- or hypointense signal relative to the gray matter from the tumor stroma, an increased signal in the central necrotic area and an area of perifocal edema. Particularly noteworthy are colorectal adenocarcinoma metastases that were characterized by a marked hypointense signal in T2-weighted image in 83% of our cases (Fig. 9.2); some of them showed signs of moderate central necrosis; the presence of perifocal edema was noted in 100% of cases.

Small metastatic lesions without the use of CA can be detected on T2-weighted images by the presence of a peritumoral edema characterized by a hyperintense signal (Fig. 9.3). In the presence of a chronic or acute hemorrhage in the metastasis stroma, hypointense areas can be observed, while the tumor tissue has a heterogeneous MR signal. However, it must be kept in mind that detection of metastases may be difficult, especially in small tumors with mild perifocal edema of the brain substance.

T2-FLAIR sequence used in the standard MR protocol in metastatic brain lesions usually has two purposes: specification, along with T2 mode, of detected small tumor lesions without the use of a contrast agent and visualization of additional signal changes in the metastatic tissue structure. Most often, in this sequence, a metastatic lesion has a hypointense MR signal relative to the gray matter. A heterogeneous signal is always detected in the presence of a hemorrhage in the tumor tissue. If an MR signal from small metastases is isointense, with a mild perifocal edema of the brain substance, it is difficult to identify the boundaries of the lesion and sometimes of the metastasis itself (Fig. 9.4).

The use of T2-FLAIR sequence is also justified in the presence of solitary metastases. One of the most common primary brain tumors is glioblastoma. It is typically slightly hyperintense relative to the cortex in this sequence, which is regarded as one of implicit signs of differential diagnosis when comparing these tumors.

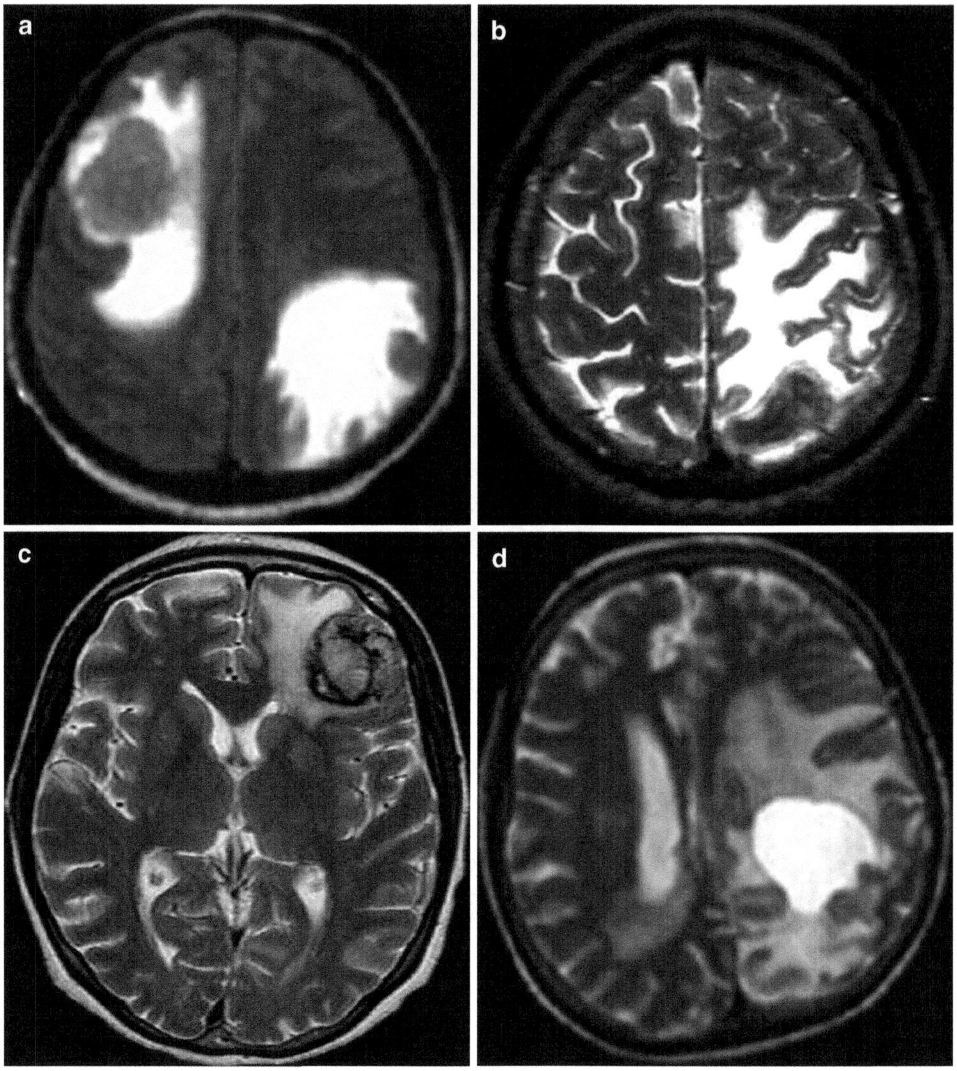

Fig. 9.3 Brain metastases from a variety of primary tumors. Variants of signal intensity on T2-weighted images in relation to the brain substance: (**a**) isointense, (**b**) hypointense, (**c**) heterogeneous, and (**d**) hyperintense

Contrast enhancement in MRI, as well as in CT, has a high diagnostic value. Structure of the lesion, spread and invasion of surrounding tissues, the number of lesions and hemodynamic characteristics of the tumor are identified best on the background of contrast enhancement. In case of brain metastases, the use of contrast agents is an obligatory link in the standard protocol of any diagnostic CT/MRI study. In literature, there is still debate over the possibilities and feasibility of the use of high doses of contrast agents for metastatic brain lesions. According to Sze et al. (1998), in 70 patients with negative results on MRI with a standard contrast agent dose out of 92 patients with confirmed or suspected metastatic brain lesions, administering a triple dose of the contrast agent did not help identify any additional lesion. Yuh et al. (1992), as well as other researchers, identified additional lesions after using a triple dose of the contrast agent in MRI only in a small number of cases (Akeson et al. 1995; Vogl et al. 1995; Tatsuno et al. 1996; Gasperini et al. 2000; Rowley et al. 2008; Attenberger et al. 2009).

A study using T1-weighted sequence with contrast enhancement can detect both large and pinpoint lesions of pathological CA accumulation not visualized with other types of contrast enhancement. However, according to Mintz et al. (2004), there is always a danger of a false-positive result. For example, in case of telangiectases or when the slice plane is perpendicular to the blood vessel, there is a possibility of erroneous interpretation of findings in favor of a nonexistent small metastasis. In such situations, it is advisable to use volumetric scanning programs. 3D FSPGR (T1-weighted sequence) allows to neutralize an increase in the signal from the blood flow; in some cases, constructing multiplane images or reformats allows to “remove” the course of the blood vessel and thus eliminate the seeming presence of a small metastatic lesion.

MRI with contrast enhancement as compared to CT allows to obtain the largest amount of diagnostic information regarding the tumor and conduct differential diagnosis between focal brain lesions similar in the standard modes by

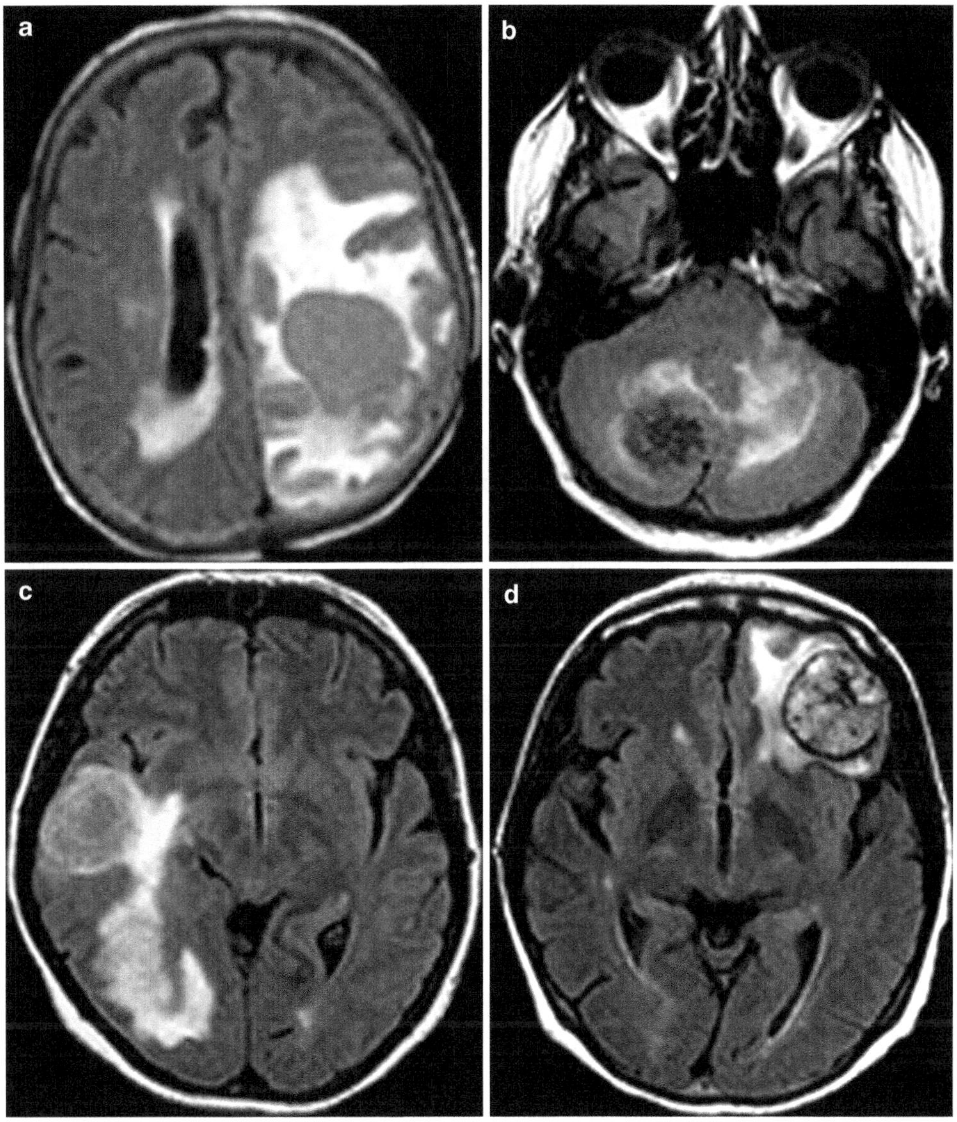

Fig. 9.4 Brain metastases from a variety of primary tumors. Variants of signal intensity on T2-FLAIR-weighted images in relation to the brain substance: (**a**) isointense, (**b**) hypointense, (**c**) hyperintense, and (**d**) a heterogeneous tumor lesion

their visualization characteristics. Metastases, meningiomas, benign astrocytomas, lymphomas, and neuromas without contrast enhancement may look similar on CT and MRI. However, when there is a massive hemorrhage in the tumor, the use of contrast enhancement is often uninformative (Fig. 9.5).

Special attention was paid in our studies of patients with metastatic brain tumors to the specifics of CA accumulation by metastases of different origins. An MRI study with contrast enhancement determined the extent, nature, and time of CA accumulation and elimination from the area of interest. The main types of CA accumulation in the tumor tissue were identified based on the analysis of findings obtained: "target," "blurred contour," "in the form of a rim with clear contours," "heterogeneous," "annular," "annular with a solid area," and "homogeneous." We will use this classification of CA accumulation hereinafter. The typical visualization features for each type of CA accumulation will be review below.

"Target": CA accumulations as "blurred contour" and "in the form of a rim with clear contours" were combined in one group—both types are ring shaped with a "clearing" in the center, indicating the presence of tumor tissue decay in the middle area of the lesion. CA accumulation in the form of "blurred contour" is characterized by the presence on the periphery of the contrast enhancement of pointed areas (protrusions) that transit into the surrounding brain tissue without any clear contours. In another type of CA accumulation ("in the form of a rim with clear contours"), MR image of the lesion is annular but with a dense homogeneous halo with a clear, sharp boundary between the CA area and the brain substance (Fig. 9.6). Perifocal edema in metastases of these types of CA accumulation is very significant. Such metastases differ by different lesion sizes and various widths of a "ring" of CA accumulation. We observed CA accumulation in the form of a "target" in 36.8% of cases of breast cancer metastases (Dolgushin 2012).

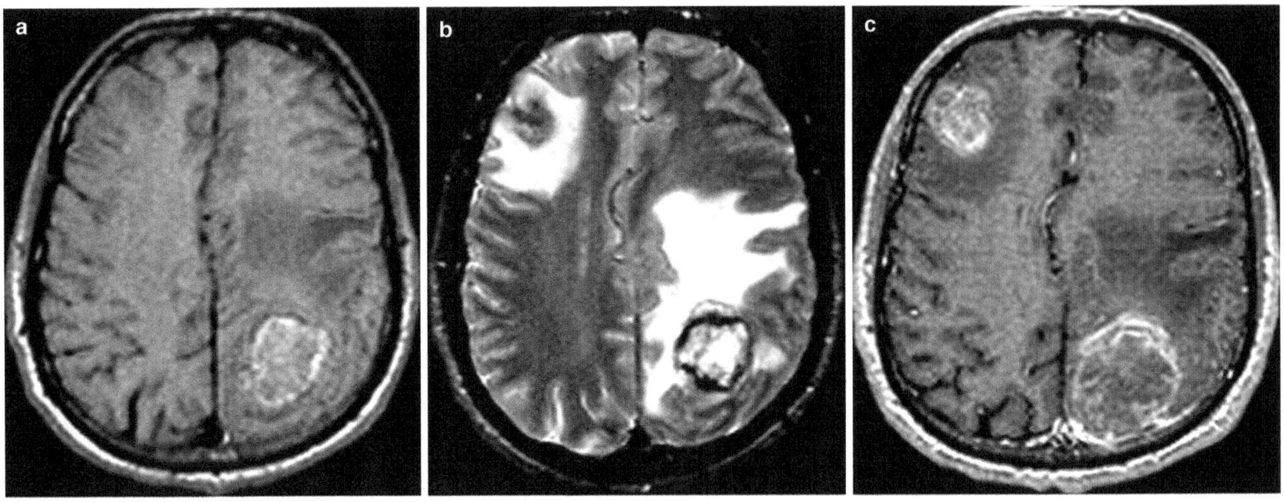

Fig. 9.5 Multiple lung cancer metastases in the brain. (**a**) T1-weighted image before injection of CA: there is a marked hyperintense (due to the hemorrhagic content) space-occupying lesion with signs of pronounced perifocal edema in the left parietal region. The lesion in the right frontal region is visualized on the background of edema in T2-weighted image (**b**) and after the administration of a contrast agent (**c**)

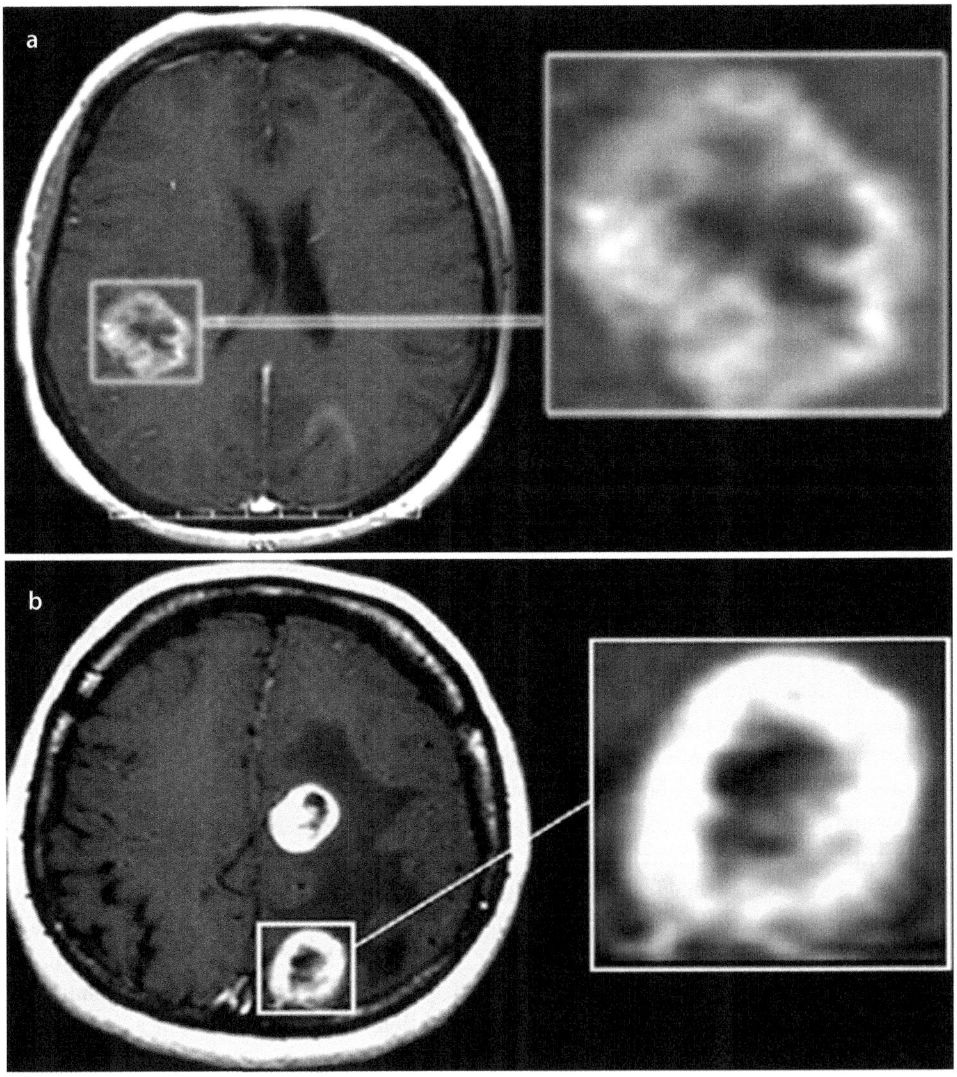

Fig. 9.6 Brain metastases. Types of contrast agent accumulation in MRI: (**a**) a rounded lesion with signs of "blurred contour" and (**b**) another rounded lesion with mostly clear contours of contrast enhancement. In both cases, there was central necrosis in the tumor

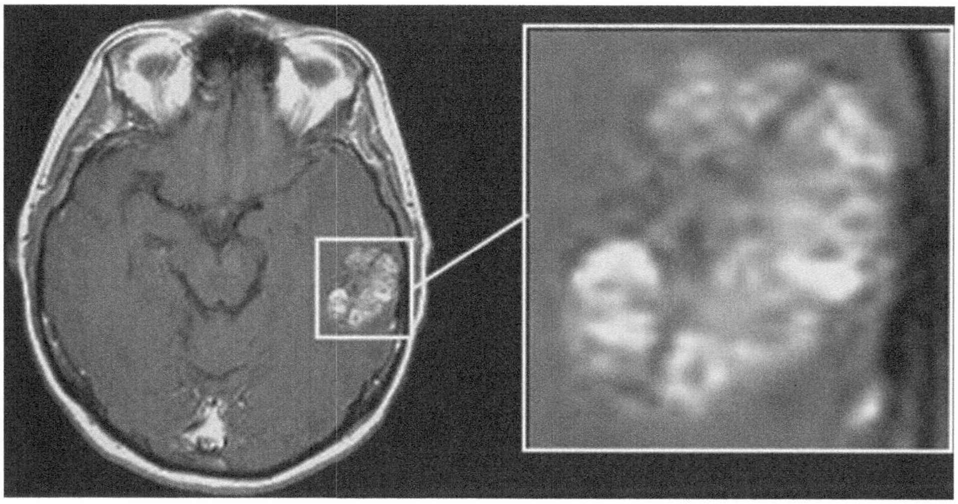

Fig. 9.7 A brain metastasis. Types of contrast agent accumulation in MRI: CA accumulation of heterogeneous type in the tumor stroma. There are no large areas of necrotic tumor decay

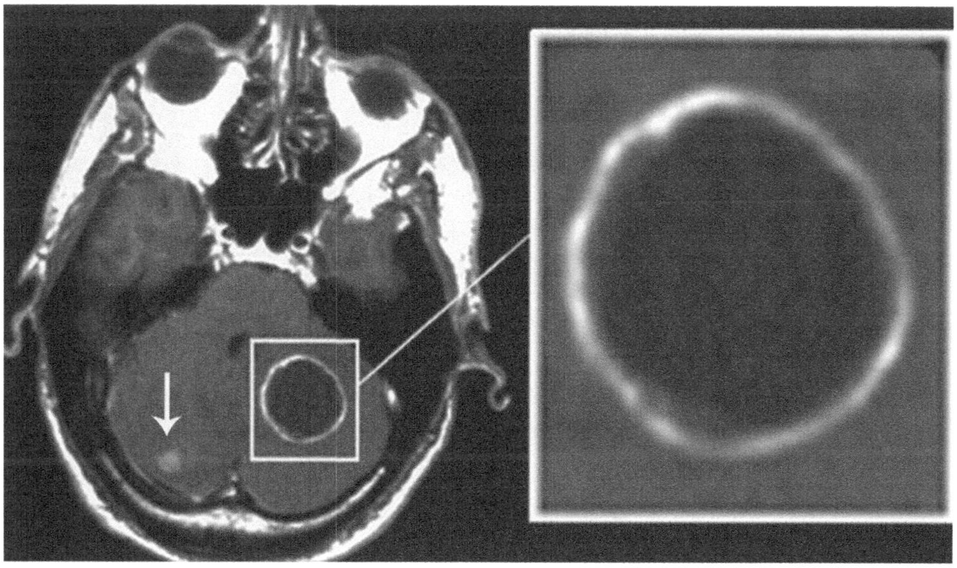

Fig. 9.8 Brain metastases. Types of contrast agent accumulation in MRI: a rounded lesion in the left hemisphere of the cerebellum with signs of annular (thin) CA accumulation. There is additionally a small, homogeneous lesion in the right hemisphere

A "heterogeneous" type is characterized by separate sites of CA accumulation with different sizes in different areas of the tumor (Fig. 9.7). In this type, in contrast to the two previous types of CA accumulation, clarification areas on the scan, corresponding to portions of necrotic tumor decay, are randomly located within the pathological focus. This type of CA accumulation is also observed in cases of hemorrhages in the tumor tissue, with the intensity of MR signal from blood clots sometimes exceeding that of the contrast-enhanced tissue. The extent of the perifocal edema varies and depends more on the characteristics of the tumor site and its size.

"A ring" is characterized by the accumulation of CA in the form of a thin, closed, annular rim, and we observed it in our clinical material in 15% of cases. This "ring," as such, can have different shapes; therefore, this definition is quite arbitrary. No hemorrhages into the tumor tissue were observed in this type of CA accumulation. The signal from the central area of metastasis in all scan sequences was almost homogeneous. In solitary or even multiple brain metastases, lesions characterized on MRI scans by a similar type of CA accumulation most often have to be differentiated from brain abscesses. Tumors characterized by CA accumulation in the form of a "ring" almost completely lack a perifocal edema surrounding the brain substance (Fig. 9.8).

"Ring + tissue" in cases where a solid part of the tumor accumulating CA is adjacent to the annular "rim": we defined this type of manifestation of metastases as "ring + tissue." An annular cystic component is not in the center but is adjacent to the solid part of the tumor. There are sometimes areas of hemorrhages (in the solid portion). A perifocal edema in cases of such MR manifestation of tumors is quite significant (Fig. 9.9).

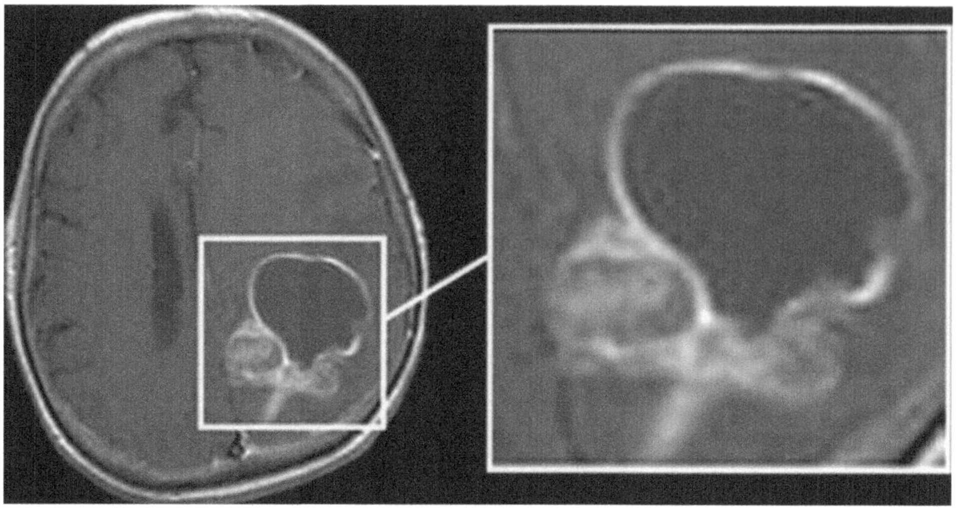

Fig. 9.9 A brain metastasis. Types of contrast agent accumulation in MRI: a rounded thin-walled lesion with annular CA accumulation in the anterior tumor fraction and with a solid portion in the posterior portion

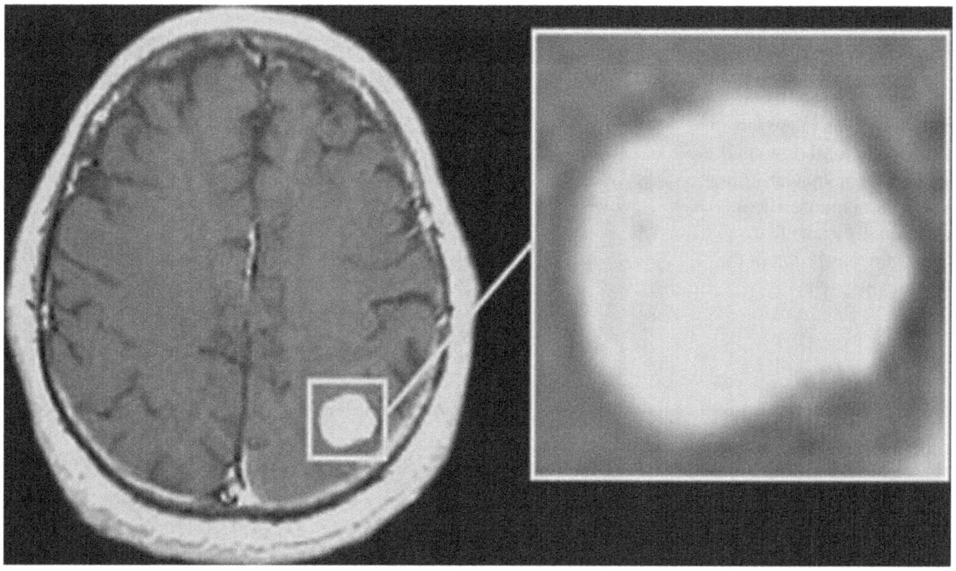

Fig. 9.10 A brain metastasis. Types of contrast agent accumulation in MRI: a rounded lesion accumulating homogeneously CA. There are no cystic or necrotic inclusions

Table 9.1 Variants of contrast agent accumulation in MRI study of focal brain lesions ($n = 130$)

Type of contrast enhancement	"Target"		Heterogeneous	"Ring"	"Ring + tissue"	Homogeneous	Total	
	"Unclear contour"	"Clear contour"					*n*	%
Amount	9.2%	17.7%	13.9%	15.3%	13.1%	30.8%	130	100

A "homogeneous" type of CA accumulation is the most frequent MRI picture of the tumor lesion (30.8%). It is characterized by uniform accumulation of contrast agent in metastases represented by a solid lesion, while the degree of CA accumulation may be different. The brain edema in this type of MRI manifestations of the tumor is significant (Fig. 9.10).

Distribution of observations based on the accumulation characteristics of contrast agent in brain metastases is shown in Table 9.1.

There is no significant relationship between the type of CA accumulation and abnormal structure of the primary tumor. Metastases of different etiologies may be contrasted in the form of a "target." The same is applicable to other CA accumulation patterns. Differences in CA accumulation by metastases, in our opinion, are due to, first of all, their size, duration of existence, intensity of the tumor growth, and metabolic activity of the tumor tissue, which manifests by the absence or presence of areas of necrosis, decay, and bleeding in the abnormal focus. The confirmation of this can be seen in one of our cases, when, in multiple brain metastases, a few different types of CA accumulation were found, as well as the detection of the same type of contrast in metastatic tumors that differed in their histogenesis (Fig. 9.11).

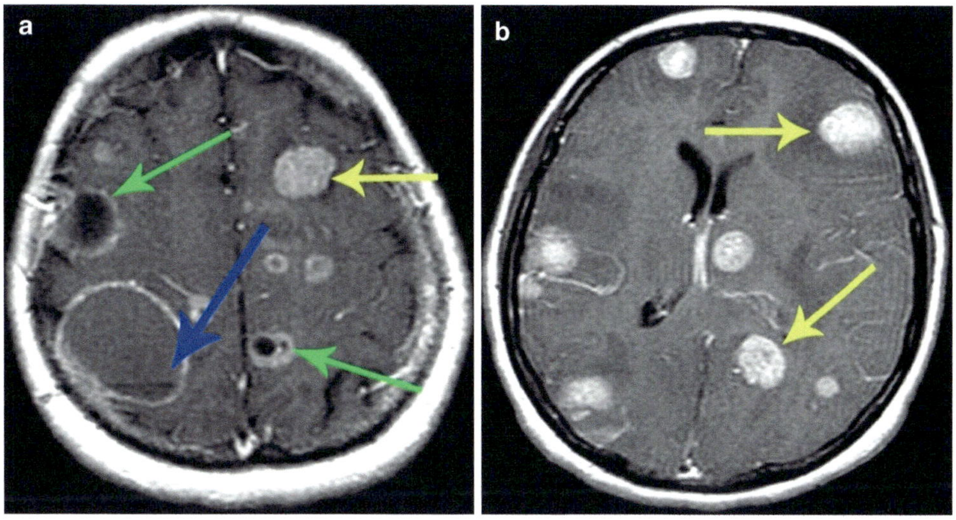

Fig. 9.11 Multiple lung cancer metastases in the brain. Brain MRI with contrast enhancement in two different patients. (**a**) Multiple brain lesions with different variants of MR manifestations of metastatic lesions. (**b**) Multiple brain lesions in the form of homogeneous similar foci with different sizes. In the first case (**a**), lesions with mixed structure are identified: solid lesions with a cystic structure and signs of central necrosis (*arrows*). The largest tumor lesion in the right frontoparietal region also has a cystic structure with the signs of hemorrhagic content and a liquid "level" (*arrow*), with the lesion size being an indirect evidence of its "age." In the second case, all lesions have a solid structure and intensely accumulate the contrast material (*arrows*)

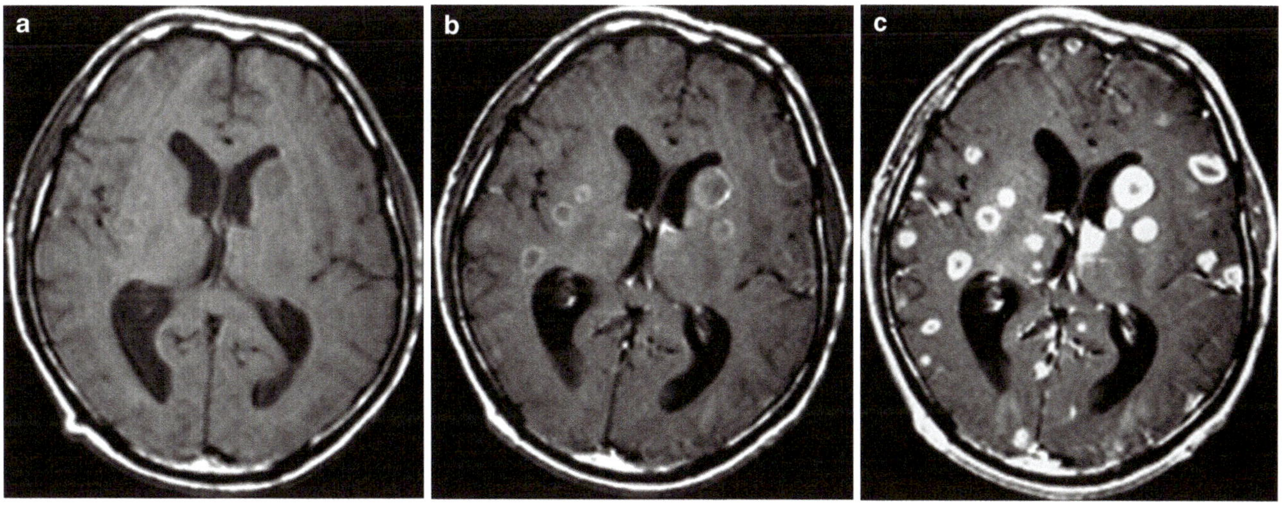

Fig. 9.12 Multiple metastatic brain lesions. T1-weighted images. Small lesions homogeneously accumulate contrast agents, with larger ones having the form of a "ring." (**a**) Before contrast enhancement, tumor lesions have a homogeneous hypointense signal. (**b**) After administration of the contrast agent at the standard dose of 0.2 ml of the product (at the concentration 0.5 mg/ml) per kg of body weight of the patient, there is a moderate increase in the signal from larger lesions. (**c**) After administration of a double dose of 0.4 ml with the concentration 0.5 mg/ml per kg of body weight of the patient, there is an expressed signal increase from the previously detected lesions and additional small metastases

9.1 A Double Dose of Contrast Agent

A standard dose of CA in the diagnosis of metastatic lesions in the brain is 0.2 ml/kg of body weight with the concentration 0.5 mg/ml. In multiple metastatic brain lesions, administration of increased doses of the contrast agent sometimes allows not only to more accurately assess the boundaries of a tumor detected under standard contrasting conditions but further identify small metastatic lesions (Figs. 9.12 and 9.13).

In case of involvement of bone structures or meninges, it is extremely important to use protocols with suppression of MR signals from fat (fat saturation), which allows to identify metastases located in the soft tissues and bones of the head in T1-weighted images with contrast enhancement (Fig. 9.14).

Increasing the concentration of administered CA can result in its increased accumulation in large brain sinuses (in particular, in transverse sinuses), which can produce artifacts on T1-weighted MRI. Areas with emerging artifacts often

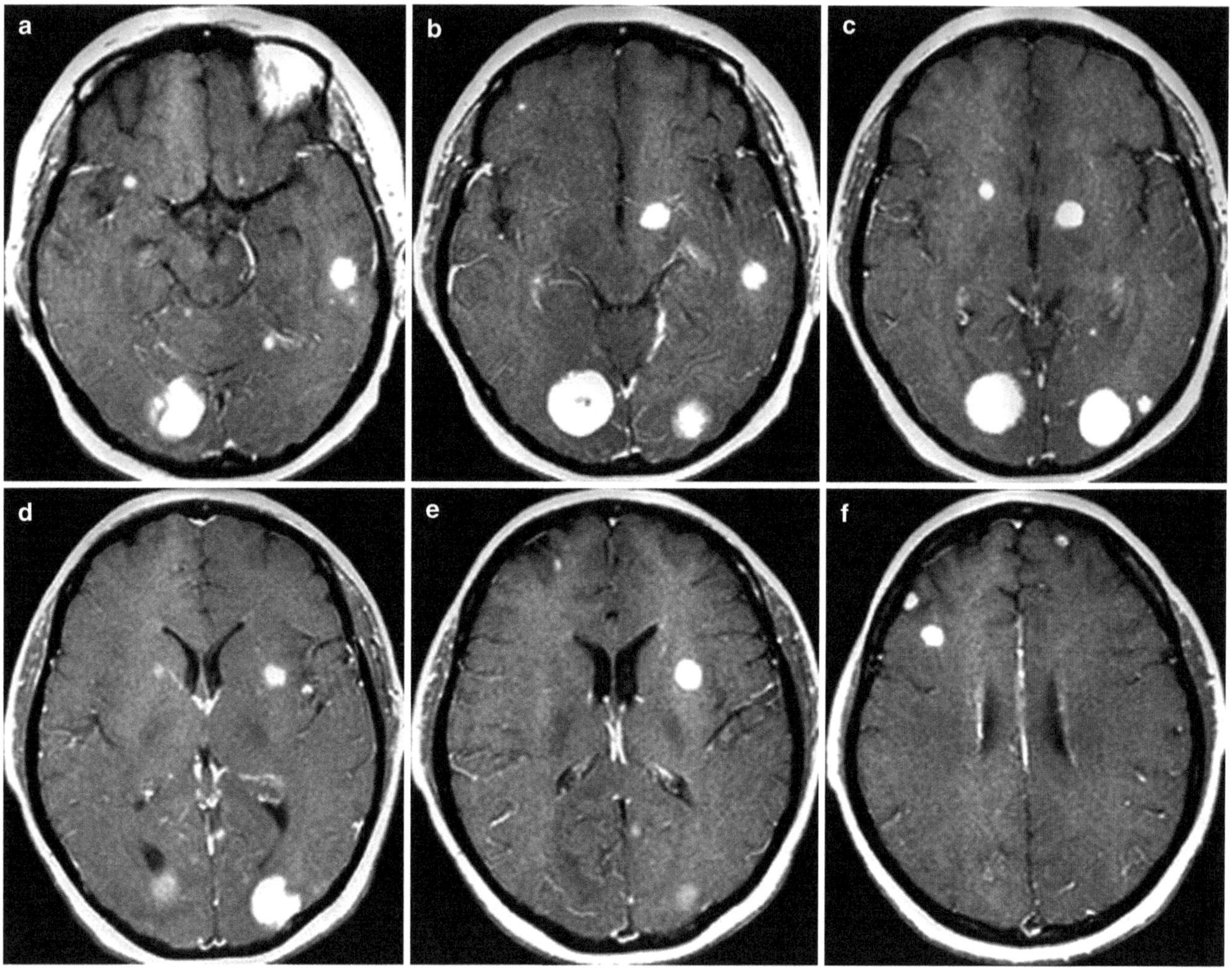

Fig. 9.13 Multiple metastases with sub- and supratentorial location. On T1-weighted MRI (**a–f**), following administration of a triple dose of the contrast agent, there are multiple tumor lesions with a solid structure on different scans. Small (less than 5 mm) metastatic lesions are also clearly visualized

follow the contours of end sections of the transverse sinuses, which may both overlap with space-occupying lesions with small sizes and mimic the latter on the background of blood pulsations and contrast enhancement (Fig. 9.15).

In the event of such a questionable matter, a follow-up study should be performed with the same positioning of the sections, but changing the direction of phase-encoding gradient pulse, so that the artifact will be seen in a different direction, or sections in other projections should be used.

Difficulties of differential diagnosis using a standard MRI study with contrast enhancement most often occur in solitary lesions, when, first of all, intracerebral tumors (usually glioblastoma) and brain abscess should be excluded.

9.2 Additional MRI Techniques

The so-called volumetric scan sequences are included in the standard MRI investigation protocols for visualization of the anatomical features of abnormalities: 3D FSPGR, BRAVO/VIBE (T1), CUBE (T2), FIESTA (T2), 3D FLAIR (T1/T2), etc. Volumetric 3D scanning sequences allow to reduce the total study duration, perform 0.6–1.0 mm sections, as well as build 2D and 3D reformats and anatomical 3D models with high anatomical resolution and isotropic voxel, which is important for navigation programs and planning the radiation treatment. Today, due to the possibility to obtain images with diverse tissue

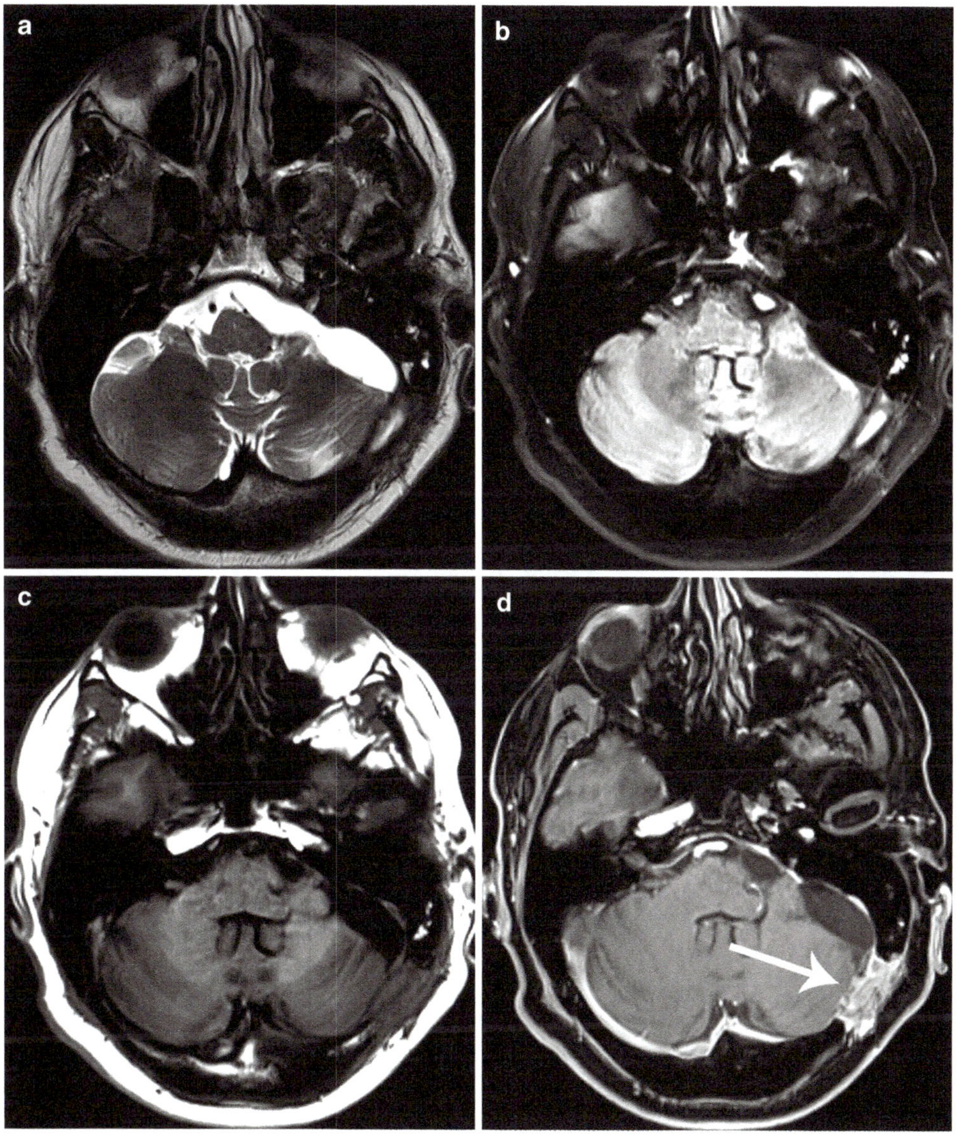

Fig. 9.14 Melanoma metastases. A relapse of the metastatic tumor after its surgical removal. MRI shows a space-occupying lesion in the occipital bone, extending to the adjacent meninges. The metastasis is characterized by a hyperintense signal on T2-weighted and T2-FLAIR MRI (**a**, **b**) and an isointense signal in T1 (**c**); after IV contrast enhancement on T1-fat sat MRI (**d**), there is intense accumulation of contrast agent in its structure (*arrow*)

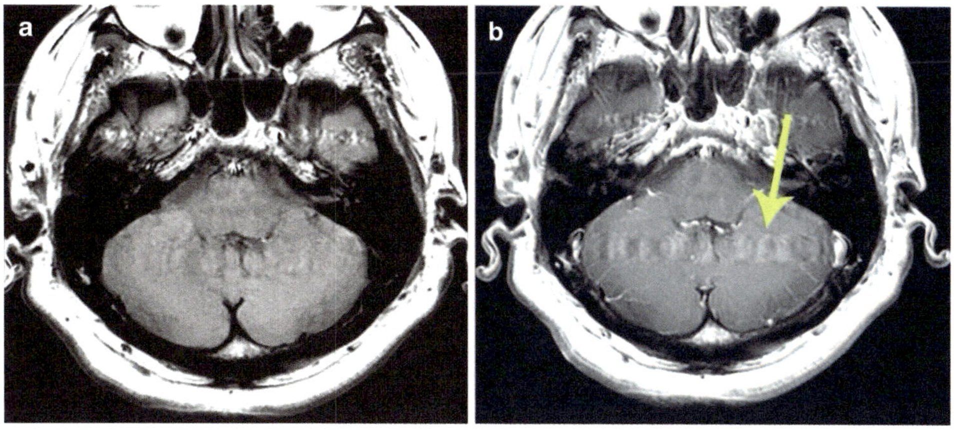

Fig. 9.15 Brain MRI in the axial projection of the patient with a suspected metastatic brain lesion before (**a**) and after (**b**) administration of CA. The patient had a history of colorectal cancer. The arrow indicates an artifact from blood pulsation in the transition region of the transverse sinus into the sigmoid one. This artifact can overlap with the lesion or mimic it

contrast, MR imaging is a highly efficient and sensitive method of detecting not only tumors but also assessing some intratumoral processes, such as hemorrhages and arteriovenous shunts.

9.3 3D T1-Weighted Sequence

The pulse sequence 3D FSPGR (or VIBE) in metastatic brain lesions produces high-resolution MR images with slice thickness of less than 1 mm. Currently, the use of 3D T1-weighted images is routine not only in the preoperative diagnosis but also in the basic protocol for radiosurgery. An appropriate dose of the contrast agent allows to detect lesions not visualized by other MR sequences (Fig. 9.16).

MRI possibilities are not limited to standard techniques and contrast enhancement. Currently, neuroimaging extensively uses additional diagnostic MR technologies, such as SWI (SWAN), MR spectroscopy, perfusion MRI, and diffusion and diffusion tensor MRI, based on the diversity of tissue contrast types in magnetic resonance imaging. Most of the additional MR technologies and investigation protocols based on them not only provide a picture of anatomical changes but also imply obtaining quantitative characteristics of a particular pathological process, associated with the specifics of its metabolism and hemodynamics.

As known, one of the most effective treatments for metastatic brain lesions, especially multiple ones, is radiological methods and, above all, Gamma Knife and CyberKnife. MRI

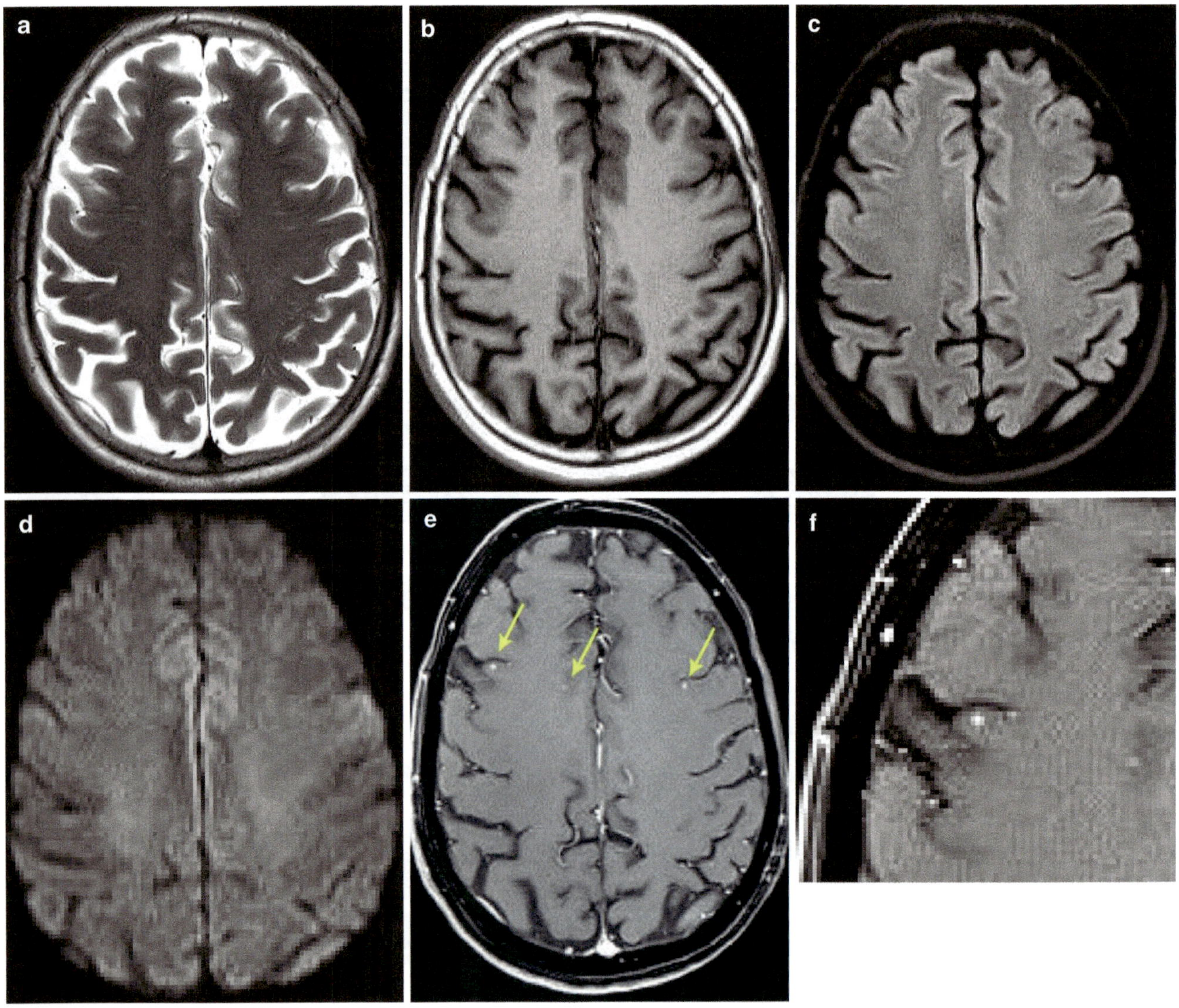

Fig. 9.16 Multiple melanoma metastases in the brain. On T2-weighted (**a**), T1-weighted (**b**), and DWI (**d**) MRI, metastatic lesions are not visualized in the brain substance. In T2-FLAIR sequence (**b**), multiple small foci are determined that are poorly visualized and mimic ischemic lesions. After contrast enhancement on T1-weighted MRI, pinpoint metastatic lesions are clearly visualized (**e**, **f**)

with contrast enhancement is a mandatory procedure to evaluate the effectiveness of the treatment of cerebral neoplastic lesions, including after radiosurgery (RS).

A favorable outcome of RS in our material (*n* = 490, 88.4%) was a reduction in the tumor volume up to a complete disappearance of regions with abnormal contrast agent accumulation, reduction of the perifocal edema, and regression of neurological symptoms. When the size of tumors decreased as a result of radiation treatment, pinpoint contrasted areas persisted without any signs of increased perfusion indicators in 95% of 490 cases. In 5% of cases, positive changes were characterized by a complete disappearance of areas of abnormal CA accumulation and regression of edema. Analysis of the extent of reduction of metastatic lesions in size in the control group (*n* = 45) showed that a pronounced and moderate decrease in the tumor size (more than 50% within the first 3 months) was identified in 85% and 15% of patients, respectively (Fig. 9.17).

9.4 SWI (SWAN)

In the 1990s of the last century, the use of SP T2* GRE for visualization of venous structures was started. Such MRI studies were called BOLD (blood oxygenation level-dependent) venography (Lee et al. 1992; Reichenbach 2001). In T2-weighted* images, venous structures were well seen; however, the images contained artifacts due to magnetic susceptibility. In 1997, a way was developed to eliminate phase artifacts at "air-to-brain" and "bone-brain" interface and display within each voxel local phases of interest in terms of tissue magnetic susceptibility (Haacke et al. 2007).

Pulse sequences SWI (SWAN) (susceptibility-weighted imaging) and SWI (SWAN) (T2 star-weighted angiography) that are based on high-resolution 3D T2* GRE with the possibility of obtaining an isotropic voxel with full compensation of flow effects, sensitive to blood products, particularly to deoxyhemoglobin of venous blood, allowed to obtain

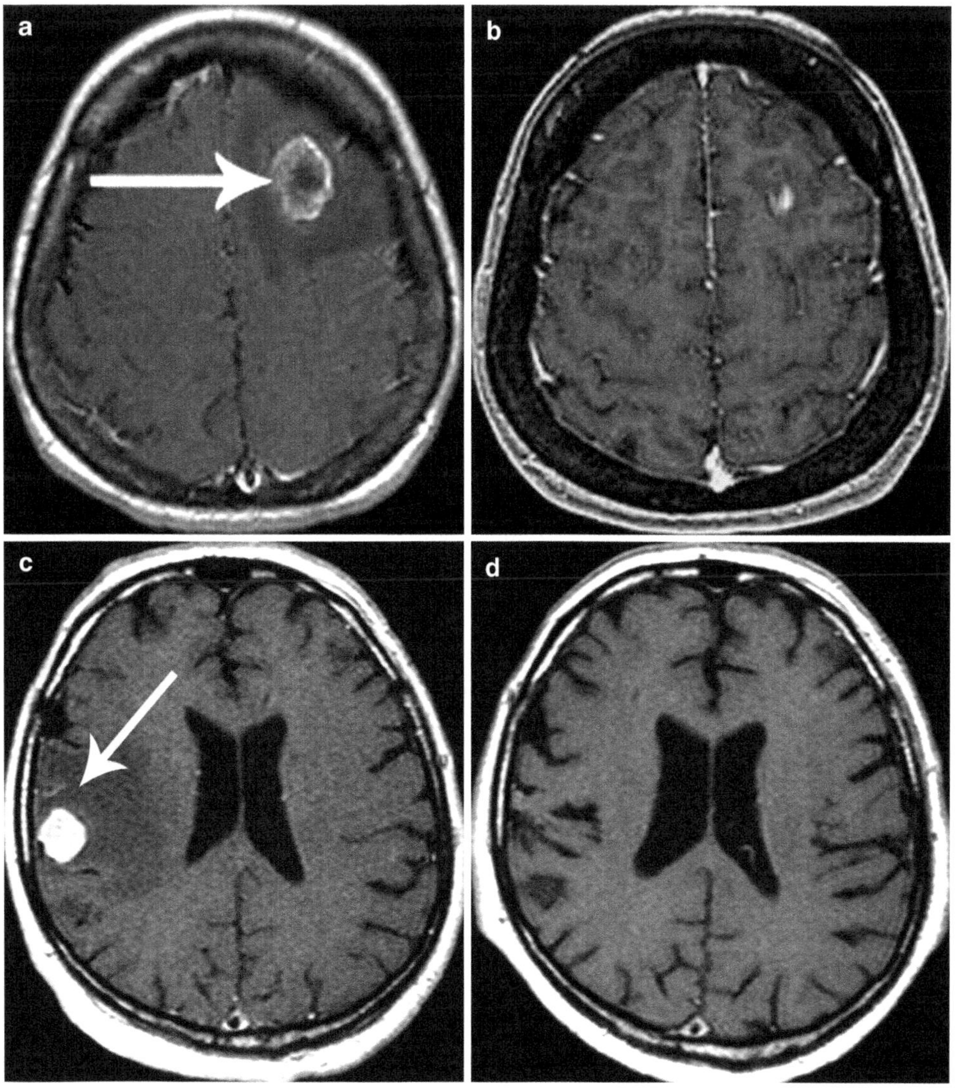

Fig. 9.17 Colorectal cancer metastases in the brain. Cases of two patients with incomplete (**a**, **b**) and complete (**c**, **d**) response to RS treatment. Partial response: (**a**) before treatment and (**b**) after treatment. Complete response: (**c**, **d**) 3 months after the radiosurgery

images "weighted" by the tissue magnetic susceptibility (Haacke et al. 2010;. Pronin et al. 2011; Dolgushin et al. 2012a, b; Zakharova et al. 2013). Local inhomogeneity of the magnetic properties of tissues (due to the differences in their magnetic susceptibility) creates dephasing of proton precession within each voxel. This dephasing manifests in the amplitude and phase images in the form of a reduction in MR signal. SWI (SWAN) uses amplitude images, and SWI (SWAN) uses both phase and amplitude images. The SWI (SWAN) sequence is most commonly used. The combination of amplitude and phase components in the data processing allows to obtain images, whose contrast is due only to the magnetic susceptibility—i.e., to map magnetic susceptibility in order to quantify the magnetic properties of tissues in terms of the chemical shift in parts per million (ppm).

A decrease in the MR signal intensity in SWI (SWAN) sequence due to the deoxyhemoglobin presence allows to visualize some anatomical and primarily venous structures. Hemosiderin deposits as the main sign of a hemorrhage can be detected in the SWI (SWAN) sequence, which allows to visualize the effects of hemorrhages, even in intervals remote from the event. SP SWI (SWAN) visualizes lesions of micro-hemorrhages with sizes up to 5 mm (Haacke et al. 2010).

The tissue magnetic susceptibility in the amplitude SWI (SWAN) images is assessed by the presence of areas of the MR signal with reduced intensity. Pinpoint hypointense areas in the parenchyma are regarded as a cross section of the deformed, abnormal vessels (the form of a "point"). Areas with the similar signal intensity but larger (>2–3 mm) are considered microhemorrhages (the form of "lumps" or "micronodules"). The lack of any hypointense inclusions is interpreted as a homogeneous solid tumor without abnormal deformed vasculature and hemorrhages. The signal constancy from hypointense areas in the SWI (SWAN) sequence after CA administration confirms the presence of a hemorrhage (Dolgushin et al. 2012a, b).

Standard parameters of the SWI (SWAN) sequence in the magnetic field of 3.0 T have the following values: TR, 82–91.5 ms; TE, 42.5 ms; flip angle, 20°, and slice thickness, 1.0 mm; size of the region of interest (slab), 60–80 mm; and study duration, 4–6 min.

For a semiquantitative analysis of the signal nonuniformity in the structure of lesions, we introduced a uniformity coefficient (UC), which is characterized as the ratio of the MR signal intensity from the tumor (affected area) to the signal strength in the area of white matter on the contralateral side. UC for a homogeneous structure is close to unity. The relative value was calculated by dividing the uniformity coefficient in the tumor by its value on the contralateral side (rSWAN = $SWAN_{tumor}/SWAN_{c/s}$). Thus, the results showed that the largest differences in the relative signal intensity MRSrel. (rSWAN) (high UC values) are identified in the structure of metastatic tumors with no evidence of a hemorrhage—a homogeneous form and a variant with tortuous vessels with MRSrel. from 0.56 to 1.09 and with MRSrel. from 0.63 to 1.09, respectively. The lowest UC values were obtained in the structure of metastatic tumors with signs of a hemorrhage with rel. 0.69–0.76 UC for a structure with inhomogeneous magnetic properties of CBS which is much lower than 1.

UC can be calculated on a workstation using an image processing software, such as FUNCTOOL (Advantage Windows, GE). Regions of interest (ROI) are set in the most hypointense tumor areas in the boundary area and the contralateral side of the brain (Fig. 9.18). For a more precise determination of the boundaries of the solid tumor, the SWI (SWAN) sequence is also repeated after administration of the contrast agent.

Based on all the findings (Dolgushin 2012), the structure of metastatic tumors in the SWI (SWAN) sequence before administration of contrast agent was homogeneously hyperintense (34%) or had signs of the presence of deformed vessels—"points" (50%). Hemorrhages ("lumps") in the structure of metastatic tumors were detected rarely in 16% of cases. The next cases of observations show these results.

As noted earlier, brain metastases from the same primary source may have different shapes and visual appearances on

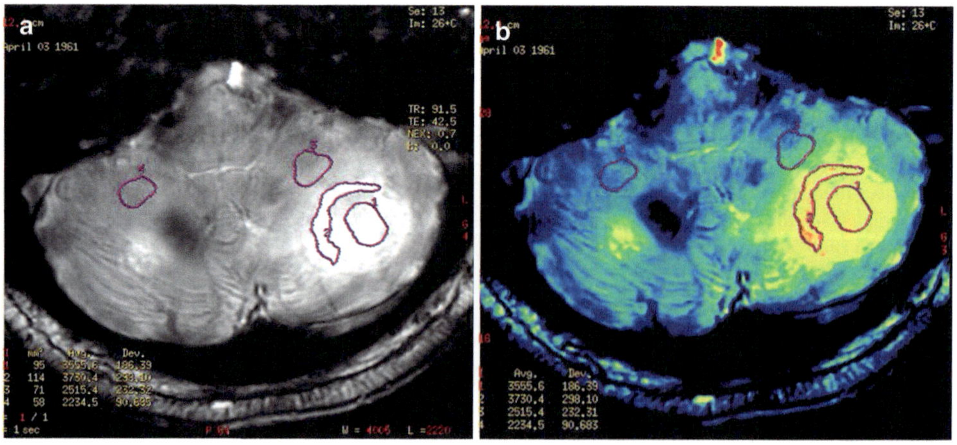

Fig. 9.18 A cancer metastasis in the left hemisphere of the cerebellum. Regions of interest in "raw" SWI (SWAN) images (**a**) and the distribution map of relative signal intensity (**b**) for quantification. (1), the central area of necrosis; (2), accumulation area of the contrast agent; (3), edema area; (4), contralateral (symmetrical) side of the cerebellum

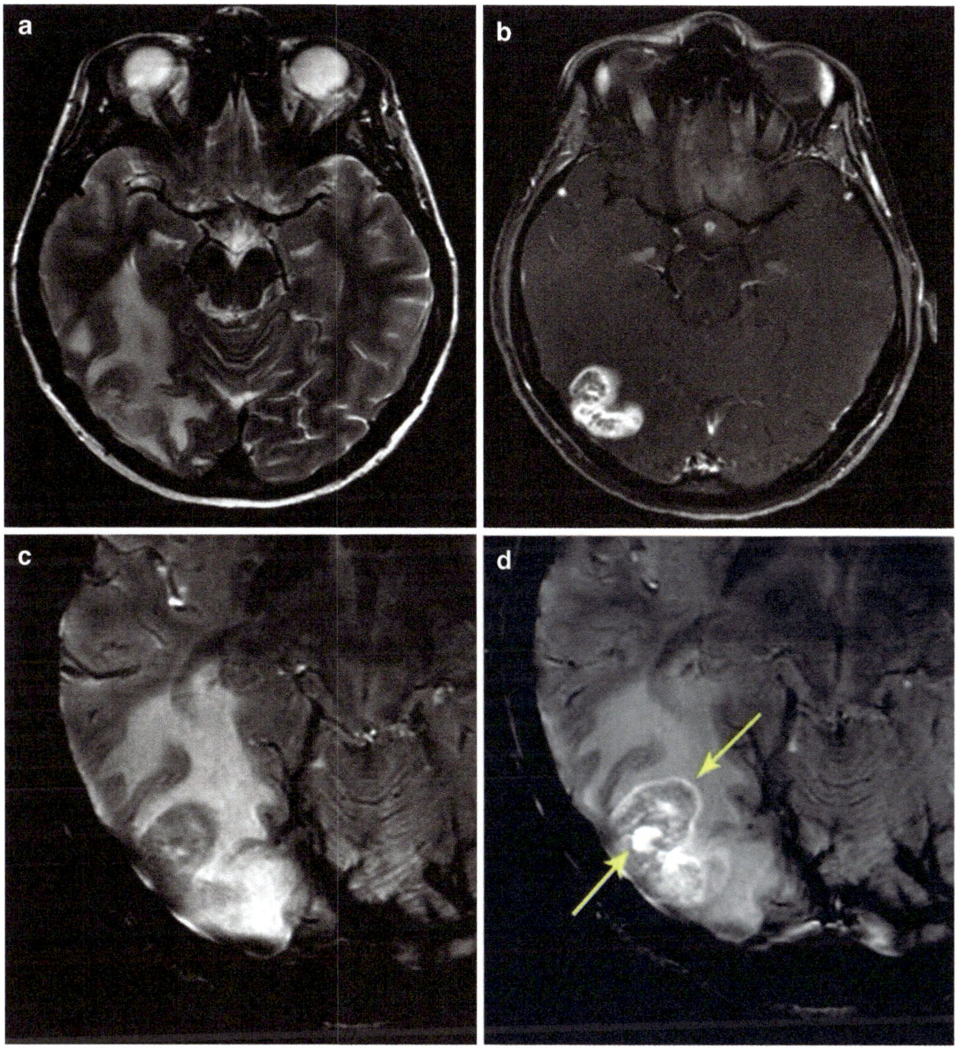

Fig. 9.19 A breast cancer metastasis in the brain. On MRI, there is a lesion in the right parieto-occipital area, characterized by an isointense signal in T2-weighted image with a pronounced perifocal edema (**a**) and intense homogeneous accumulation of the contrast agent on T1-weighted WI with fat suppression (**b**). In the SWI (SWAN) sequence, hypointense inclusions are not detected (**c**), while the accumulation of the contrast agent (**d**) is most pronounced on the periphery and in the center of the lesion (*arrows*)

CT and MR images. At the same time, despite the rapid, aggressive growth with severe dislocation of brain structures and perifocal edema, metastatic lesions may have a homogeneous structure. In such cases, hypointense inclusions are absent in T2 and SWI (SWAN) images; in other words, hemorrhages and deformed vascular microstructures remain undetected. After administration of a contrast agent in such cases, an increase in MR signal in the SWI (SWAN) sequence is most pronounced on the periphery and in the central parts of metastatic lesions, although, in T1-weighted images, accumulation of the contrast agent can be more intense in the peripheral parts of the lesion (Fig. 9.19).

Figure 9.20 presents a case of a patient with glioblastoma characterized by an isointense signal in T2-weighted images and a pronounced perifocal edema (a). On MRI, there is a tumor with hypointense signal in T1-weighted images before contrast enhancement and intensive CA accumulation on the periphery (b, c) after its administration. On SWI (SWAN) MRI (d), a quite large hypointense fragment (bleeding station) is indicated by the arrow on the background of multiple point areas with low density (altered blood vessels), which is not visualized in T1- and T2-weighted images and does not accumulate a contrast agent.

Using the SWI (SWAN) sequence to verify vascular changes in the tumor structure provides additional visual information regarding the properties of the blood vessels in the tumor and allows to obtain semiquantitative (UC) and quantitative (magnetic susceptibility maps) estimates.

Thus, the results of the studies on the use of the SWI (SWAN) sequence in preoperative diagnosis show a great potential and high sensitivity in demonstrating abnormal capillary network and microhemorrhages in secondary malignant brain tumors. This opens up new possibilities for the study of angiogenesis of not only metastatic but primary tumors.

The SWI (SWAN) sequence has worked well in controlled studies after radiotherapy, since the occurrence of hemorrhages in the metastasis tissues after radiotherapy is naturally associated with damage to the vascular wall (Mitomo et al.

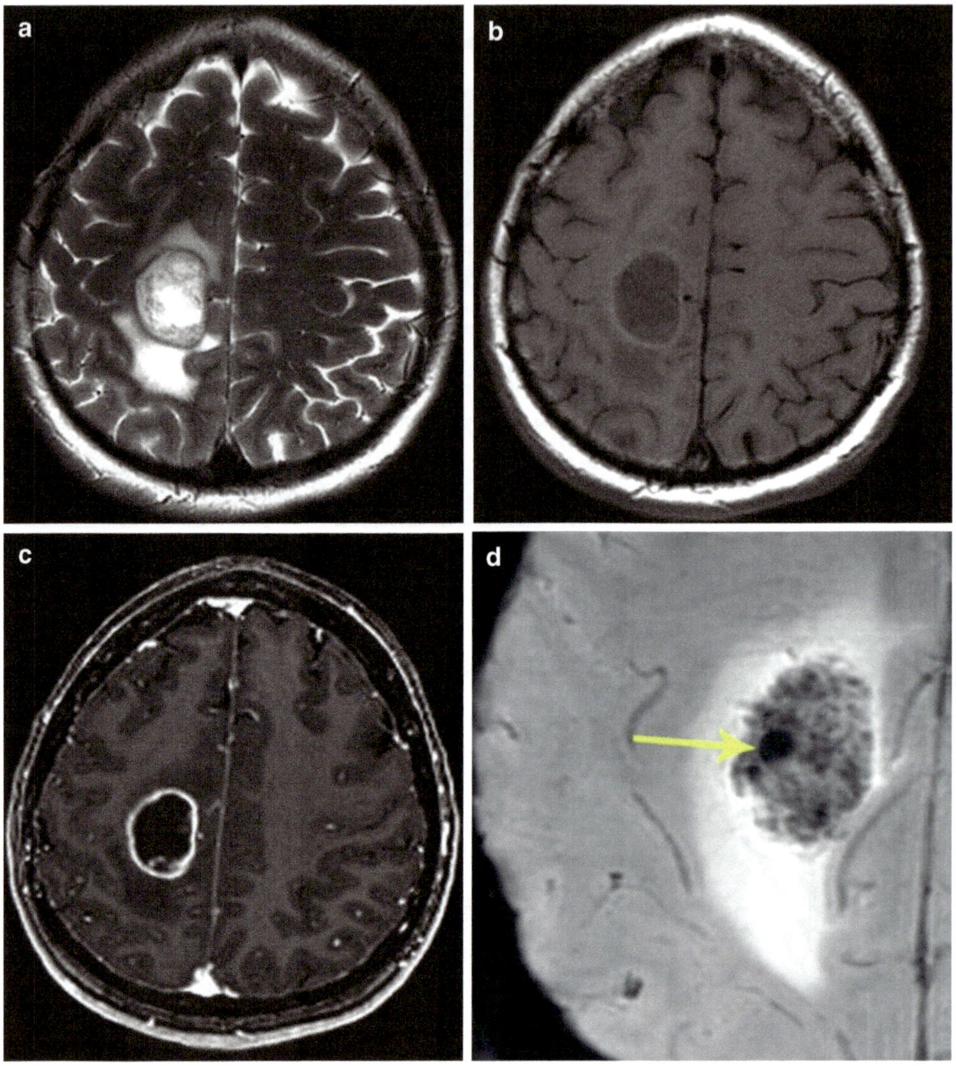

Fig. 9.20 Glioblastoma of deep portions of the right frontal region. On T2-weighted MRI (**a**), there is a lesion surrounded by peritumoral edema; on T1-weighted MRI (**b**) and after intravenous contrast enhancement (**c**), there is an annular opacification. On SWI (SWAN) MRI (**d**), in infiltrative and necrotic parts of the tumor, multiple hypointense lesions are visualized—small hemorrhages in the form of lumps (the arrow), as well as deformed blood vessels in the form of small "points" throughout the lesion with a bright area on the periphery of the edema

1986; Remler et al. 1986). The so-called radiation vasculitis develops, which is accompanied by an increase in the vascular permeability and vasogenic edema, proliferation of endothelial cells occurs, and then hyalinosis and fibrinoid necrosis of the arterioles develop. As a result of damage to vasa vasorum (microvessels supplying the vascular endothelium), telangiectasia may be formed, and hemorrhages from them may occur. In a morphological study, necrotic changes are detected in the area of radiation necrosis and microhemorrhages from telangiectatic blood vessels (Werner et al. 1988; Yamaguchi et al. 1991). The SWI (SWAN) sequence allows to detect these microscopic changes as hypointense areas with various shapes (Fig. 9.21). A comparative analysis of T2-weighted MRI in the control group of patients with metastases after radiotherapy did not allow to visualize any specific changes in the MR signal in the said sequences (4545), which would imply the presence of hemorrhagic inclusions, while SWI (SWAN) images clearly visualized small hypointense inclusions (microhemorrhages) in all cases.

Perfusion magnetic resonance imaging methods allow to obtain a more detailed visualization and quantitative characteristics of cerebral hemodynamics.

9.5 Perfusion MRI Techniques (DSC, DCE, ASL)

It is known that malignancies are characterized by active growth and have a high demand for an intensive blood supply, which occurs already when the tumor reaches 2–4 mm^3 (Leenders et al. 2003). This condition can be provided only by an active formation of a well-developed vasculature in the tumor (angiogenesis). The rapid growth of the tumor, causing hypoglycemia and hypoxia, stimulates endogenous synthesis of angiogenic cytokines, with the vascular endothelial growth factor (VEGF) being the main. Several investigators have shown that newly formed blood vessels differ from normal brain vessels (Cascino T. et al. 1983; Roberts 1997;

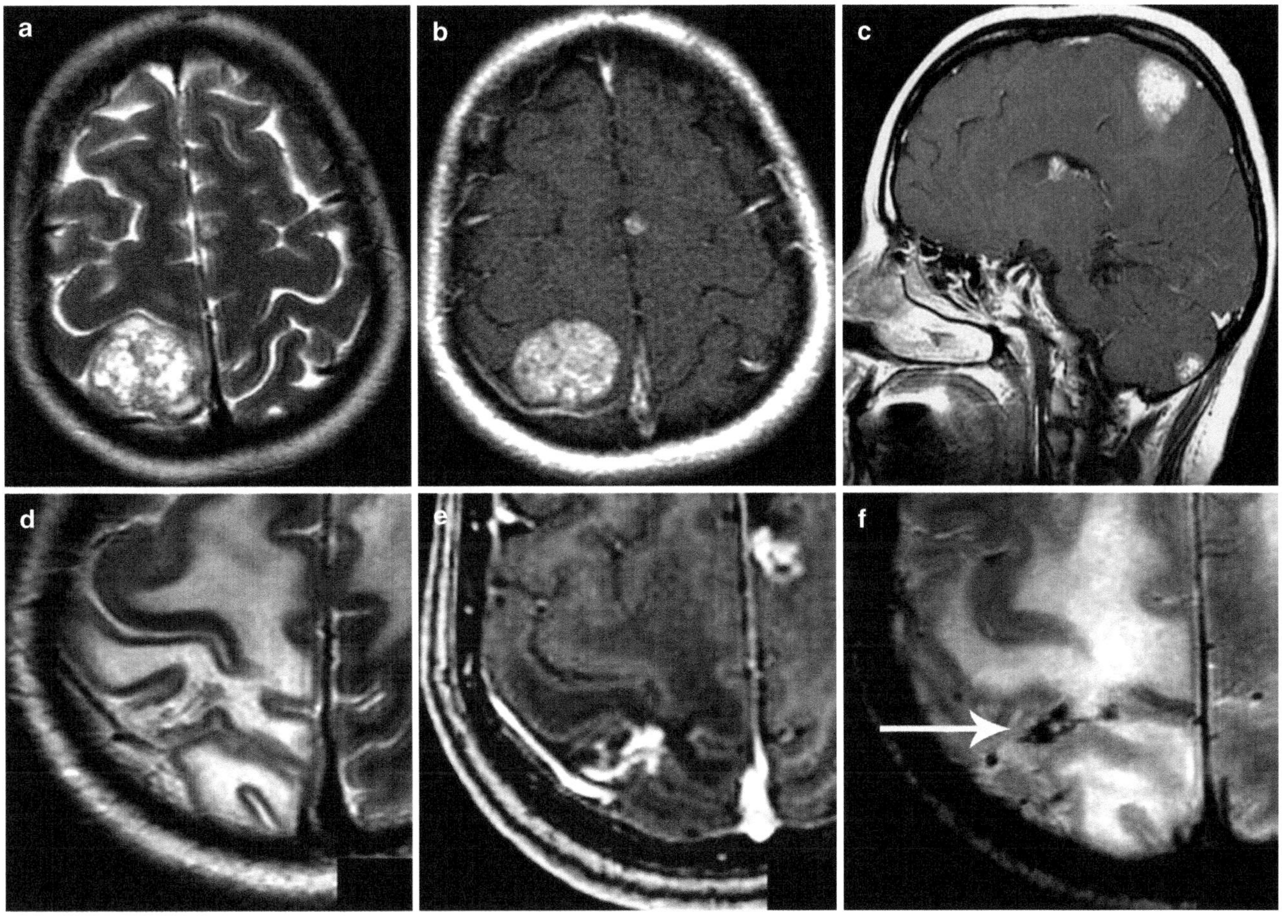

Fig. 9.21 Multiple breast cancer metastases in the brain. MRI before and after radiation therapy. Before treatment, on T2-weighted MRI (**a**) and T1-weighted contrast-enhanced MRI (**b, c**), there is a large space-occupying lesion in the right parietal region that rapidly accumulates contrast agent. Follow-up scans 2 years after the radiotherapy. There is a marked reduction in the lesion size. On T2-weighted MRI (**d**), an irregularly shaped fragment with moderately low signal is identified. After administration of the contrast agent, a small portion of its accumulation persists on T1-weighted MRI (**e**). On SWI (SWAN) MRI (**f**), there are hypointense (hemorrhagic) inclusions (the *arrow*)

Blouw et al. 2003): they are characterized by an extreme degree of heterogeneity; presence of a plurality of capillaries with indirect, curved course and fragile walls; presence of arteriovenous shunts and closely spaced vessels; and alternating areas of brain tissue hypoxia and active neoangiogenesis. The walls of the newly formed capillaries are characterized by high permeability due to the presence of extended gaps between endothelial cells, partial absence of the basement membrane, etc. (Nussbaum et al. 1996). The complex of these factors results in a degradation and increase in the BBB permeability. The above morphological differences in normal and tumor blood vessels also determine the differences in perfusion (hemodynamic) properties of normal and abnormal tissue.

Different methods are used to assess the hemodynamic parameters in the cerebral blood flow: positron emission tomography (PET) with 15O, $H_2{}^{15}O$, and $C^{15}O$, single-photon emission computed tomography (SPECT) with ^{99m}Tc-HMPAO and ^{133} Xe, computed tomography (CT) with xenon (Xe) and iodine-containing CA (so-called CT perfusion), and magnetic resonance imaging (MRI perfusion). There are three main technologies evaluating hemodynamic changes in the tissues by MRI: arterial spin labeling (ASL), T2-*weighted perfusion MRI (DSC, dynamic susceptibility contrast), and T1-weighted perfusion MRI (DCE, dynamic contrast enhanced). Perfusion techniques, being highly informative in assessing the structures and functions of microvasculature, allowed to evaluate the architecture of the tumor vasculature, suggesting its probable histological structure (Baert and Sartor 2005; Cha et al. 2007; Wang et al. 2011; Nechipay et al. 2015; Griffith and Jain 2015; Pizzinni et al. 2015; Gaddikeri et al. 2016).

MRI perfusion techniques are based on the change in the intensity of the MR signal on T1-, T2-, or T2-*weighted MRI during the transit of a bolus of contrast agent through the bloodstream (Sorensen and Reimer 2000; Tofts 2004; Ostergaard 2005; Saremi 2015).

Concentration of MRCA in the bolus is usually 0.1 mmol/kg of body weight, the volume of semi-molar MRCA bolus is 10–15 ml, and the administration rate is 4–5 ml/s. Following bolus administration of MRCA, the buffer solution (20 ml saline) is administered at 4.5 ml/s. In perfusion MRI, similar to perfusion CT, images of each slice (10–15 layers) are repeatedly recorded during the MRCA bolus transit through the vasculature. Scanning takes 4 to 60 s in T2-/T2-*weighted MRI (DSC) and 3.2 min in T1-weighted MRI (DCE). The MRCA bolus transit on successive slices corresponds to a sharp decrease in the MR signal intensity on T2/T2-*weighted MRI and a sharp increase in the MRCA concentration (Fig. 9.22). The curve of intensity changes as MRCA bolus passes provides the "signal intensity to time" dependence in each pixel of the slice.

The form of this relationship in pixels of brain arteries, veins, and tissues (tumor, normal substance) gives, respectively, arterial, venous, and tissue function by which the tissue hemodynamic parameters are calculated: time to peak concentration (TTP), cerebral blood volume (CBV), cerebral blood flow (CBF), and mean transit time (MTT). Stages of transformation of dynamic DSC data when constructing parametric perfusion maps are shown in Fig. 9.23.

The cerebral blood volume (CBV) and time to peak concentration (TTP) can be estimated from the concentration curve—C(t)—but cerebral blood flow (CBF) and mean transit time (MTT) are calculated using "deconvolution" algorithms (SVD, etc.) as well as by processing the perfusion CT data. In contrast to perfusion CT, values of cerebral blood volume and flow in DCS are presented in relative units:

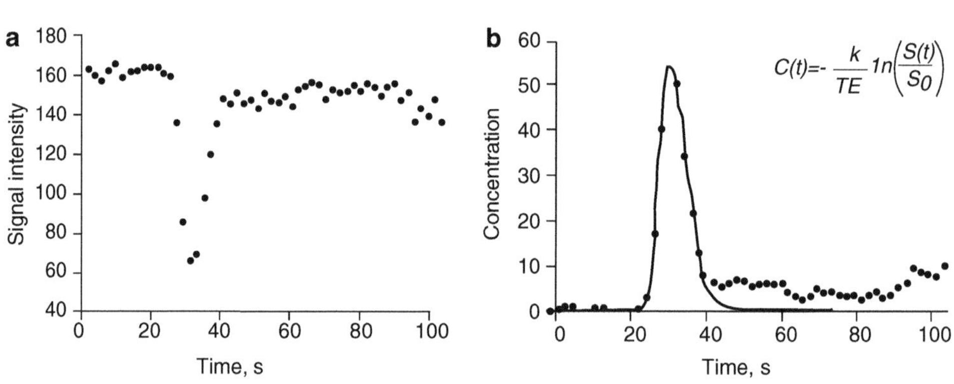

Fig. 9.22 A decrease in MR signal intensity on T2/T2-*weighted MRI (**a**) and a sharp increase in the MRCA concentration in the tissue (**b**) as bolus passes

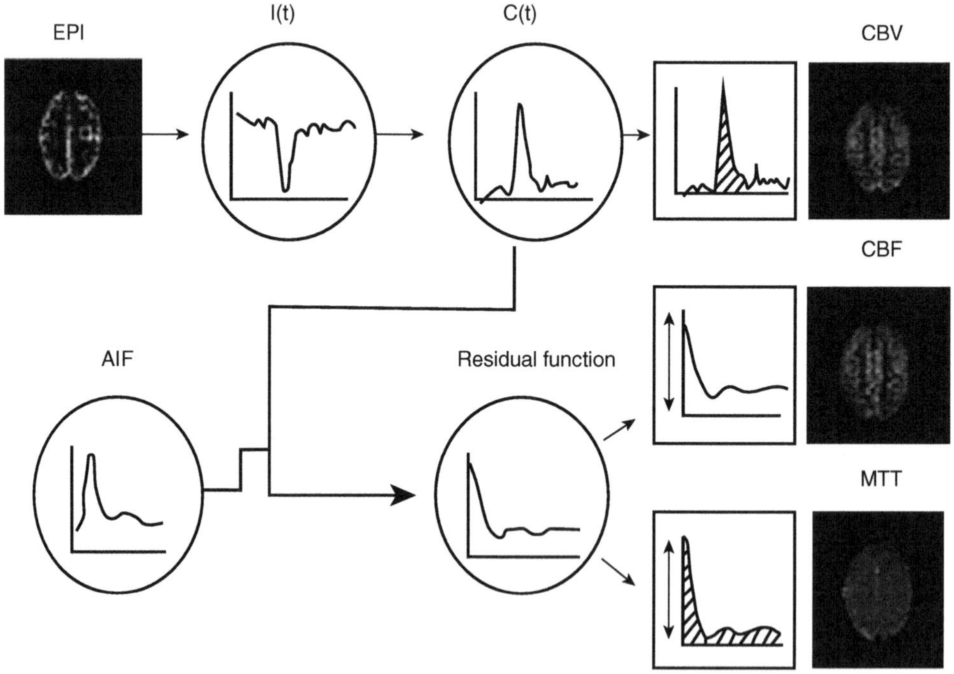

Fig. 9.23 A schematic description of perfusion data processing algorithm in DSC MR perfusion (from Shiroishi et al. 2015). AIF—arterial input function, residual function

rCBF and rCBV with normalization for the respective values in the brain substance on the contralateral side with respect to the tumor (Wetzel et al. 2002; Shiroishi et al. 2015). Parametric maps constructed in an "off-line" mode on workstations allow to visually assess the hemodynamic of a metastasis or other brain tumors.

On perfusion T2-*weighted MRI, an ideal situation is believed to be an intravascular spread of CA. In this case, echo planar pulse sequences (SE, GRE) are used that can provide temporal resolution of 1–2 s in the curves of intensity change in the MR signal. CA leakage outside the vascular bed in an impaired BBB affects the shape of the "signal intensity to time" curve, as the presence of CA in extravascular spaces results in a reduction in the T1 relaxation time constant and an increase in the MR signal intensity due to the T1 effect. In such cases, dynamic perfusion T1-weighted MRI (the DCE) or MR DC (dynamic contrast enhancement) are used.

Dynamic T1-weighted contrast enhancement is also performed using a bolus intravenous injection of the standard amount of CA with the construction of "signal intensity to time" curves. This is based on the two-component Tofts and Kermode model that considers the CA distribution in both intra- and extravascular space and the kinetics of the contrast agent transition from one space to another and back (Tofts and Kermode 1991; Tofts et al. 1999). This allows to calculate the vascular permeability parameters and the extent of CA spread, K^{trans}, V_e, and K_{ep}, and construct relevant parametric maps. Figure 9.24 schematically shows tissue components and direction of CA movement in them. A two-component Tofts and Kermode model of pharmacokinetic exchange includes several components, each of which is represented by the complex of tissues with their characteristics: intravascular bed and extracellular, extravascular (EES—extravascular extracellular space), and intracellular space (Weidner 1998; Tofts et al. 1999). The MR dynamic contrast enhancement characterizes them as a whole: CA exchange occurs only between the intravascular and intercellular spaces (constant K^{trans}).

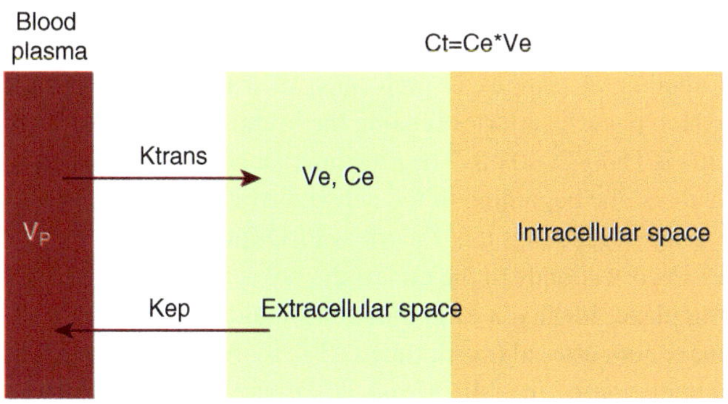

Fig. 9.24 MRCA kinetics. Two-component model (Tofts and Kermode 1991)

- K^{trans} (transfer constant) is the CA diffusion constant between the blood plasma and extracellular extravascular space. The K^{trans} value depends on the total surface area and permeability of the capillary walls per unit of tissue volume, as well as the blood flow velocity. This parameter reflects the value of the product of microvascular permeability by the area of vascular damage—PS for its minor damage. In the normal brain tissue, K^{trans} is almost zero; however, in a tumor, this parameter may be much higher than in the surrounding tissues (Bisese 1992).
- V_e (EES) is the volume fraction of the interstitial extracellular space.
- K_{ep} is the constant of reflux from the extravascular extracellular space to the blood plasma ($K_{ep} = K^{trans}/V_e$).

These parameters were recommended in 1999 by a group of researchers, who developed the methodology of dynamic contrast enhancement (Weidner 1998).

A DCE study involves obtaining "native" maps of T1 relaxation of tissues and dynamic scanning with IV bolus administration of contrast agent on T1-weighted MRI, for example, pulse sequences FSE (General Electric Healthcare) and TWIST (Siemens Healthcare) (Haacke et al. 2005). The dynamic scan data processing is performed in an *off-line* mode on workstations. On a workstation syngo MR (Siemens Healthcare), the program Mean Curve calculates "signal intensity/time" curves, and the program Tissue 4D calculates parameters of vascular permeability (K^{trans}, V_e, K_{ep}) with construction of relevant parametric maps. Perfusion parameters are calculated in regions of interest (ROI) in the solid portion of tumors (a region that corresponds to homogeneous accumulation of contrast agent). Any cystic, necrotic components, areas of hemorrhagic change, and vessels passing in the tumor depth should be excluded from the region of interest.

Thus, the data received by MR T1 DK (DCE) method can be evaluated both qualitatively and quantitatively. Quantitative estimates allow to isolate substrates that are associated with the distribution and kinetics of the injected contrast agent in the tumor. Figure 9.25 shows an example of CA distribution in the lung cancer metastasis.

Along with MR perfusion studies, based on changes in T1, T2, and T2* relaxation times of blood with bolus CA administration (DCE, DSC), there is a non-contrast-enhanced MRI method of imaging the capillary cerebral blood flow.

The advantage of cerebral blood flow studies by arterial spin labeling (ASL) is the use of endogenous contrast enhancement. Arterial spin labeling is performed using special radio-frequency pulses that change the magnetization of the blood in the supplying brain arteries. Labeled spins of arterial blood inflowing into the brain tissue act as an endogenous marker. This blood forms a small bolus volume of water molecules with modified magnetization, which inflows

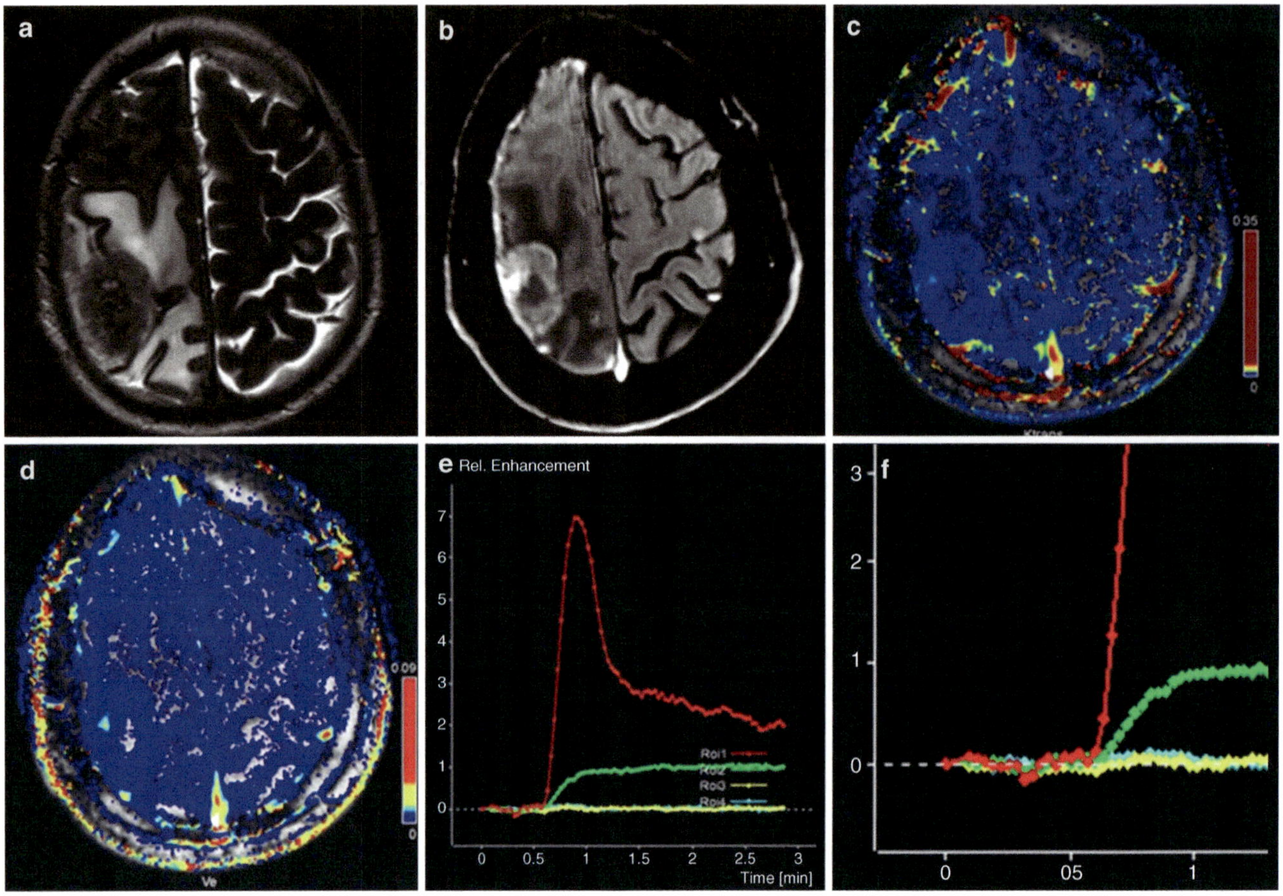

Fig. 9.25 A lung cancer metastasis in the brain. MRI in the right parietal lobe in T2-WI (**a**) and T1-VIBE (**b**) sequences after IV administration of contrast agent shows a space-occupying lesion with a necrosis area in the central parts, pronounced perifocal edema, and uneven CA accumulation. (**c**, **d**) Parametric maps of K^{trans} and V_e (**e**) "concentration/time" curve (*red* artery, *green* metastasis, *yellow and blue* the intact brain matter on the affected and contralateral sides, respectively). (**f**) The slope of the leading edge of the "signal intensity to time" curve is proportional to CBV

with the bloodstream into the capillary network of the brain tissue with a certain delay—δ. Brain scans performed after the inflow of s bolus of the endogenous marker produce an image, whose contrast enhancement will be formed in the presence of labeled spins. Such an image is called labeled. The second scan of the same brain region is performed without a previous inversion or saturation of the spins of water molecules in arterial blood. In this case, the image is called a reference image and is used to determine the baseline tissue contrast enhancement. By subtracting the reference image from the labeled one, slices with tissue contrast enhancement can be obtained, corresponding to the distribution of labeled spins in the brain tissue, i.e., perfusion images.

Currently, two versions of the ASL method are used—continuous and pulse labeling. We used a pseudo-continuous arterial spin labeling—pCASL (T1)—recommended for clinical use (Kornienko et al. 2012; Alsop et al. 2015). Figure 9.26 shows a layout of the labeling plane (red line) and regions of flow mapping (green contour).

Registration of reference and labeled images is repeated sequentially several times, just as it is done in fMRI, averaging the signal intensity for each voxel in the image using the corresponding screens.

A pseudo-continuous (pseudo-continuous ASL) method of spin labeling of arterial blood protons using several radiofrequency and gradient pulses—pcASL—was proposed by Alsop et al. (2015). It combines high values of labeling efficiency and signal/noise ratio in the perfusion images. Labeling of protons is performed in a thin layer, through which pass the arteries feeding the brain. The labeling duration is 1500–2000 ms. The time interval between the labeling end and the beginning of the data registration affects the efficiency of labeling; it is known as PLD (post-labeling delay). PLD corresponds to the end of the bolus transit in the labeling plane. Ideally, a PLD duration should be longer than the maximum arterial transit time (ATT) to the brain tissues, but attenuation of the MR signal in the arterial blood with T1 time constant makes to search for a compromise solution.

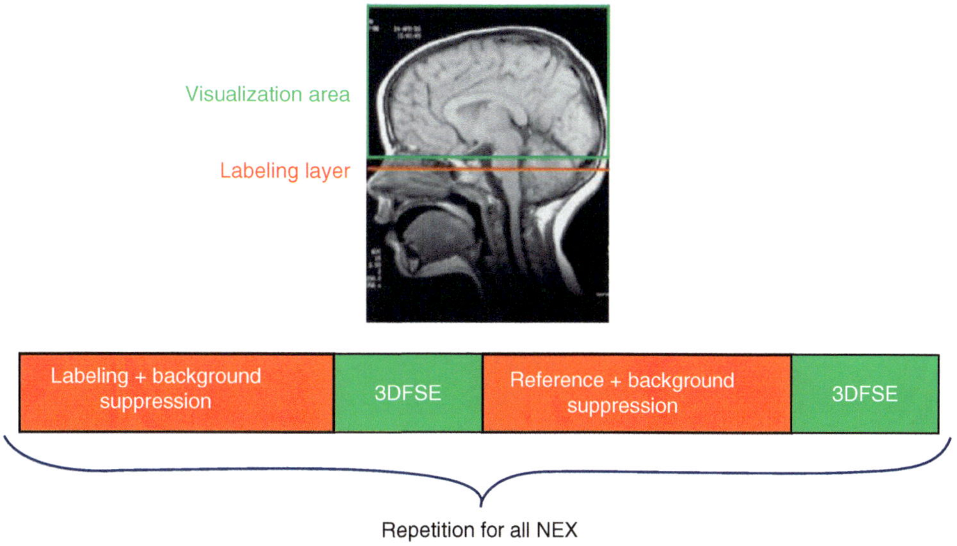

Fig. 9.26 The scheme for obtaining reference and labeled images

The recommended value for healthy adults is 1800 ms (3.0 T). The MR signal is registered in 3D mode almost from the entire brain. The scanning trajectory is an eight-start helix; a delay between the labeling and registration of reference data is 1025–1525 ms. The study duration is 5–6 min.

Cerebral blood flow (CBF) maps are constructed in an off-line mode on a workstation or directly on the MRI scanner. CBF (mean and standard deviation) is measured in regions located symmetrically in the tumor and the contralateral side, and the ratio of CBF values obtained is calculated. Figure 9.27 demonstrates the case of multiple lung cancer metastases in the brain. MRI with contrast enhancement (d) demonstrates multiple lesions with different sizes, with a marked contrast enhancement. An ASL SVF map (e) shows an inhomogeneous moderate increase in the blood flow in the metastatic lesions.

The comparisons of the results of CBF measurement by the ASL and DSC methods showed a high degree of correlation of the data obtained by these methods (Järnum et al. 2010). The ASL perfusion method, counterbalancing the limitations of CT perfusion (radiation exposure, iodine-based CAs), allows to obtain quantitative measures of the cerebral blood flow velocity with a broad anatomical capture in any region of interest (Fig. 9.28): in areas of the tumor, a central necrosis, and normal brain tissue (Wolf and Detre 2007; Tourdias et al. 2008; Kornienko et al. 2012; Lowther et al. 2015). MRI perfusion studies without CA have become an important feature of modern neurodiagnosis.

At present, the development of neuroimaging methods transforms into a new quality—from the structural to molecular imaging to study the functional features of the brain. One of such methods is magnetic resonance spectroscopy.

Magnetic resonance spectroscopy (MRS) is a method of in vivo determination of the presence in the brain tissues of chemical compounds involved in metabolic processes in normal and abnormal conditions. The MR spectrum provides information on the chemical composition of tissues. The positions of the MR spectrum peaks characterize the chemical composition, the peak width reflects the value of T2 relaxation time of compounds, and the peak height and area under the peak are proportional to the compound concentration. Thus, MRS provides the possibility of determining the concentrations of chemical substances present in the tissues. MRS is a powerful noninvasive method of obtaining in vivo information on the chemical composition of the brain matter on the metabolic level.

The MRS is based on the difference in resonance frequencies of identical nuclei in different materials, caused by the fact that these nuclei are surrounded by various chemical bonds that affect the local value of the magnetic field strength and determine the resonant frequency of the nucleus in the compound. The difference of the nucleus resonant frequencies in a chemical compound from the resonant frequency of a "free" nucleus is called the *chemical shift*. The difference of the resonant frequencies of different compounds is dependent on induction of the external magnetic field and typically is of the order of tens to hundreds of Hz, while the resonant frequencies are of the order of tens to hundreds of MHz. Therefore, the chemical shift is usually measured relative to the fundamental resonant frequency in parts per million (ppm). Spectroscopy is based on this difference in chemical shift of the resonance frequency of the nuclei of different chemical compounds. MR spectroscopy evolved from an analytical method of high-resolution NMR spectroscopy that appeared in the 1950s of the last century. It should be noted that the emergence of MR imaging was encouraged by the works of Damadian on spectroscopy of benign and malignant tumors in the early 1970s. Currently MRI scanners

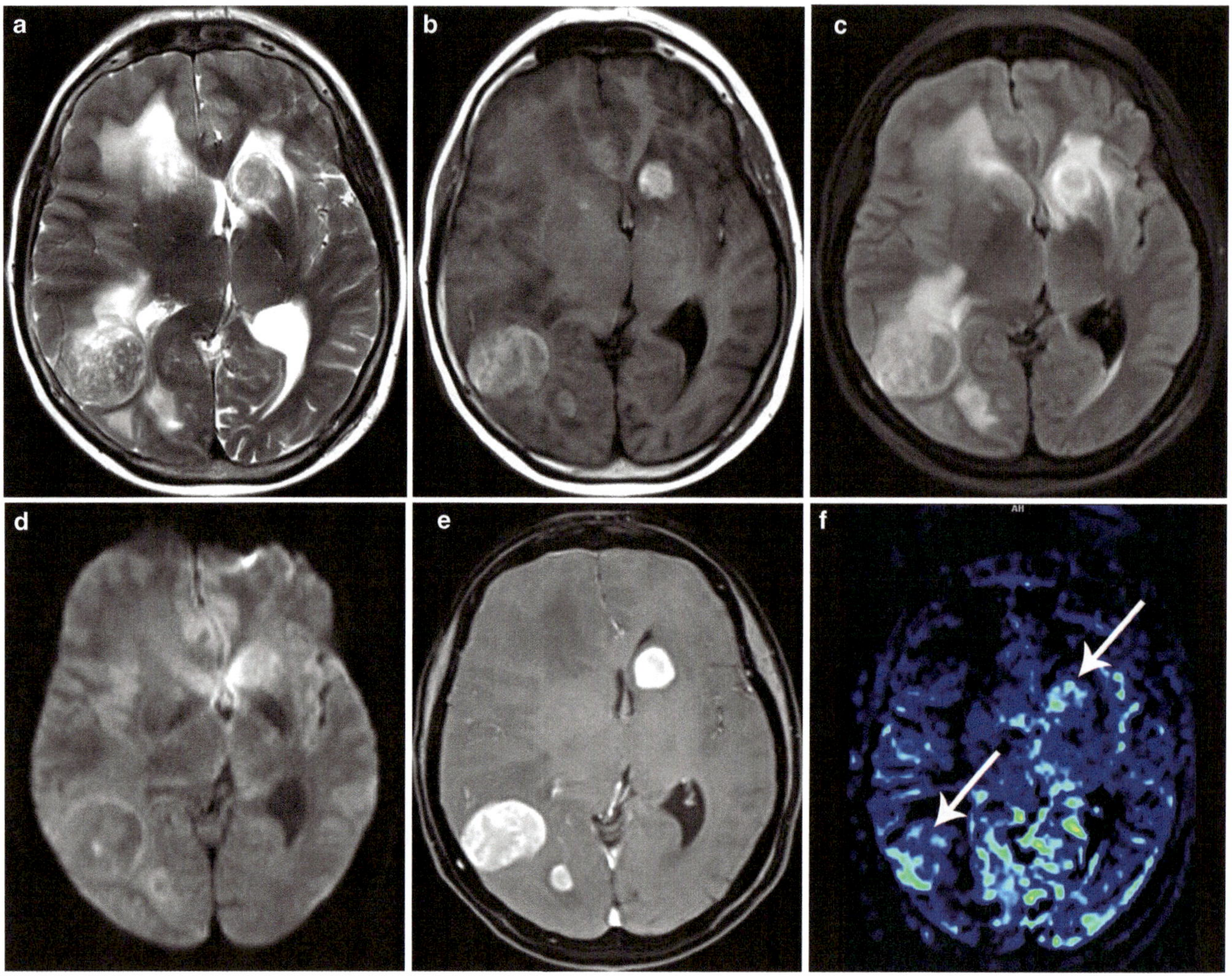

Fig. 9.27 Multiple lung cancer metastases in the brain. On T2-weighted (**a**), T1-weighted (**b**), and T2-FLAIR (**c**) MRI, multiple lesions are observed with a moderate perifocal edema and hemorrhagic impregnation—an increased signal in T1-weighted sequence (**b**). In DWI image (**d**), the signal from the lesions is mostly isointense. On contrast-enhanced T1-weighted MRI (**e**), there is a pronounced accumulation of the contrast agent in the lesions. The CBF map in the ASL sequence (**f**) shows a heterogeneous weak nature of the blood flow increase in metastases (*arrows*)

allow to obtain MR spectra based on the resonance frequencies of the nuclei of hydrogen (^{1}H), phosphorus (^{31}P), fluorine (^{19}F), sodium (^{23}Na), and potassium (^{39}K). In clinical practice, proton ^{1}H MRS is the most widely used, as almost all organic compounds include hydrogen atoms and proton nuclei in water molecules have a high magnetic moment and form a sufficiently high MR signal.

Proton MRS is the most sensitive method for determining the presence of metabolites in the nervous tissue even in small concentrations. The proton MR spectrum has peaks of compounds such as NAA (*N*-acetylaspartate) with a peak of 2.0 ppm; Cho, choline (3.2 ppm); Cr, creatine (3.03 and 3,94 ppm); mI, myoinositol (3.56 ppm); Glx, glutamate and glutamine peaks (2.1–2.5 ppm); Lac, lactate peak (1.32 ppm); and Lip, lipid complex (0.8–1.2 ppm).

Currently, MR spectroscopy uses two main approaches: single-voxel (SV) MRS and multi-voxel MRS (2D/3D MRS or chemical shift imaging). Multi-voxel MRS allows to obtain spectra for multiple parts of the brain with a single scan.

Figure 9.29 shows a proton spectrum of the white matter of the brain in a healthy person, obtained in single-voxel MRS in a magnetic field of 3.0 T. The highest peak is NAA. *N*-acetylaspartate is a form of aspartate accumulation in neuronal cells; it is synthesized in the mitochondria. Creatine, phosphocreatine (Cr), is involved in the cell energy metabolism; it is a supplier of phosphate groups for the conversion of ADP to ATP. Choline (Cho), a cell membrane component, displays the total reserves of choline in the brain tissue. Myoinositol (mI) is contained in glial cells and participates in the osmolar status

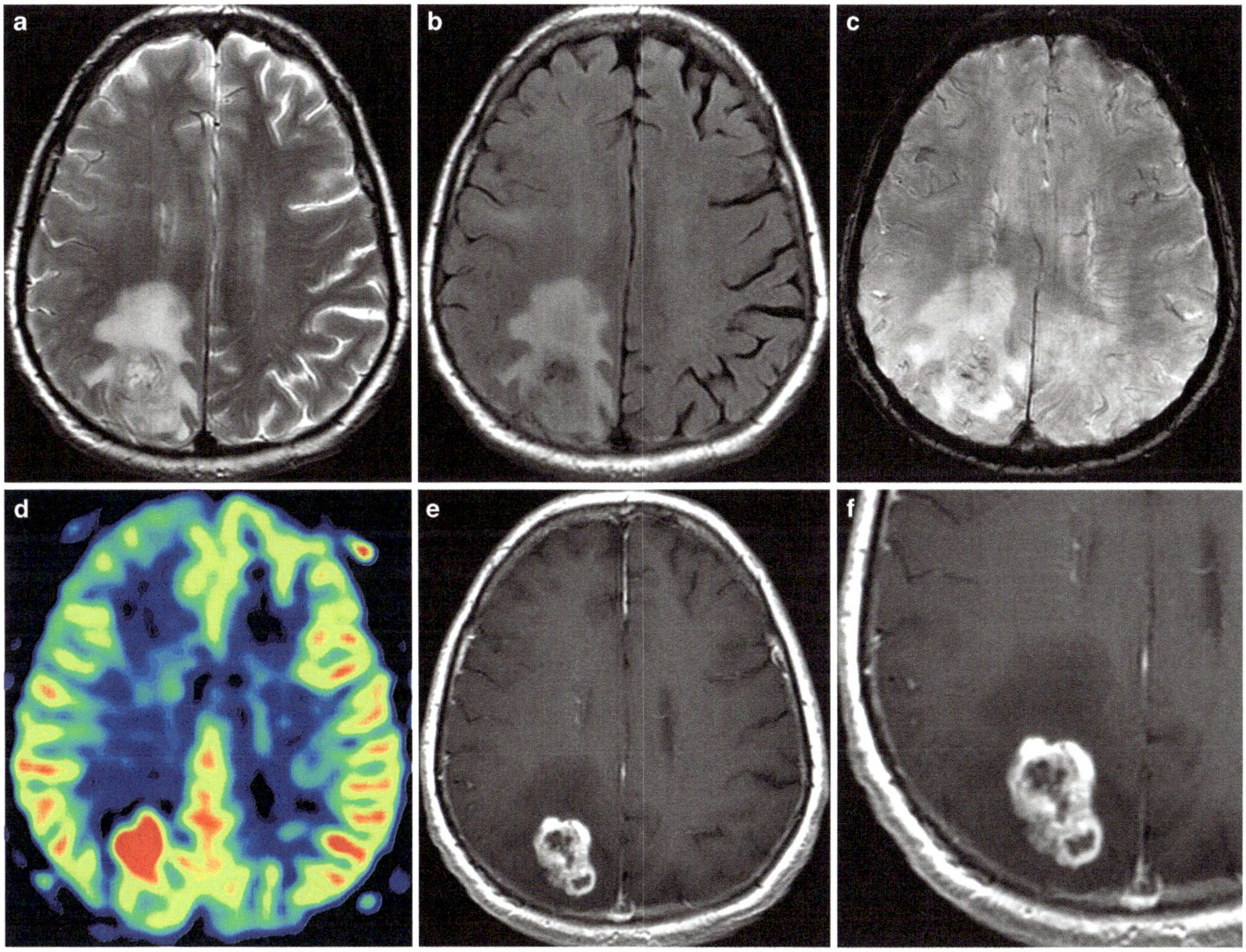

Fig. 9.28 A cancer metastasis from an unidentified primary source. On MRI, in the right parietal region, there is a space-occupying lesion with an irregular shape, with signs of a pronounced perifocal edema. In T2-weighted (**a**) and T2-FLAIR (**b**) images, the signal from the metastasis is mainly isointense. In SWI (SWAN) (**c**) images, there are marked isolated hypointense inclusions in the solid part of the metastasis that is characterized by a sharp increase in the blood flow values on the ASL (**d**) maps. After the administration of contrast agent (**e**, **f**), its intense accumulation in the tumor occurs, and another small necrotic lesion is further visualized

regulation. Glx is a total peak of glutamate and glutamine. Glutamine, an amino acid and a precursor of glutamate in astrocytes, is an excitatory neurotransmitter. Low peaks of glutamine and glutamate are present in the spectra in case when MRS uses short times TE = 30–35 ms. Lactate (Lac) is an anaerobic glycolysis product absent in a healthy tissue.

When selecting a region for MR spectroscopy, the tumor location relative to the bone structures, great vessels, and cerebrospinal fluid spaces should be taken into account. Incorporation of these structures in the study region brings additional local inhomogeneity of the magnetic field, which results in a reduction in the signal/noise ratio. Excitation of nuclear substances that make up the body fat is one of the main issues in MR spectroscopy, since the signals of these nuclei introduce interferences and noise in the MR spectrum of the region of interest. Various methods, including manually setting the saturation bands, are used to suppress the signal from the fat. During registration of spectroscopy data, the area under saturation bands does not receive excitatory impulses. A standard MRS protocol allows the use of 10–12 saturation bands. Six of them have standard positions in the anterior, posterior, right, left, top, and bottom planes around the region of interest. Four additional bands are set manually by the operator around the study region of the brain through their rotations and translations. It is recommended to position these bands in regions adjacent to the adipose tissue, bone structures, and blood products.

Since the concentration of the studied metabolites is 10,000-fold lower than the concentration of water in the brain tissue, the high MR signal from the water is masking weaker signals from metabolites. Therefore, before registering the spectrum, it is necessary to suppress the signal from water.

a

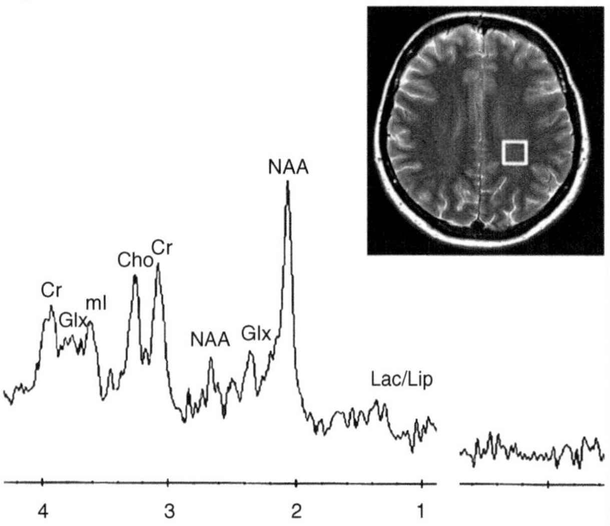

b

Metabolite	Name	Chemical shift, ppm
NAA	N-acetylaspartate	2.0
Cr	phosphocreatine	3.2
Cho	Choline	3.03; 3.94
mI	Myo-inositol	3.56
Glx	Glutamate and glutamine	2,1 -2,5
Lac	Lactate	1.32
Lip	Lipid complex	0.8-1.2.

Fig. 9.29 Single-voxel PMRS of a brain region in the normal white matter. The NAA peak is most pronounced. Lip and Lac peaks are virtually indistinguishable at the noise level

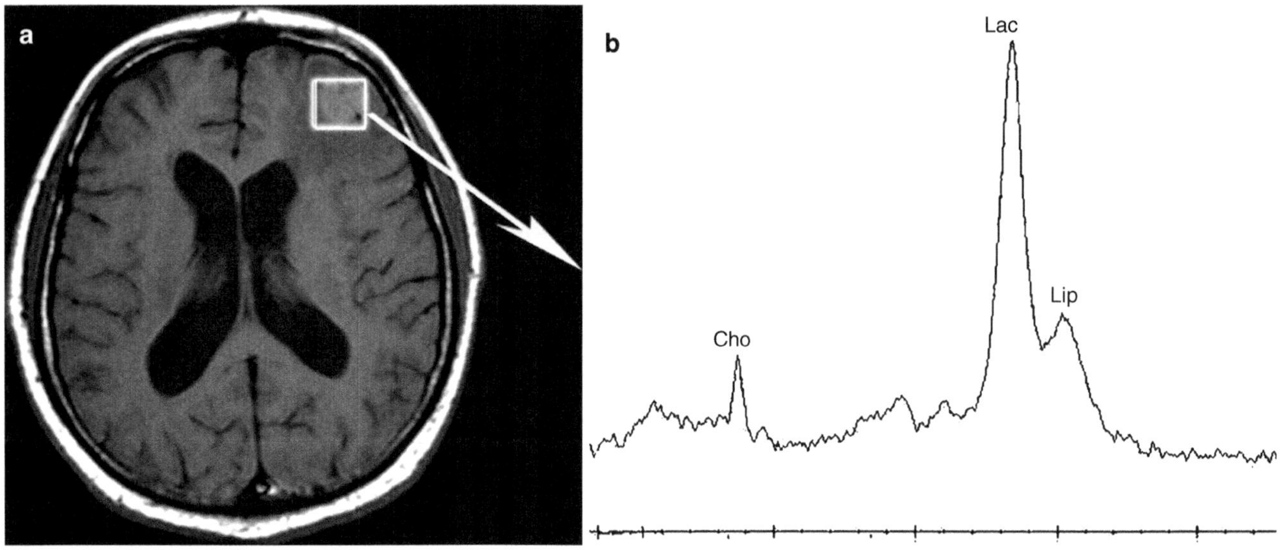

Fig. 9.30 A kidney cancer metastasis in the brain. On T1-weighted MRI (**a**), there is a rounded lesion in the left frontal lobe of the brain. On PMRS (**b**) there is a decrease in major peaks characteristic of normal brain tissue and a sharp increase in peaks of the Lip-Lac complex

This suppression is performed automatically when setting up the apparatus before MRS (PreScan).

An important criterion for setting the apparatus before MRS, in addition to the correct choice of a square of study, is the value of the spectral line width that should not exceed 4–7 Hz in the field of 1.5 T and 15–25 Hz in the field of 3.0 T.

Figure 9.30 shows the MR spectrum of a renal cell carcinoma metastasis. The lesion is characterized by an a low raised signal on T1-weighted MRI. On PMRS, there is a marked decrease in peak heights from major metabolites of normal nervous tissue, while the spectrum contains a pronounced peak of the Lip-Lac complex.

On PMRS, there is an increase in peaks of lactate (Lac) and lipids (Lip) and in 10% of cases a moderate peak of choline (Cho) in the central part of metastases (usually, an area of tumor decay). In our opinion, the presence of Cho is most likely related to an error in the study, since the voxel volume in small lesions may involve the adjacent brain substance.

Multi-voxel MR spectroscopy (MMRS) allows to perform a differentiated study of the ratio of metabolites in various elements of the tumor, in the boundary area, and in an intact part of the brain using a single scanning. This approach allows to perform a more accurate assessment of tumor areas with necrotic changes and identify their solid part, which can be used for a biopsy. Figure 9.31 shows the results of multi-voxel MR spectroscopy in a patient with colon cancer metastases in the brain. The lesion is characterized by a reduced signal on T2-weighted MRI (a) and intensely and unevenly accumulates the contrast agent (b). The graphs of multi-voxel spectroscopy show a pronounced peak of the Lip-Lac complex in the central portions of the lesion, and the Cho peak appears in the peripheral portion of the latter. In the peritumoral area, the peak height of the Lip-Lac complex decreases and reaches the Cho peak level.

The spectra obtained in multi-voxel and single-voxel spectroscopy are not crucially different. In order to determine the concentrations of metabolites present in the MR spectra, a specialized processing of spectroscopy results is required. The form of the spectrum allows to qualitatively compare the composition of metabolites in normal and abnormal tissues. For the semiquantitative analysis, the peak height ratios of major metabolites are used.

Multi-voxel spectroscopy is often accompanied by expressed "noise" due to local inhomogeneity of the magnetic field. It is not always possible to obtain the quantitative information of the necessary quality. Artifacts emerging in such cases are provoked by hemorrhagic inclusions with paramagnetic properties that accompany the post-radiation response, as well as plenty of free water in the edematous area and leukoencephalopathy.

The metabolite peak ratios in the solid structure of metastatic tumors in the brain are shown in Table 9.2. As can be seen, the Lac peak can be almost ninefold higher than the

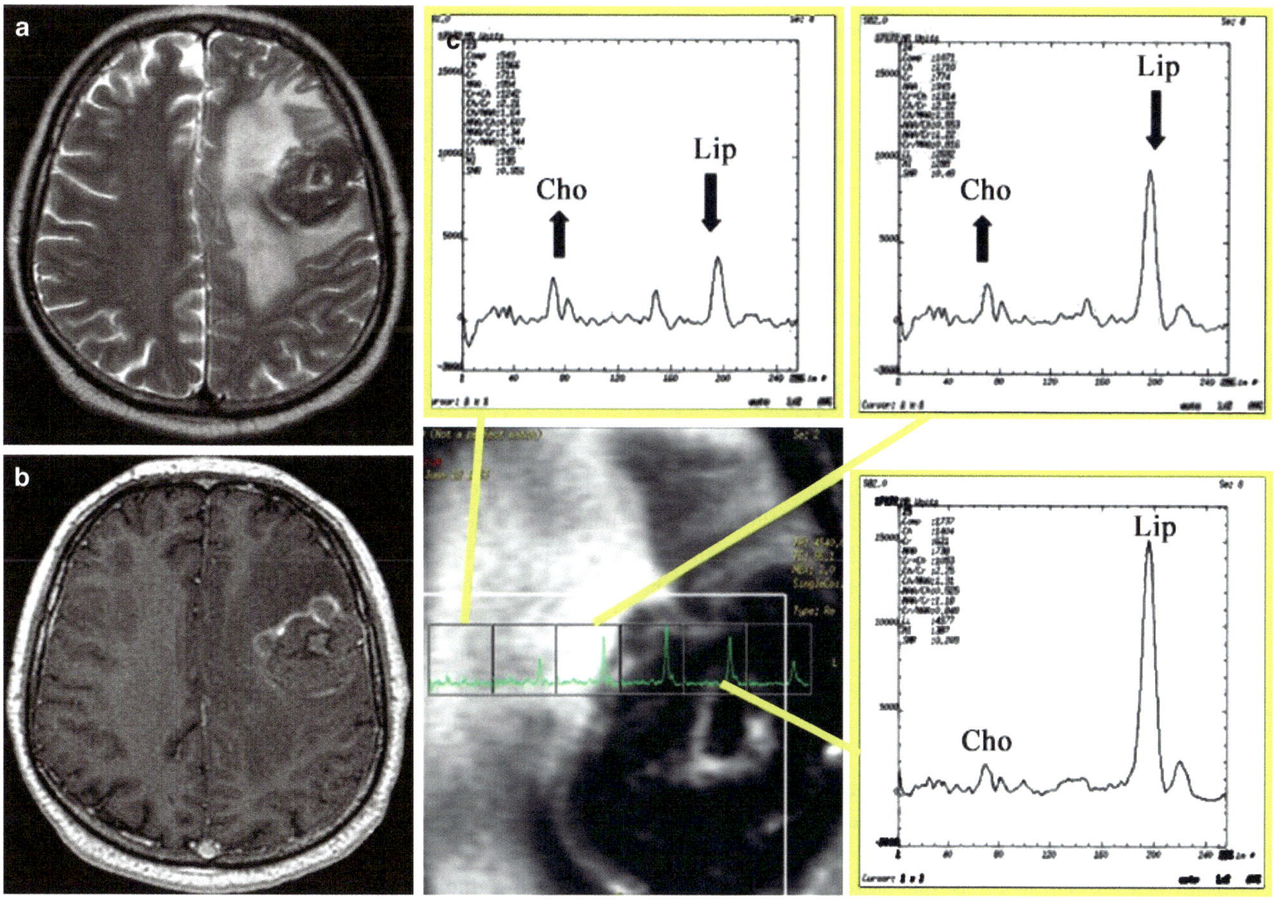

Fig. 9.31 A colorectal cancer metastasis in the left frontal region of the brain. On T2- (**a**) and T1-weighted contrast-enhanced MRI (**b**), a large lesion with a pronounced perifocal edema and the typical reduction in the T2-weighted signal are detected in the left frontal region. On MMRS (**d**), there is a pronounced Lip-Lac complex in the central portions of the lesion. In the perifocal area, there is a decrease in the Lip peak and occurrence of the Cho peak

Table 9.2 Mean values of metabolite ratios in proton magnetic resonance spectroscopy of metastases ($n = 78$)

Metabolite ratio	Cho/Cr	NAA/Cr	mI/Cr	Lac/Cr
Mean, standard deviation	2.82 ± 0.37	1.71 ± 0.37	1.47 ± 0.37	8.82 ± 1.47

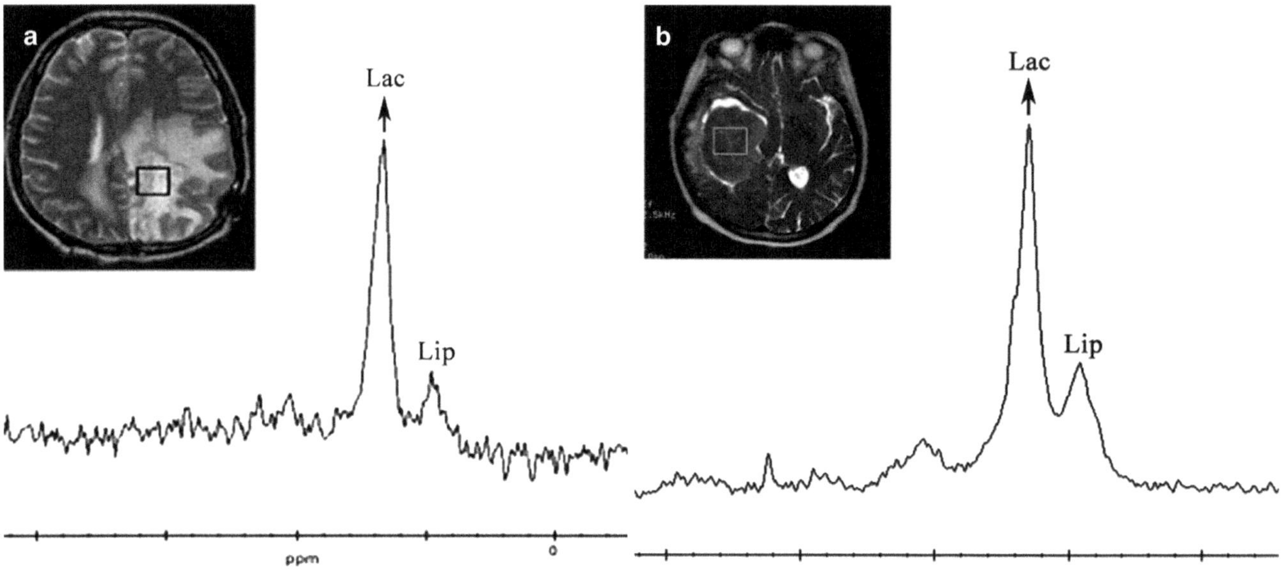

Fig. 9.32 MRI scan and the spectrum of the radiation necrosis area in the left parietal-occipital region (**a**) and a large solid metastasis of lung cancer in the right temporal region (**b**). The spectra show similar signs—a pronounced Lac and Lip peak—while peaks of other metabolites are not determined

creatine peak, while the choline peak is almost threefold higher than the creatine peak. The peaks of NAA and mI are not pronounced, and their height is slightly higher than that of the Cr peak.

MR spectroscopy showed no significant specificity for differentiation of metastatic brain lesions of various etiologies. Changes similar to PMR spectra in metastases were observed in glioblastoma and other tumors with necrotic decay (Fig. 9.32). Thus, the use of single-voxel PMRS does not allow to differentiate MTSs from malignant glial tumors as characteristics of single-voxel PMR spectra and images of both are similar in standard MR sequences.

9.6 Diffusion-Weighted MRI

A distinctive feature of MRI is the possibility to visualize not only the movement of blood through the capillary network but also thermal or Brownian motion of water molecules in the brain tissues. Diffusion is the basic physical process occurring in the metabolic cell reactions. Chaotic (Brownian) motion of molecules (thermal motion, speed of the order of 10^{-3} mm^2/s) ensures their kinetic energy. Phenomenologically, diffusion properties in an isotropic medium are characterized by Fick's law that relates the vector of molecule flow with their concentration gradient (Murase 2015). The diffusion coefficient D acts as a proportionality coefficient. The higher the diffusion coefficient, the faster the solution mixing. The higher the value of the diffusion coefficient, the greater the distance that the average molecule can move within the same time. The unit of measurement of the diffusion coefficient is mm^2/s—a circle area—where the molecule may be present for 1 s.

The movement of water molecules in living tissue occurs both within a single cell (restricted diffusion) and in the intracellular spaces among the structures that limit the movement of molecules, leaving some freedom for maneuvering between obstacles (free and hindered diffusion). In general, the magnitude of the diffusion coefficient depends on the composition and microstructure of the material in which water molecules diffuse. At body temperature, in a large volume of water (free diffusion) as compared to the size of a water molecule (2 nm), the diffusion coefficient is (2–2.5) × 10^{-3} mm^2/s. In real biological environment, the following natural barriers hinder free movement of protons: cell membranes and large protein molecules, which water molecules can encounter over time. Therefore, in practice, the actual value or apparent diffusion coefficient (ADC) is calculated, which is less than the magnitude of the diffusion coefficient for pure water at body temperature.

The first diffusion-weighted MR image was obtained in 1985 (Le Bihan and Breton 1985); however, DWI came in clinical practice with generation III MR scanners (Le Bihan et al. 1991). In order to obtain diffusion-weighted DWI MRI scans, modern scanners use echo planar pulse sequences "spin echo" with two additional diffusion gradients (DG) (before and after the 180-degree RF pulse). The first DG in SP adds a phase to precessing protons in the slice; the second one reads the changes since the precession direction changes after the 180-degree RF pulse. Phase changes in stationary protons in macromolecules, caused by the action of two DGs, are fully compensated by the time of data registration. The MR signal from these protons at the time of registration corresponds to the tissue T2 and is equal to the signal recorded in the same SP SE EPI in the absence of DG, i.e., when b = 0 s/mm^2. Protons involved in the diffusion motion of water molecules receive different phase addendums by action of two DGs, and, at the time of registration, the MR signal from them will be reduced in comparison to the MR signal of T2-weighted images. Regions of tissue with slow diffusion on DWI will look brighter than the regions of tissue with a high rate of diffusion movement. A marked decrease in the visual MR signal intensity occurs when the signal phase changes by two- to threefold.

When b = 500/mm^2, the diffusion of protons can be visually assessed with an average diffusion coefficient of 5.0 × 10^{-3} mm^2/s. For b = 1000 s/mm^2, the optimum conditions for measuring the MR signal reduction will be slower in diffusing protons with ADC of about 2.5 × 10^{-3} mm^2/s, i. e., almost as in water-free. Using even higher b values, the rate of diffusion movement in cell compartments can be estimated (Le Bihan and van Zijl 2002). In our studies, we used the value of the diffusion factor = 1000 s/mm^2. As a result of each DW MRI study, a series of T2-weighted MRIs (without DG) and several series of T2- and diffusion coefficient-weighted MRIs are obtained (Basser and Pierpaoli 1998; Pronin et al. 2000). The extent of weighing by the diffusion rate is determined by the value of a so-called diffusion factor—b—that is dependent on the DG duration and the time delay between the two:

$$b = \gamma^{2*} G^{2*} \delta^{2*} \left(\Delta - \delta / 3\right), \tag{9.1}$$

where γ is the gyromagnetic ratio, Gisthe amplitude of the diffusion gradient, δ is the length of each diffusion gradient, Δ is the interval between the two diffusion gradients.

The unit of measurement for b is s/mm^2. The b value is a parameter of the DWI pulse sequence protocol. The MRI signal value depends on the direction along which DG acts. In diffusion MRI, for each DG direction, the first measurement is performed without DG, i.e., for b = 0 s/mm^2 (A), and with DG, for b = (500–7000) s/mm^2. In this case, DW MRI measures the MR signal, whose intensity is dependent on T2 in the tissue –$S(0)$ and simultaneously on T2 and the speed of diffusion of water molecules along the movement direction of the diffusion gradients $S(b)$. Taking the logarithm of the measured MR signals, the value of the diffusion coefficient can be obtained directly along the DG direction:

$$\ln S\left(b\right) = \ln S\left(0\right) - bD. \tag{9.2}$$

For biological tissues, $S(b)$ is typically measured for three directions of DG action (R-L, A-P, S-I), and the diffusion coefficient values calculated using three equations are averaged (summed up and divided by 3). This average value of the diffusion coefficient in the standard DW MRI is called an apparent diffusion coefficient (ADC). Thus, the standard DW MRI allows to calculate for each voxel the average diffusion coefficient for three directions, i.e., to map ADC. Using the map of the average diffusion coefficient or ADC, the ADC in the region of interest is measured (Fig. 9.33).

Based on the feasibility of using DWI in the differential diagnosis of cerebral metastases, we sought to identify those areas of the tumor that would have a marked qualitative difference and allowed to differentiate the metastases from primary brain tumors. For example, it is known that cells of glial tumors diffusely grow into the normal brain tissue, in contrast to metastases that normally grow expansively and only mechanically affect the brain tissue. Therefore, in all studies performed, we focused not on the features of the tumor stroma diffusion but on the area adjacent to the edge of the abnormal lesion (the edema region not accumulating the contrast agent).

Figure 9.34 shows the regions of study of the diffusion coefficient with factor b = 1000, the central area of necrotic changes, the area of contrast agent accumulation, the edema area directly adjacent to the tumor, and the vasogenic edema area and contralateral (symmetrical) side of the brain.

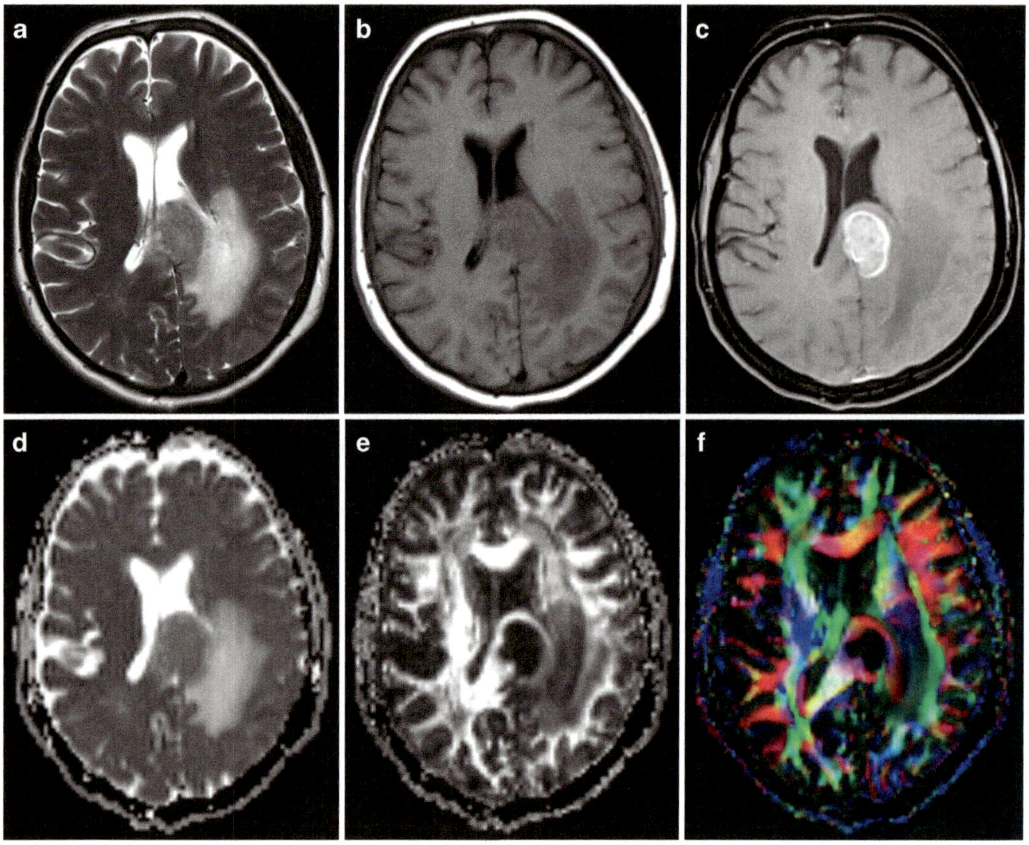

Fig. 9.33 A metastasis of colorectal cancer. On T2-weighted (**a**), T1-weighted (**b**), and T1-weighted contrast-enhanced (**c**) MRI, there is an oval-shaped space-occupying lesion with a pronounced perifocal edema and intense accumulation of contrast agent in the posterior segments of the corpus callosum. Parametric diffusion maps: ADC or average diffusion coefficient (**d**), the fractional anisotropy map (**e**), and the color structural anisotropy map (**f**) show a deformation of the tracts of the corpus callosum

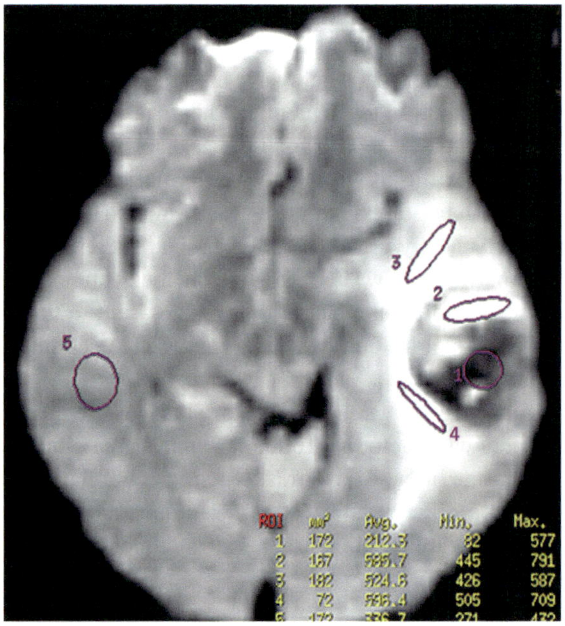

Fig. 9.34 Regions of interest ADC in DWI images of metastases in the brain. (1), the central area of necrosis; (2), the area of the contrast agent accumulation; (3), the vasogenic edema area; (4) the edema area, directly adjacent to the tumor; and (5), the contralateral (symmetrical) side of the brain

Table 9.3 Average values of DWI MRI in brain metastases (ADC × 10^{-3} mm²/s)

Region of study	Tumor stroma	The nearest peritumoral area	Vasogenic edema area
Obtained ADC values (in 10^{-3} mm²/s)	1.15 ± 0.2	1.37 ± 0.2	1.56 ± 0.2

On diffusion MRI, metastatic tumors are characterized by heterogeneous changes on DWI and ADC maps. Solid lesions usually have an increased and homogeneous MR signal on DWI, and ADC values are significantly lower than those for glial tumors. Table 9.3 shows the results of measuring ADC in the stroma of metastases in the near peritumoral area and in the area of vasogenic edema. Metastases, unlike glial tumors, have a lower DWI signal in the edema area, which is likely due to the denser structure of the brain tissue and less free movement of water molecules in the edema area around the primary tumor site.

In case of hemorrhagic inclusions in the metastatic lesion, the intensity of the MR signal may increase from iso-hyperintense to hyperintense (in our material—27% and 9%, respectively), Fig. 9.35.

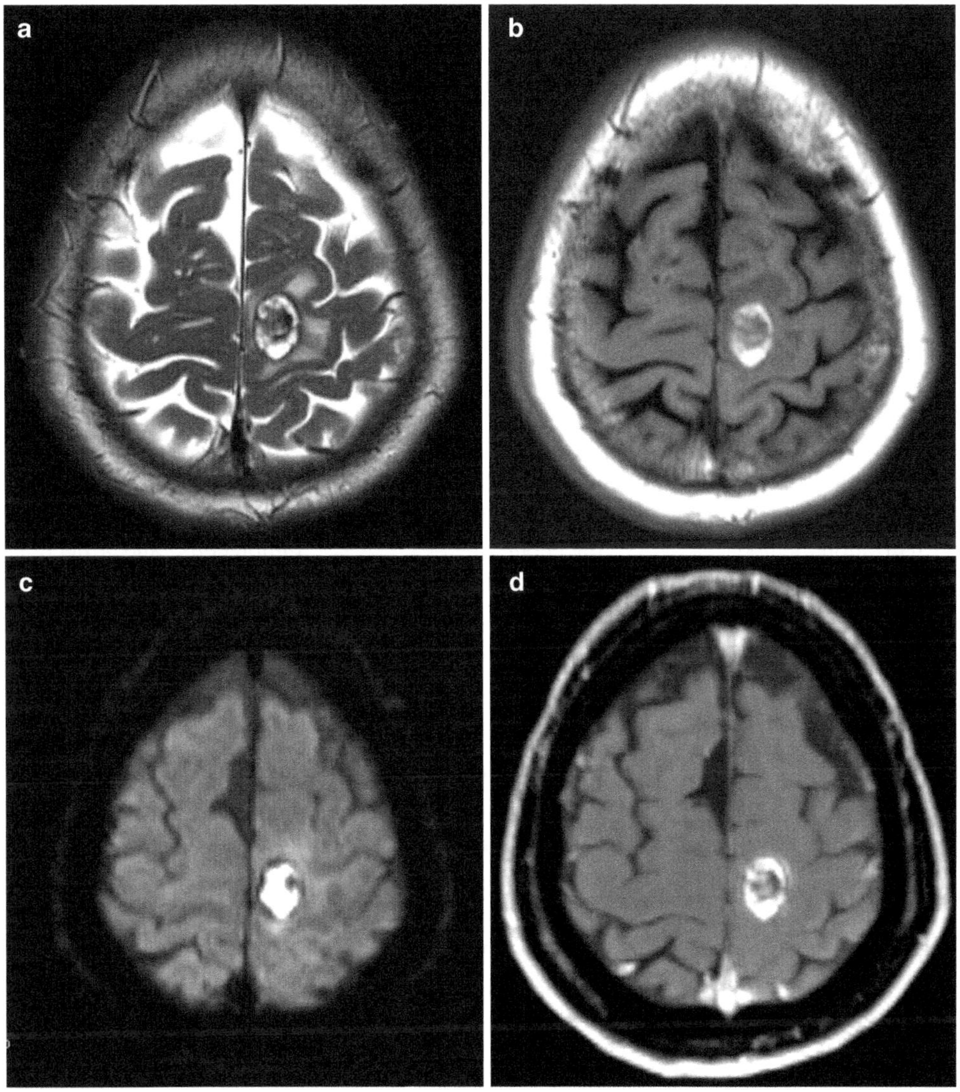

Fig. 9.35 A lung cancer metastasis in the brain. On MRI, there is an oval-shaped space-occupying lesion with signs of mild perifocal edema in the left frontal region. On T2-weighted MRI (**a**), the tumor is heterogeneous with hypo- and hyperintense inclusions. On T1-weighted (**b**) and DWI (**c**) MRI, the signal from the formation is primarily increased due to a hemorrhagic content. After the administration of contrast agent in T1-fat sat sequence, its fragmentary accumulation along the medial contour of the tumor (**d**) is observed

In such a situation, it is impossible to differentiate the metastases based on DW MRI.

Further information can be obtained by diffusion tensor MRI (Lu et al. 2003). The authors noted the difference in the diffusion values in the area of perifocal edema, suggesting a different degree of diffusion of extracellular water molecules and probably of various degrees of infiltration of the surrounding tissues by tumor cells. In addition, the expansive growth of metastases results in a displacement (dislocation) of adjacent white matter tracts, while in glioma they undergo destruction.

9.7 Diffusion Tensor MRI (DT MRI)

The dependence of the diffusion speed on the direction is called *diffusion anisotropy*. Water molecules in the white matter of the brain easily diffuse along the nerve fibers, but their movement across the fibers is limited by an impermeable myelin sheath. In order to visualize the anisotropy of water diffusion in the tissue, diffusion tensor MRI is used. The mathematical apparatus of tensors is used to describe the diffusion properties that change with the direction.

Diffusion isotropy means that the diffusion motion of molecules does not depend on the orientation of the medium and the molecule does not go beyond the sphere with radius D, where $D = (D_{xx} + D_{yy} + D_{zz})/3 = \mathrm{ADC}$, during the observation.

Diffusion anisotropy suggests that due to the orientation of the elements of the medium during the observation, the molecule does not go beyond the boundaries of the "diffusion ellipsoid" with semiaxes.

The degree of "organization" of the conductive tracts into a single tract is assessed using anisotropy factors or indices, for example, by a fractional anisotropy ratio—FA (Basser and Pierpaoli 1996; Pronin et al. 2011; Zakharova et al. 2013). The values of anisotropy coefficients or indices range from 0 to 1.

On the maps of fractional anisotropy, the diffusion pixel brightness corresponds to FA. FA values allow for color coding and codirectional diffusion movement of water molecules, wherein the preferential direction of the movement in each pixel of a slice corresponds to the direction of the eigenvector of diffusion tensor: red, on the *x*-axis; green, on the *y*-axis; and blue, on the *z*-axis.

Diffusion tensor MRI is the means for detection of structural links between the brain regions, which is especially important to establish in space-occupying processes and diseases that distort the anatomic structure or destruct the white matter. The movement of water molecules along axons can be shown as a line connecting the eigenvectors of individual voxels, which corresponds to the nerve fibers. There are different algorithms for constructing paths, varying from a simple regression algorithm (FACT) to quite complex ones (HARDY, Q-ball). However, they allow to "draw" the course of a plurality of nerve fibers that make up the nerve tract. Therefore, tensor MRI is often referred to as tractography, a visualization method of the nerve tract course.

Simple algorithms of tractography well draw single large tracts, for example, the corticospinal tract, and do not require a large number of different DG directions during the data registration (minimum—six directions). More sophisticated algorithms allow to track the area of a tract intersection or branch points, but, for this, the diffusion data for a large number of DG directions and higher values of the diffusion factor should be obtained in order to achieve a high angular resolution of directions (60–200 and above). In clinical practice, a relatively simple algorithm FACT (fiber assignment by continuous tracking) is commonly used. The data acquisition time for tractography in this case is 3–5 min.

All diffusion studies are conducted without the administration of a contrast agent, which is important for critically ill patients. DW and DT MRI provides additional qualitative (visualization) and quantitative tissue characteristics that assess the extent of the damage to the gray and white matter in disease (diffusion coefficients and anisotropy).

The specifics of structural organization of some brain tumors, in particular, meningiomas, schwannomas, and gliomas, allow to predict with a high degree of confidence a histological type of a tumor even before the surgery by using diffusion-weighted images (Moritani et al. 2004; Kornienko and Pronin 2008a, b, 2010). Figure 9.36 shows a large metastasis of breast cancer with the cystic structure and a mild perifocal edema. Tractography visualizes a significant dislocation of the conductive tracts by the lesion.

When brain metastases are detected, it is important to establish their primary source. Positron emission tomography (PET) identifies metastatic lesions by accumulation of radiopharmaceuticals (RP) in them and allows to construct a three-dimensional model of the radiopharmaceutical distribution in the body. Studies by Takahara et al. (2004) showed that DWI MRI allows to construct a 3D model of distribution of areas with an increased cell density for the whole body, similar to that in PET.

9.8 Whole-Body DWI MRI

In order to perform the whole-body DW, Takahara et al. (2004) added the echo planar pulse sequence for DWI and a complex of radio-frequency pulses to suppress the signal from fat—STIR. This method is called whole-body diffusion-weighted MRI with suppression of the background signal (DWIBS). Malignant tumors are known to have higher metabolic parameters, a compact structure of tumor cells, and a decreased volume of the intercellular space (Koh and Collins 2007). This allows to visualize the tumor structure on the background of unaffected tissues on the whole-body DWI MRI (Guo et al. 2002; Yamasaki et al. 2005; Nemeth et al. 2007). This study is carried out using a spinal multichannel coil. The data registration time is 430 s with obtaining 80 axial 4 mm slices with a 1 cm overlapping. The obtained axial DW MRI simultaneously weighted by diffusion and T2 are processed on a workstation using a multiplanar reconstruction algorithm (MPR or REFORMAT) with the inverted shades of gray scale. As a result, a three-dimensional model is constructed, similar to the one obtained by PET (Fig. 9.37). Figure 9.38 shows the results of PET and whole-body DW MRI studies of a patient with peripheral lung cancer. The projection of the upper lobe of the left lung on PET shows an increased signal area (arrow A); in addition, the central sections of the right lung additionally contain a pinpoint region with similar signal intensity (arrow B). The whole-body DWI in similar planes (D, E, F) detects a large tumor with an increased signal in the right lung, similar to the lesion intensely accumulating RP. In addition, the whole-body DWI body identified multiple affected paratracheal lymph nodes.

Noninvasiveness and minimal time to obtain DWI are an advantage of whole-body DW MRI in the diagnosis of the primary source of metastatic brain lesions. Along with whole-body DW MRI, the study protocol includes obtaining T1- and T2-weighted MRI of the "region of interest" to clarify the origin of findings, although, in fact, the purpose of the study is not so much an accurate histological diagnosis, as the determination of "targeted" abnormal sites to facilitate a subsequent tumor search and disease verification.

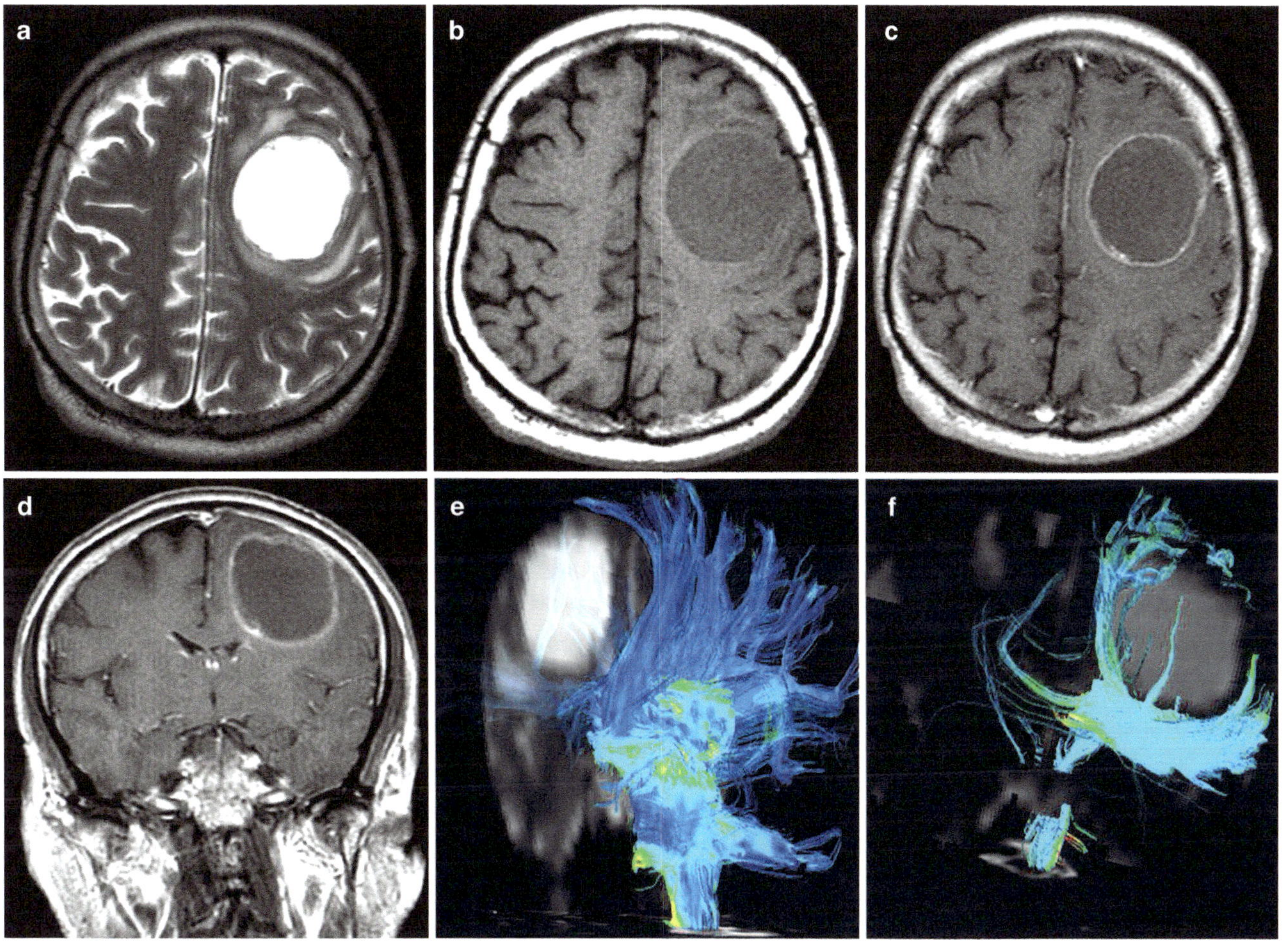

Fig. 9.36 A breast cancer metastasis in the brain. In the left frontal region, there is a large cystic lesion with an increased signal on T2-weighted MRI (**a**). Noteworthy is a mild edema on the background of the large tumor. On T1-weighted MRI before the administration of contrast agent (**b**), the lesion is homogeneous and hypointense, while after the administration of contrast agent (**c**, **d**), there is a thin rim of its intense accumulation. The MR tractography (**e**, **f**) shows a severe dislocation of the tracts

The methods aimed to investigate the internal organs and body structures, such as ultrasound and X-rays, do not give an overall picture of the "whole body." This picture can be obtained by MRI and nuclear medicine: scintigraphy, SPECT, and PET. It is generally accepted that PET with ^{18}F-FDG is the gold standard in the evaluation of tumor dissemination, but these studies cause an ionization burden and their cost is quite high. Therefore, there is a constant search of alternative diagnostic methods that could be referred to as screening methods. Whole-body DWI studies are called PET simulation or PET-like images as whole-body DW MRI results are similar to those in radiologic diagnosis, including PET (Fig. 9.38). The patient with Hodgkin's lymphoma on an osteogram has lesions with an increased RP accumulation in the thoracic vertebrae and rib IX on the right on PET with ^{18}F-NaF (sodium fluoride), and additional lesions are visualized in the pelvis and the spinous process of vertebrae L1 and rib 2 on the right. On PET with ^{18}F-FDG, tumor lesions are visualized in the mediastinum; these are also seen on DWI. Thus, whole-body DW MRI allows to suspect a space-occupying lesion in the upper lobe of the left lung, similar to PET with ^{18}F-FDG.

The size, shape, and number of lesions on MRI and PET are generally not identical, differing in the direction of both an increase and a decrease. A decrease in the size of lesions may be associated with chest excursions during respiration and a partial loss of changes on MRI. An increase in high-signal areas on whole-body DW MRI may be affected by a

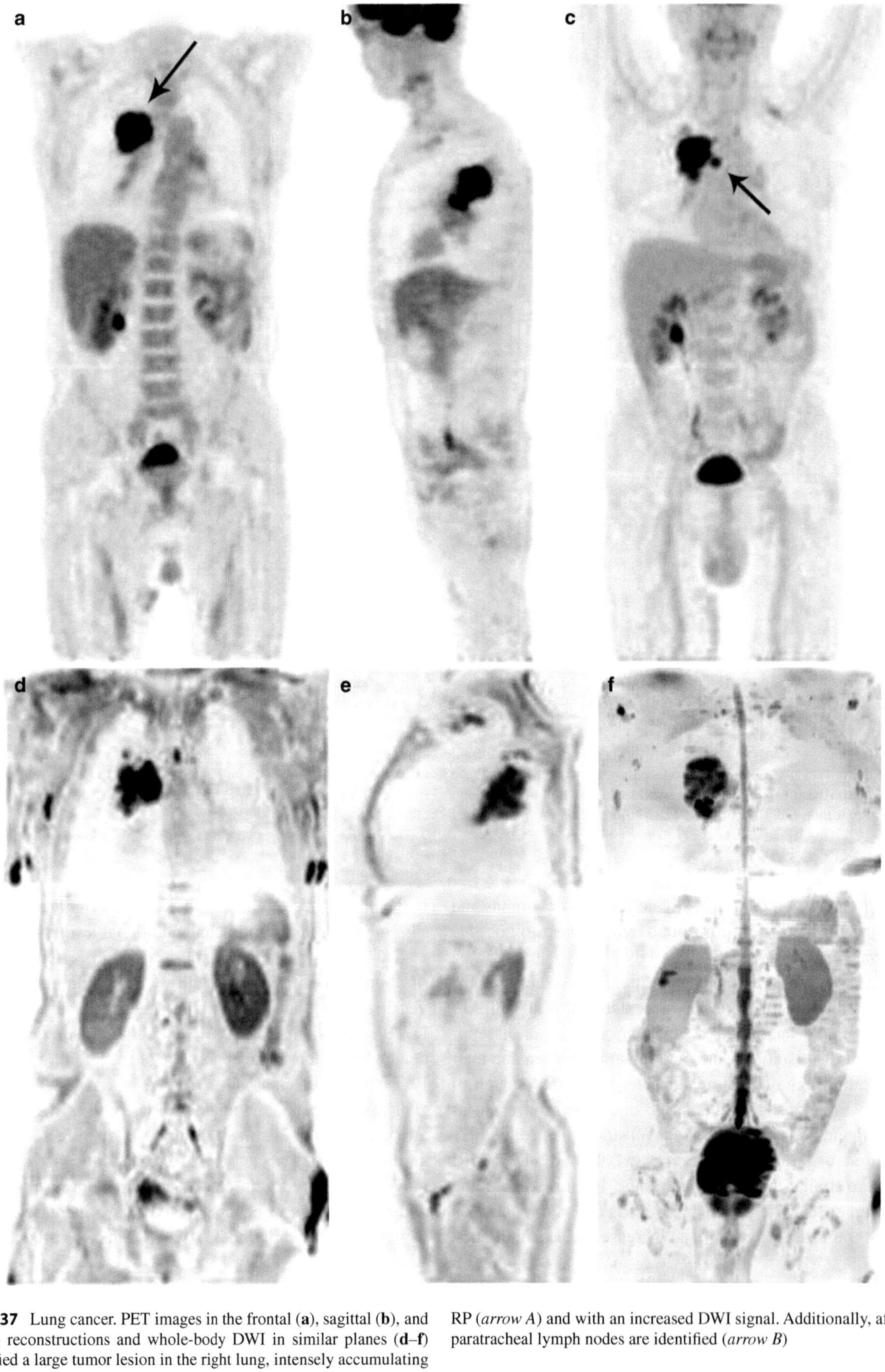

Fig. 9.37 Lung cancer. PET images in the frontal (**a**), sagittal (**b**), and 3D (**c**) reconstructions and whole-body DWI in similar planes (**d**–**f**) identified a large tumor lesion in the right lung, intensely accumulating RP (*arrow A*) and with an increased DWI signal. Additionally, affected paratracheal lymph nodes are identified (*arrow B*)

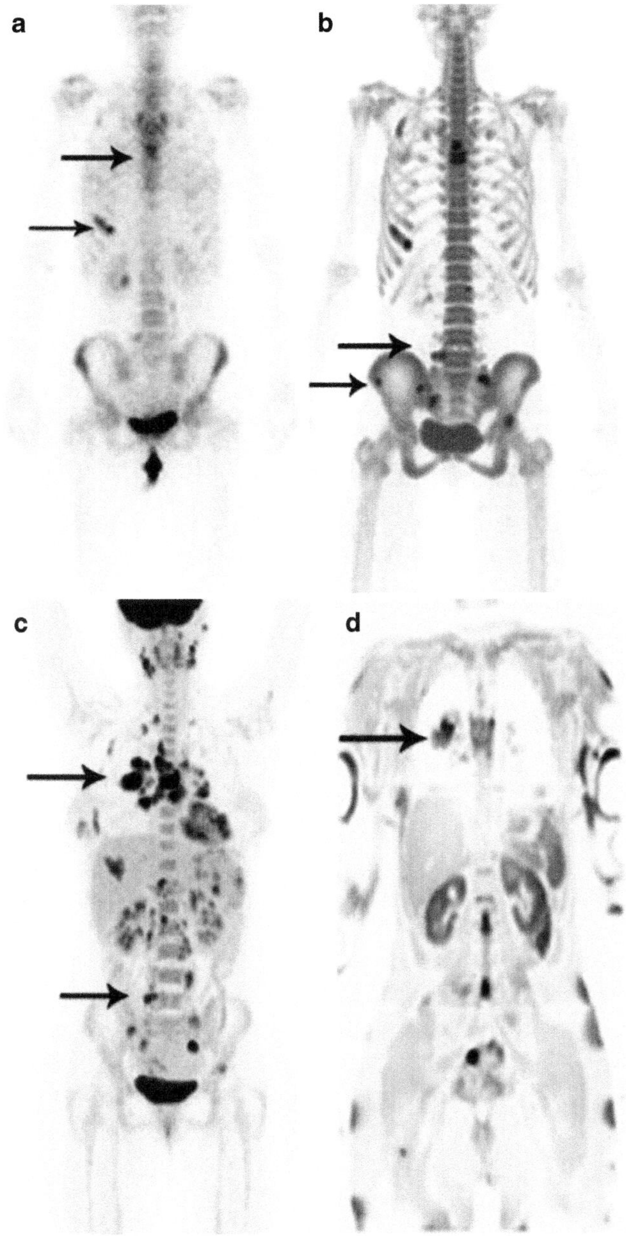

Fig. 9.38 Hodgkin's lymphoma. A bone scan (**a**), PET with ^{18}F-NaF (**b**), ^{18}F-FDG (**c**), and whole-body DWI MRI (**d**) of a Hodgkin's lymphoma patient with multiple lesions in the bones. On the osteogram, there are lesions with an increased RP accumulation in the thoracic vertebrae and rib IX on the right on PET with ^{18}F-NaF, and additional lesions are visualized in the pelvis and the spinous process of vertebrae L1 and rib 2 on the right. On PET with ^{18}F-FDG (**c**), tumor lesions are visualized in the mediastinum that are also determined on DWI (**c**)

perifocal edema, atelectasis, the presence of cysts, and hemorrhages in the lesion stroma. However, DW MRI is performed without CA and without breath holding. The study duration is 10–15 min.

Using standard flexible coils for a study of the body allows, if necessary, to investigate the "region of interest" on standard T1- or T2-weighted MRI for verifying the origin of abnormalities.

In general, the analysis of our own material has shown that, in order to adequately assess abnormalities on whole-body DWI MRI, a number of features of this technology should be taken into account. Thus, it is possible to wrongly interpret a visualized fluid accumulation in the intestine and peritoneal "pouches" of the abdominal cavity, perineural spaces along the exit of the roots from the intervertebral foramen, ureters, filled bladder, and stomach contents. Postoperative changes, such as "fresh" scars, blood congestion, edema of the postoperative area, and exudative pleurisy, also cause an increase in the signal on DWI MRI. These findings can be misinterpreted as metastases. In our study, in 24% of cases, in addition to the above changes, false-positive results were also observed in the form of hyperintense areas in the projection of the axillary and inguinal lymph nodes (manifestations of non-tumor hyperplasia) and venous structures (a slow blood flow in the valve area).

The main issue in the study of the internal organs using any method is artifacts from the physiological movements (breathing, peristalsis, heartbeat, blood flow). Standard MR sequences are most sensitive to such artifacts; in addition, they require duplicate scanning with contrast enhancement. At the same time, they are considered to be the most informative in assessing the tissue characteristics. DWI MRI does not provide the same quality of the anatomical picture that may be obtained in standard CT and MR studies; however, this method can visualize the movement of water molecules at the cellular level. Thus, the DWI method allows for visualization of the tissue with a high water content, characterized by a high ADC. As with PET, DW MRI of the body evaluates molecular changes in the affected tissues.

One of the advantages of this method is the ability to track changes over time and quickly change the treatment strategy and combining scans of the brain and whole body. In view of the time and cost of the study, the whole-body DWI MRI can be regarded as a screening method.

10 Positron Emission Tomography (PET)

A distinctive feature of radionuclide methods, including positron emission tomography (PET), is their initial focus on a visual and quantitative assessment of biological processes within the cell (Shinoura et al. 1997; Chen 2007; Kumar et al. 2010; Granov and Tiutin 2013). Thus, if MR or CT perfusion indirectly suggests a degree of malignancy or viability of the tumor tissue by its structural characteristics or hemodynamic parameters, PET with ^{18}F-choline, for example, estimates the intensity of the formation of cell membranes, including endothelial cells, long before the formation of the abnormal vasculature. An assessment of biochemical processes in the brain is of particular interest both in the differential diagnosis of intracranial tumors and in the differentiation of therapy-induced residual tumor necrosis and edema (Dolgushin 2008). Important is the fact that, in PET studies, a metal or other foreign bodies do not give artifacts in images, in contrast to CT or MRI, and their presence in patients is not a contraindication for the study.

Positron emission tomography (PET) using a variety of radiopharmaceuticals (RP) provides unique information about the functional state of tumors by a number of biological processes, such as glucose metabolism, protein/DNA synthesis, rate of cell membrane synthesis, angiogenesis, hypoxia, etc. (Weidner 1995; Hara et al. 1997). The first PET studies with ^{18}F-FDG were conducted on the brain and were directed to the study of functional disorders in dementia, epilepsy, Parkinson's disease, and Alzheimer's disease. However, the use of PET with ^{18}F-FDG in brain tumors is limited because of the intense physiological accumulation of the drug in the gray matter. The isotopes that emit positrons generally have expressed specific radioactivity, and, as a rule, only a small amount of RP is needed to obtain the necessary information. The relatively short half-life of the isotopes used in PET helps reduce the radiation dose and allows for repeated measurements at short intervals. Due to the specifics of the primary diagnosis of brain tumors, PET with ^{18}F-FDG is inefficient as compared to MRI. However, ^{18}F-FDG helps visualize tumors with high metabolic activity, such as metastases, glioblastoma, some types of meningiomas, and gray matter lesions, resulting in a decrease in metabolic activity. A simultaneous scanning of the "whole body" and brain with ^{18}F-FDG PET significantly reduces the information value of the study because of the high background RP accumulation in the brain deteriorating the relative contrast of extracranial lesions. This is why the so-called "whole-body" study with ^{18}F-FDG is limited to the level of the skull base.

PET diagnosis identifies tissues by varying degrees of glucose consumption. Since most tumors have a higher metabolism than intact tissues and the glucose consumption by the tumor tissue is higher, PET images display areas of abnormally high tissue metabolism. On the scans, there are foci with increased accumulation of glucose labeled with the isotope ^{18}F. The detection of increased accumulation areas on the background of areas with the normal RP accumulation indicates an increase in metabolic processes in this area, which may be caused by a tumor, inflammation, etc. An area with enhanced metabolism allows to judge with high reliability about the presence and extent of a tumor. In addition to determining the extent of the tumor process and the early detection of its manifestations due to progression, evaluating the effectiveness of cancer treatment, diagnosis of iatrogenic (postoperative) damage, and post-radiation scarring, PET is effective in the differential diagnosis of malignant tumors from benign tumors and non-tumor diseases.

10.1 Radiopharmaceuticals (RP) for PET and the PET Facility Structure

Obtaining RP is a knowledge-intensive, technologically complex, and expensive procedure, which is carried out in specialized laboratory units. The main machines for the production of radionuclides for nuclear medicine are nuclear reactors, radionuclide generators, and particle accelerators (typically cyclotrons). The reactor method is the most common in the preparation of radiopharmaceuticals for

M. Dolgushin et al., *Brain Metastases*, DOI 10.1007/978-3-319-57760-9_10

scintigraphy and SPECT, but it does not allow to produce a number of important PET radioisotopes. Production of isotopes for PET is carried out in a cyclotron by "bombing" the target with accelerated charged particles.

A PET facility must include cyclotron radiochemical complex for production of radionuclides and radiopharmaceuticals, a positron emission tomography machine (with an experimental laboratory), and workstations for processing the information obtained from the PET study. Figure 10.1 shows an external view of a horizontal cyclotron and a laboratory for synthesis of radiopharmaceuticals and quality control.

The cyclotron accelerates charged particles (protons, deuterons) H/D to an energy of 18 MeV (protons)/9 MeV (deuterons), after which the accelerated particles bombard the target material. The beam energy is one of the key parameters of an accelerator, since with its increase the possibility to obtain a larger number of radionuclides occurs. For routine production of medical radionuclides, a beam energy of the order of several tens of MeV is sufficient. For producing ^{18}F, the N.N. Blokhin Russian Cancer Research Center uses a cyclotron *Cyclone 18/9* (IBA, Belgium) with a beam energy of 18 MeV for protons and 9 MeV for deuterons. Another important indicator for producing radionuclides is a beam current: the higher it is, the more intense is the production. For a mid-sized target (MV) with the volume of 1.2 ml, a working current value is 25 mA; for larger (XXL) volume of about 3.0 ml, it is as high as 80 μA. In order to prevent possible accidents, there is a safety system provided in the cyclotron, since the excess of the permissible value of the current during irradiation can cause a failure of the entire target.

Isotopes of chemical elements presented in live biological samples in large amounts are used as the target substance, water-enriched isotope ^{18}O, nitrogen gas N^2, natural water H_2Or, and gas xenon ^{124}Xe, as well as solids tellurium ^{124}Te, thallium ^{203}TI, zinc ^{68}Zn, cadmium ^{112}Cd, etc., which may substitute stable isotopes, normally available in biological molecules, without altering their physiological properties. As a result of the bombardment and nuclear reactions (p, n), radionuclides F-^{18}, C-^{11}, N-^{13}, I-^{123}, TI-^{201}, Ga-^{67}, and In-^{111} are formed and used subsequently to label radiopharmaceuticals (RP) administered to a patient in the PET study. An example of a chemical analogue may be ^{18}F-fluorodeoxyglucose (FDG), in which hydrogen in glucose is replaced by isotope ^{18}F.

An example of a natural substrate is water labeled with ^{15}O ($H_2{}^{15}O$). Properties of chemical ligands that bind to ions of a radioactive isotope provide a high accumulation of RP in the studied organ with a minimal accumulation in other tissues. The main factors affecting the biodistribution of radiopharmaceuticals (RP) include a strong binding to blood proteins (e.g., to HSA), lipophilicity, and ionizing properties of (since lipophilic and nonionic compounds are involved in the rapid membrane transport), as well as the type of elimination (preferably excretion via the liver and kidneys).

Table 10.1 lists some of radiopharmaceuticals used in PET and presents their basic properties.

^{18}F-FDG has one of the longest half-life and a wide range of applications, so it is most commonly used in PET studies. In oncology, a number of radiopharmaceuticals based on ^{18}F are used to assess various aspects of tumor metabolism.

Although radionuclide ^{18}F produced by a cyclotron is radioactive, it exhibits the same properties as the stable isotope of fluorine (^{19}F). The technological process of RP synthesis involves a minimum number of steps and processes to reduce the synthesis time, which in turn can significantly increase the yield of the radiopharmaceutical, given a short half-life of ^{18}F (less than 110 min). The synthesis process is carried out in an automatic mode on the compact synthesis modules allowing to perform multistep chemical processes (Fig. 10.2). The automated synthesis modules are arranged in special airtight boxes designed to work with the activities of 15 Ci for ^{18}F and supporting "B" class of cleanliness inside. Facilities for synthesis and packaging of radiopharmaceuticals are equipped with a special system of supply and exhaust ventilation, ensuring a pressure drop that supports the purity class "C" at the premises and gateways and class "B" in microbiological laboratories. The process of synthesis starts with the preparation of all raw materials by an engineer radiochemist. Before starting the procedure, the engineer radiochemist collects all the necessary materials and reagents in the warehouse and delivers them to the preparatory synthesis

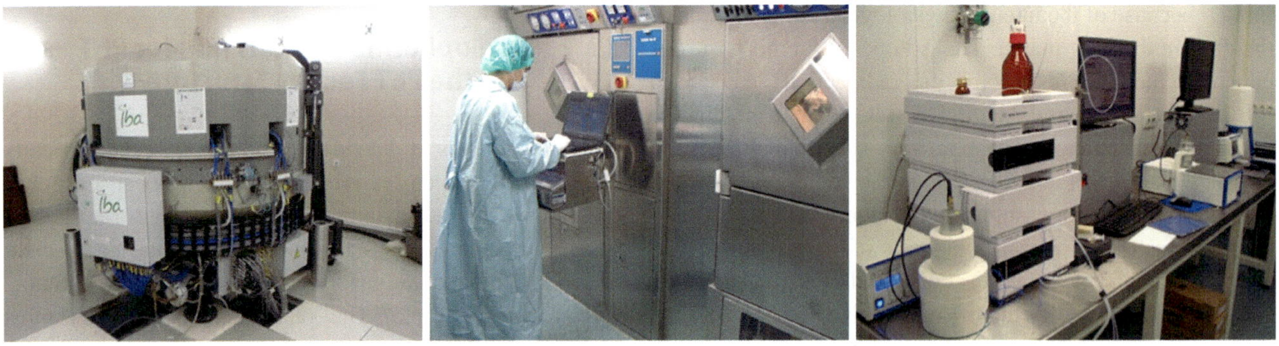

Fig. 10.1 From left to right: an open horizontal cyclotron, radiopharmaceutical synthesis laboratory, and RP quality control laboratory

Table 10.1 Examples of the most commonly used radiopharmaceuticals and their properties

Radioisotope	Half-life	Predecessor	RP	Application
F-18	109.7 min	[^{18}F]Fluoride nucleophilic substitution	[^{18}F] FDG fluorodeoxyglucose	GLA metabolism
			[^{18}F] FTHA fluorine-substituted fatty acids	β-oxidation
			[^{18}F]-misonidazole	Hypoxia
			[^{18}F] *N*-metilspiperon	D_2 receptors
			16α-[^{18}F]-fluoroestradiol	Breast cancers
			[^{18}F]-fluorocholine	Prostate cancer and its metastases; brain tumors
			[^{18}F]-thymidine	Proliferative activity rate
		[^{18}F]F_2 electrophilic substitution	6-[^{18}F]-fluoro-L-dopa	Dopaminergic function
			2-[^{18}F]-fluoro-L-*m*-tyrosine	Protein synthesis, amino acid transport
			5-[^{18}F]-fluorouracil	Tumor treatment control
C-11	20.38 min	[^{11}C] CH_3I (methyl iodide)	[^{11}C]-methionine	Protein synthesis, brain tumors
			[^{11}C] methoxy-ephedrine	Adrenergic innervation of the heart
			[^{11}C]raclopride	D_2 receptors
			[*N*-methyl-^{11}C]flumazenil	Benzodiazepine receptors
		[^{11}C] CO_2	[^{11}C]acetate	Consumption of O_2 by myocardium
			[^{11}C]palmitic acid	β-oxidation
N-13	9.96 min	[^{13} N]NH_3	[^{13}N]NH_3	Regulation of cardiac and cerebral blood flow

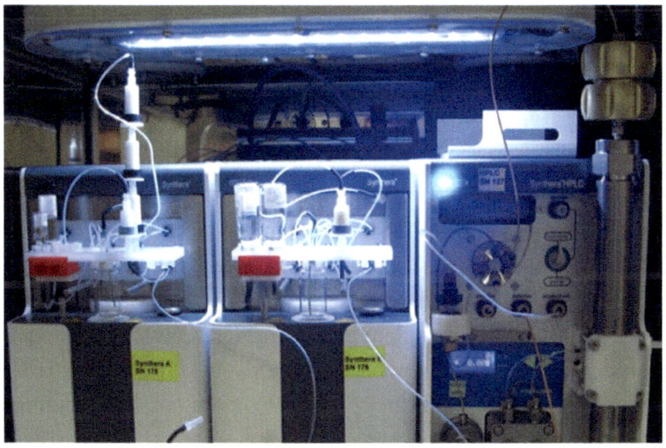

Fig. 10.2 The latest generation of synthesis modules: *IBA SynthERA II* (*left* and *center*), *SynthERA HPLC* module (*right*)—a HPLC system

room through an active pass-through window. The preparation for synthesis involves assembling a disposable fluid processor and preliminary testing. Before this, the functional activation of disposable columns is performed, required for the separation of ^{18}F from enriched water, conducting chemical reactions, as well as purification of synthesized radiopharmaceuticals from by-products and impurities.

The synthesis time depends on the type of the radiopharmaceutical synthesized and can range from 15 (for sodium fluoride) to 70 min (for fluoroethyl tyrosine). Upon completion of the synthesis, the synthesized radiopharmaceutical is automatically transmitted to the dispensing module, located in the same room. The dispensing module is an automated robotic system (*Theodorico* with an autoclave option). The radiopharmaceutical is dispensed into open vials in a sterile laminar airflow. Due to a multistage filtration system of the supplied air, the cleanliness class A is achieved in the chamber. The radiopharmaceutical can be dispensed both into sterile glass vials and sterile syringes. Dispensing is performed using sets of disposable sterile lines, vessels, and 220 nm filters used to filter radiopharmaceuticals. The first prefilled vial from each batch of the radiopharmaceutical in a protective container is transferred to the quality control laboratory. The vial is opened in a fume hood with a lead shielding; samples are taken in compliance with all the required procedures. RP is tested with respect to the following parameters: radiochemical purity, chemical purity, radionuclide purity, half-life, osmotic pressure and pH, endotoxin test, and sterility of the product (testing is performed by a random selection method a few times a month). After quality control, the radiopharmaceutical safety data sheet is issued. One vial is a retain sample and shall be kept for 3 years. The remaining vials with the radiopharmaceutical together with the safety data sheet that guarantees the safety of the produced batch are transferred to the procedural space of the PET unit.

During a PET study, the radiopharmaceutical is injected into the cubital vein, and the drug enters the tumor with the bloodstream, where it is selectively absorbed. Decomposing, the radiopharmaceutical emits a positron that, in a collision with an electron of the tissue (annihilation), generates two photons with an energy of 511 MeV, flying in the opposite directions. Such photons are called annihilation quanta. These photons are recorded by a multiple ring system of the PET scanner detectors. The computer calculates the coordinates of an area with a high frequency of annihilations, i.e., the areas of RP accumulation, and the reconstruction algorithm builds an isotope image of the tumor. In other words, the method is based on identification of areas with radiopharmaceutical accumulation specific for consumption of, for example, glucose. Since the metabolism of most tumors is more "aggressive" than that of normal tissue, therefore, the consumption of glucose and other metabolites is higher. Thus, images visualize lesions with increased tissue metabolism.

Performing PET with different, highly specific radiopharmaceuticals, "tropic" to certain types of tumors, provides valuable information about the state of metabolism in tumor lesions. This also allows for a semiquantitative estimate of metabolism by calculating the standard level of the radiopharmaceutical uptake (*standard uptake value* (*SUV*)), which is the ratio of the RP radioactivity in the region of interest (Bq/g) to the introduced activity of the radiopharmaceutical (Bq) per unit of patient's body weight (Strauss and Conti 1991).

The issues of anatomical spatial visualization in radionuclide studies have been solved by the creation of a combined *PET/CT* system (and subsequently PET/MRI systems). The advantages of such diagnostic systems are obvious: regions of functional disorders identified by radionuclide imaging with spatial resolution of 5–7 mm are localized with the maximum accuracy based on anatomical references on the tomographic slices with the spatial resolution of 0.5 mm (Khmelev 2016). Possibilities of hybrid PET/CT or PET/MRI systems are not limited to spatial coregistration of PET and CT/MRI images, including 3D reconstruction of bone structures or the major arteries, but allow to investigate in one study, for example, hemodynamic changes in tumors using PET and CT perfusion protocols. Since 2004, mono-PET scanners have been no longer manufactured; they were replaced by the so-called hybrid PET/CT and PET/MRI systems, whose number is growing steadily worldwide. An extremely important aspect is the fact that the studies are performed in the format of a single procedure, under condition of patient stability. PET-CT is a hybrid system, where the CT scanner provides high-resolution anatomical images and a PET scanner provides functional, "molecular" images. Both scanners are used sequentially, in one diagnostic study. The result is combined (coregistred) CT and PET images. CT sections allow for a correction of the X-ray attenuation in the body tissues, needed for PET. Molecular PET images showing the spatial distribution of biochemical, metabolic activity in the body's tissues are "tied" to the anatomical structures on CT slices. Figure 10.3 shows a PET/CT scanner with automatic devices for administration of radiopharmaceuticals and iodine-containing contrast agent, installed at the N.N. Blokhin Russian Cancer Research Center.

PET studies were performed after 6 h fasting with the so-called water load—excessive drinking of pure water before the study. In our studies, we used the most available for us radiopharmaceuticals—^{18}F-fluorodeoxyglucose (^{18}F-FDG), ^{18}F-choline (*N*, *N*-dimethyl-*N*-^{18}F-fluoromethyl-2-hydroxyethylammonium), and ^{18}F-fluoroethyl tyrosine. Due to their properties (half-life), these products can be used in clinic (especially in oncology) even in the absence of a cyclotron.

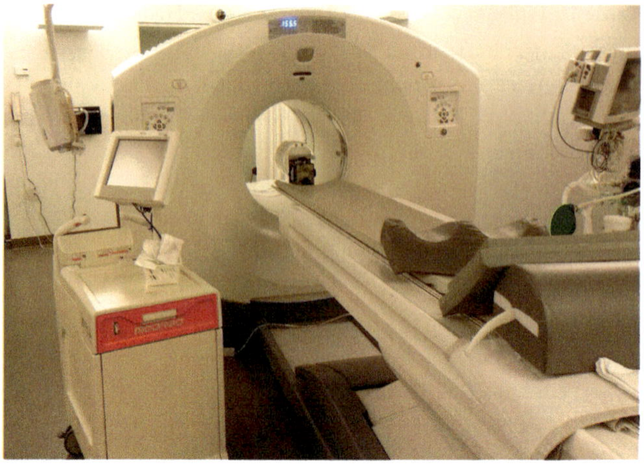

Fig. 10.3 A PET/CT scanner with automatic injectors for administration of radiopharmaceuticals and iodinated contrast agents

10.2 ^{18}F-FDG

The most common radiopharmaceutical in oncology today is ^{18}F-FDG—"the molecule of the Twenty first century." The contribution of PET with ^{18}F-FDG to the diagnosis of cancer cannot be overestimated. Differing from glucose only by a substitution of a hydroxyl group of the second carbon atom with a fluorine atom, 2-fluoro, ^{18}F-2-deoxy-D-glucose administered intravenously follows the initial portion of the glucose metabolic path, entering from the vasculature into the intercellular space and subsequently into cells, where it is phosphorylated by hexokinase. The reaction product is [^{18}F]deoxyglucose-6-phosphate that, unlike glucose phosphate, does not enter into further reactions and remains in the cells during the study, which allows to measure the concentration of radionuclide ^{18}F in the tissue. The administered dose is 122 MBq per 1 m^2 of body surface area, which is determined based on the height and weight of the subject and is on average 370–400 MBq for the whole-body study and 200 MBq for the brain.

FDG is used in PET diagnosis to assess the glucose metabolism in the heart, lungs, and brain. It is mainly applied (90%) in oncology, tumor imaging (Ruhlmann et al. 1999; Alazraki et al. 2007; Granov and Tyutin 2008; Luna et al. 2014). ^{18}F-FDG is accumulated in the cells using glucose transport systems, phosphorylated by hexokinase into FDG-6-phosphate, which is not a substrate for subsequent glycolysis, and enters cells proportionally to the glycolysis rate. This accumulation of ^{18}F-FDG-6-phosphate forms the backbone of brain tumor metabolic imaging (due to the increased glucose metabolism as compared to the normal tissue) (since glucose is a metabolic substrate for the brain cell functioning). Furthermore, the method allows to diagnose and determine the spread of colorectal cancer, breast cancer, lung cancer, melanoma, non-Hodgkin's lymphoma, Hodgkin's lymphoma, and other tumors (Ginsberg et al. 1988; Ruhlmann et al. 1999; Rohren et al. 2003; Alazraki et al. 2007; Granov and Tyutin 2008; Luna et al. 2014). In psychoneurological practice, ^{18}F-FDG allows to diagnose and perform differential diagnosis of a variety of neurodegenerative diseases, including Alzheimer's disease, diffuse Lewy body disease, frontotemporal dementia, as well as Parkinson's disease, and multisystem degeneration (multisystem atrophy, progressive supranuclear palsy, corticobasal degeneration, Huntington's chorea, etc.), and identify (in combination with EEG data and the analysis of clinical symptoms) an epileptic focus in patients with epilepsy.

Despite a rather wide application of ^{18}F-FDG in oncology, PET sensitivity in the diagnosis of brain metastases is significantly lower than the sensitivity of MRI with contrast enhancement (75% vs. 90%) (Broadwell and Sofroniew 1993; Nieder et al. 1997). The main issue is the relatively low resolution of PET in differentiation of small tumor lesions on the background of high natural metabolism of the brain substance. Therefore, PET is more appropriate for detection of a primary tumor lesion, with the proof of its presence in patients with focal brain lesion(s) suggesting the metastatic nature of intracerebral changes (Rohren et al. 2003). The ^{18}F-FDG PET findings are considered to be a tumor if ^{18}F-FDG shows an increased accumulation in the brain and other parts of the body (SUV > 3.0), where such accumulation should not be observed. The radiopharmaceutical accumulation in any portion of the brain is interpreted as a primary tumor. For an independent and more accurate verification, two radiologists visually analyze the images obtained.

PET [^{18}F] FDG in brain metastases can be carried out as an independent investigation and in addition to the whole-body PET scan. We came to the conclusion that using PET with [^{18}F] FDG (if MRI and CT are available) for the diagnosis of metastatic brain lesions is not feasible—the sensitivity as compared to MRI does not exceed 70%; the low resolution of PET (5–6 mm) does not allow to visualize small lesions (Fig. 10.4). This procedure is advisable in assessing the effectiveness of treatment of MTS with various histogeneses.

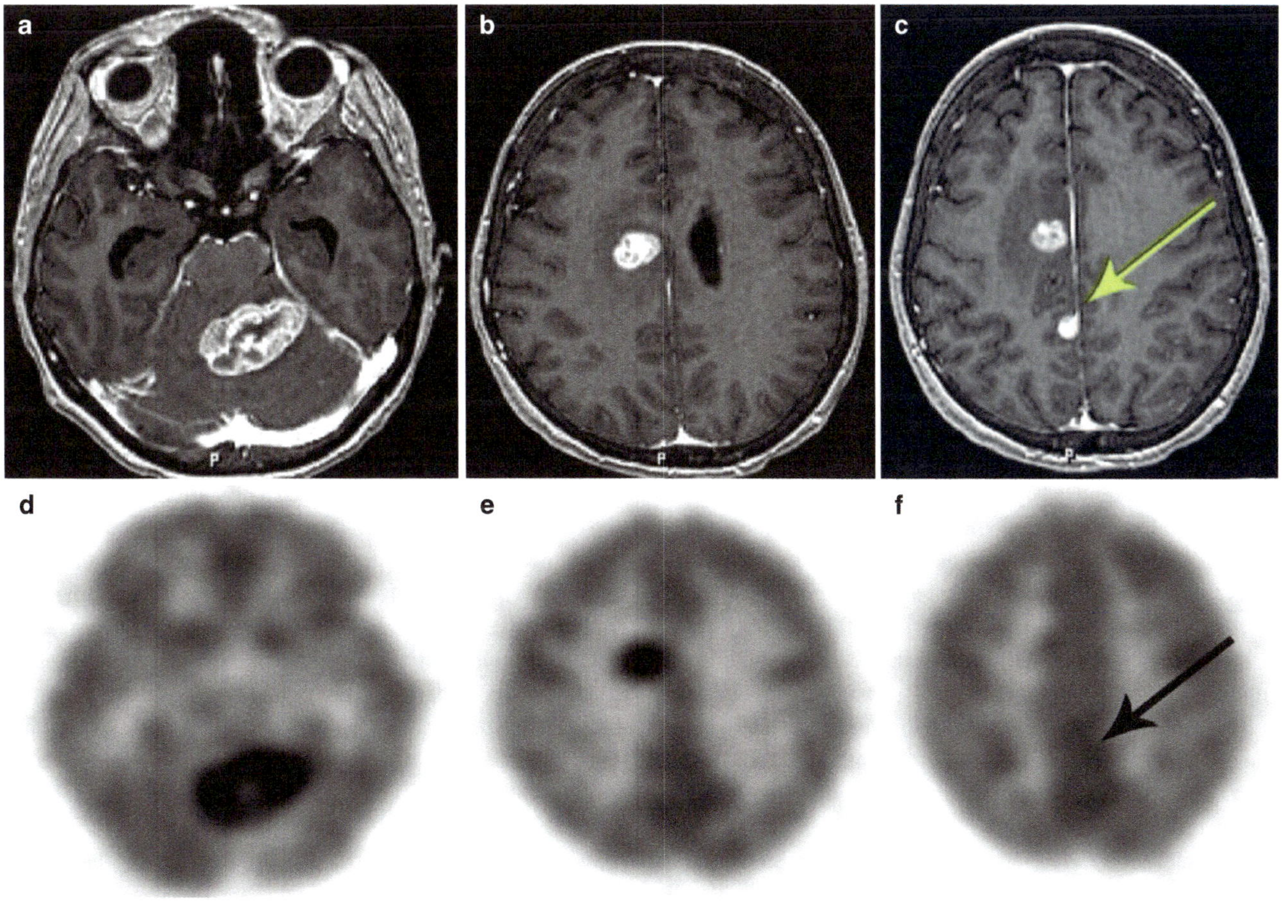

Fig. 10.4 Multiple colorectal cancer metastases in the brain. T1-weighted MR images show multiple abnormal lesions that intensely accumulate CA (**a**–**c**). The perifocal edema is mild. PET ^{18}F-FDG shows an increased RP registration in the largest lesions (**d**, **e**). A small node with parasagittal location is not visualized on PET ^{18}F-FDG (**f**) (arrows)

10.3 ^{18}F-Choline

In recent years, in the PET diagnosis of tumors, choline-based radiopharmaceuticals are of interest (*N*, *N*-dimethyl-*N*-18F-fluoromethyl-2-hydroxyethylammonium). This is a membrane marker that allows to evaluate the activity of the cell membrane formation. Choline is included in membrane phospholipids in the form of phosphatidylcholine, which is a major lipid component of plasma membranes in mammalian cells and is important for the structural stability of the membrane and cell proliferation. As known, brain cells of an adult human practically do not divide. This is also true for the formation of their nuclei and membranes; probably, due to this, ^{18}F-choline or ^{11}C-choline practically does not accumulate in the intact brain matter. This was first discovered by Gauthier et al. (1985); however, their study did not evaluate intracerebral tumors. At the same time, any processes associated with the formation of "new" cells and their components in the brain matter, like inflammation or a tumor, result in an increased accumulation of ^{18}F-choline (Amane et al. 1987; Hamel et al. 1987; Estrada et al. 1990).

The cell membrane is usually composed of a phospholipid bilayer. Phospholipid or phosphatidylcholine has a hydrophilic "head" and a hydrophobic "tail." Hydrophilic heads are oriented toward the outer layers of the membrane (both internal and outer cell surfaces), while hydrophobic tails are oriented inside the membrane itself. One of the most common elements of cellular membranes is choline. Choline is incorporated in the composition of phospholipids in the form of phosphorylcholine. One of the first reactions of ATP-dependent phosphorylation in the choline incorporation chain is catalyzed by the enzyme choline kinase (Nakagami et al. 1999; Ramirez de Molina et al. 2002). Fluorocholine is a fluoromethylated choline analogue consisting of flyuorometil-dimethyl-2-hydroxyethylammonium labeled with radioactive ^{18}F. In the brain, besides membrane complexes, choline is a part of acetylcholine involved in the transmission of impulses in the cholinergic nerve endings. Also, a number of studies have noted that quite a large amount of choline accumulates in the cerebral vascular endothelium. Therefore, the "background" drug accumulation includes all of the above structures (Slack et al. 1972; Katz-Brull and Degani 1996).

A cell requires choline not only for cell proliferation and as a building membrane component but also to maintain vital functions, such as the transport of substances through the cell wall. Thus, PET studies can also evaluate the activity of transport of substances through the membrane, which may not necessarily be associated with cell proliferation.

According to some authors, an increased accumulation of ^{18}F-choline is observed in inflammatory changes (including vasculitis of various etiologies) (Langen et al. 2003; Provenzale et al. 2004). We assume that the radiopharmaceutical accumulation is relatively stable in the areas of inflammatory changes (in granulocytes and macrophages) and should not result in an increase in SUV. In benign intracranial tumors, absolute SUV values and their changes with time should not be high. In malignant neoplasms, whose cells actively divide and constantly experience a need for structural elements of the membranes, in particular, phosphatidylcholine, SUV values should be high and increase over time. The first PET images of tumors using choline-containing radiopharmaceuticals have been presented in an example of brain and prostate tumors using ^{11}C-choline; however, the short half-life (20 min) significantly limits its use in practice. The first studies on the use of choline-containing tracers in the diagnosis of brain tumors were published in 1997 (Ohtani et al. 2001; Goebell et al. 2006). The authors noted that the radiopharmaceutical concentration at the 10:1 ratio in a tumor and cortical regions of the brain is achieved as early as 5 min after the administration of ^{18}F-choline, which, from a diagnostic point of view, is much superior to ^{18}F-FDG. The first use of ^{18}F-choline with a long half-life (110 min) was demonstrated in the papers by Hara et al. (1997) and DeGrado et al. (2001) in prostate cancer. Of great interest is the work on the use of ^{18}F-choline in the differential diagnosis of metastatic and intracerebral tumors. It was shown that metastatic tumors were characterized by higher SUV values, while glioblastomas had signs of peritumoral accumulation exceeding the area of abnormal accumulation of a contrast agent in MRI, confirming the theory of infiltrative growth of gliomas (Shinoura et al. 1997; Vanpouille et al. 2009; Tan et al. 2011).

A PET/CT study with ^{18}F-choline was carried out in two stages on 43 patients. The first and the second phases of the scanning were performed immediately after an intravenous injection of the radiopharmaceutical to the patient and 45–55 min after the administration, respectively. The drug was administered by an automatic injector for radiopharmaceuticals Intego 2010. The administered activity was 300 MBq. Quantification of SUV (max) was performed off-line on a workstation SyngoVia using the oncology protocol. Two parameters of RP accumulation were evaluated: maxSUV1 values registered at the first phase (5 min after the administration) and changes of maxSUV2 with time (in 45–55 min after the intravenous administration of radiopharmaceutical). We studied the following areas: a solid part of the tumor, the central necrosis area, and the contralateral side of the brain.

Quantitative analysis of the level of RP accumulation in the intact white matter of the cerebral hemispheres showed that the mean maxSUV1 values were 0.34 at stage I, while stage II maxSUV2 values either slightly decreased or remained stable—0.24 (Table 10.2).

Table 10.2 Average maxSUV values (normal) of ^{18}F-choline in the intact brain tissue ($n = 43$)

The mean maxSUV1 values and standard deviations in the intact white matter of the brain at stage 1	The mean maxSUV2 values and standard deviations in the intact white matter of the brain at stage 2
0.34 ± 0.11	0.24 ± 0.08

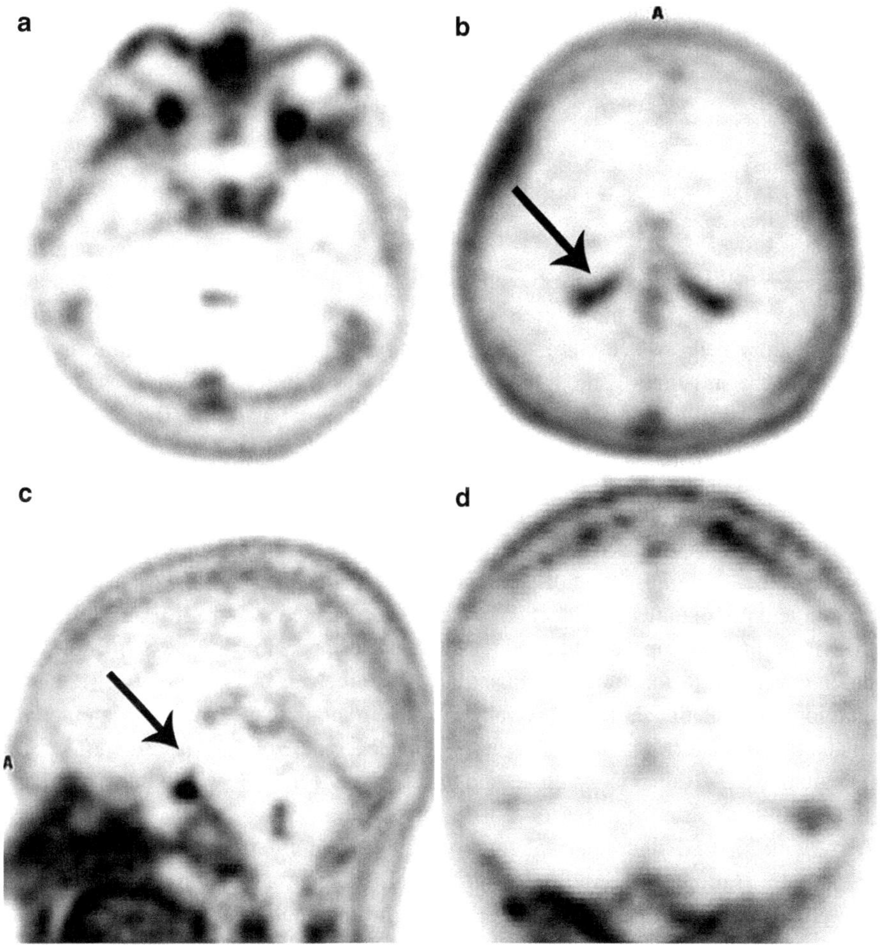

Fig. 10.5 Normal PET of the head with ^{18}F-choline in axial (**a**, **b**), sagittal (**c**) and coronal (**d**) projections. A physiological, increased RP accumulation in the pituitary gland and choroidal plexus of the brain (*arrows*)

In all cases of patients ($n = 43$) included in the analyzed group, there was a decrease in maxSUV2 in the intact white matter (0.18). The maxSUV1 values in the cerebellum and brainstem (subtentorially) with respect to the cerebral hemispheres were lower (0.3 and 0.37, respectively), which was probably due to the less active blood supply to the posterior fossa structures (Fig. 10.5).

10.4 Amino Acids

Subsequent evolvement of radiopharmacology was aimed at the development of radiopharmaceuticals with tumor tropism, allowing to visualize only the affected brain structures. In PET diagnosis of glial tumors, radiopharmaceuticals based on labeled amino acids are commonly used. These include ^{11}C-methionine (MET), ^{18}F-tyrosine (FET), and ^{18}F-thymidine (FLT) (Wester et al. 1999; Langen et al. 2003). These products help determine the velocity of transport of amino acids involved in the nucleus division and formation of DNA strands, which provides a possibility to evaluate the proliferative activity of tissues. In addition, low levels of amino acid uptake in the normal brain tissue using these radiopharmaceuticals in PET allow to clearly distinguish a tumor from the normal brain tissue.

To date, ^{11}C-methionine is the most widely used. Its accumulation allows to distinguish glial tumors by their malignancy grade, to determine their boundaries on a background of the brain substance edema, as well as to identify residual tumors after the treatment. The specificity of the product is high and reaches 90% (Hara et al. 1997; Tan et al. 2011; Skvortsova et al. 2014).

The next-generation products with the diagnostic value similar to that of ^{11}C-methionine are ^{18}F-FET (fluoroethyl tyrosine) or *O*-(2[^{18}F]fluorophenyl)-L-tyrosine labeled with fluorine and having a longer half-life, which significantly expands the scope of their application (Langen et al. 2003; Kwee et al. 2007; Wyss et al. 2007). Another advantage of these radiopharmaceuticals is that they are not uptaken by macrophages and granulocytes and, as a result, do not accumulate in altered inflammatory tissues, including after surgery or various types of radiation therapy. PET with ^{18}F-FET in some cases allows to make a differential diagnosis with nonspecific (non-tumor) lesions (Table 10.3).

As can be seen from the table, ^{18}F-FET is superior by its diagnostic characteristics to both ^{11}C-MET and ^{18}F-FDG. In our study, we evaluated the information value of ^{18}F-tyrosine (D-2- {18} F-fluoroethyl-L-tyrosine) in the detection of metastatic brain lesions ($n = 24$). FET is not included in the metabolic processes in cells but is transported through the epithelium

Table 10.3 Sensitivity (%), specificity (%), and diagnostic accuracy (%) of amino acids as compared to ^{18}F-FDG in the diagnosis of metastatic brain lesions

	Sensitivity	Specificity	Diagnostic accuracy
^{18}F-FDG PET	80–86	80–93	80–92
^{11}C-MET PET	80–94	80–91	80–94
^{18}F-FET PET	93–95	96–99	97–98

and the epithelial blood barrier by subtypes of the transport system L (LAT2). This transport system is not identified in inflammatory cells, which eliminates the possibility of FET uptake in the inflamed tissue, and potentially makes it even more tumor specific than MET. Unlike ^{11}C-MET, ^{18}F-FET is not involved in the protein synthesis and is a marker of amino acid transport. The ^{18}F-FEE accumulation in tumors depends on the extent of angiogenesis and density of tumor cells.

The study was conducted in three phases: immediately after the intravenous administration of the radiopharmaceutical and 10 min and 45 min after the injection; we defined a change in the RP accumulation in the tumor and intact brain substance. In order to reduce an inaccuracy of quantitative parameters, in addition to calculating the true SUV values in these regions, the calculation of TBR (tumor-to-brain ratio) was made—a ratio of quantitative SUV values in the tumor and intact substance.

Figure 10.6 shows images of a three-phase brain PET study with ^{18}F-FET under normal conditions: 1–2 min after the administration of the radiopharmaceutical, there is an expressed accumulation in the venous sinuses; the accumulation in the brain substance is plumiform, probably due to the predominant presence of RP in the vessels. Ten minutes after the administration of the radiopharmaceutical, there are a more pronounced diffuse and homogeneous accumulation in the brain matter and a decrease in the SUV values in the sinuses. Forty five minutes after the intravenous administration of the radiopharmaceutical, venous sinuses are not differentiated; a marked increase in the accumulation in subcortical nuclei and a homogeneous accumulation in the white and gray matter are observed. Usually, the key steps for evaluating the tumor activity are the first 15 min after the administration of a radiopharmaceutical, subsequently, a plateau or a moderate increase in SUV is observed in the normal brain tissue, a decrease in values by 45 min is observed in the tumor, while the values increase in post-radiation changes.

Thus, in our material, the method does not identify any abnormal RP accumulation outside the brain in 17% of 170 cases with ^{18}F-FDG PET. Moreover, the assessment of the total diagnostic information including CT, MRI, and PET findings gave a reason to consider primary brain lesions in only 10% of cases (a false-negative result), while the histological examination confirmed the secondary nature of brain lesions. It should be noted that a tumor search using ultrasound, CT, MRI, etc. did not allow to identify abnormal changes even with a further in-depth investigation of the patients in question.

The analysis of the results of PET with ^{18}F-FDG in patients with brain metastases before the treatment showed that the majority of tumors (70%) are characterized by high SUV values: average values are 5.3 (2.8–8.6). In the remaining 30% of cases, metastases were not visualized despite an intense accumulation of the contrast agent in MRI. From our point of view, the use of PET with [^{18}F] FDG for the diagnosis of metastatic brain lesions (if MRI and CT are available) is not justified. The low PET resolution of 5–6 mm does not allow to visualize small lesions.

A brain PET study may be performed to assess the effectiveness of the treatment, while the SUV analysis provides quantitative indicators reflecting a decrease in the metabolic activity or an increase as a negative response to treatment.

It also should be kept in mind that a one-time scan of the whole body and brain with [^{18}F] FDG has its technical specifics, since physiological hyperfixation of RP in the cerebral cortex "hides" its accumulation in tumor lesions; additional time is required for a decrease in the drug activity in the brain structures, which changes the study process and the logistics of movement of "active patients."

Comparison of the high cost of whole-body PET as one of the main disadvantages of the study with a total cost of a standard set of diagnostic procedures (ultrasound, X-ray, endoscopic diagnosis, CT and MRI scans of the chest or abdomen, etc.) aimed at achieving the same goal (identification of the primary tumor) showed that a PET study is cheaper and, just as importantly, allows to solve diagnostic issues in a much shorter time. However, despite its clear advantages, the method still has some significant limitations that do not allow to use it as a screening method. First of all, it is a technically complicated procedure. A need for producing a radiopharmaceutical (RP), its transportation, and use require, in addition to medical staff, involvement of additional staff. Another important aspect is a rather high cost of the study. Long scanning time, limitations associated with comorbidities (diabetes), also restricts the possibilities of the use of this method.

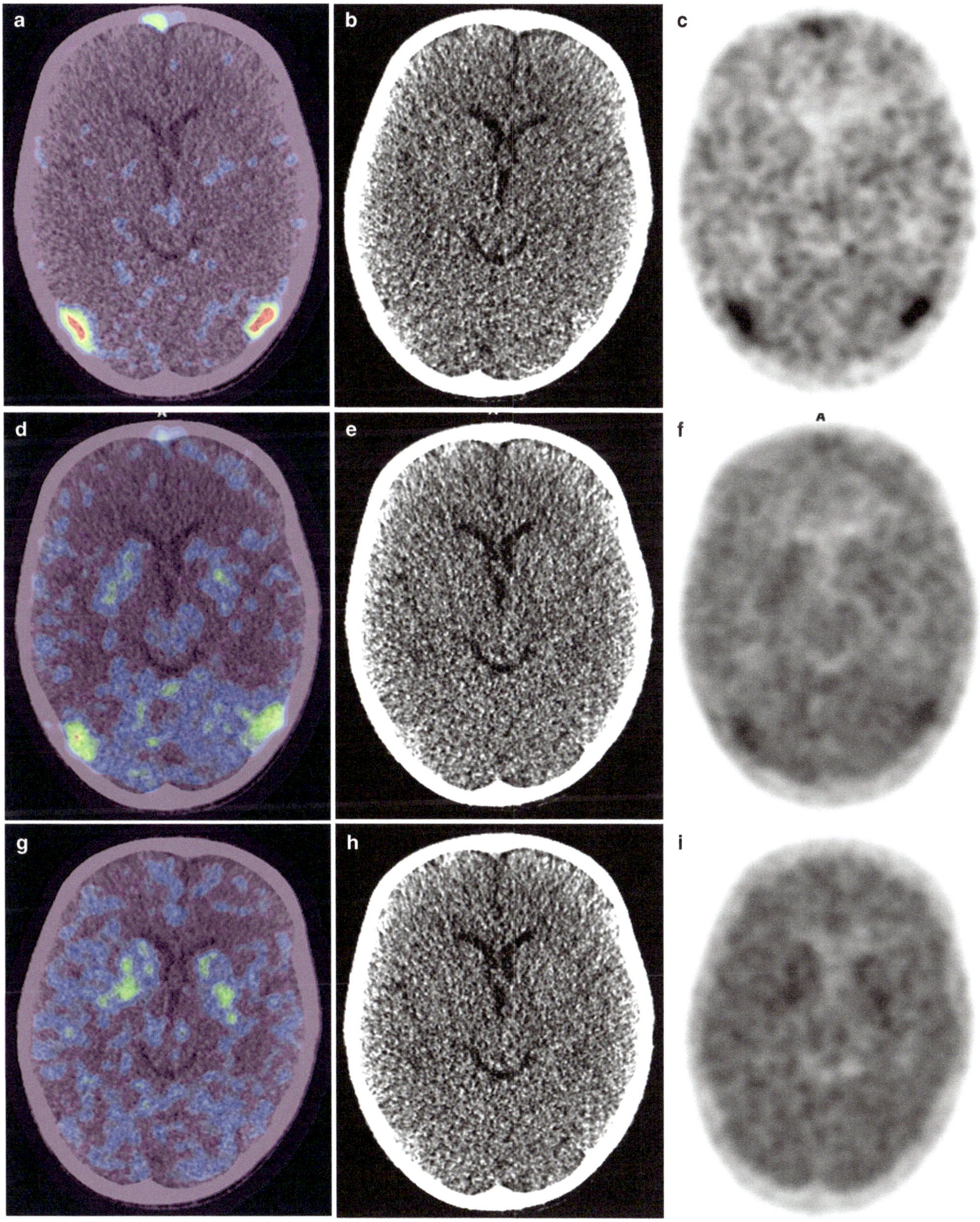

Fig. 10.6 A three-phase brain PET with ^{18}F-FET under normal conditions. CT/PET (**a**), CT (**b**), and PET (**c**) images in the axial projection at the level of subcortical nuclei 1 min after the administration of the radiopharmaceutical by an automatic injector show an intense in the product accumulation in the cerebral sinuses. (**d**–**f**) 10 min after the administration of the radiopharmaceutical and (**g**–**i**) 45 min after the intravenous administration of the radiopharmaceutical: a gradual RP elimination from the major blood vessels and an increase in its accumulation in the brain matter

Part III

Metastases of Malignant Tumors in the Brain

11 Introduction to Metastases of Malignant Tumors in the Brain

In this chapter, we sought to illustrate the possibilities of the most modern neuroimaging methods and compare their diagnostic capabilities in relation to metastases based on their primary source. Before illustrations in each nosological group, some background information is presented, while manifestations of metastases are described by their primary source. The findings allowed not only to carry out a visual assessment of the size and extent of the pathological process but also to quantify the intensity of biological processes that occur in the tumor tissues and the surrounding brain structures, as well as to evaluate changes induced by the treatment.

Before proceeding to the analysis of materials we have accumulated over 15 years, we would like to define the terminology. Metastasis is a malignant tumor or an inflammatory lesion transferred to any organ or a tissue from another affected organ or tissue. The term "metastasis of the brain" often used in practice erroneously implies a focus of an intact brain tissue in any organ. For example, the concepts of "lung cancer metastases in the brain" or "lung cancer metastases to the brain" appear to be correct.

Changes of the MR signal in different modes, degree, and character of the contrast agent accumulation by the tumor, intensity and extent of edema, hemorrhage into the tumor, and presence of its necrotic changes—all of these affect the selection of study areas and regions in MR spectroscopy, DBU, ASL, SWI (SWAN), and CT perfusion imaging. For example, the proximity of the identified tumor to the bone structures of the skull in CT perfusion forced us to change the projection (from axial to oblique) when selecting the region of interest and exclude the subsequent spectroscopic examination from the diagnostic algorithm when searching for hemorrhagic changes due to an increased "noise" caused by the presence of hemosiderin. When the sizes of MRI contrast agent accumulation areas in the regions of suspected radiation necrosis were small (up to 5 mm), we did not perform CT perfusion or PET.

Mandatory basic images studied before applying the above additional methods were scans obtained using T1-weighted, T2-weighted, T2-FLAIR, DWI, and T1-weighted with contrast enhancement (usually a 0.7 mm slice) MRI in the axial projection using fat saturation. This set of pulse sequences should be considered standard in the diagnosis of metastatic brain tumors. In some cases, it is advisable to add studies in sagittal and frontal projections using T1-weighted sequences after contrast agent administration.

It is advisable to perform a whole-body study as often as possible both in case of a suspected metastatic brain tumor and in cases of known history of cancer. This is a justifiable tactic that allows to adjust the therapy. Of course, the main criterion in this case is the patient's radiation exposure during these studies. A PET/CT method is the method of choice today as the most specific; however, it is associated with high patient's radiation exposure. An alternative method of whole-body scanning for patients with metastatic brain tumors can be considered DWI MRI. The method is becoming more common in the diagnosis of cancer; however, due to a significant proportion of false-positive results, it requires an extremely careful application. Therefore, at the primary stage of diagnosis, we aimed to use a set of whole-body MRI DWI and PET/CT. Follow-up scans were primarily performed using MRI, with MRI supplemented by a PET/CT scan only in difficult differential diagnostic cases.

M. Dolgushin et al., *Brain Metastases*, DOI 10.1007/978-3-319-57760-9_11

This monograph is based on the analysis of patient's history; visual and quantitative evaluation of CT, MRI, and PET images; and histological studies in more than 3000 patients. Table 11.1 shows the distribution of clinical cases with metastatic brain lesions by the primary tumor site.

As shown in Table 11.1, the most common sources of metastatic tumors were lung cancer (25.8%), breast cancer (22.4%), melanoma (18.2%), kidney cancer (13.9%), colon cancer (5.4%), uterine cancer (3.7%), and ovarian cancer (1.8%). The source of metastases in the brain from other malignant tumors was found in the thyroid (0.8%), stomach (0.4%), larynx (0.2%), pancreas (0.2%), prostate (0.3%), and others (0.2%), which in total amounted to 2.1%. The primary source of metastases in the brain verified during the surgery could not be identified in 6.3% of cases.

Table 11.1 Distribution of cases with metastatic brain lesions by the site of the primary tumor ($n = 2650$)

#	Primary tumor	Cases of patients with metastases in the brain (%)	
1.	Lung cancer	25.8	*93.7*
2.	Breast cancer	22.4	
3.	Melanoma	18.2	
4.	Renal cancer	13.9	
5.	Colorectal cancer	5.4	
6.	Uterine cancer	3.7	
7.	Ovarian cancer	1.8	
9.	Others	2.1	
10.	Metastases of unknown primary in the brain	*6.3*	
	Total	100%	

12 Lung Cancer (LC)

Lung cancer (LC) is the most common malignant neoplasm in the world's population and, as a cause of cancer mortality, amounts to almost 1.6 million people annually. More than 1.8 million of new cases of lung cancer are registered each year worldwide. In Russia, lung cancer is diagnosed each year in more than 55,000 patients (43.4 per 100 thousand). According to Davydov and Axel (2014a, b) the incidence of lung cancer, taking into account all age groups, was 18.7% in 2012 and put lung cancer at the first place in the structure of prevalence of malignant neoplasms in Russia among men. There are two major forms of lung cancer—small cell (SCLC) and non-small cell lung cancer (NSCLC): the latter accounts for up to 80% of total cases. Both forms of lung cancer have different degrees of biological activity, which are reflected in the approaches to the selection of diagnostic and treatment methods (Spencer 1977; Trachtenberg 1987; Davydov and Polotsky 1994; Jänne et al. 2002; Ramazanova and Kislichko 2012; Peters et al. 2012; Rossi et al. 2014; Folkert and Timmerman 2015). The development of lung cancer is believed to be associated with smoking: approximately 90% of affected men and 80% of affected women. At the time of diagnosis, the disease in most patients has common forms.

By the incidence of metastases to the brain, lung cancer is on the first place among all malignant tumors: according to different data, it accounts for 30–60% of all metastases in the brain (to our knowledge, not less than 25%). Up to half of lung cancer patients have a high risk of developing metastatic brain lesions (Takakura et al. 1982; Sen et al. 1998). Based on the study of case records in 2410 patients with lung cancer, brain lesions were identified in 790 (32.9%) patients, with solitary metastases being more common in adenocarcinoma than in poorly differentiated cancer (Martynov and Idrisova 1981). Alperovich (1975) noted that poorly differentiated cancer metastasizes more often. The time interval from the diagnosis of lung cancer to the detection of MTSs in the brain is on average 2–9 months, which is slightly shorter than with cancers from other sites (Sundaresan and Galicich 1985; Nussbaum et al. 1996). The median survival rate of untreated patients with lung cancer MTSs in the brain ranges from 6 to 12 weeks (Carney 1999). Lung cancer metastases in the brain appear to be more common in men.

According Chute et al. (1985), SCLC accounts for 18–30% of all cases of lung cancer. This type of tumor is characterized by an early and rapid spread of metastases via intrathoracic lymph nodes, mediastinal lymph nodes, as well as to the brain, liver, skeletal bone, and adrenals. Jereczek et al. (1996) noted that an autopsy found distant metastases in 143 (82%) cases in the group of 174 patients who died from SCLC, including in the liver (49%), adrenal glands (25%), peripheral lymph nodes (21%), kidneys (18%), brain (17%), and pancreas (12%). This is why a brain MRI study with contrast enhancement in confirmed SCLC is included in the mandatory investigation protocol.

NSCLC comprises several groups: adenocarcinoma (40%), squamous cell carcinoma (30%), and large cell cancer, bronchoalveolar cancer, and other subtypes which account for up to 30% of cases. The proportion of cases of metastatic squamous cell carcinoma was found to increase to up to 80% with the 2-year survival of patients. Literature describes cases of simultaneous presence of different morphological NSCLC forms and neuroendocrine variants, which greatly complicate an accurate diagnosis. In stage IV NSCLC, the overall prognosis is unfavorable: a 1-year survival rate in such cases does not exceed 20% (Riquet et al. 1997). Metastases in the brain occur in one third of NSCLC patients and often manifest by multiple lesions, while the latter can be located both sub- and supratentorially.

Metastatic lesions in the meninges (carcinomatosis) in patients with lung cancer are less common than, for example, in breast cancer (Grossman et al. 1993; Grossman and Krabak 1999); however, according to Mahajan et al. (2002), the source of metastases was lung cancer in 50% of 101 patients with confirmed meningeal involvement.

Clinical symptoms in intracranial metastases of lung cancer include headache, vomiting, motor and sensory deficits, seizures, behavioral and mental disorders, and aphasia. However, these symptoms can often be "subdued," which

M. Dolgushin et al., *Brain Metastases*, DOI 10.1007/978-3-319-57760-9_12

complicates the early clinical diagnosis of the lesion. Thus, according to Jena et al. (2008) in 46.7% of cases of 62 patients with lung cancer metastases in the brain, there were no neurological symptoms.

The method of choice for primary diagnosis of metastatic brain lesions of any etiology is MRI; if it cannot be performed, a viable alternative is CT.

Lung cancer metastases in a CT study performed without contrast enhancement often look like isodense lesions or lesions with a reduced (in the cystic form) density. The size of a perifocal edema area relative to the sizes of the lesion varies greatly up to the absence of edema as such.

Administration of a contrast agent in a CT study is a must, because a solid part of lung cancer metastases rapidly accumulates the contrast agent. Small, convexitally located lesions not always are visualized even after the CA administration.

A CT perfusion study in lung cancer metastases in the brain allows to obtain mean values (CBV = 11.27 ± 3.21 ml/100 g) of the blood flow volume similar to those in metastases of breast cancer, colon cancer, and uterine cancer in the brain. CBF values representing the blood flow velocity in the depth of a metastatic tumor in lung cancer have similar mean values (CBF = 85.03 ± 19.56 ml/100 g/min) as compared with the mean CBF values detected in patients with MTSs of other origin. A solid part of lung cancer metastases in the brain is characterized by relatively low (8.83 ± 2.85 s) MTT as compared to MTT in other metastatic lesions.

Despite the large number of conducted MRI studies, we were unable to establish any MR trends in manifestations of lung cancer metastases in the brain, although we identified a number of pathognomonic MRI manifestations in cases of metastatic brain lesions of another origin (melanoma, kidney cancer, colon cancer). The MR picture of metastatic brain lesions in lung cancer is similar to MRI manifestations of MTSs of tumors from other sites.

Metastatic brain lesions in lung cancer in most cases have a cystic nature with the presence of an area of moderate perifocal edema and are characterized by an increased signal on T2-weighted MRI. However, in our material, metastatic lesions with both a solid and cystic-solid structure with a small area of perifocal edema were identified. In cases where there is an acute hemorrhage in the metastasis stroma in T2-weighted images, there are small hypointense areas, and the tumor tissue becomes heterogeneous. In cases where the metastatic lesion has a solid structure, T2-weighted images show an iso-hypointense MR signal.

T1-weighted MRI allows to display manifestations typical for the active tumor growth. A hyperintense and heterogeneous MRI signal on T1-weighted images is generally caused by the presence of a hemorrhage in the metastasis.

In lung cancer, in cases of multiple metastatic lesions, tumor lesions can be located in a chaotic fashion throughout the brain, both sub- and supratentorially. We did not identify any site "characteristic" for solitary lung cancer metastases in our clinical material. At the same time, multiple microfoci were noted in the brain parenchyma with lung adenocarcinoma. In such cases, a perifocal edema is usually insignificant, which can be partly attributed to the typical manifestations of multiple parenchymal metastases in this morphological type of lung cancer.

Metastases to the skull bones and vertebral bodies can occur not only via the systemic blood flow but also along the vertebral venous plexuses, a valveless system of venous anastomoses running along the spine from the brain to the lesser pelvis. Particular attention in the analysis of diagnostic images should be paid to the occipital bone. The analysis of bone structures in a CT study is mandatory, as metastases to the skull bones in lung cancer occur in up to 30% of cases. In typical cases, a characteristic area of bone destruction in combination with the soft tissue component is visualized. In case of small lesions in the cranial bones, especially its vault, it is difficult to differentiate the metastases from emissary veins.

When the bony structures of the skull base are affected, there is typically a combination of a bone destruction focus with a soft tissue tumor component that is intensely enhanced after intravenous administration of a contrast agent. In such cases, T1-weighted MRI with fat suppression should be used before and after administration of gadolinium preparations. In dural dissemination of metastatic lesions, the symptom of a "dural tail" can be visualized. It is observed on MRI in case of local invasion of the dura mater on the periphery of the main lesion.

We successfully used proton MR spectroscopy (PMRS) as a supplementary option in protocols of differential diagnosis of brain metastatic lesions from primary lesions of tumor and non-tumor origin. However, the prevalence of the Lip-Lac complex characteristic of the tumor lesions, displaying the fact of necrotic changes in the tumor tissue, due to its resemblance to chronic post-radiation changes also accompanied by necrosis and an increased Lip-Lac complex does not allow to consider MR spectroscopy as a method of reliable differential diagnosis of metastases in the brain from formed radiation necrosis after radiotherapy. This statement is fully true for lung cancer metastases in the brain.

SWI (SWAN) images in lung cancer metastases showed a small or moderate number of abnormal vessels, which generally did not result in a significant decrease in the MR signal in this sequence.

In patients diagnosed with primary metastatic tumor in the brain, a one-study whole-body DW MRI provided information on the primary tumor site and extent of the disease in general. Thus, in our studies, whole-body DW MRI in patients with peripheral lung cancer usually clearly detected a primary site of the tumor (both on PET and DWI). Furthermore, besides the primary lesion in the lungs, small metastases with sizes of about 7 mm were identified in some cases. This demonstrates the high diagnostic sensitivity of DW technology.

When analyzing the results of these studies, we observed that the size and shape of lesions on DWI MRI and whole-body PET were often not the same, differing both in the direction of an increase and a decrease. A decrease in the size of lesions may be associated with chest excursions during respiration and a partial loss of changes on MRI. From our point of view, an enlargement in high-signal areas on MRI may be caused by concomitant atelectasis, the presence of cysts and hemorrhages in the lesion stroma.

The whole-body DW MRI has high sensitivity in malignant lung lesions—85% of lesions detected with PET. However, this method has insufficient (76%) specificity due to a large number (24% in our material) of false-positive results.

A whole-body FDG-PET study by Yap et al. (2002) in patients with bronchoalveolar lung cancer showed a fairly high (95%) specificity of the method as compared to CT. However, it was noted that the use of PET with the superficial location of the tumor in the bronchus lumen (without any signs of significant invasion) was less effective. Similar results, confirming the superior specificity of PET, were shown by Vansteenkiste and Stroobants (1998) in a comparative study of the diagnostic efficiency of PET and CT in relation to distant NSCLC metastases in the lymph nodes.

According to our data, the use of PET/CT with ^{18}F-FDG in lung cancer is justified only to assess extracranial lesions. Due to mostly cystic and microfocal brain lesions, the drug accumulation foci in the solid part of lung cancer metastases merge with the physiological accumulation of ^{18}F-FDG. Products with low accumulation in the brain parenchyma, such as ^{18}F-thymidine, ^{18}F-Tyrosine, and ^{11}C-methionine, are significantly superior to ^{18}F-FDG in investigation of intracranial lesions. Hara and Inagaki (2000) investigated the possibility of PET diagnostics with ^{11}C-choline and ^{18}FDG in patients with NSCLC. ^{11}C-choline sensitivity appeared to be 100%, while that of FDG was 75%, which indicates higher efficiency of ^{11}C-choline in the diagnosis of NSCLC and its distant metastases.

12.1 Clinical Observations

See Figs. 12.1, 12.2, 12.3, 12.4, 12.5, 12.6, 12.7, 12.8, 12.9, 12.10, 12.11, 12.12, 12.13, 12.14, 12.15, 12.16, 12.17, 12.18, 12.19, 12.20, 12.21, 12.22, 12.23, 12.24, 12.25, 12.26, 12.27, 12.28, 12.29, 12.30, 12.31, 12.32, 12.33, 12.34, 12.35, 12.36, 12.37, 12.38, 12.39, 12.40, 12.41, 12.42, 12.43, and 12.44.

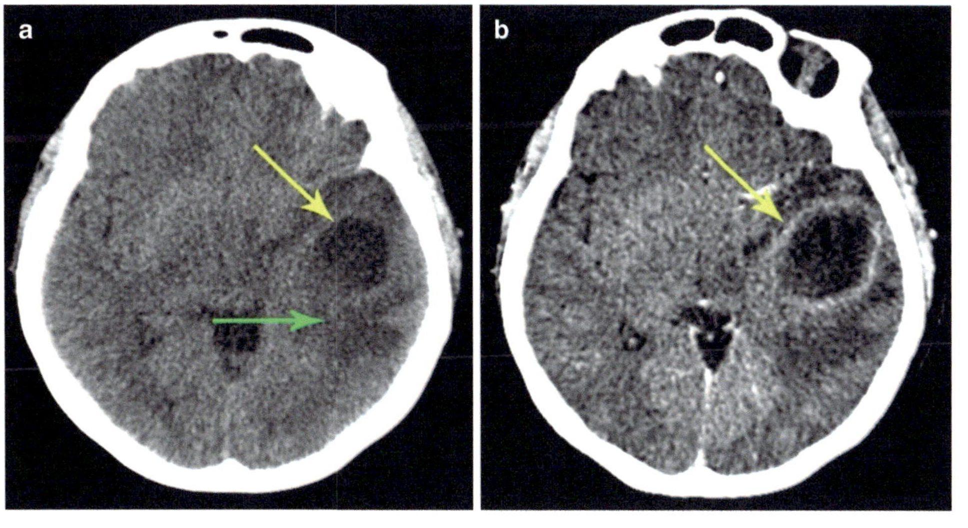

Fig. 12.1 (**a**, **b**) A lung cancer metastasis in the brain. Brain CT before (**a**) and after (**b**) the administration of the contrast agent. There is a rounded hypodense area (*bottom arrow* **a**) in the projection of the left temporal region before the administration of the contrast agent (**a**) on the background of edema. After the administration of the contrast agent (**b**), a thin ring-shaped accumulation of the contrast agent in the solid part of the tumor (*upper arrows* **a**, **b**) is identified

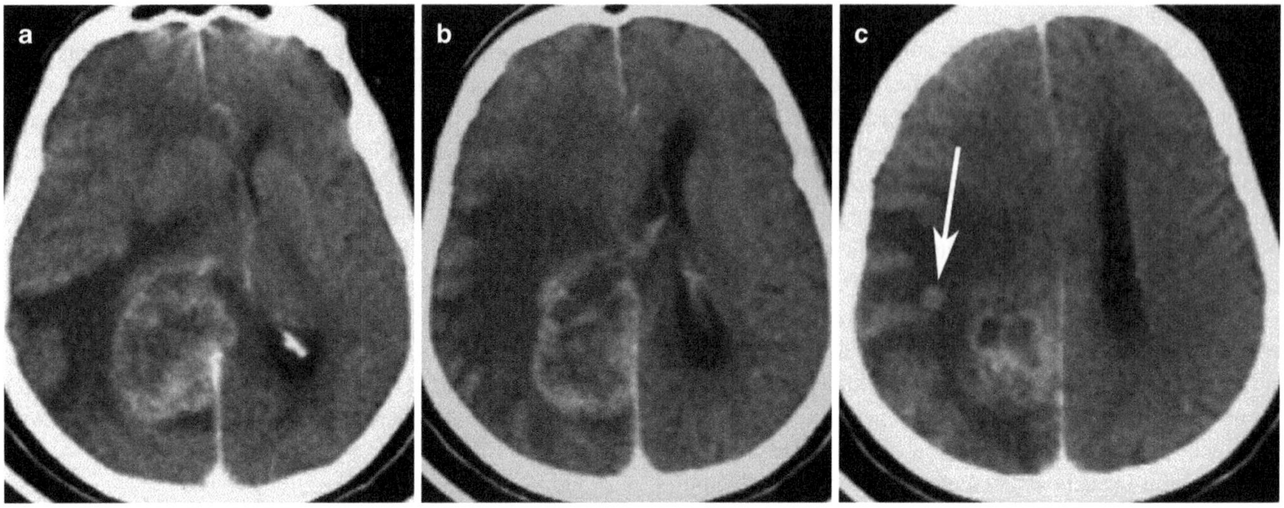

Fig. 12.2 Multiple lung cancer metastases in the brain. On a CT scan after intravenous contrast enhancement (**a**–**c**), there is a large lesion with marked, heterogeneous contrast enhancement in the right parietal region and the second lesion (*arrow*) anteriorly to it (**b**)

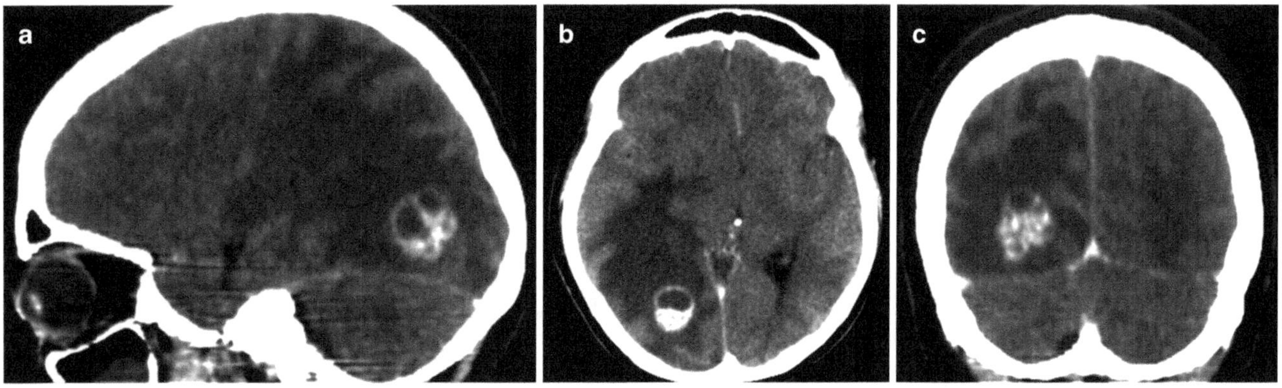

Fig. 12.3 A metastasis of lung cancer in the right occipital region of the brain. On a CT scan after intravenous contrast enhancement (**a**–**c**), a small-sized tumor site surrounded by an area of pronounced perifocal edema is visualized

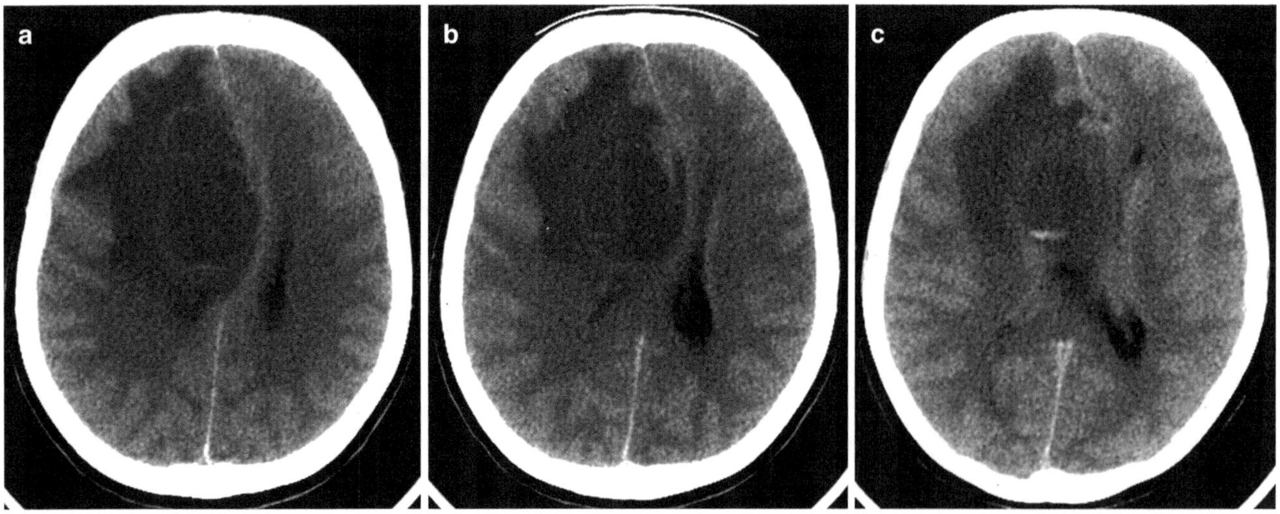

Fig. 12.4 Multiple lung cancer metastases in the brain. CT before (**a**–**c**) and after (**d**–**f**) intravenous contrast enhancement. There are two tumor sites with contrast enhancement in the form of a thin rim (**a**, **d**). Metastases have a centrally located area of necrosis with signs of a pronounced perifocal edema and a midline shift to the left

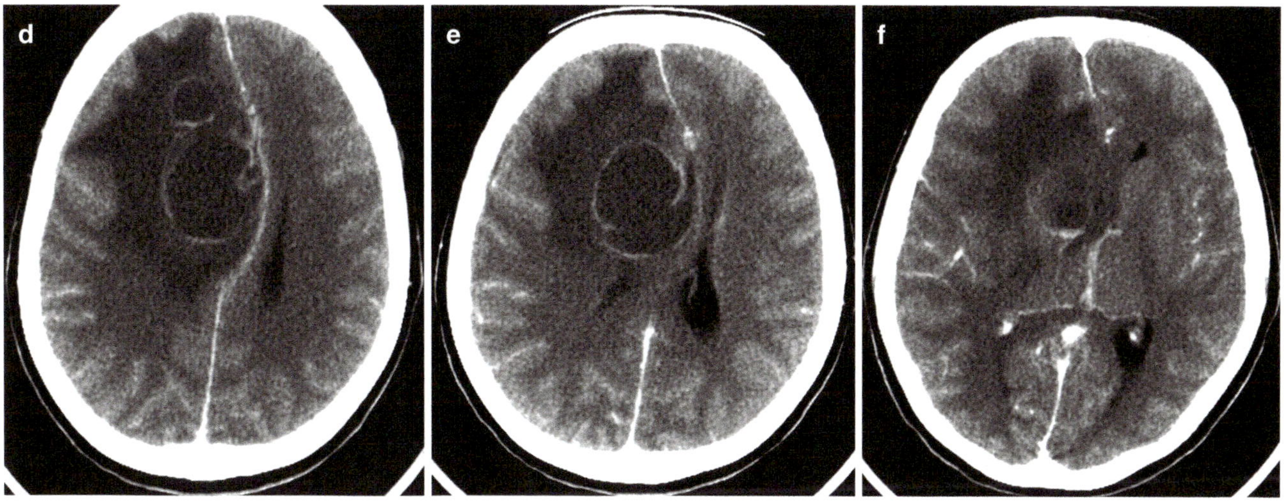

Fig. 12.4 (continued)

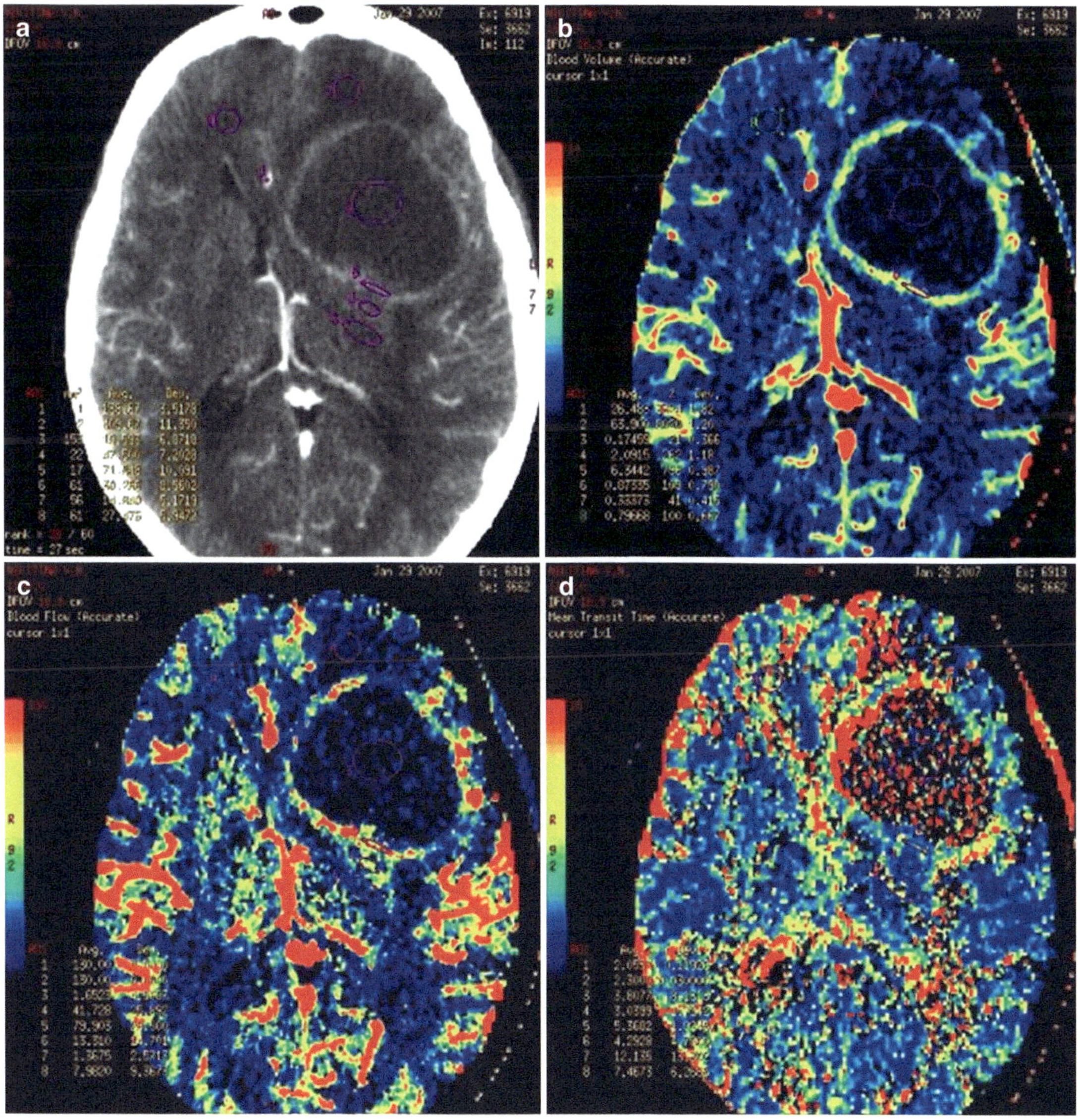

Fig. 12.5 A lung cancer metastasis in the brain. CT perfusion. In the left frontal lobe, there is a space-occupying lesion, predominantly with a cystic structure, accumulating the contrast agent on the periphery (**a**), CT perfusion shows a marked decrease in perfusion in the cystic component and a pronounced uneven increase in CBV (**b**), CBF (**c**), and MTT (**d**) along the contour of the cavity

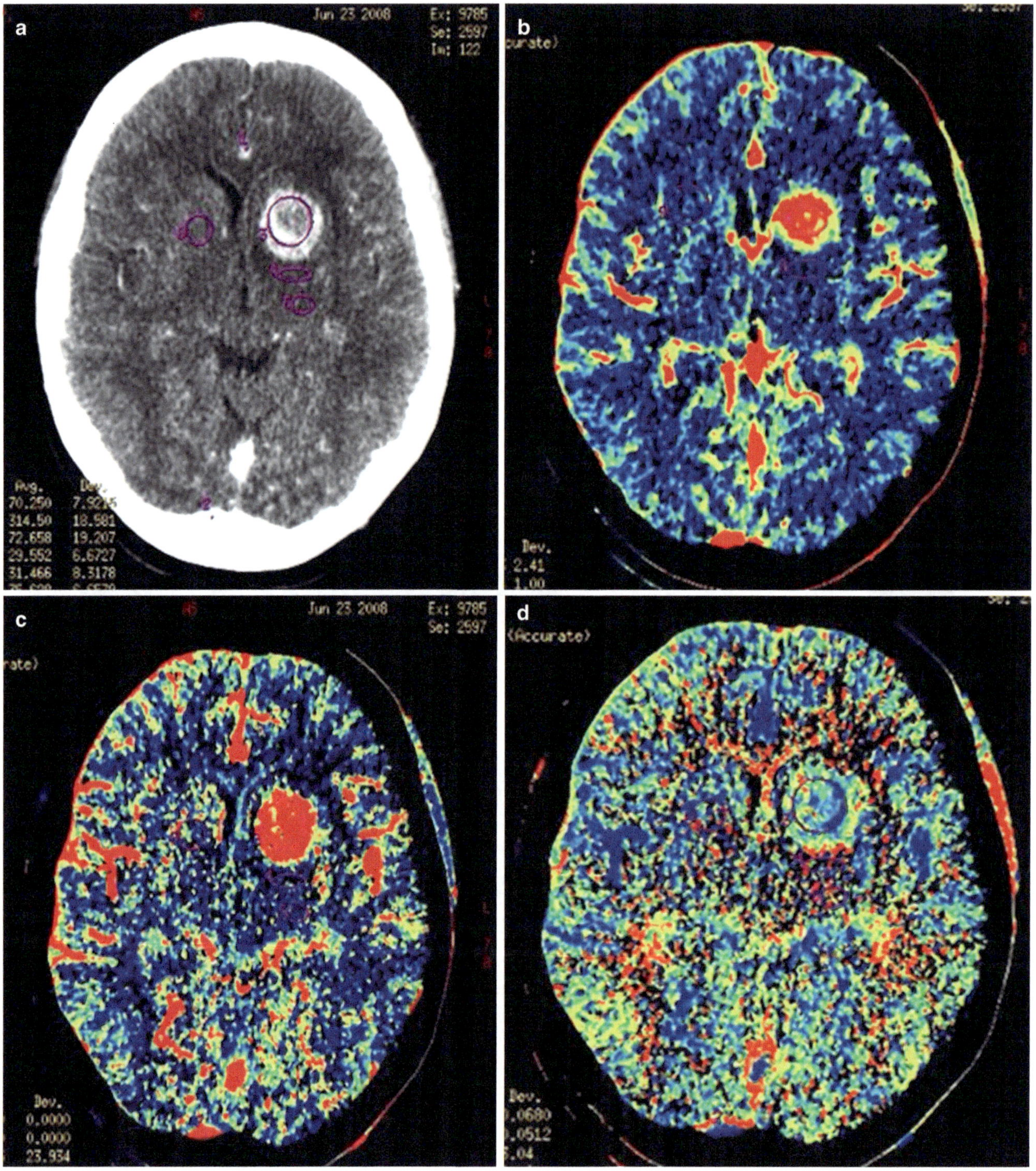

Fig. 12.6 A lung cancer metastasis in the brain. In the subcortical nuclei on the left, there is a richly vascularized space-occupying lesion, rapidly accumulating the contrast agent on CT (**a**) and characterized by higher perfusion parameters CBV and CBF relative to the intact brain substance (**b**, **c**), and MTT values (**d**) are increased to a lesser extent

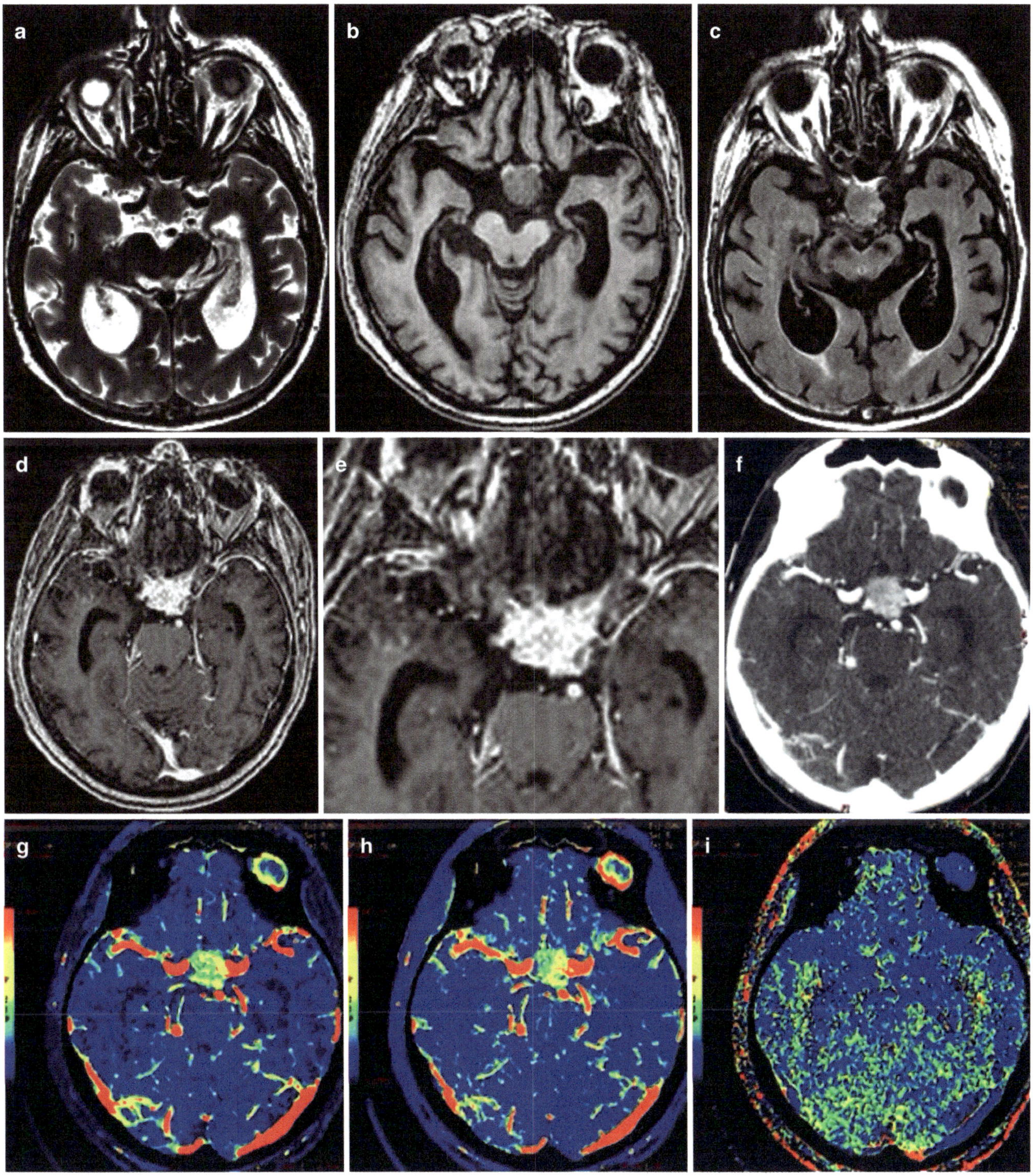

Fig. 12.7 A lung cancer metastasis in the brain. Intra- and suprasellarly, there is a space-occupying lesion with isointense MR signal in T2-weighted (**a**), T1-WI (**b**), and T2-FLAIR (**c**) images that uniformly and intensely accumulates the contrast agent both in MRI (**d**, **e**) and CT (**f**). On CT perfusion maps, there is a marked asymmetrical increase in CBV (**g**) and CBF (**h**), while MTT (**i**) values are slightly increased

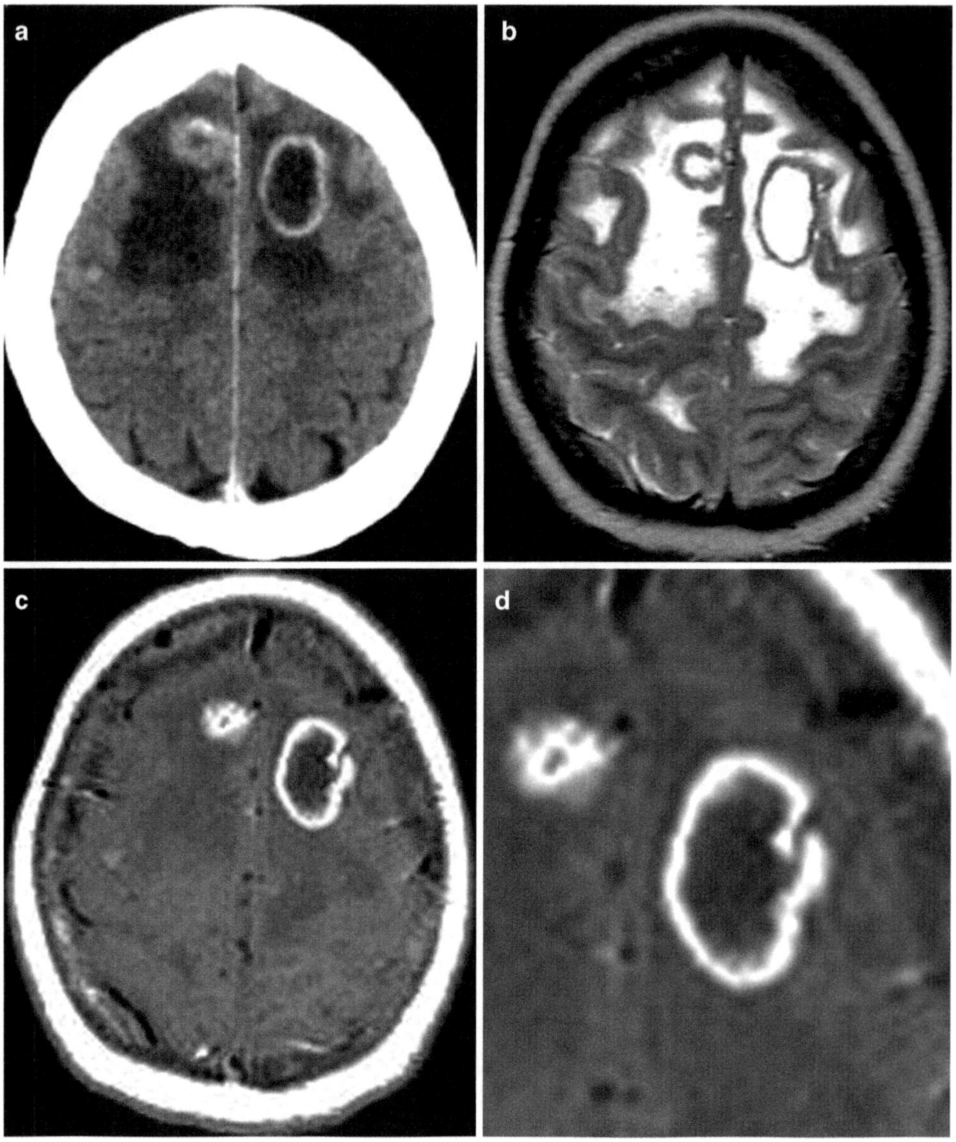

Fig. 12.8 Multiple lung cancer metastases in the brain. In frontal areas, two space-occupying lesions with different diameters are identified. The lesions intensely accumulate the contrast agent both on CT (**a**) and T1-weighted MRI (**c**, **d**). The signal from the central part of the lesions on T2-weighted MRI (**b**) is increased. The symmetry of the perifocal edema enhancement stands out, despite the differing sizes of tumors

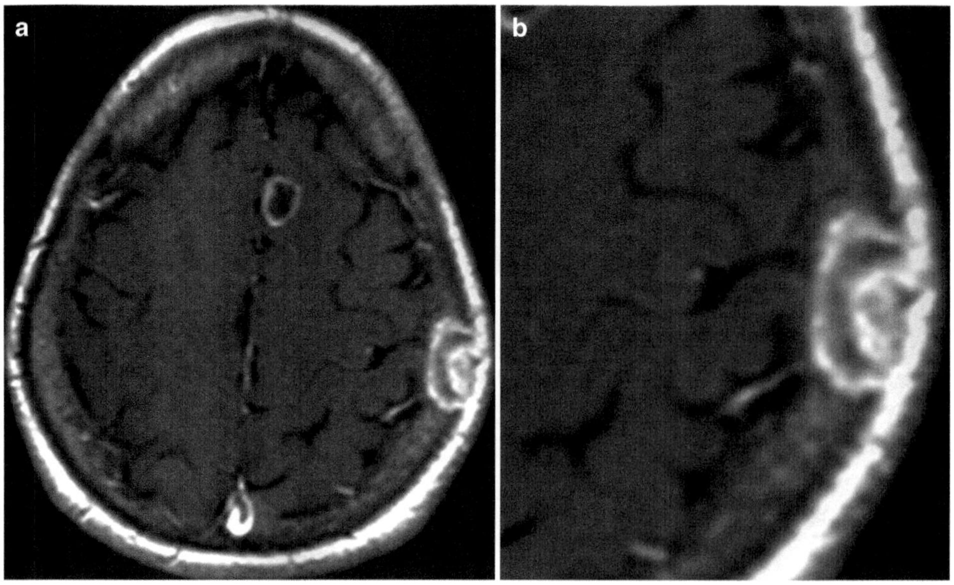

Fig. 12.9 Multiple lung cancer metastases in the brain. On a series of MRI images with contrast enhancement in the axial (**a**, **b**, **c**) and sagittal (**d**) projections, there are multiple tumor lesions located supra- and subtentorially, with no signs of perifocal edema. In the squama of the frontal bone on the left (**a**, **b**), there is a large lesion with uneven contrast enhancement. Metastases in the brainstem and cerebellum (**d**) are characterized by a cystic structure

Fig. 12.9 (continued)

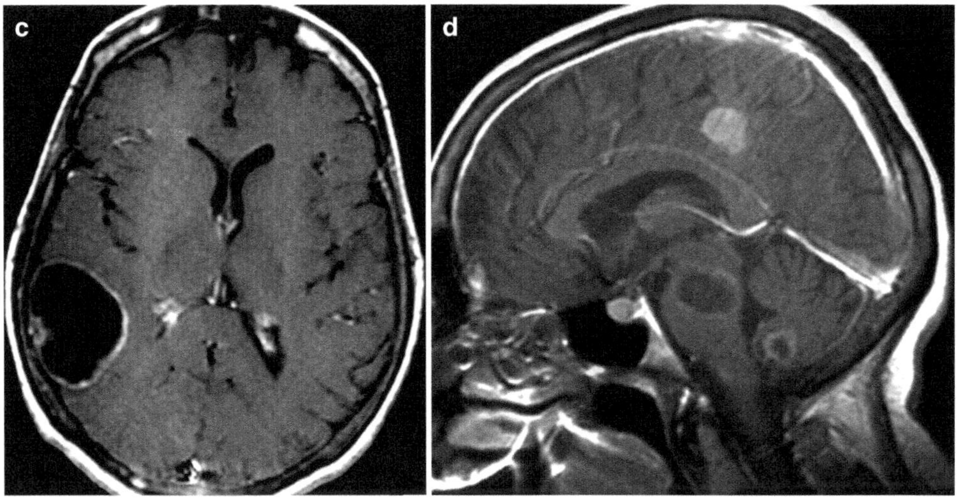

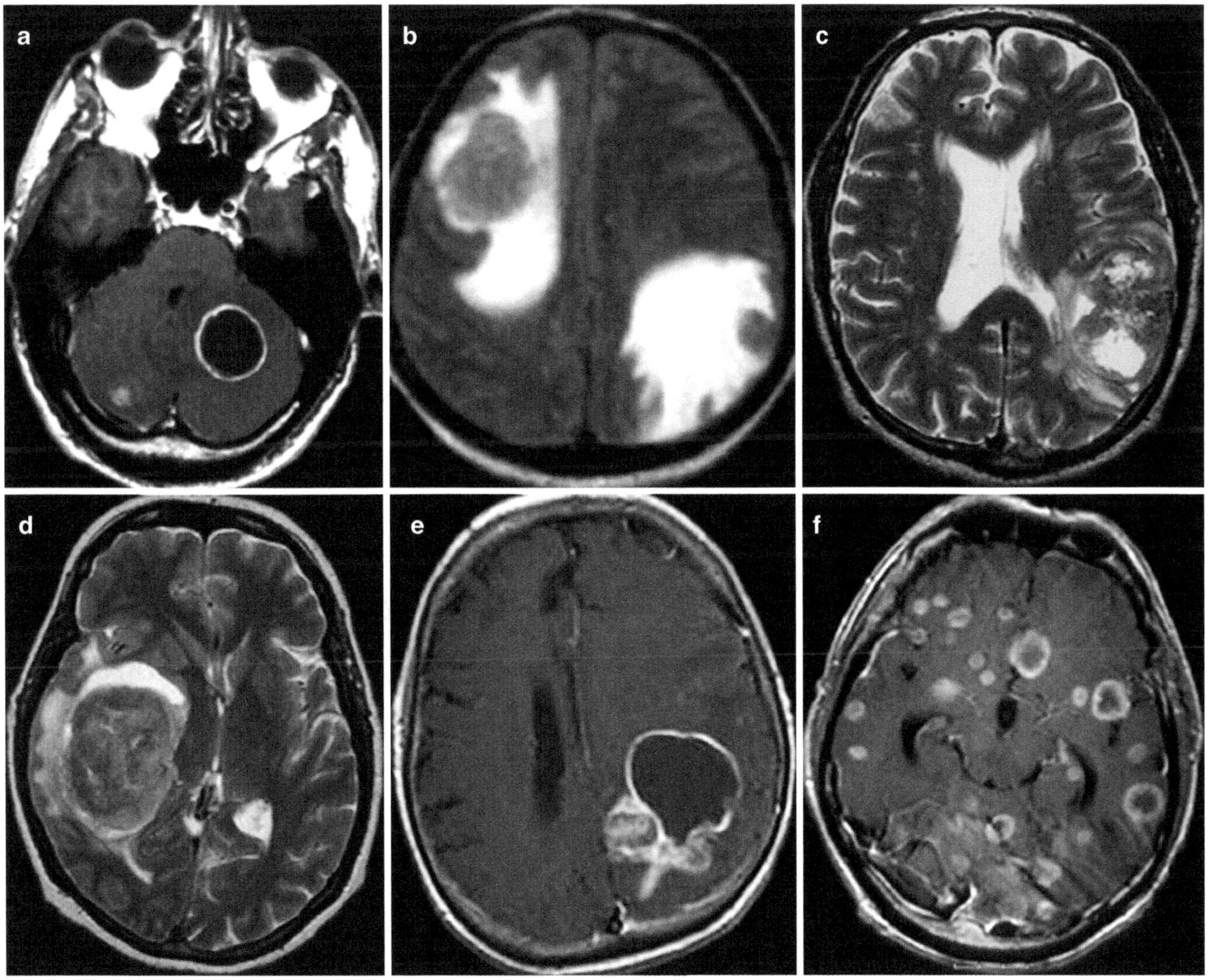

Fig. 12.10 Lung cancer metastases in the brain. Different types of MR manifestations of metastases: (**a**) cystic subtentorial metastases, (**b**) multiple solid lesions with a pronounced perifocal edema, (**c**) a lesion with the mixed structure without a perifocal edema, (**d**) a lesion with the solid structure with a minimum perifocal edema, (**e**) a lesion with the mixed structure, and (**f**) multiple lesions with necrosis in the center

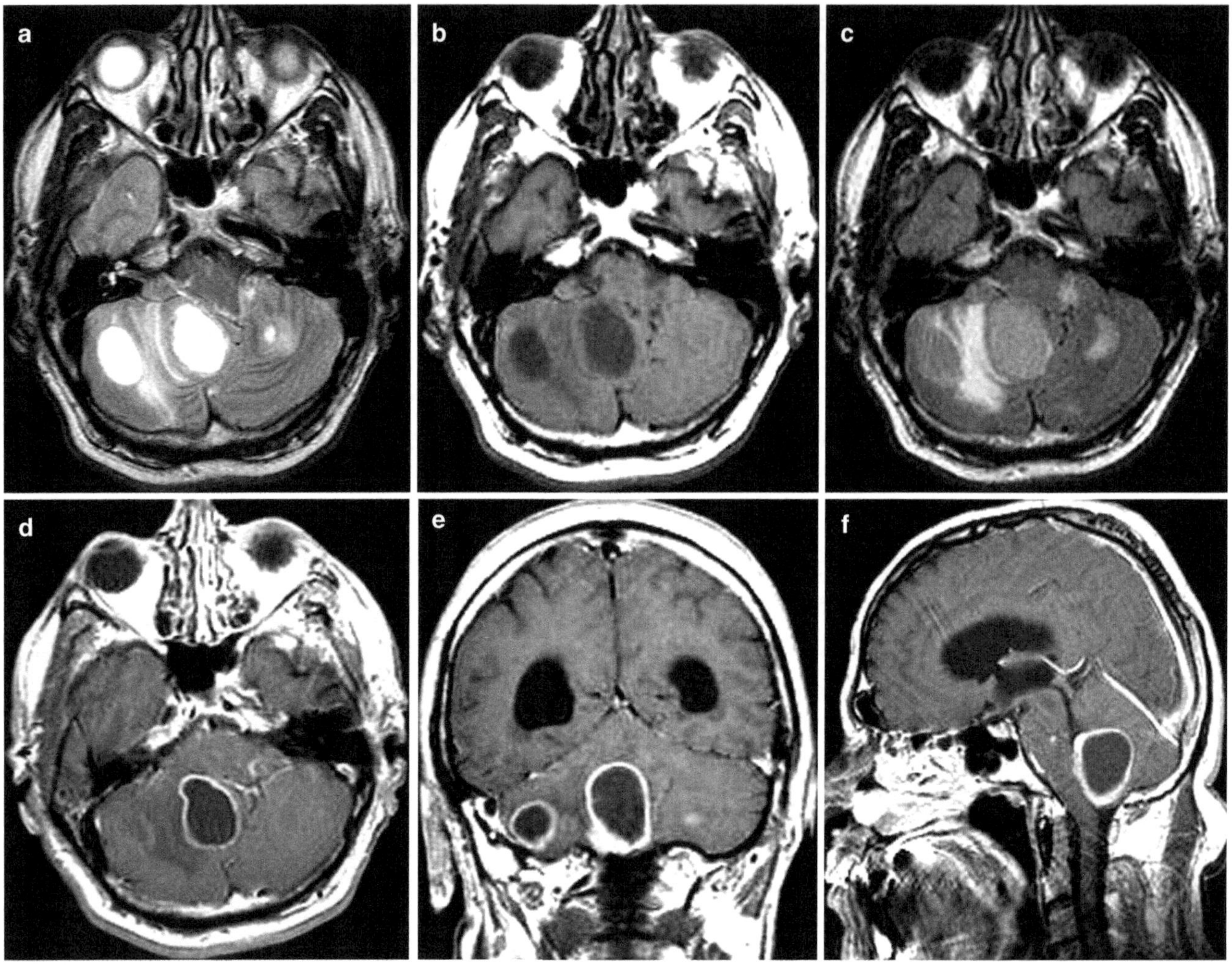

Fig. 12.11 Multiple lung cancer metastases in the brain. In both cerebellar hemispheres, there are solid cystic lesions with a moderate perifocal edema (**a**–**c**). After the administration of the contrast agent, its intense accumulation is noted mainly on the periphery of the lesions (**d**–**f**). On frontal sections (**e**) in the area of the cerebellar vermis, along the lower contour of the metastasis, a solid tumor fragment is well visualized

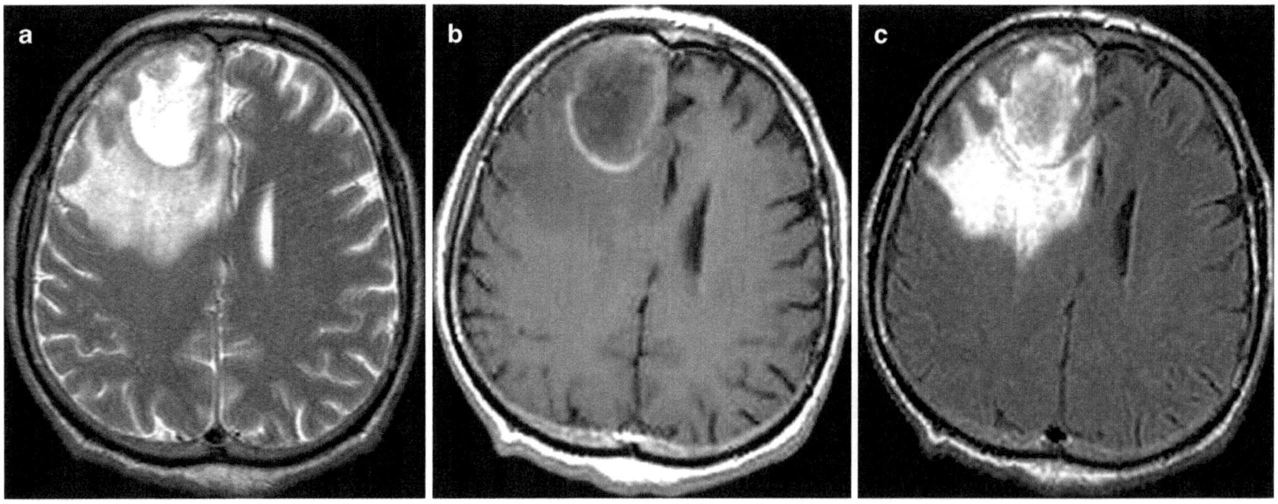

Fig. 12.12 A lung cancer metastasis in the brain. In the right frontal area, there is a solitary cystic lesion with a pronounced perifocal edema (**a**, **b**, **c**) with a hemorrhage area along the contour (**b**) and a hyperintense signal in T1-weighted MRI. No apparent signs of an increased T1-weighted signal after intravenous CA injection on a background of hemorrhagic changes were identified (**d**–**f**)

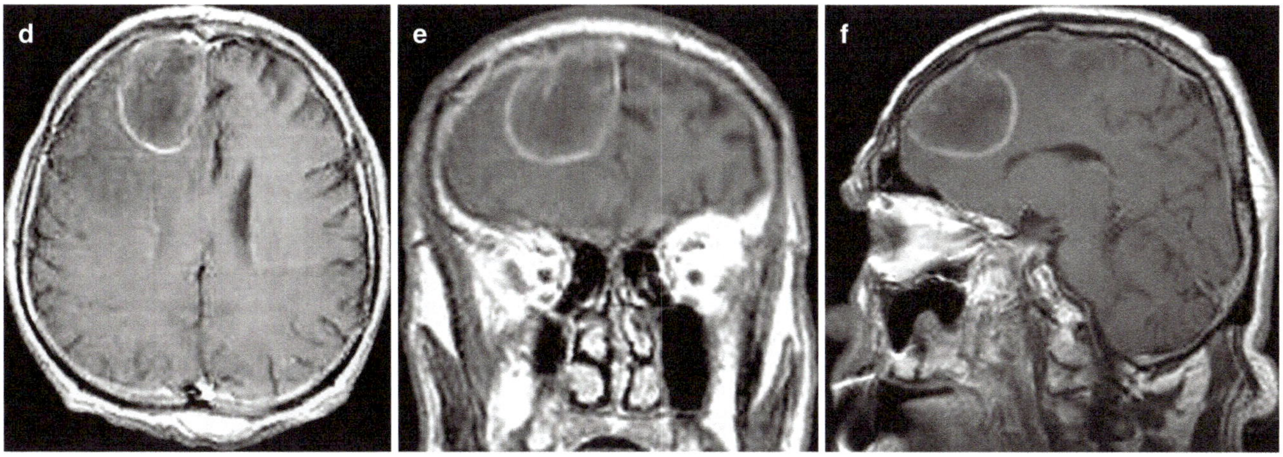

Fig. 12.12 (continued)

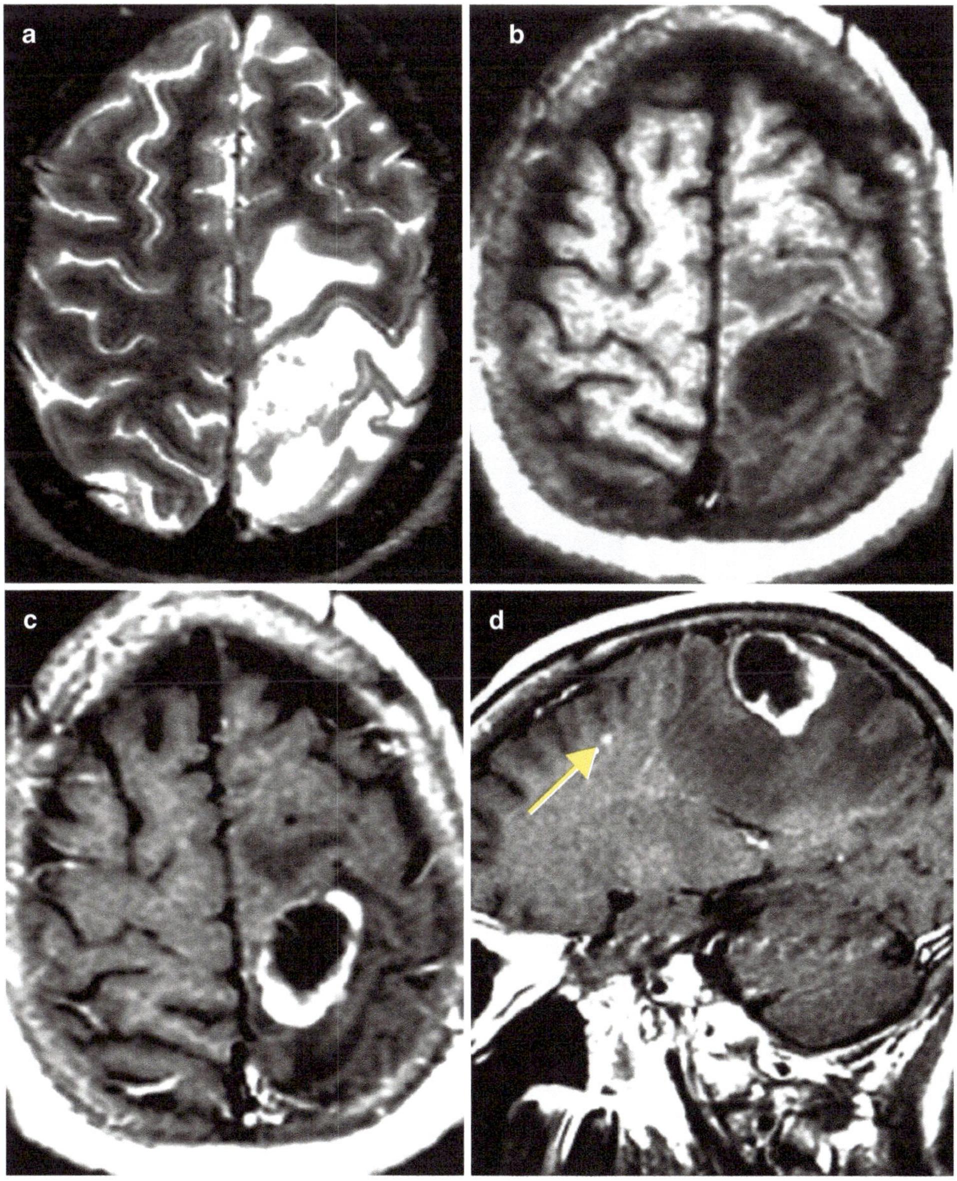

Fig. 12.13 Multiple lung cancer metastases in the brain. In the left parietal region, there is a rounded cystic lesion with a pronounced perifocal edema (**a**). The cystic part of the tumor has a hypointense signal on T1-weighted MRI (**b**), while the solid one (an iso-hypointense signal) merges with the brain substance. After the CA administration, its intense accumulation along the contour of the lesion (**c**, **d**) with a more pronounced thickening at its posteroinferior pole is observed. In addition, the contrasting allowed to visualize a pinpoint metastatic lesion (the *arrow*) in the sagittal projection, anteriorly to the above (**d**) lesion

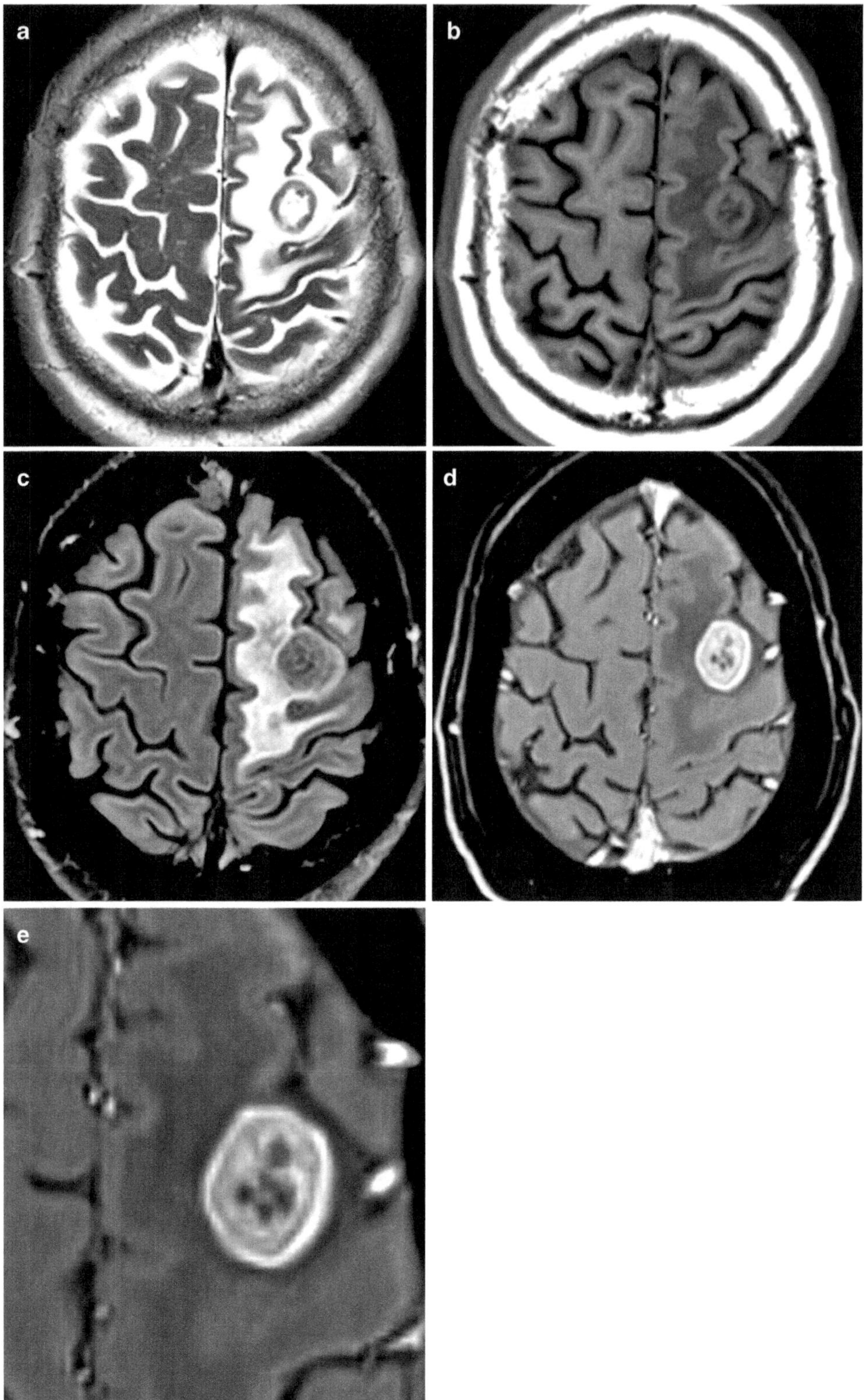

Fig. 12.14 Lung cancer metastasis in the brain. In the left frontal area, there is a rounded space-occupying lesion with the solid structure, clear, smooth contours, and an area of a pronounced perifocal edema (**a**). On T1-weighted and T2-FLAIR MRI, the signal from the metastasis is isointense (**b**, **c**). After IV CA administration, its intense accumulation (**d**, **e**) is noted in the lesion, with a more pronounced CA accumulation being observed in the marginal parts of the tumor

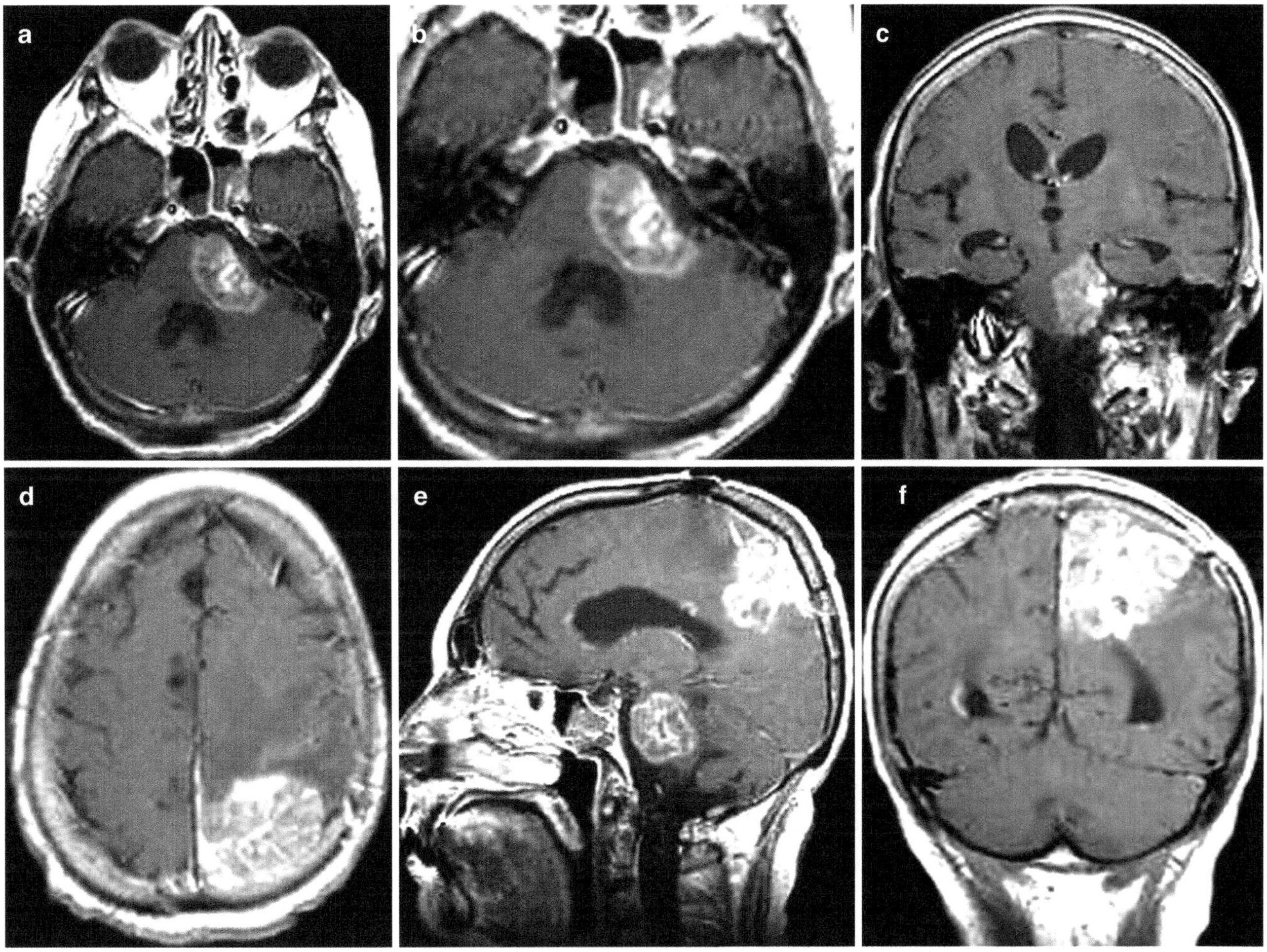

Fig. 12.15 Multiple lung cancer metastases in the brain. A two-level study after the surgical removal and radiation therapy. There are large metastases in the pons (**a**, **b**, **c**, **e**) and a recurrent tumor in the left parietal region (**d**, **e**, **f**). Metastases intensely accumulate CA and have a solid structure

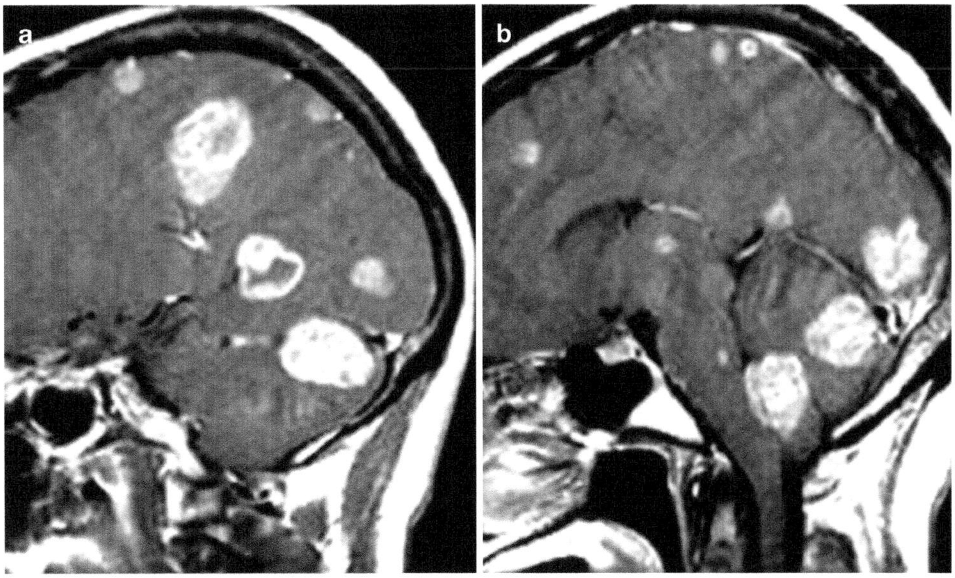

Fig. 12.16 Multiple lung cancer metastases in the brain. There are multiple solid-cystic lesions intensely and unevenly accumulating CA in the brain matter, both sub- and supratentorially, as well as in the brain stem, in the sagittal (**a**, **b**) and frontal (**c**, **d**) projections. Lesions, regardless of their size, have both a cystic-solid and solid structure

Fig. 12.16 (continued)

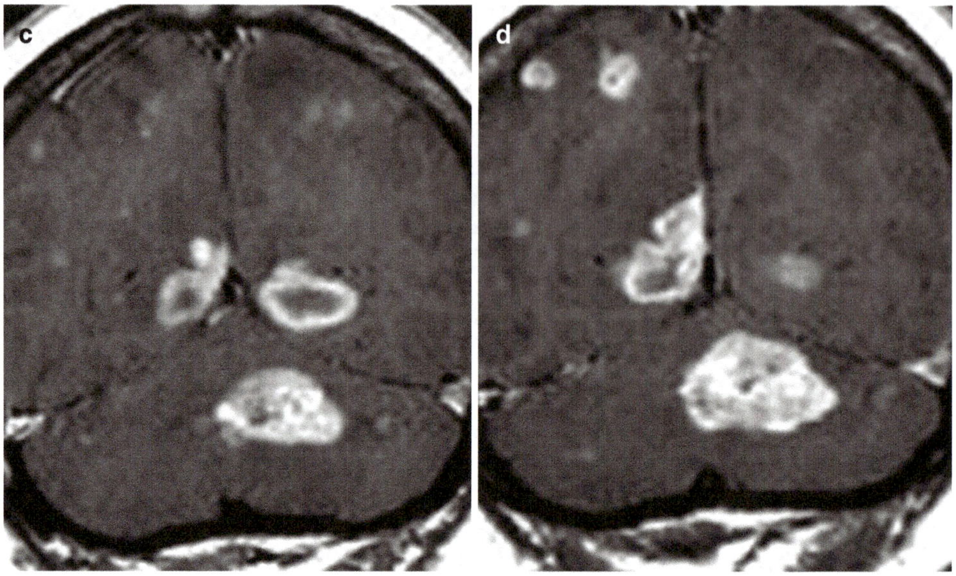

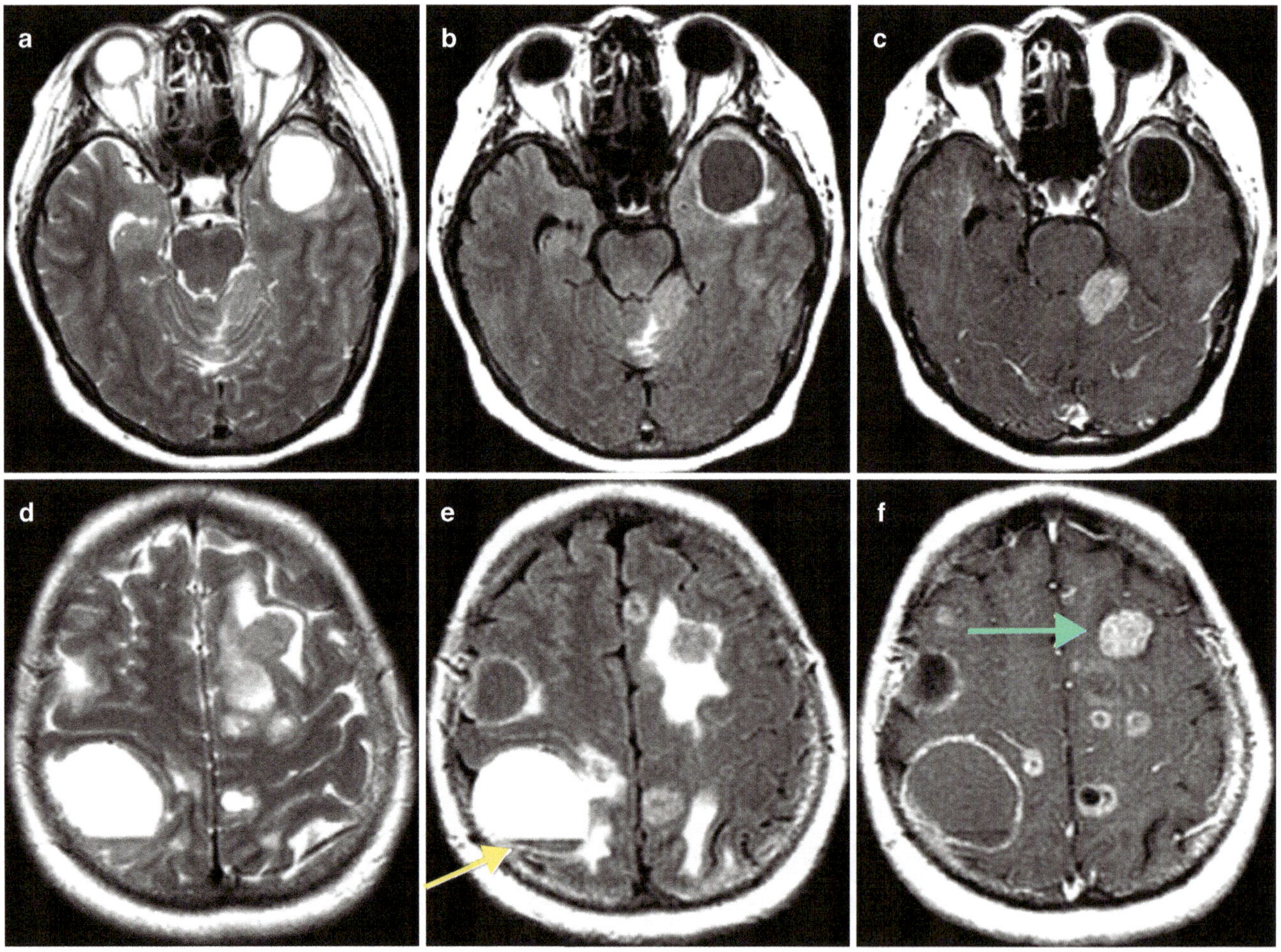

Fig. 12.17 Multiple lung cancer metastases in the brain. A three-level study. In all parts of the brain, there are multiple lesions with solid, cystic, and solid-cystic structure with signs of heterogeneously expressed perifocal edema (**a**, **b**, **d**, **e**). Following intravenous administration of CA, all the lesions intensely and unevenly accumulate the contrast agent (**c**, **f**, **g**–**i**). The largest lesion (**e**) has a cystic form with the "level" of hemorrhagic content (the *arrow*), and others (**f**), in spite of their superior size, have solid structures (the *arrow*)

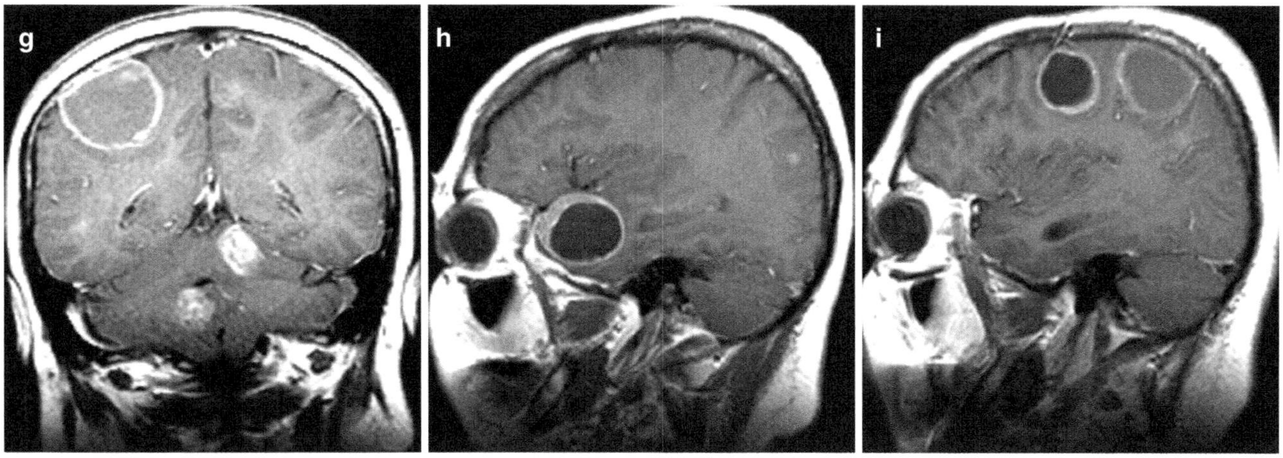

Fig. 12.17 (continued)

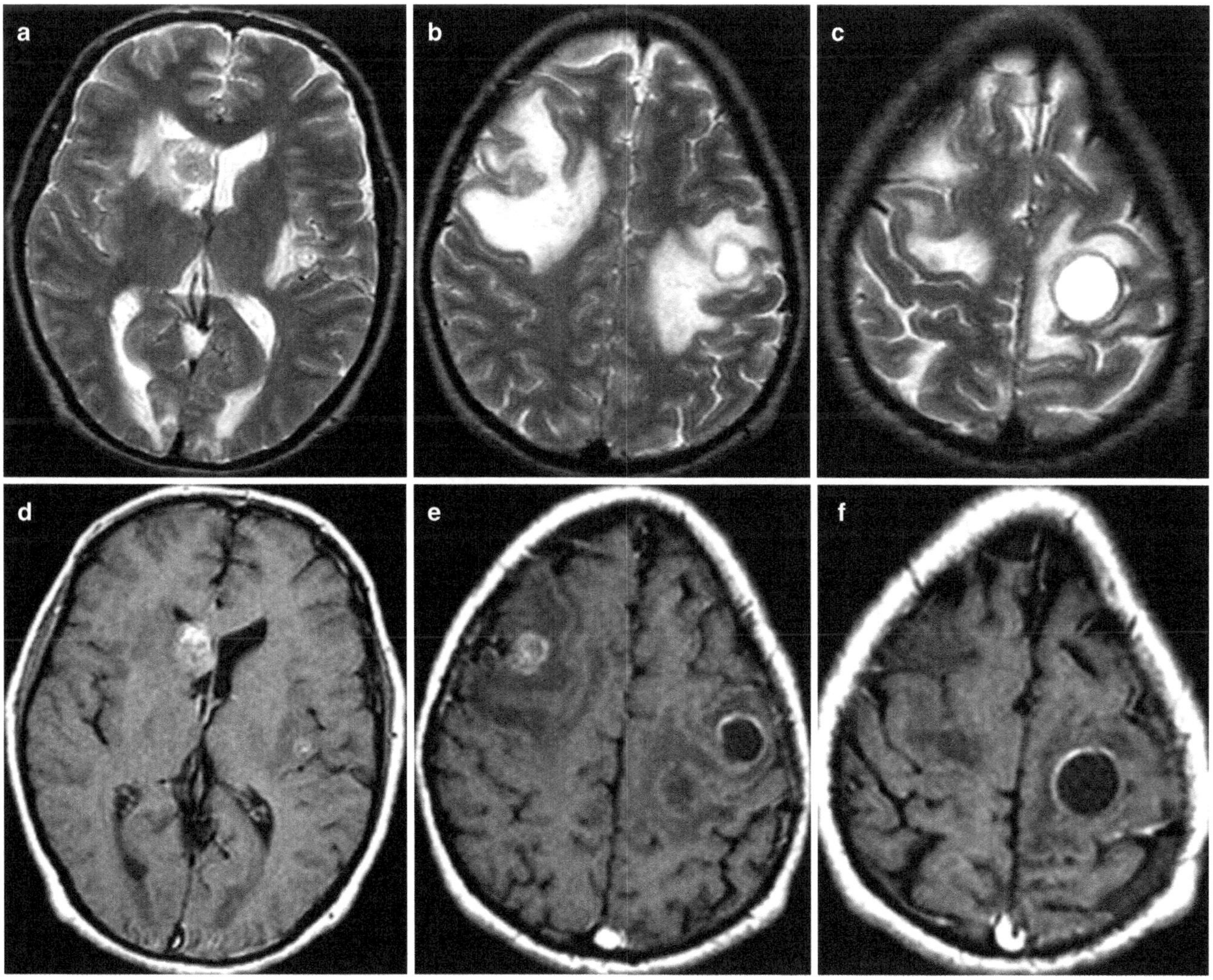

Fig. 12.18 Multiple lung cancer metastases in the brain. A three-level study. In the brain matter, there are multiple space-occupying lesions, some of which have solid structures, while others are predominantly cystic (**c**–**h**) and have a pronounced perifocal edema (**a**–**c**). After administration of CA, the solid lesions accumulate it intensely and unevenly, while the cystic ones accumulate it along their contours (**e**, **f**, **i**)

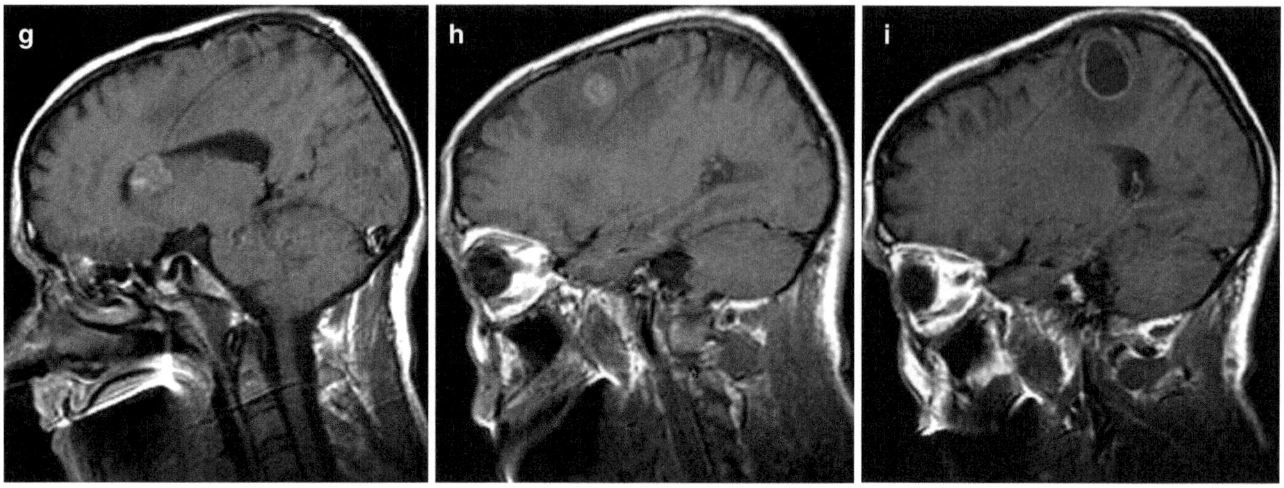

Fig. 12.18 (continued)

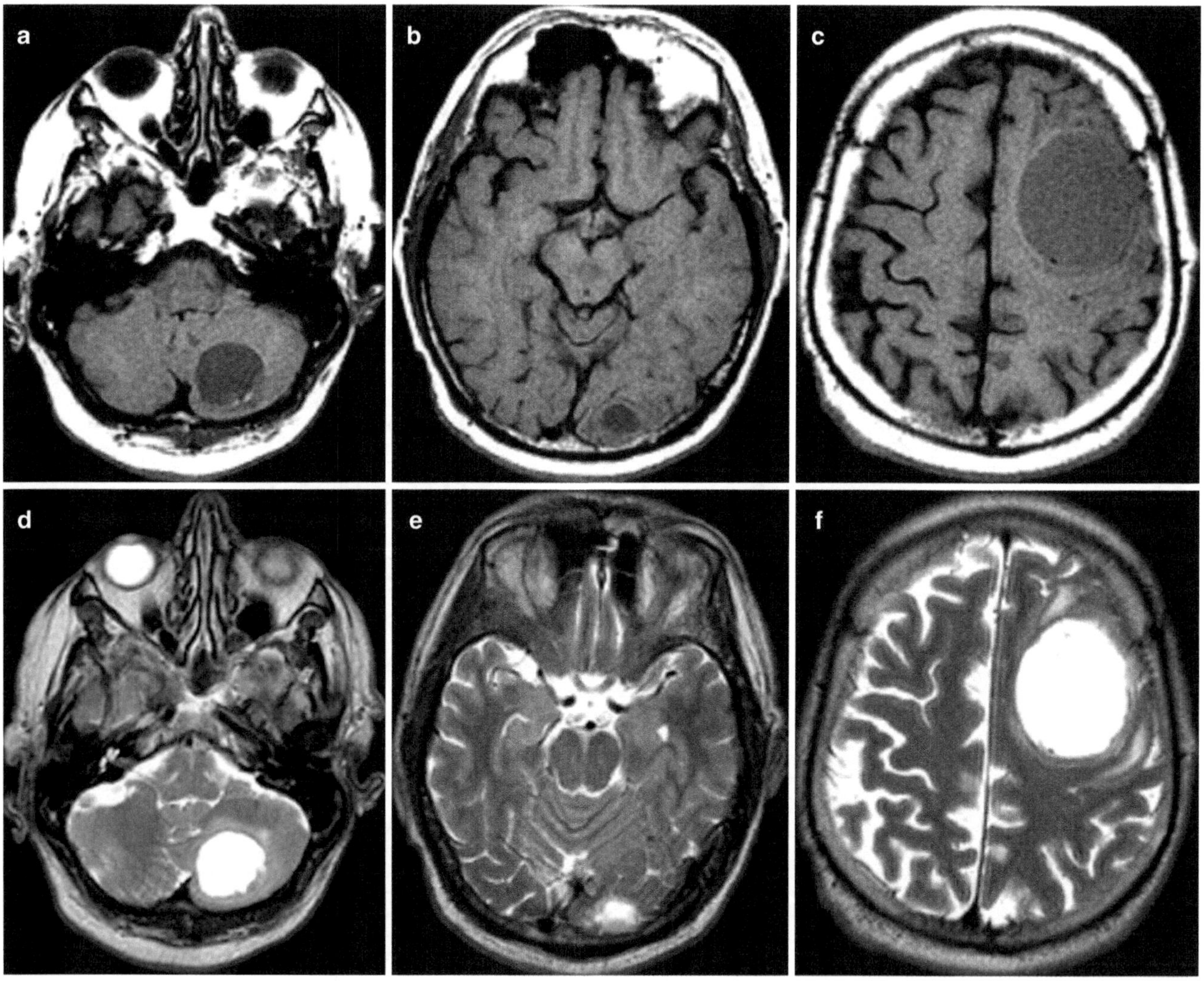

Fig. 12.19 Multiple lung cancer metastases in the brain. A three-level study. In the left cerebellar hemisphere (**a**), in the left occipital region (**b**), and the left frontal lobe (**c**), there are solid-cystic lesions, while the accompanying perifocal edema is mild despite their large size (**d**, **e**, **f**). After administration of CA, its accumulation along the contour of the cavities with the formation of nodules in most solid tumor fragments is observed on T1-weighted MRI in the axial (**g**, **h**, **i**) and frontal (**j**, **k**, **l**) projections

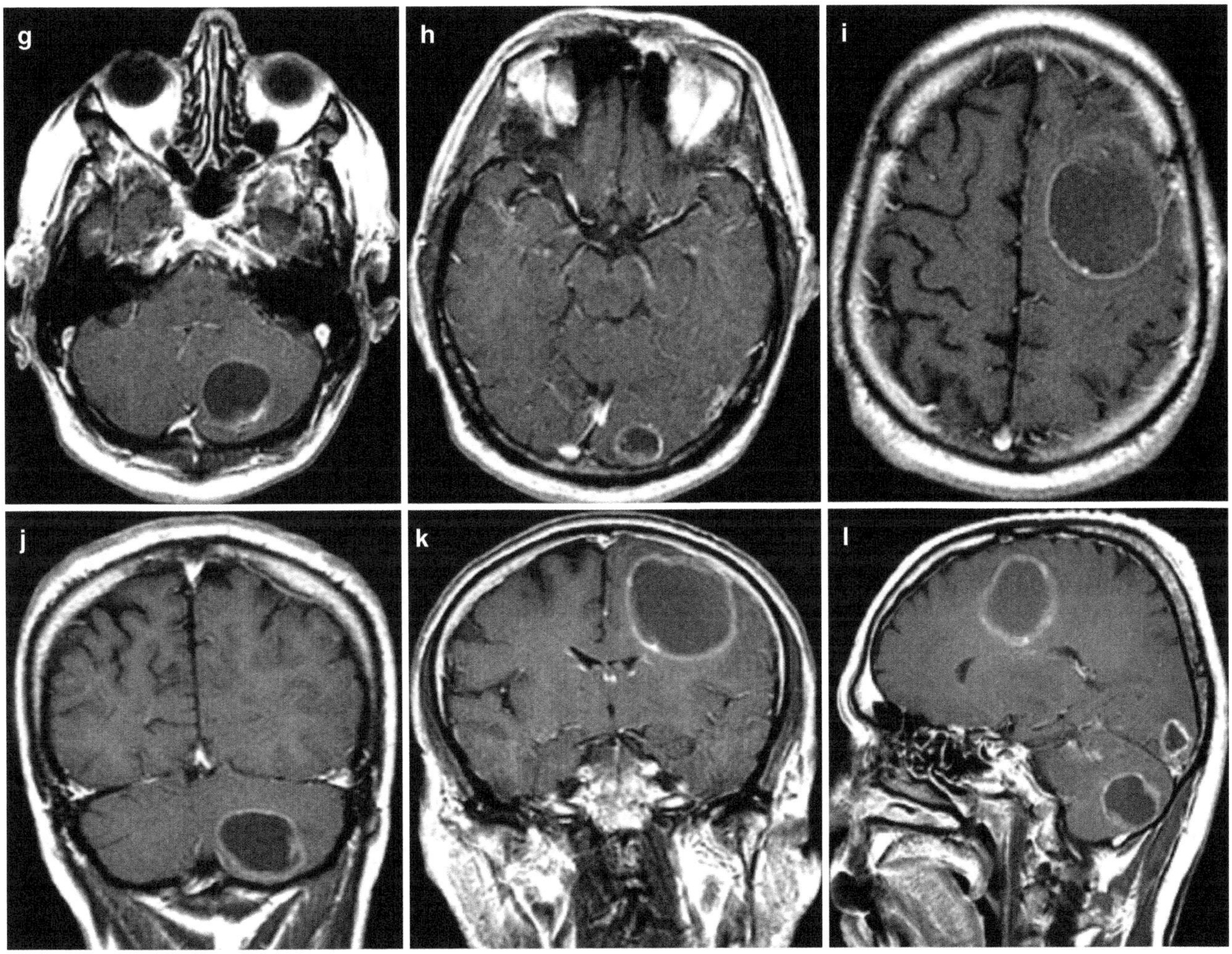

Fig. 12.19 (continued)

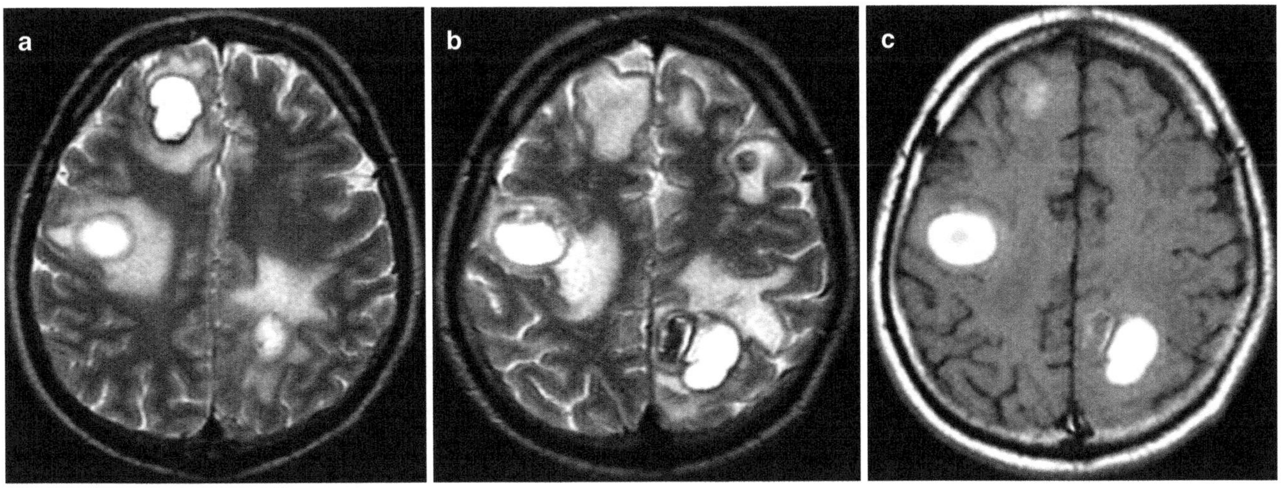

Fig. 12.20 Multiple lung cancer metastases in the brain. A two-level study. In both hemispheres of the brain, there are multiple lesions with a solid-cystic structure and a pronounced perifocal edema (**a**, **b**). Without intravenous contrast agent, there is an intense, uneven increase in the signal from lesions in T1-weighted images, which displays a hemorrhagic component of the tumor: axial (**c**, **d**) and sagittal (**e**, **f**) projections

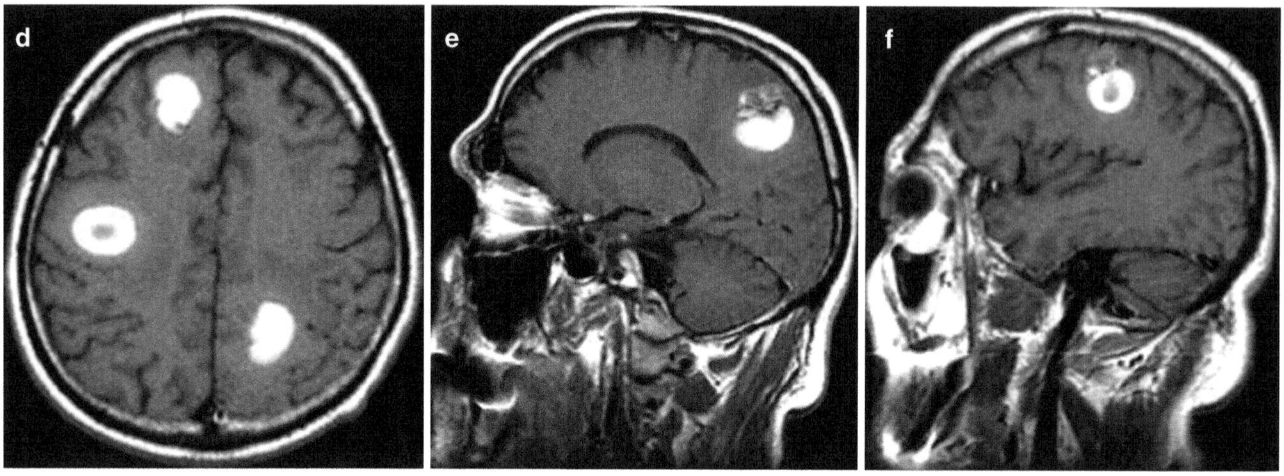

Fig. 12.20 (continued)

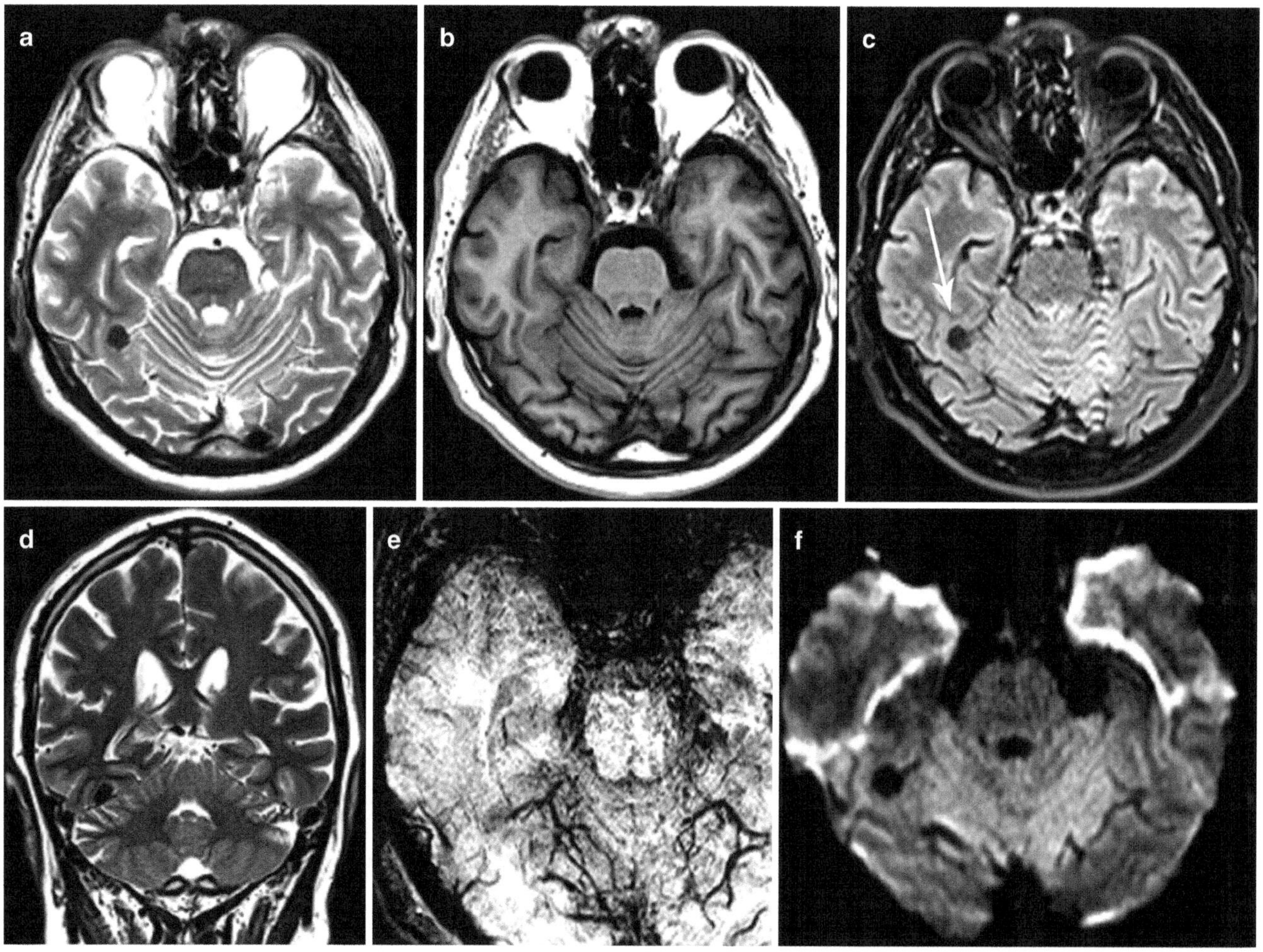

Fig. 12.21 A lung cancer metastasis in the brain. In the right posterior temporal region, there is a small rounded lesion closely adjacent to the cerebellar tentorium. The metastasis is characterized by a low MR signal on T2-weighted (**a**, **d**), T2-FLAIR (**c**) (the *arrow*), and DW (**f**) images with no signs of perifocal edema and an isointense signal on T1-weighted images (**b**). There are no hypointense inclusions in the tumor structure in SWI images (**e**). The lesion intensely accumulates the contrast agent (**g**, **h**, **i**)

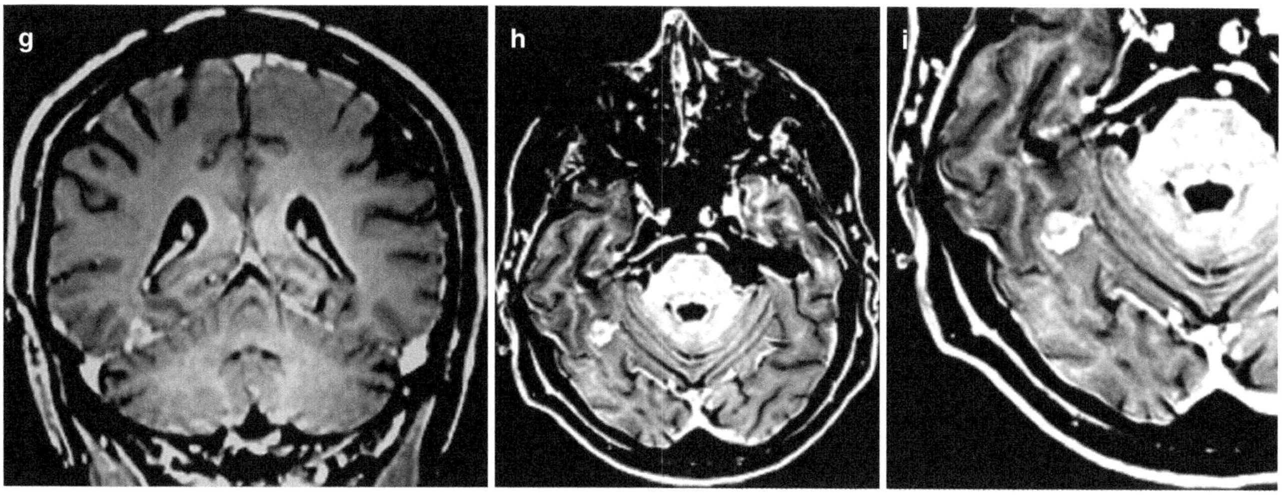

Fig. 12.21 (continued)

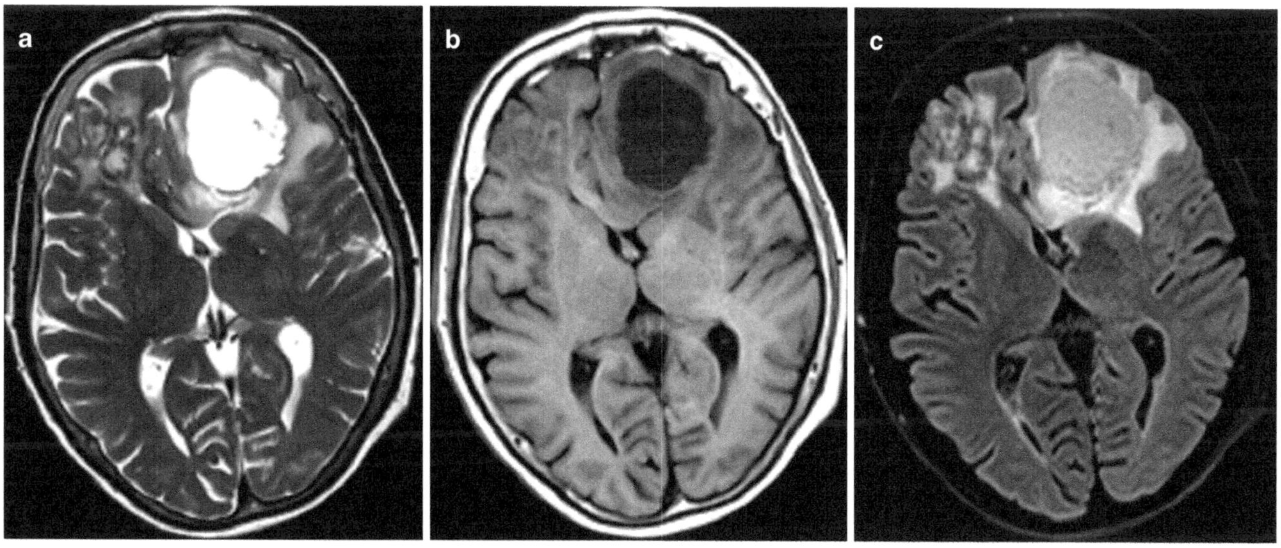

Fig. 12.22 Multiple lung cancer metastases in the brain. In the substance of the cerebral hemispheres, there are multiple lesions with various sizes, with heterogeneously hyperintense signal in T2-weighted and T2-FLAIR (**a**, **c**) images and hypointense in T1-weighted images (**b**). After IV administration of CA on T1-weighted fat suppression MRI (**d**, **e**), its intense accumulation is observed on the periphery of the lesions. The largest metastasis is located in the left frontal lobe with a significant mass effect manifested in the form of the compression of the anterior horn of the left lateral ventricle and displacement of the midline structures; however, the perifocal edema is mild. On SWI MRI (**f**, **g**), a small number of hypointense inclusions are detected only along the lateral contour of the large lesion. On ASL MRI (**h**), the solid part of lesions is characterized by a poor blood flow. On MR tractography (**i**), the conductive pathways are not differentiated in the area of the large lesion in the left frontal lobe

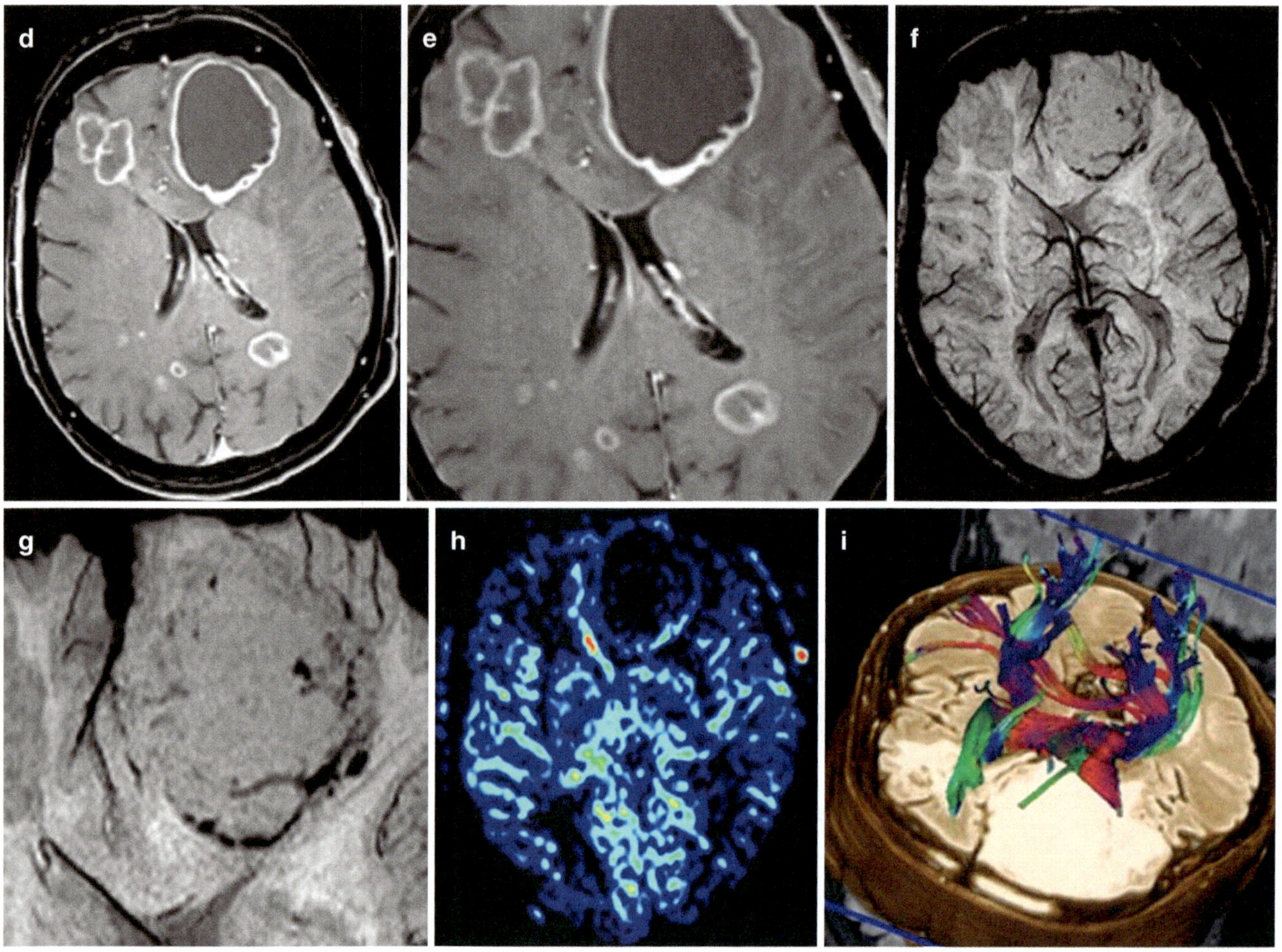

Fig. 12.22 (continued)

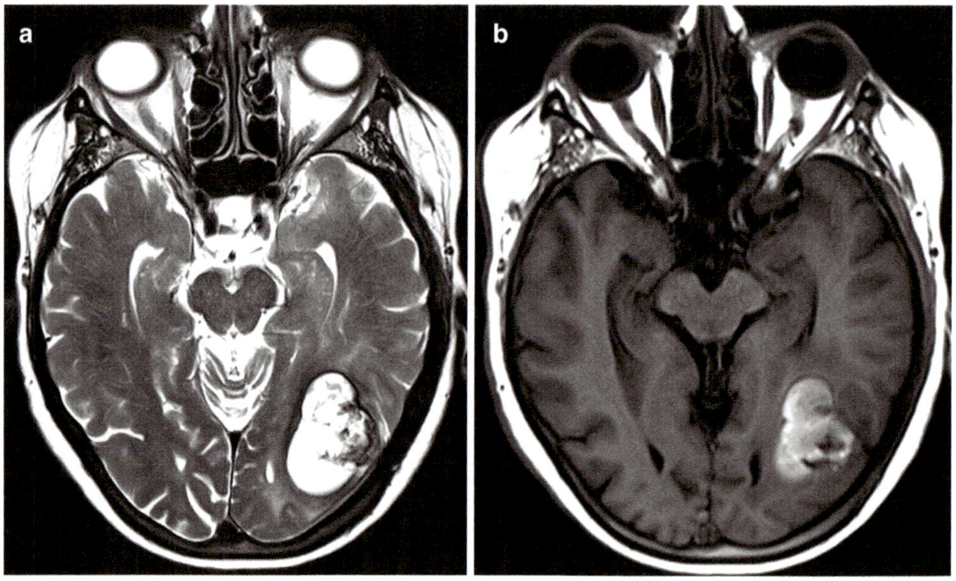

Fig. 12.23 A lung cancer metastasis in the brain. In the left occipital region, there is a heterogeneous lesion on T2-weighted (**a**), T1-weighted (**b**), and T2-FLAIR (**c**) MRI due to an expressed hemorrhagic component. The lesion unevenly accumulates the contrast agent predominantly along the lateral contour (**d**). The perifocal edema is minimal

Fig. 12.23 (continued)

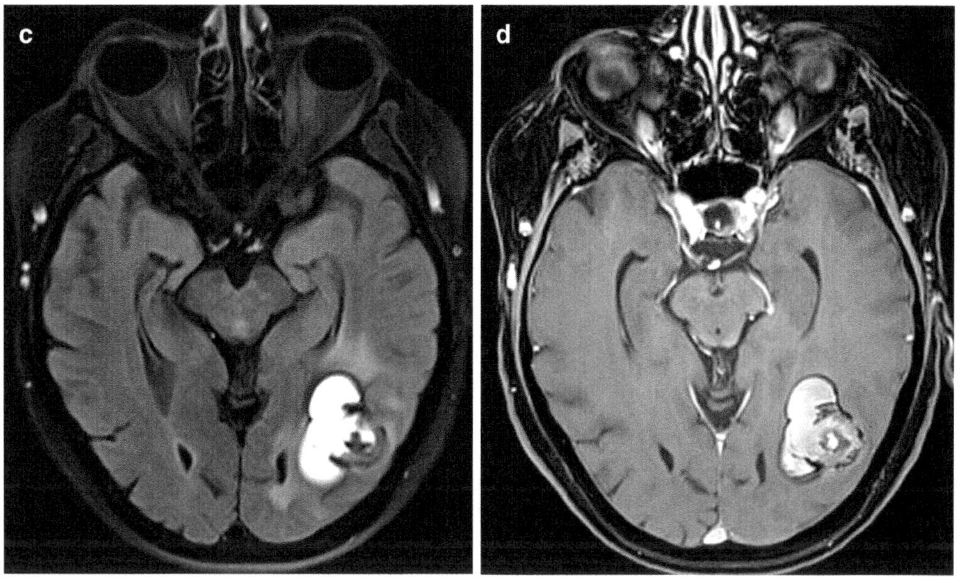

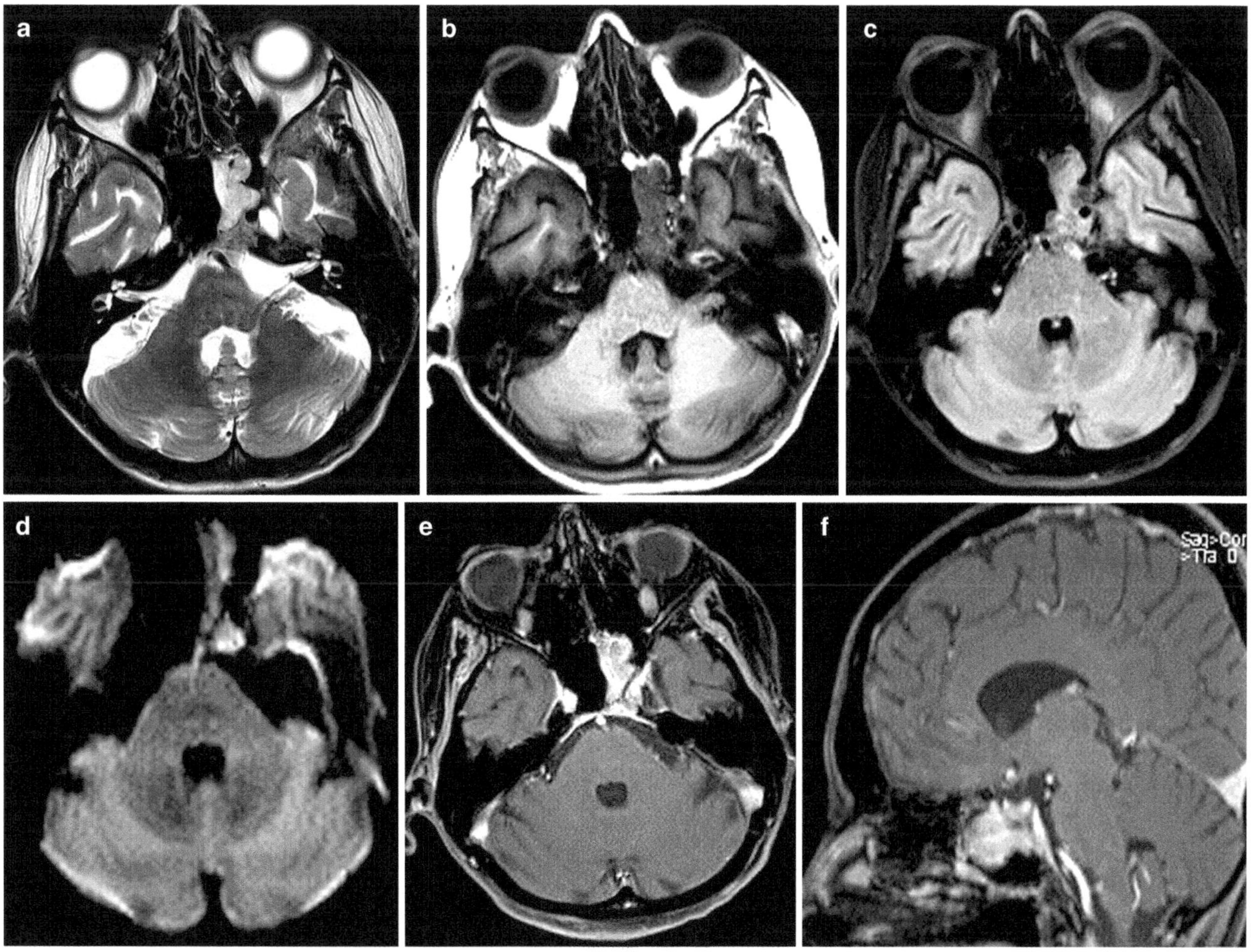

Fig. 12.24 A lung sarcoma metastasis in the brain. In the left half of the sphenoid sinus, there is a soft tissue lesion with an increased signal in T2-weighted (**a**) images, iso-hypointense signal on T1-weighted (**b**) images, and moderately high in T2-FLAIR (**c**) and DWI (**d**) images. Following intravenous administration of CA, an intense, uniform accumulation of the contrast agent (**e**, **f**) is observed. The lesion extends posteriorly to the sphenoid bone and cavernous sinus and partially envelops the left ICA

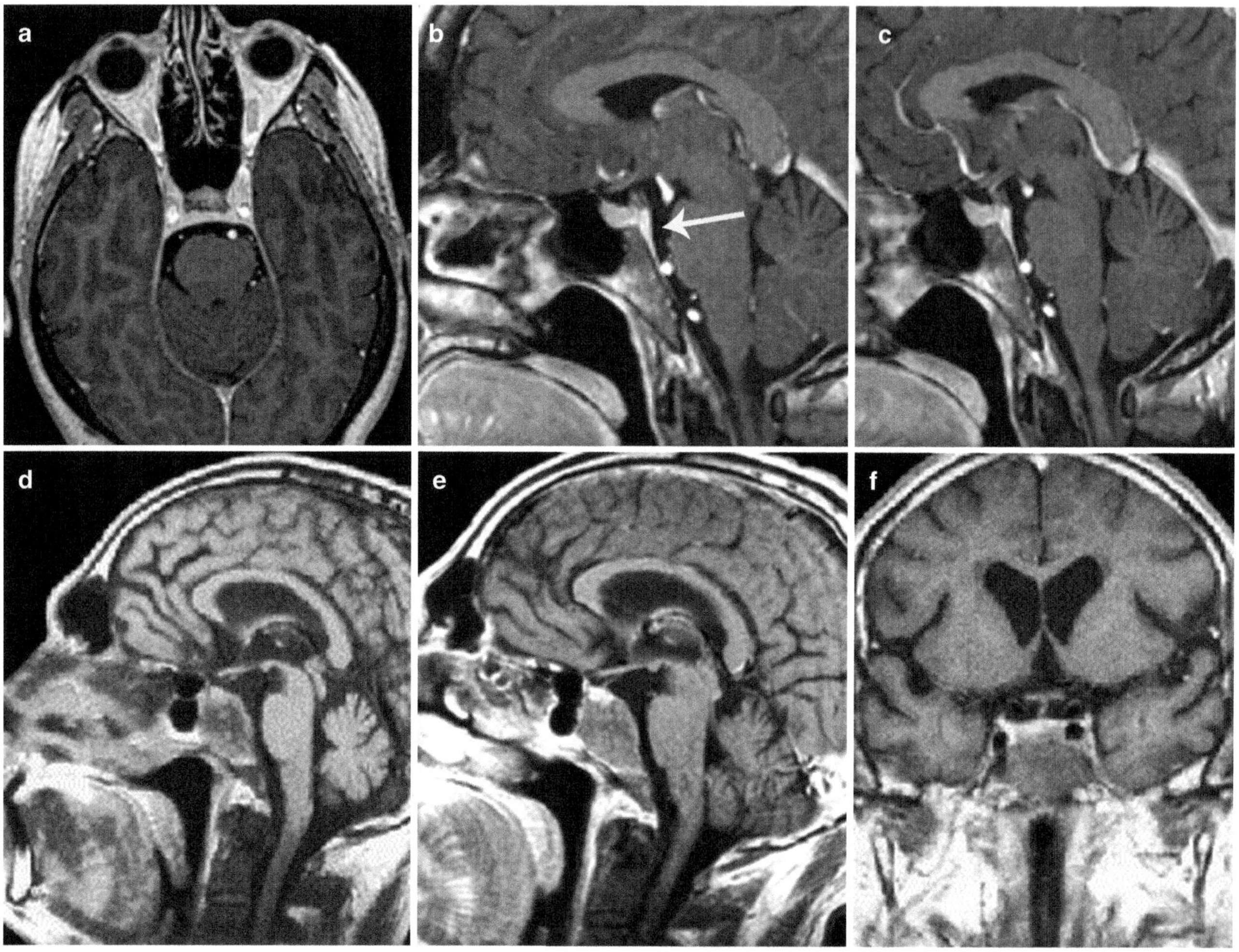

Fig. 12.25 Lung cancer metastases in the brain. *Case No. 1* (**a**–**c**). MR scans in the axial (**a**) and sagittal (**b**, **c**) projections after the administration of contrast agent show a change in the MR signal from the clivus of the sphenoid bone, a local thickening, and expressed contrast enhancement of the dura posteriorly and downward from the Turkish saddle (the *arrow*). *Case No. 2*. Metastatic lesions of the clivus with a decrease in the MRI signal intensity from its structure and with a change in the form (**d**). After the contrast agent administration (**e**, **f**), its accumulation is moderately expressed and diffuse. The absence of boundaries between the adenohypophysis and the affected bone tissue of the clivus indicates a destruction of the cortical bone

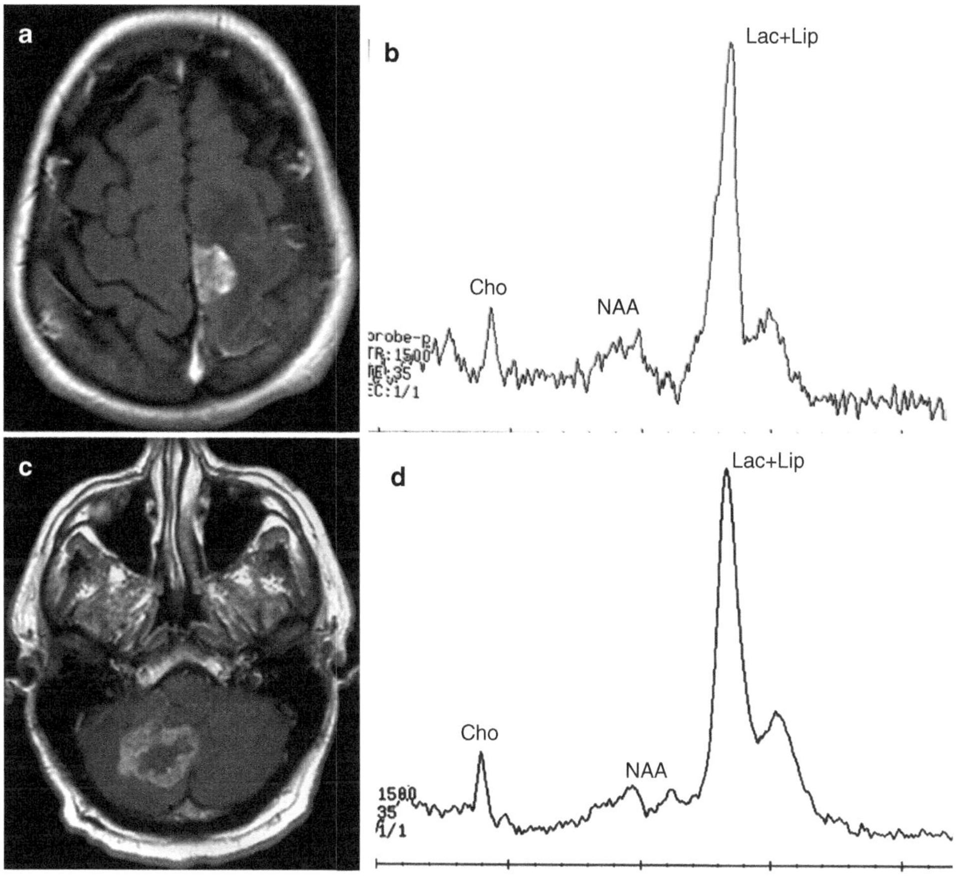

Fig. 12.26 Cancer metastases in the brain. (**a**) and (**b**) a parasagittal metastasis of lung cancer in the left frontoparietal region: MRI with contrast enhancement (**a**) and MR spectrum (**b**). On the MR spectrum, there is an increased Lip-Lac complex and a moderate Cho peak. (**c**) and (**d**) a kidney cancer metastasis in the right hemisphere of the cerebellum: MRI with contrast enhancement (**c**) and MR spectrum (**d**). MR spectrum shows peaks identical to those in image (**b**)

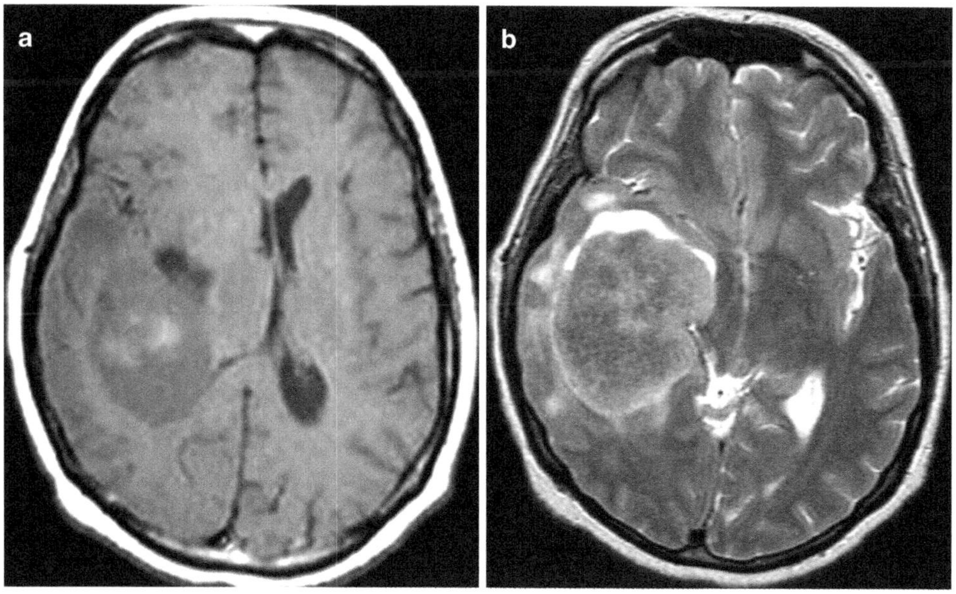

Fig. 12.27 A lung cancer metastasis in the brain. In the right temporofrontal area, there is a space-occupying lesion with a heterogeneous structure (**a**), causing the displacement of the midline structures, without an expressed perifocal edema, characterized by a moderately hypointense signal on T2-weighted MRI (**b**) and unevenly accumulating the contrast agent (**c**–**e**). MR spectroscopy determined a significant increase in the Lip-Lac complex and a decrease in other peaks (**f**) in the lesion structure

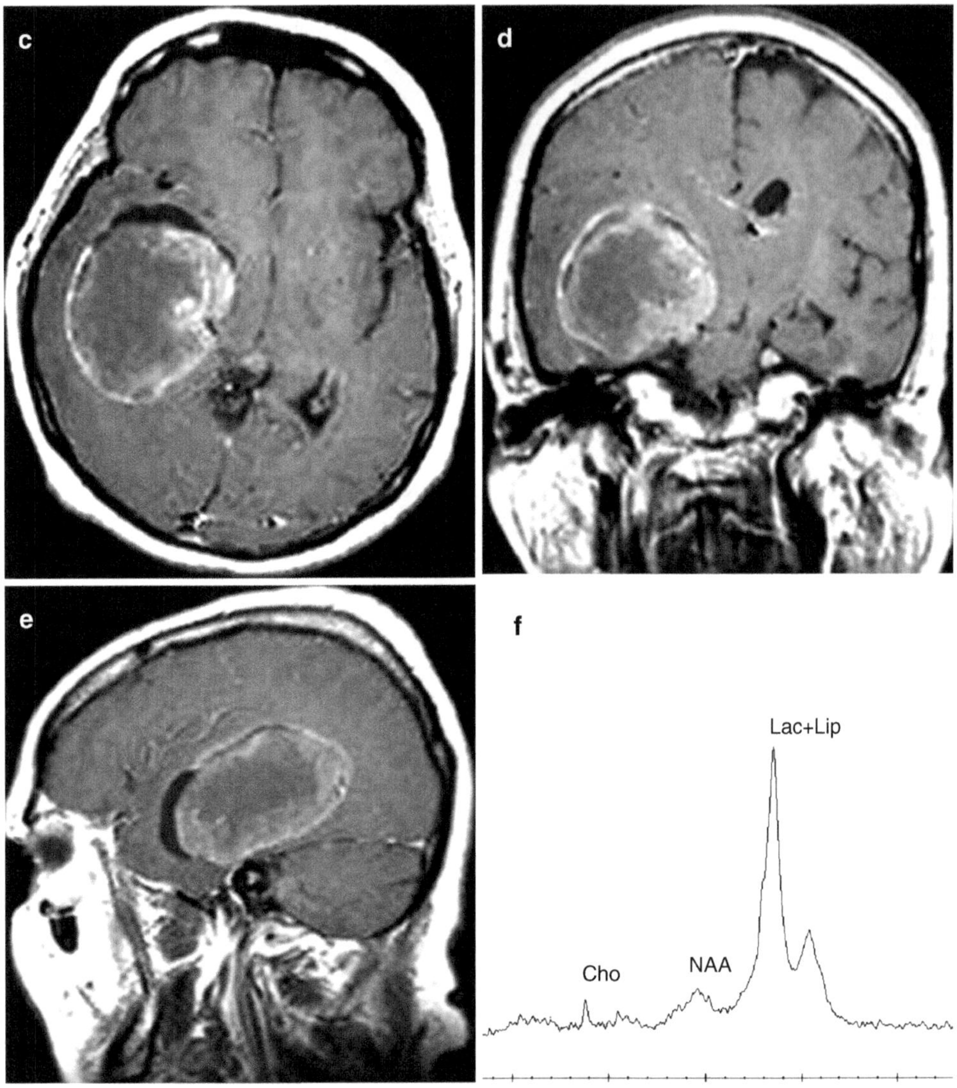

Fig. 12.27 (continued)

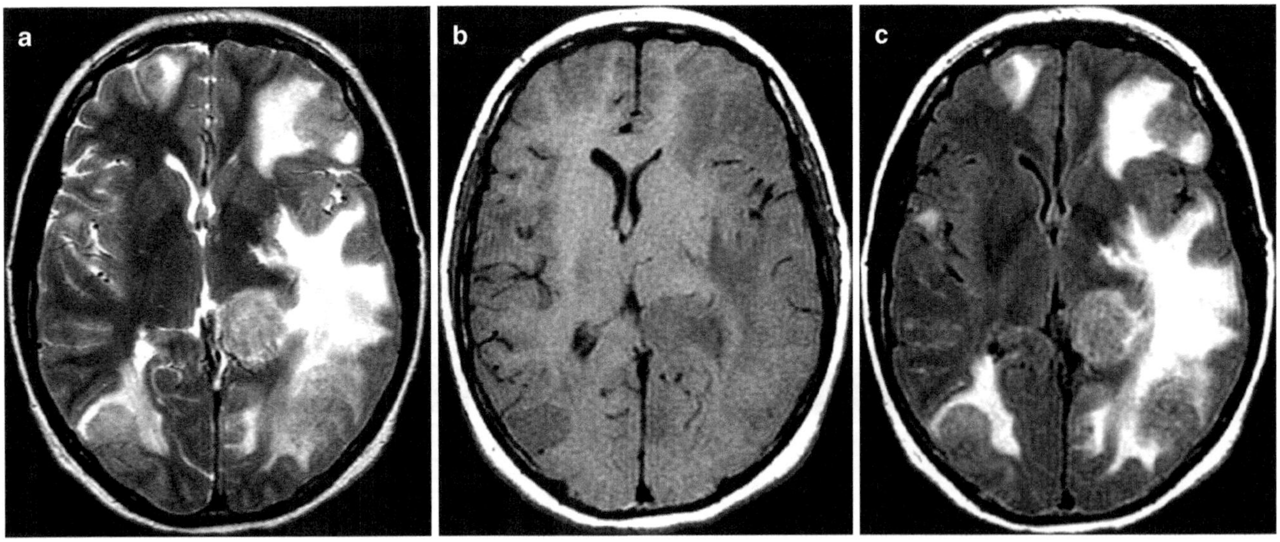

Fig. 12.28 Multiple lung cancer metastases. In the brain matter, there are multiple solid lesions with an area of expressed perifocal edema (**a**, **c**). The lesions have a mildly reduced signal on T1-weighted MRI (**b**) and an increased signal on DWI MRI (**d**). After intravenous administration of the contrast agent, all lesions intensely, evenly accumulate the contrast agent (**e**, **f**). On MR spectroscopy, a marked increase in the Lip-Lac complex with a simultaneous reduction in the height of other peaks (**g**, **h**)

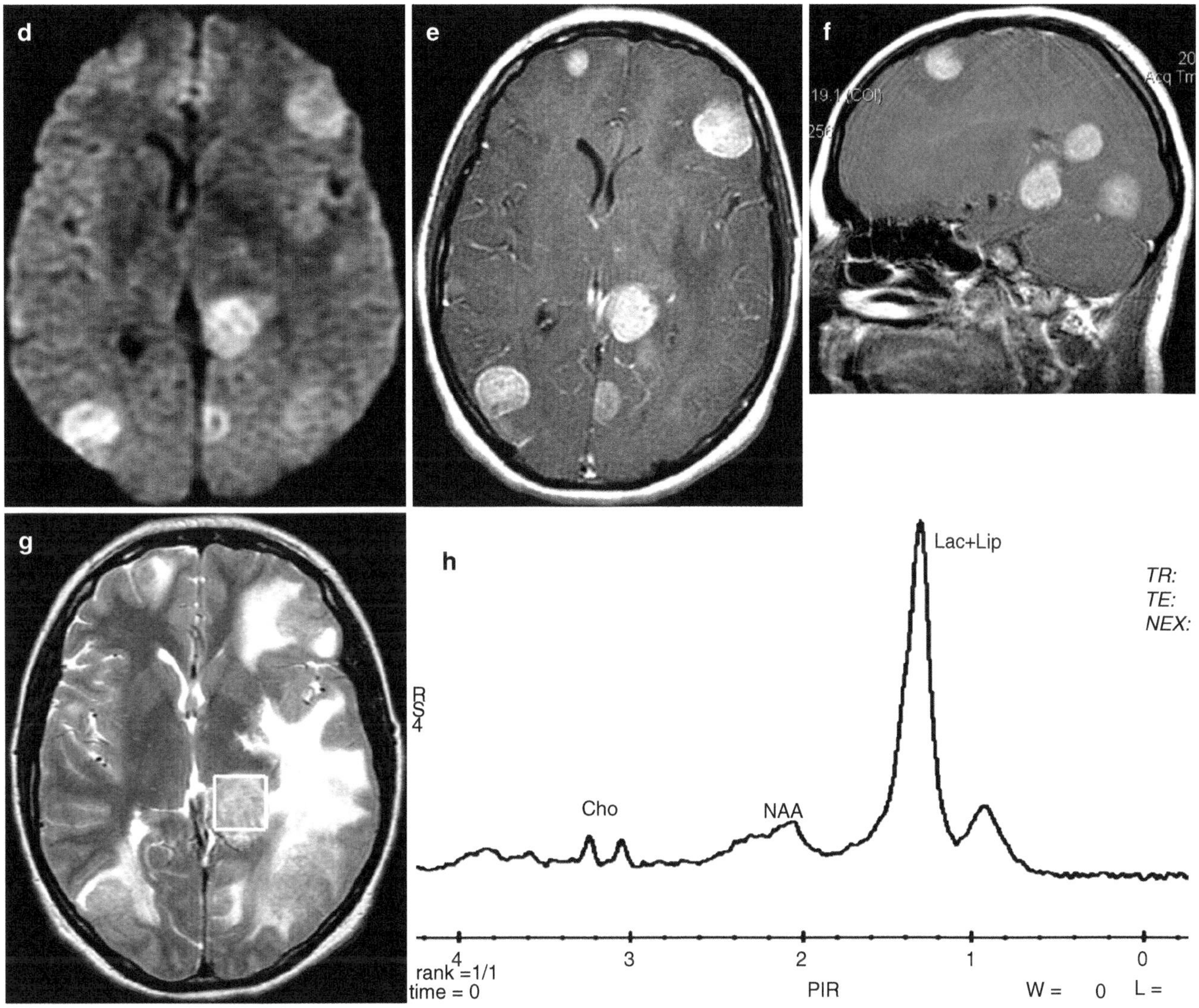

Fig. 12.28 (continued)

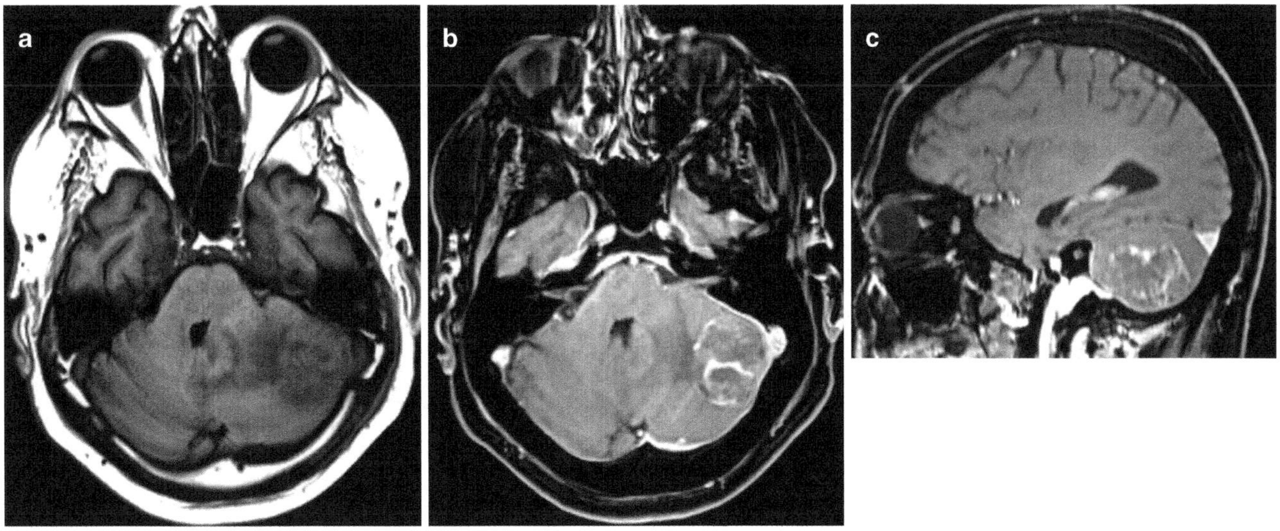

Fig. 12.29 A lung cancer metastasis. In the left cerebellar hemisphere, there is a lesion with a hypointense MR signal on T1-WI MRI (**a**), with signs of uneven accumulation of the contrast agent (**b, c**). On SWI MRI, individual pinpoint inclusions with a hypointense MR signal (**d, e**) are observed in the tumor structure. On DWI MRI, the signal from the tumor is heterogeneously increased (**f**). On MR tractography, there is a marked displacement of the conductive pathways upward and medially with respect to the tumor (**g–i**)

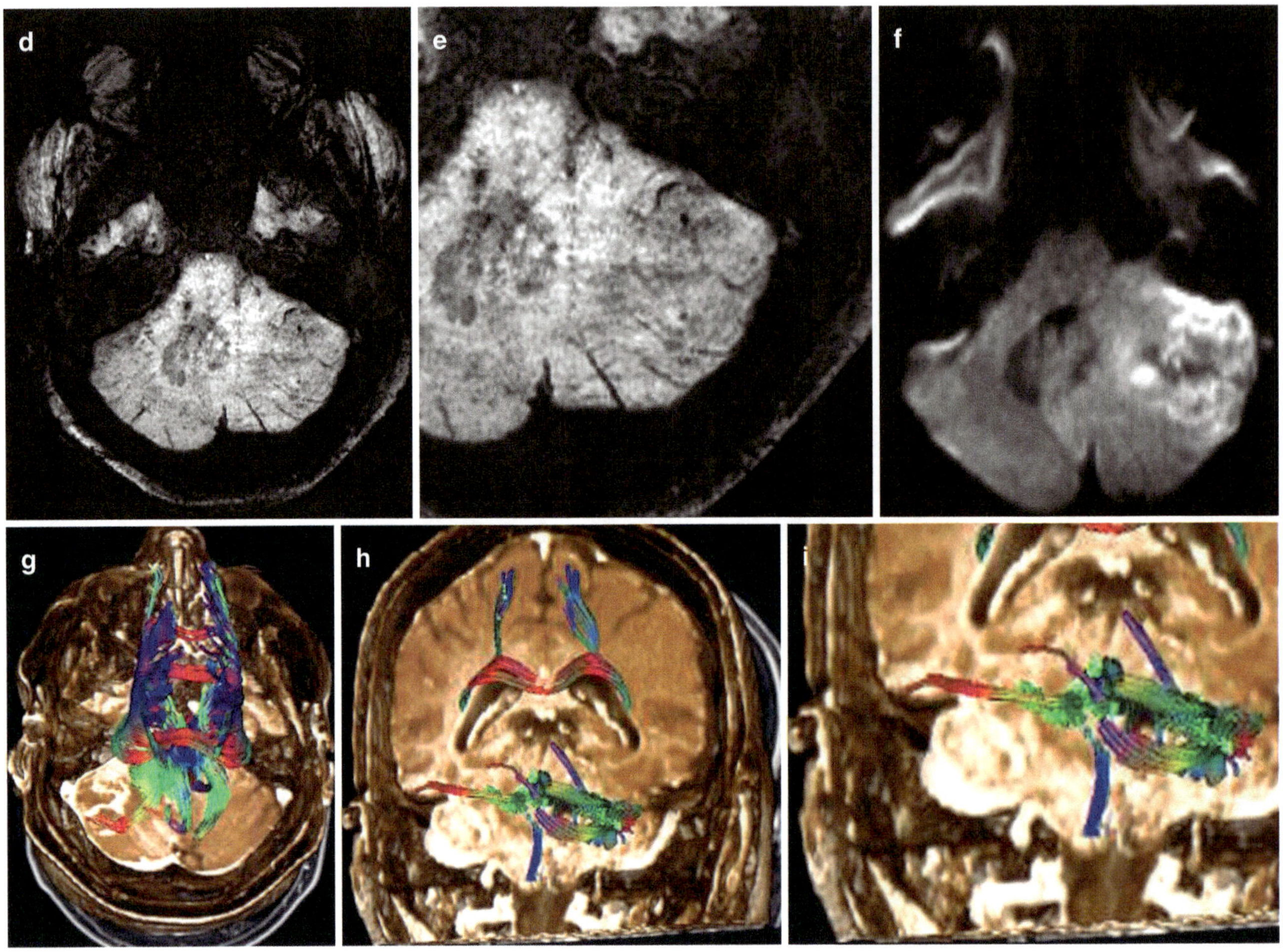

Fig. 12.29 (continued)

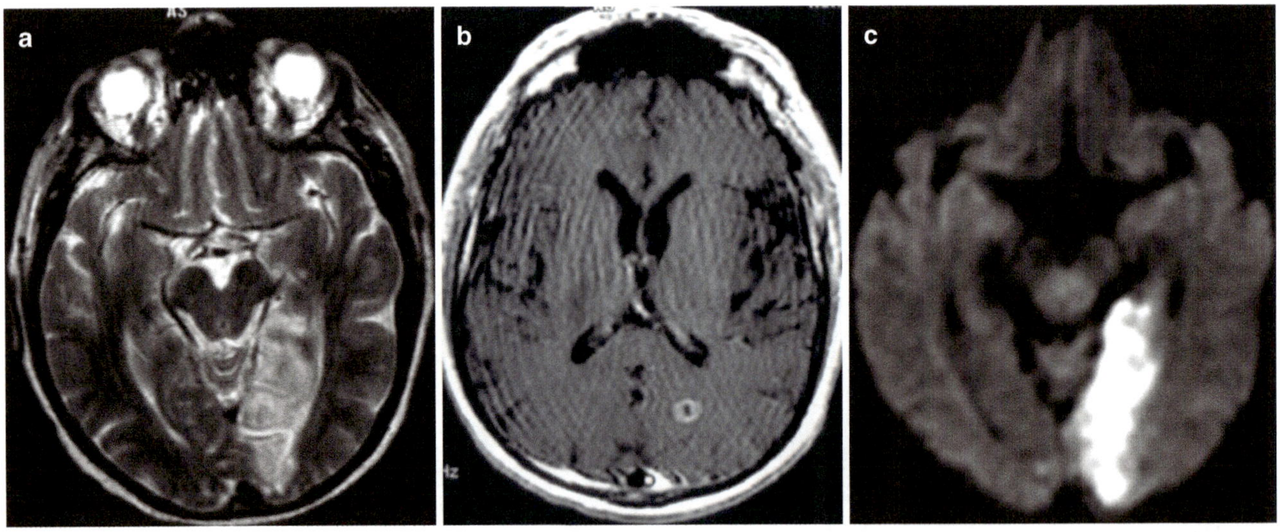

Fig. 12.30 A lung cancer metastasis in the brain. On T2-weighted MRI (**a**), in the left area of the occipital lobe, there is an abnormal increase in the MR signal. After contrast enhancement, a small ring-shaped metastasis (**b**) is identified in the occipital lobe. On DWI MRI (**c**), an area with an increased MR signal on T2-weighted MRI is consistent with a focus of acute ischemia in the left posterior cerebral artery system and is not a perifocal edema around the metastatic lesion

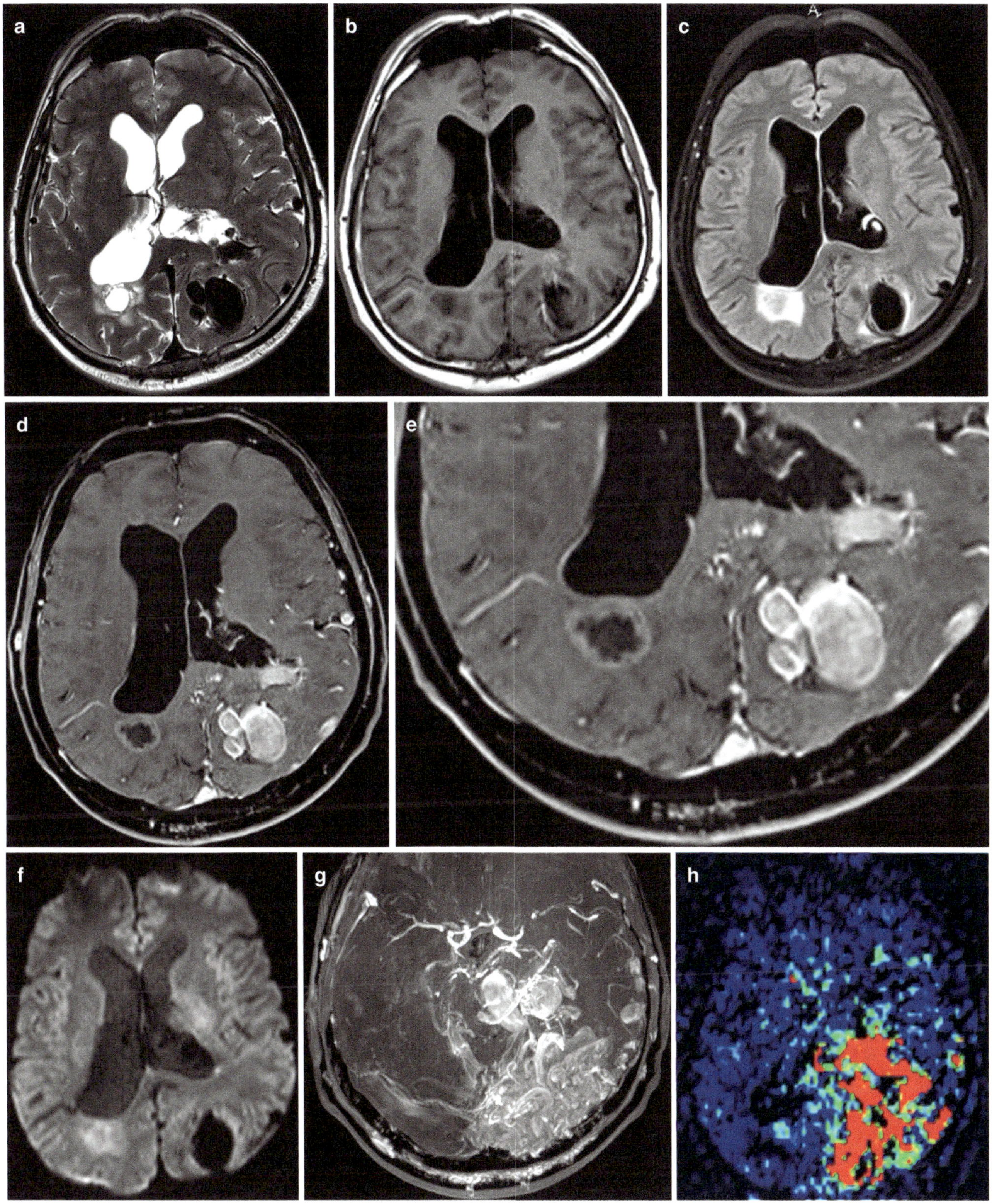

Fig. 12.31 A lung cancer metastasis in the brain. An arteriovenous malformation in the left parietal-occipital region and a venous angioma in the right temporoparietal region. Posteriorly to the posterior horn of the right lateral ventricle in the right occipital region, there is a solid-cystic rounded lesion with an increased signal on T2-weighted (**a**) and T2-FLAIR MRI (**c**), with an area of a moderate perifocal edema. The lesion moderately accumulates the contrast agent (**d**, **e**), mostly on the periphery. In the left occipital region, there is a giant AVM, hypointense in all the "standard" sequences (**a**–**c**), intensely accumulating the contrast agent (**d**, **e**). Venous angioma in the right temporoparietal region—in the form of a linear region intensely accumulating the contrast agent (**d**, **e**). On DWI MRI, the metastasis has an increased signal, while AVM and venous angioma have decreased signals (**f**). A MIP reconstruction visualizes the entire AVM volume intensely accumulating CA (**g**). On ASL MRI, there is a large area with an increased blood flow in the AVM projection and a moderate increase in the metastasis (**h**)

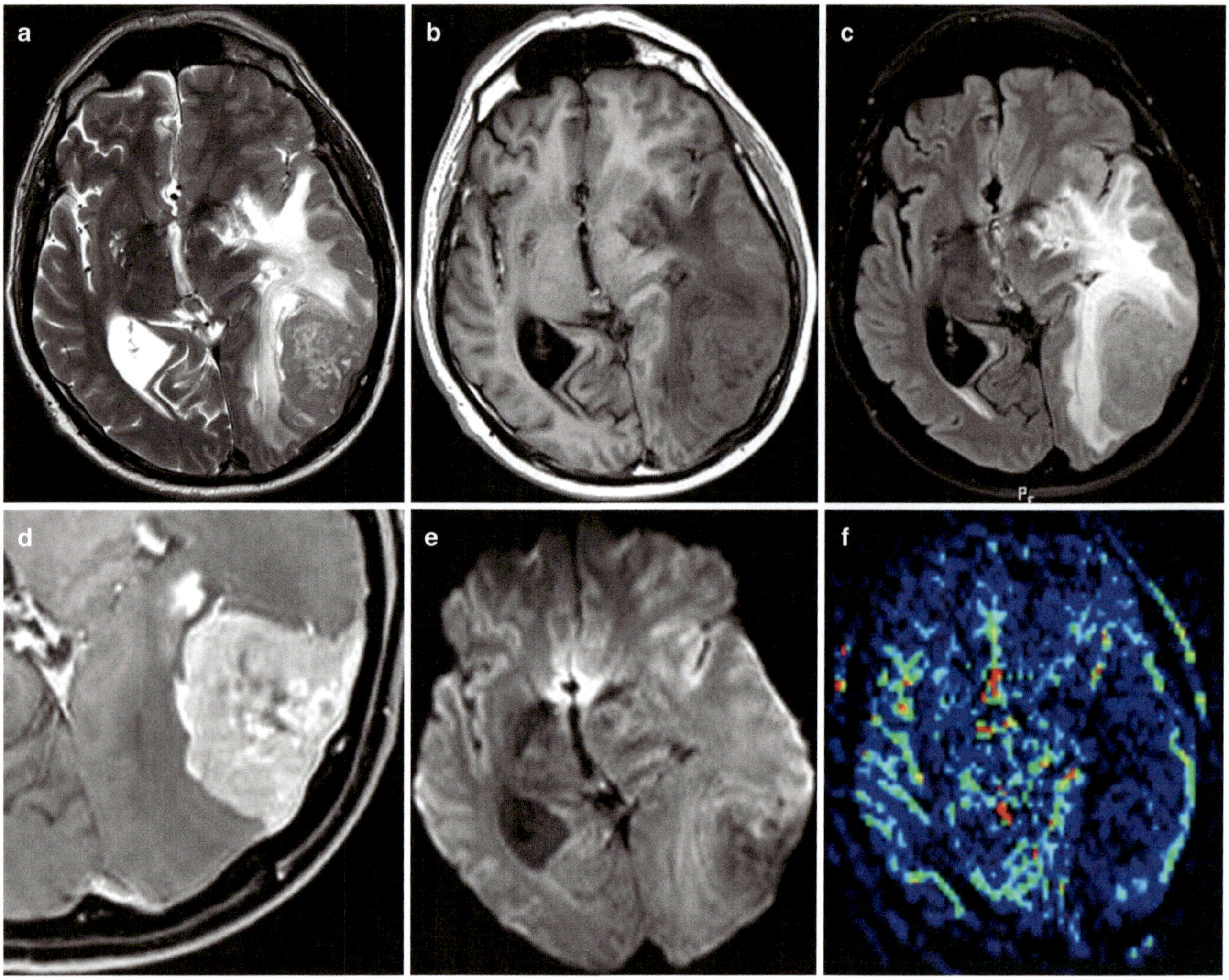

Fig. 12.32 A lung cancer metastasis. In the left occipital region, there is a space-occupying lesion closely adjacent to the dura mater, with a small area of necrosis in the central parts, surrounded by a pronounced perifocal edema (**a**–**c**). After CA administration, its intense, uneven accumulation is noted in the tumor and adjacent brain membranes (**d**). On DW images (**e**), the lesion is characterized by a decreased signal. On ASL MRI, no findings indicative of an increase in the tumor blood flow were obtained (**f**)

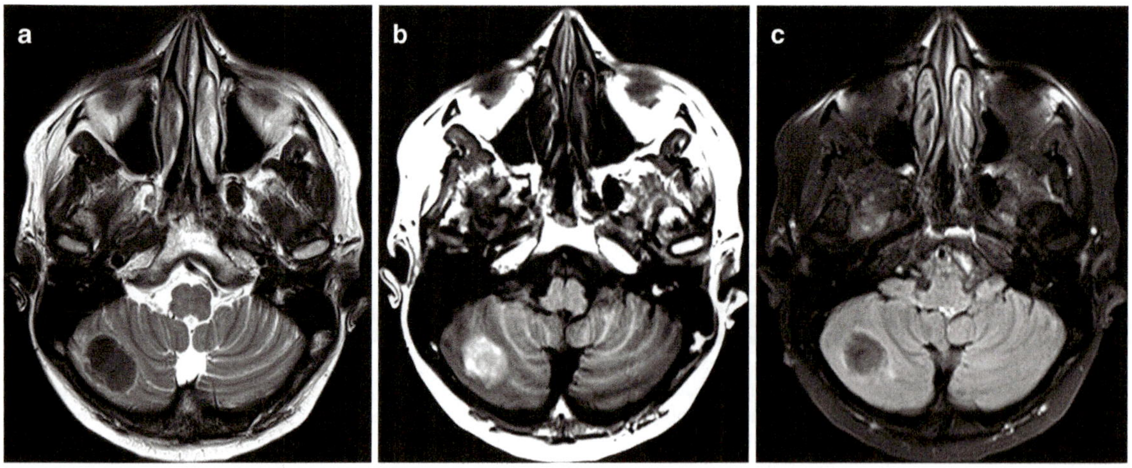

Fig. 12.33 Multiple lung cancer metastases in the brain. MR images at two levels of the brain. Tumor lesions in the right cerebellar hemisphere and the right frontal lobe with a moderate perifocal edema are characterized by a low signal on T2-weighted (**a**, **d**) and T2-FLAIR (**c**, **f**) MRI and a high signal (hemorrhagic inclusions) on T1-weighted MRI (**b**, **e**). On DWI MRI, the signal from the central parts of metastases is reduced (**g**, **j**). There is uneven accumulation of CA in the lesions, mostly on the periphery (**h**, **k**). On ASL MRI, these lesions have reduced CBF values (**i**, **l**) with respect to the intact brain substance

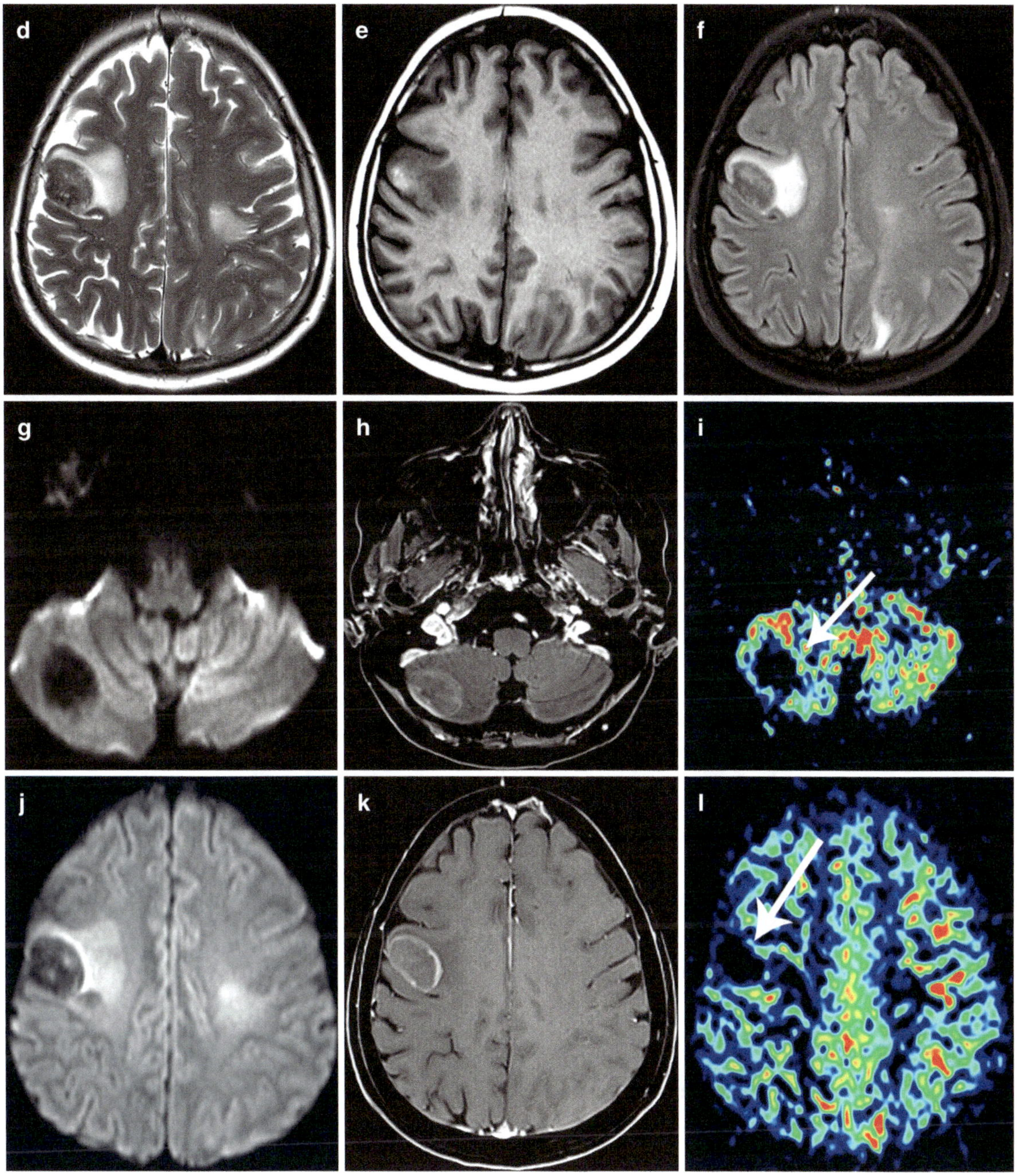

Fig. 12.33 (continued)

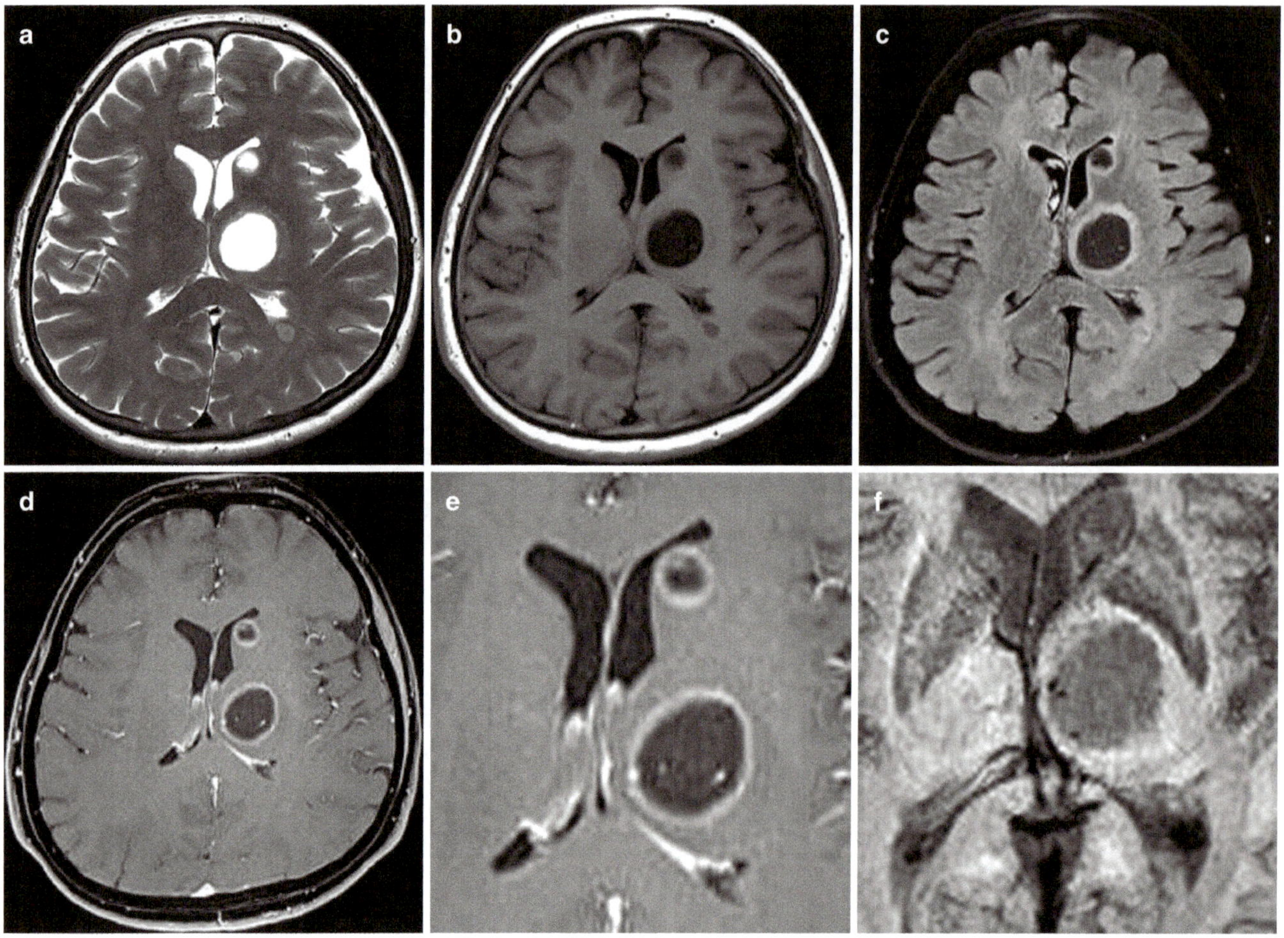

Fig. 12.34 Multiple lung cancer metastases in the brain. In a series of MR scans, multiple cystic, rounded lesions without signs of perifocal edema and high signal on T2-weighted MRI are identified (**a**) in the subcortical nuclei on the left. The lesion is characterized by a hypointense signal (**b**) on T1-weighted MRI and a hyperintense rim on T2-FLAIR MRI (**c**). After CA administration, its intense accumulation along the tumor contour is observed (**d**, **e**). On SWI MRI after intravenous CA administration, there are individual, pinpoint, hypointense inclusions (**f**) along the medial contour of the large lesion.

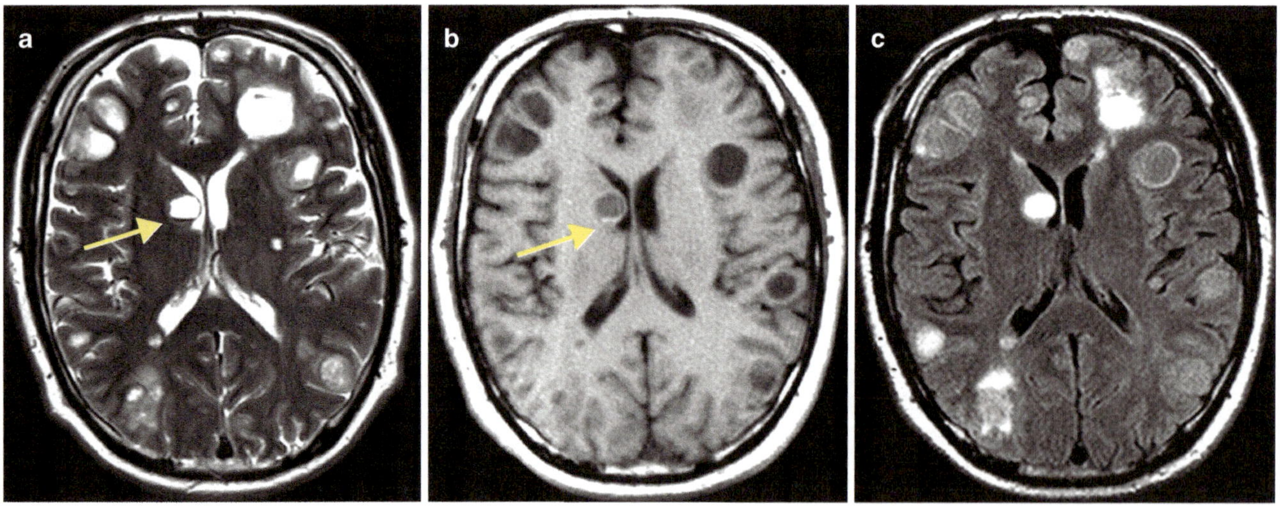

Fig. 12.35 Multiple lung cancer metastases in the brain. In the brain matter, there are multiple lesions with a solid-cystic structure, characterized by an increased signal on T2-weighted MRI (**a**), the formation of hemorrhagic "levels" (**a**, **b**, **f**—*arrows*), and a mild perifocal edema (**c**) in the area of individual lesions. Following intravenous CA administration, its uneven moderate accumulation in the solid structure of lesions is observed (**d**). On non-contrast-enhanced MR perfusion, separate lesions with increased CBF values are identified (**e**, *arrow*). On SWI MRI, the lesions have a hyperintense MR signal, with some of them (**f**) having inclusions with a hypointense contour (hemorrhagic) (the *arrow*)

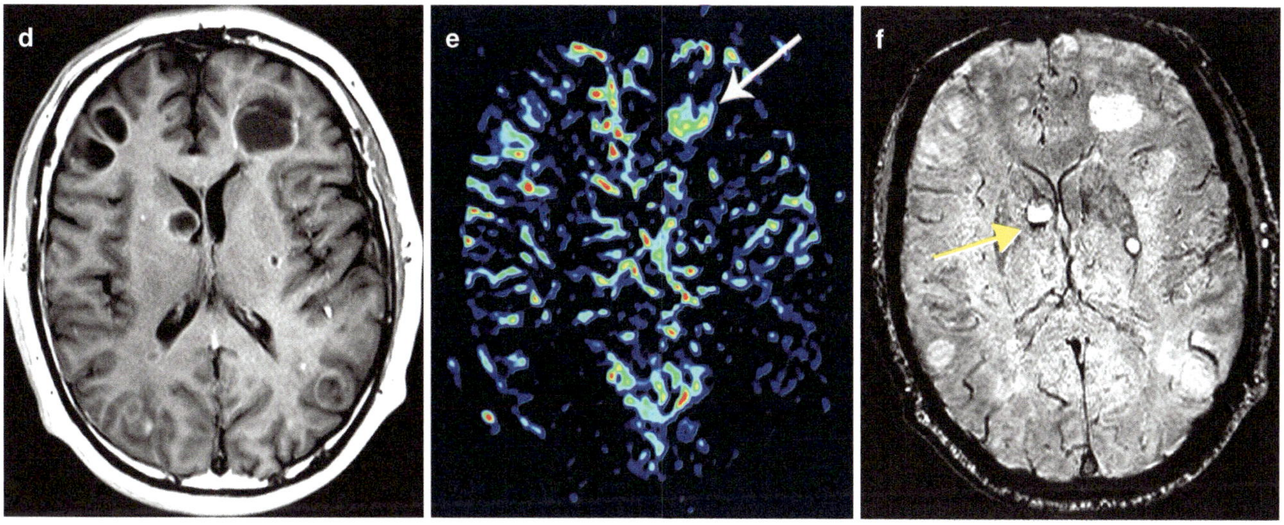

Fig. 12.35 (continued)

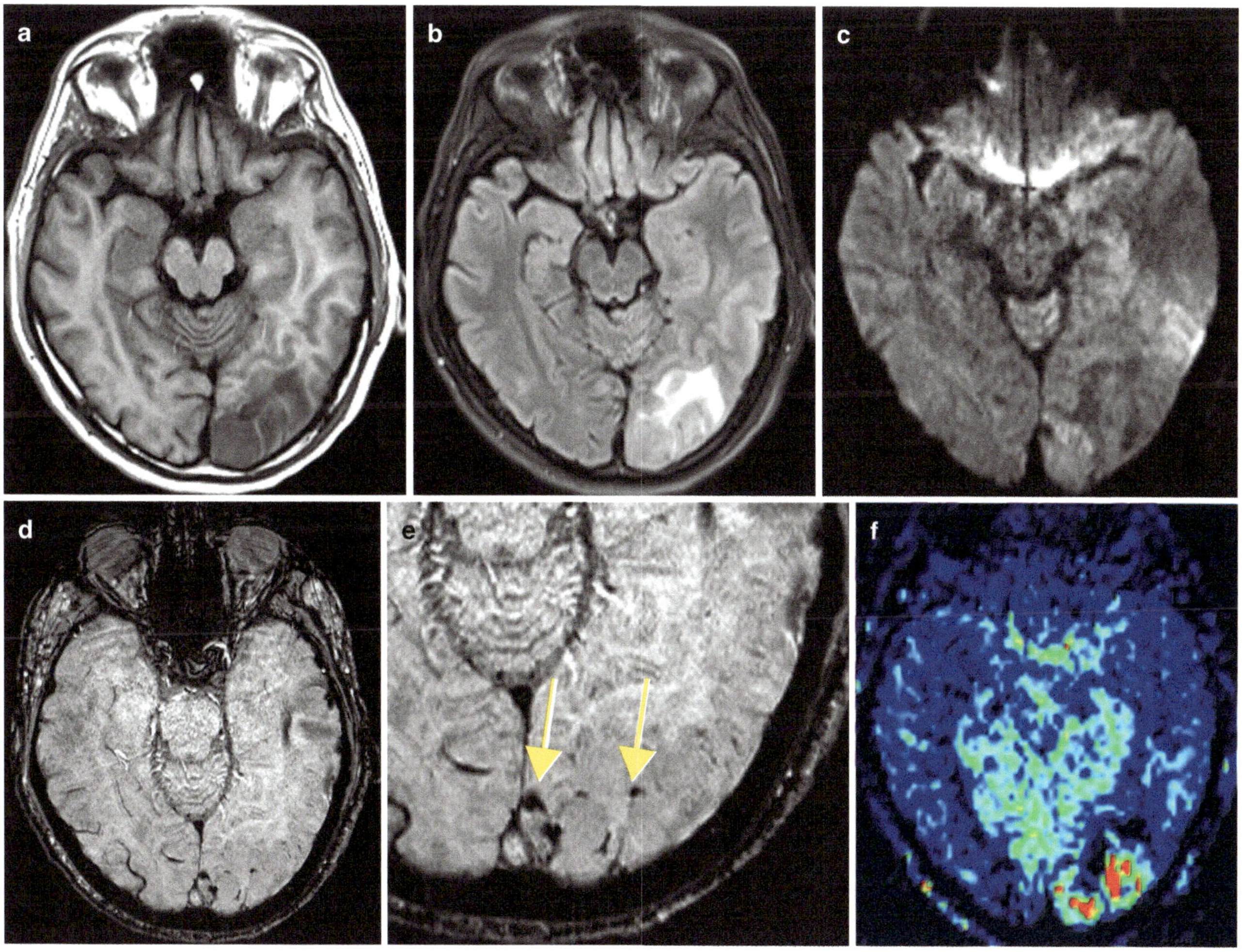

Fig. 12.36 A lung cancer metastasis in the brain. In the left occipital region, there are two confluent tumor lesions with an MR signal hypointense on T1-WI MRI (**a**), isointense on T2-FLAIR MRI (**b**), and hyper-hypointense on DWI MRI (**c**). On SWI MRI (**d**, **e**), no hypointense inclusions in tumors are identified; however, dilated veins (the *arrows*) are well differentiated along their contours. On ASL MRI, there are multiple sites with a significantly increased blood flow (**f**). Following intravenous CA administration, metastatic lesions are intensely enhanced (**g**). Tractography does not show any involvement of optic radiation in the pathological process (**h**, **i**)

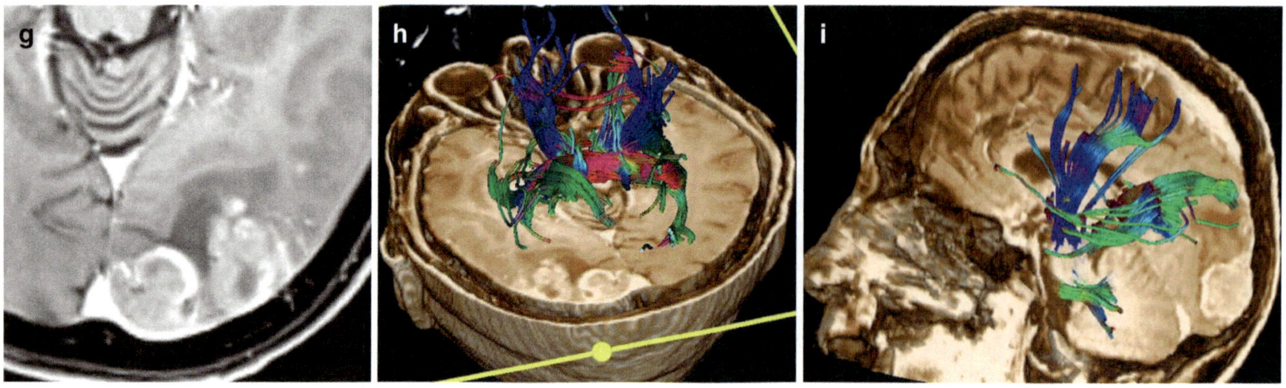

Fig. 12.36 (continued)

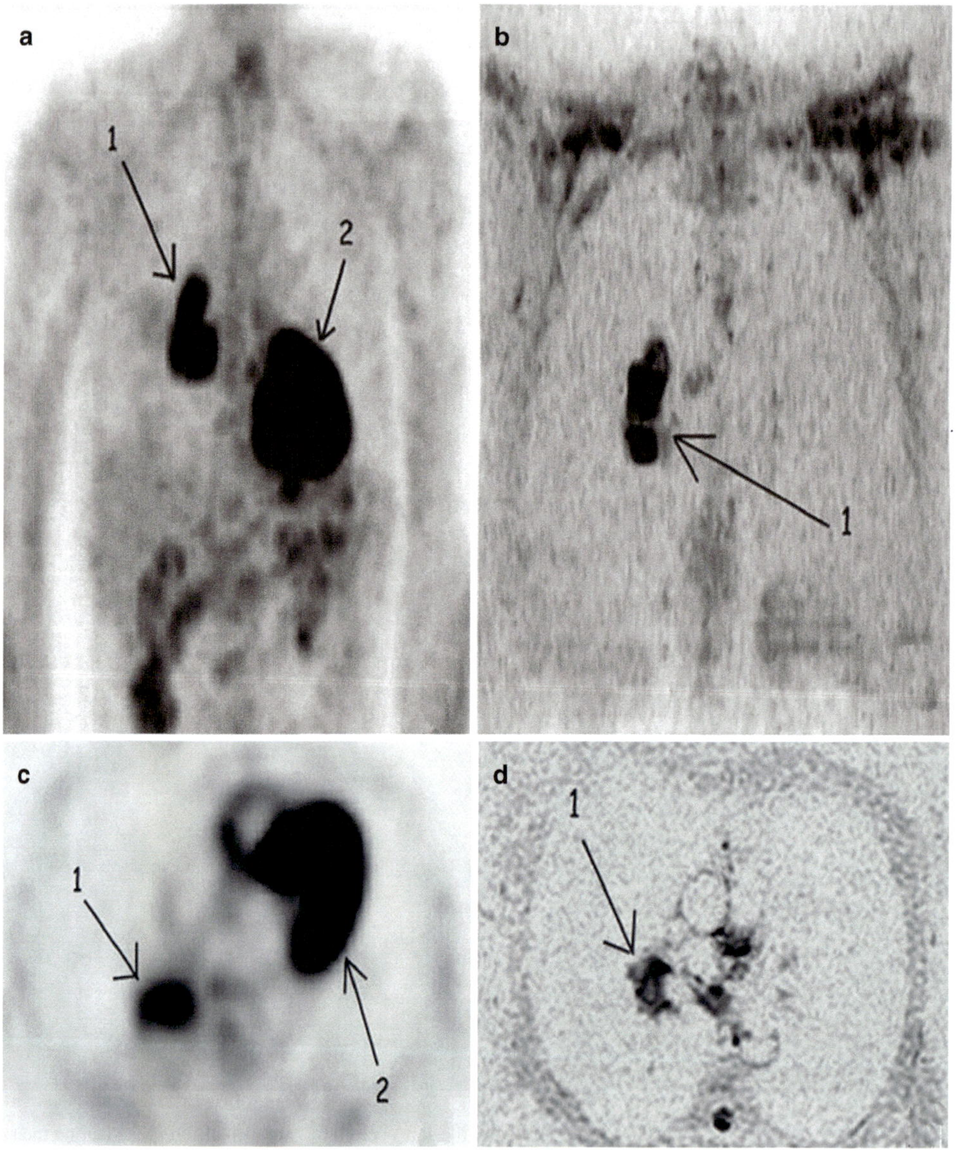

Fig. 12.37 Central lung cancer. ^{18}F-FDG PET (**a**, **c**) and whole-body DW MRI (**b**, **d**). In the projection of the right lung hilum, there is a portion with radiopharmaceutical hyperfixation on PET and an increased signal on MR scans (*arrow 1*). On PET images, there is a marked accumulation of RP in the heart area (*normal*), which is not visualized on MRI (*arrow 2*)

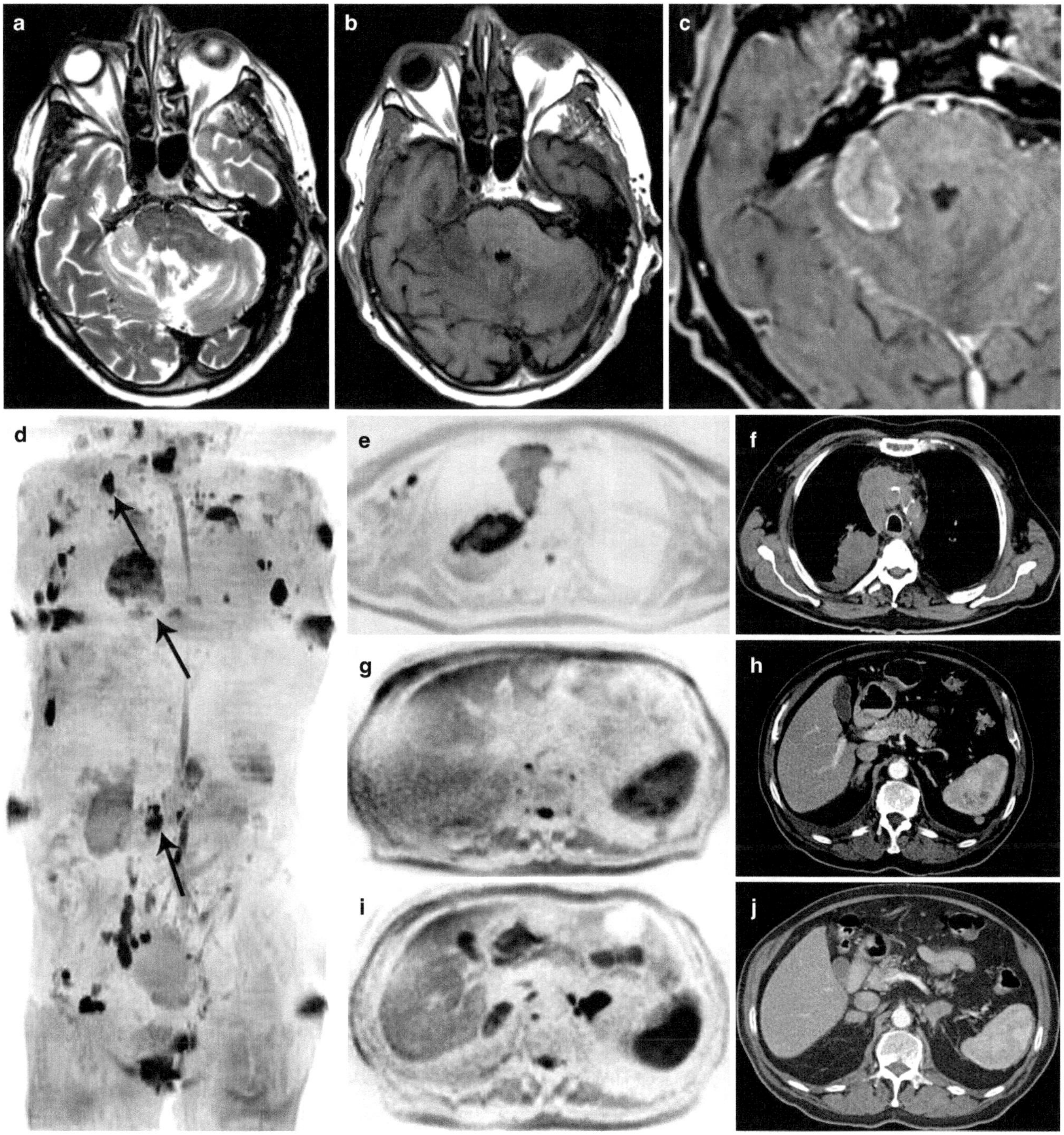

Fig. 12.38 Lung cancer metastases. In the area of the right cerebellopontine angle, there is a space-occupying lesion with an increased signal on T2-weighted MRI (**a**) and iso-hypointense signal on T1-weighted MRI (**b**), intensely accumulating the contrast agent (**c**). On the whole-body DW MRI (**d**, **e**, **g**, **i**), there is an increased signal in the submandibular area on the right, in the supraclavicular areas, a large area in the parenchyma of the right lung, multiple areas in the mediastinum, in the adrenal glands, and along the course of the main vessels of the abdominal cavity, consistent with the findings confirmed by a CT study (**f**, **h**, **j**)—a tumor of the right lung and multiple metastases

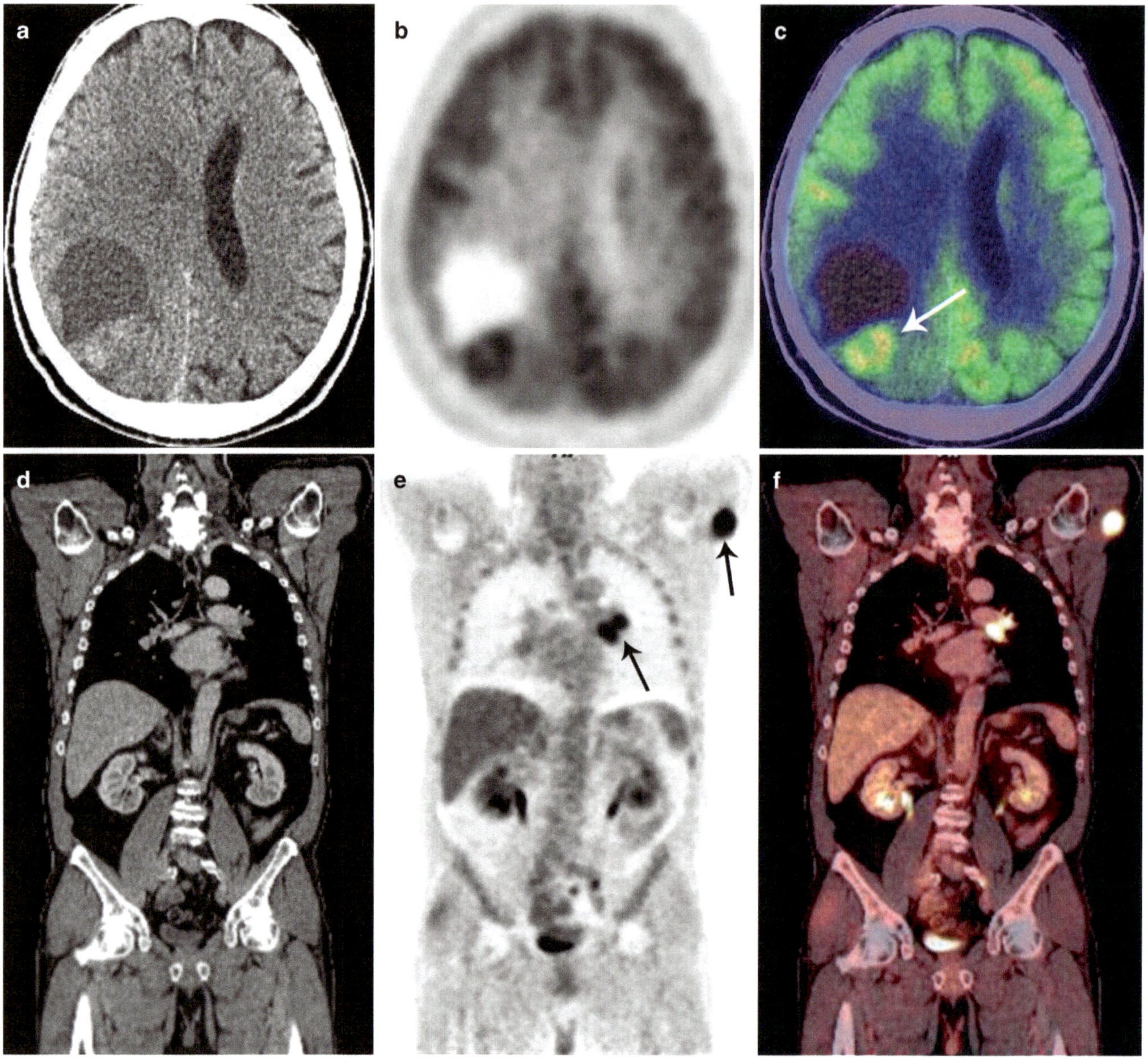

Fig. 12.39 Lung cancer metastases. In the right occipital parietal region, there is a cystic-solid lesion with signs of weak accumulation of the contrast agent on CT (**a**) in the posterior parts of a metastasis. On PET with ^{18}F-FDG, there is an intense RP accumulation in the solid component of the tumor (**b**, **c**–*arrow*). In the whole-body PET/CT study, there are also areas with increased RP accumulation (**d**–**f**) (*arrows*) in the hilum of the left lung (central cancer) and left axilla (metastases)

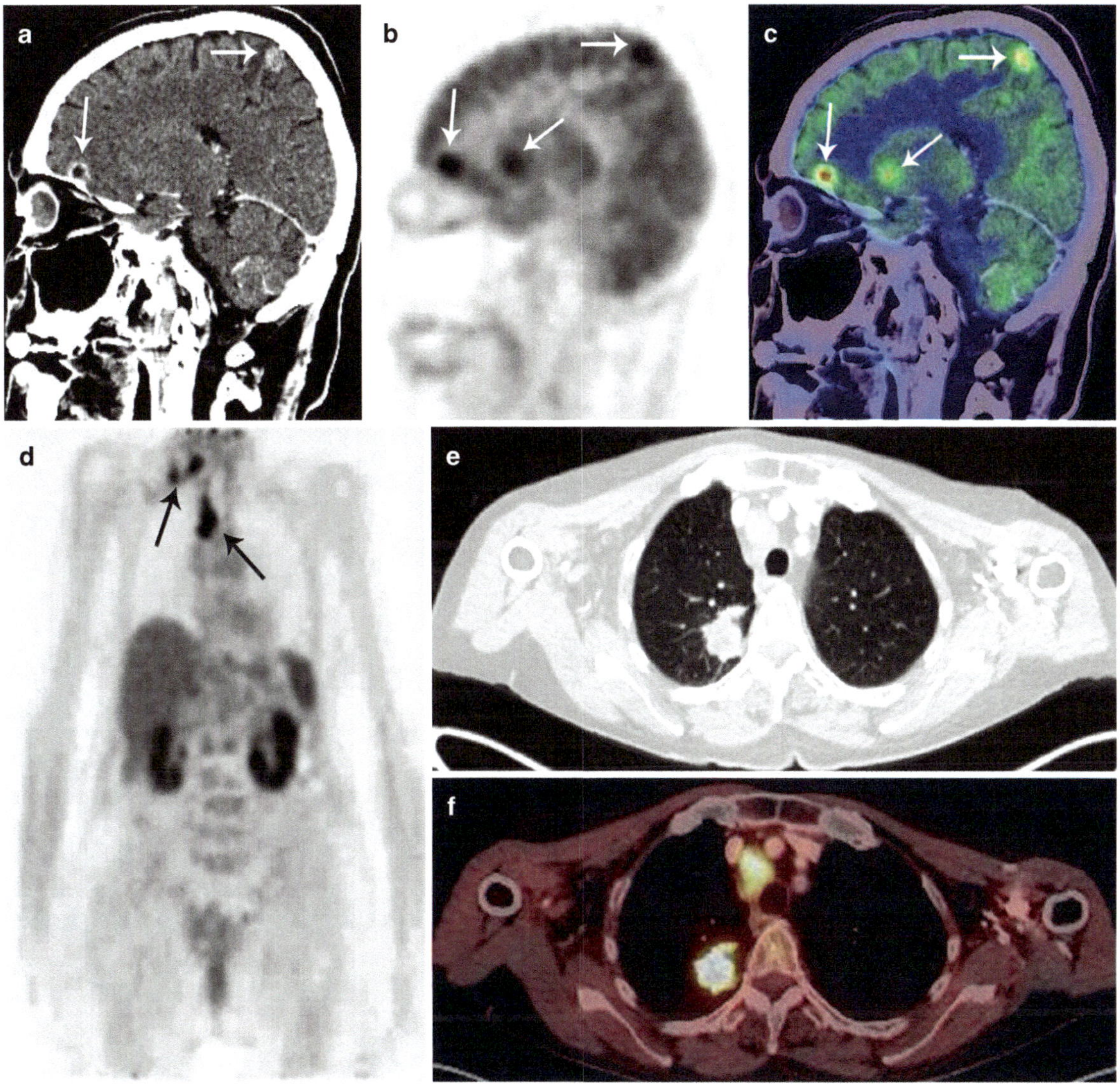

Fig. 12.40 Multiple lung cancer metastases. In the CT image, in the sagittal projection (**a**), there are multiple, rounded lesions (the *arrows*) intensely accumulating CA. On PET (**b**) and PET/CT with ^{18}F-FDG (**c**), in the sagittal projection, there is a pronounced accumulation of the radiopharmaceutical by the metastatic lesions (*arrows*). On whole-body PET/CT scans, there is a large tumor lesion in the apex of the right lung and multiple large lesions in the anterior mediastinum and supraclavicular area on the right (**d**, **e**, **f**) (*arrows*)

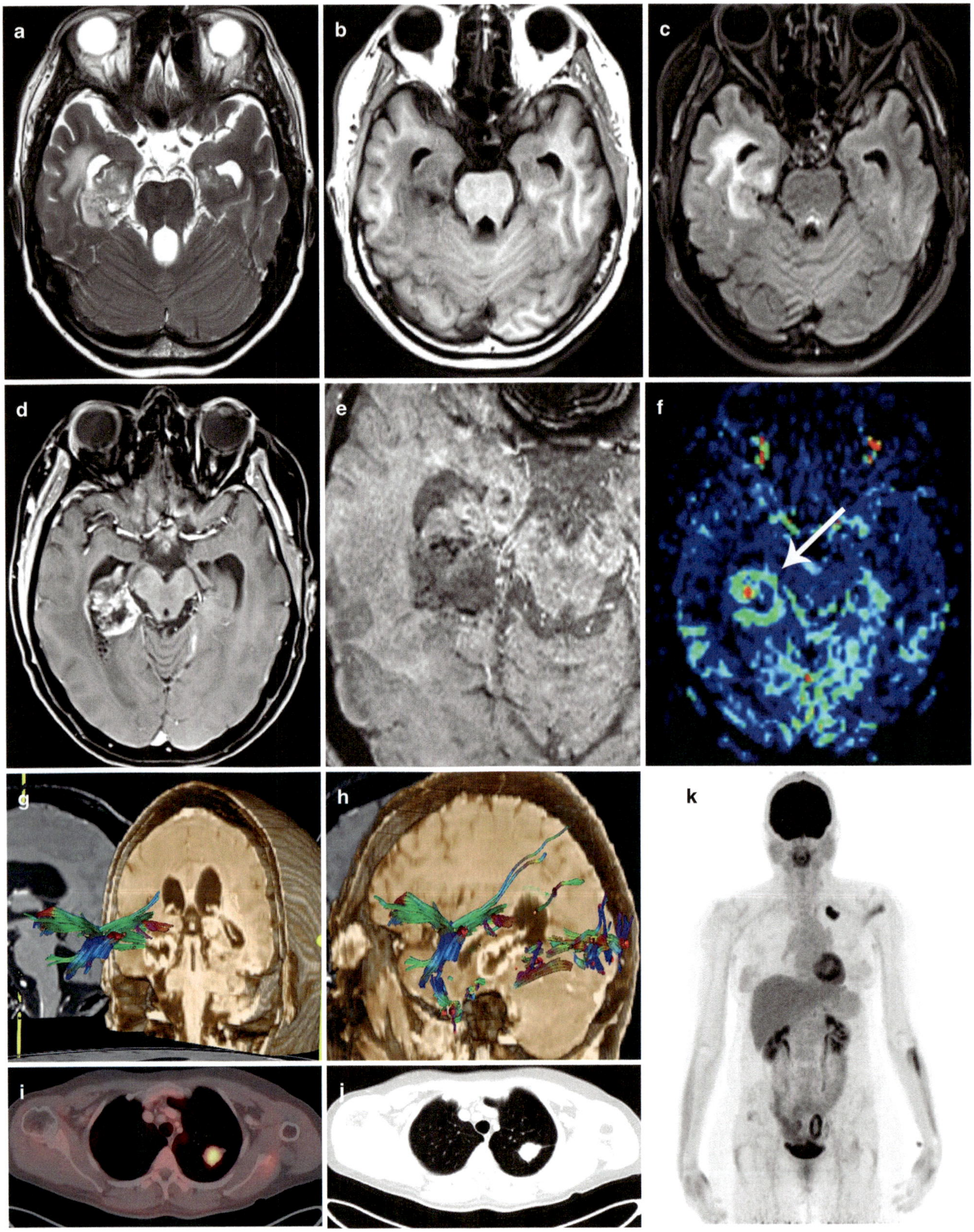

Fig. 12.41 A lung cancer metastasis in the brain. Posteriorly and medially to the anterior parts of the temporal horn of the right lateral ventricle, there is a space-occupying lesion with an increased signal on T2-weighted and T2-FLAIR MRI (**a**, **c**) and moderately hypointense signal on T1-weighted MRI (**b**). Following intravenous CA administration, the lesion with decay in the center accumulates it intensely and unevenly (**d**). There are individual pinpoint areas with a low MR signal in the structure of the tumor on SWI MRI (**e**). On ASL MRI, increased perfusion values (**f**) (*arrow*) are observed. On MR tractography, there is a marked displacement of the conductive pathways upward with respect to the tumor (**g**, **h**). On whole-body PET/CT with ^{18}F-FDG in the upper lobe of the left lung, there is intense RP accumulation corresponding to the nodule area in the lung tissue on a PET/CT and CT study (**i**, **j**, **k**)

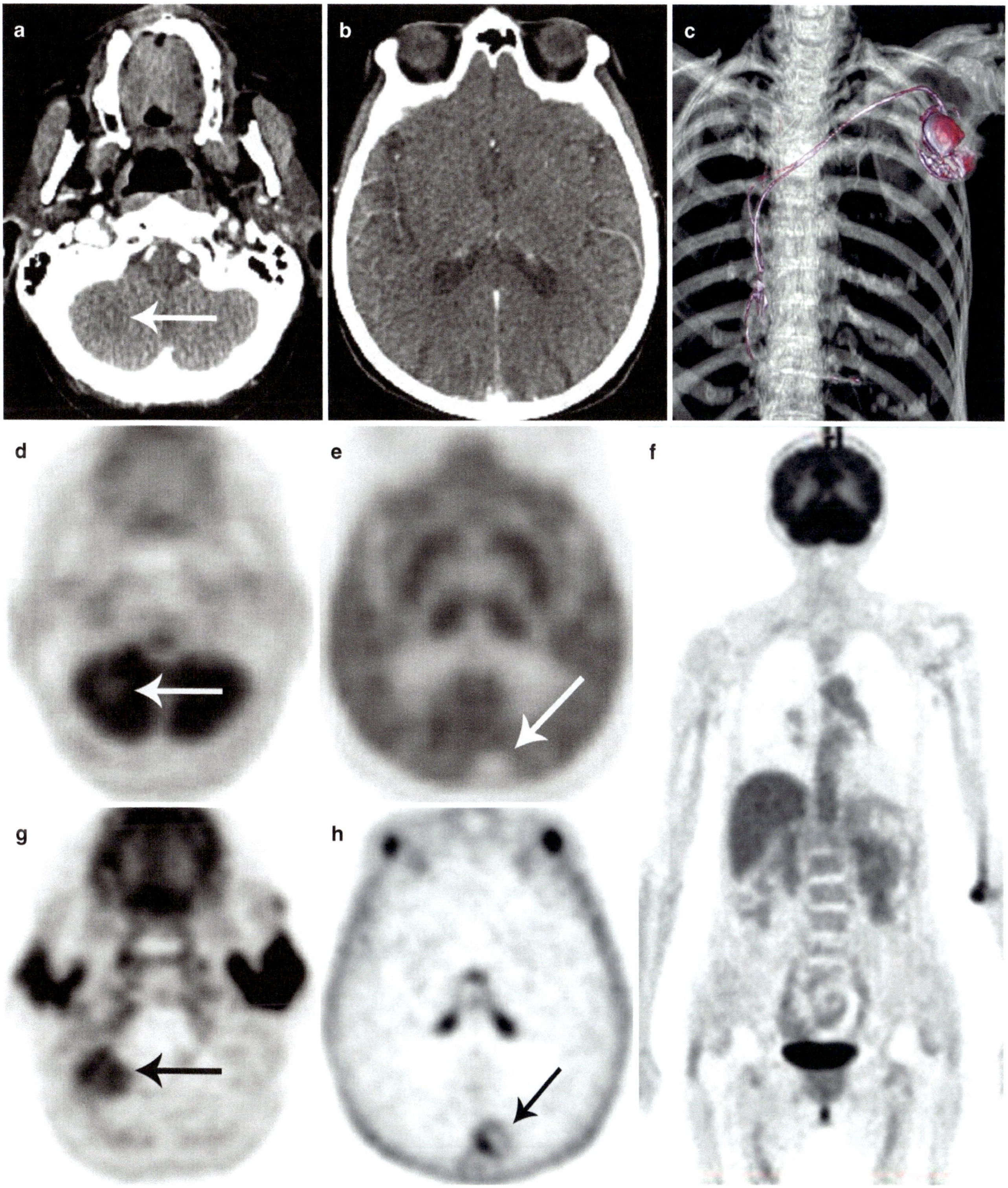

Fig. 12.42 Multiple lung cancer metastases. A two-level study. On CT, in the right hemisphere of the cerebellum, there is a poorly differentiated area with moderately low density (**a**, **b**) (the *arrow*). In 3D reconstruction images, structural components of the installed pacemaker (**c**) can be seen in *red color*. It did not allow to perform an MR study. On brain (**d**, **e**) and whole-body (**f**) PET/CT with ^{18}F-FDG, ametabolic areas (the *arrows*) are observed in the right hemisphere of the cerebellum and parasagittal sections of the left occipital region. No indication of abnormalities in the extracranial structures was identified (**f**). On PET with ^{18}F-choline, the lesions with increased CA accumulation in the above brain areas are clearly visualized (**g**, **h**) (the *arrows*)

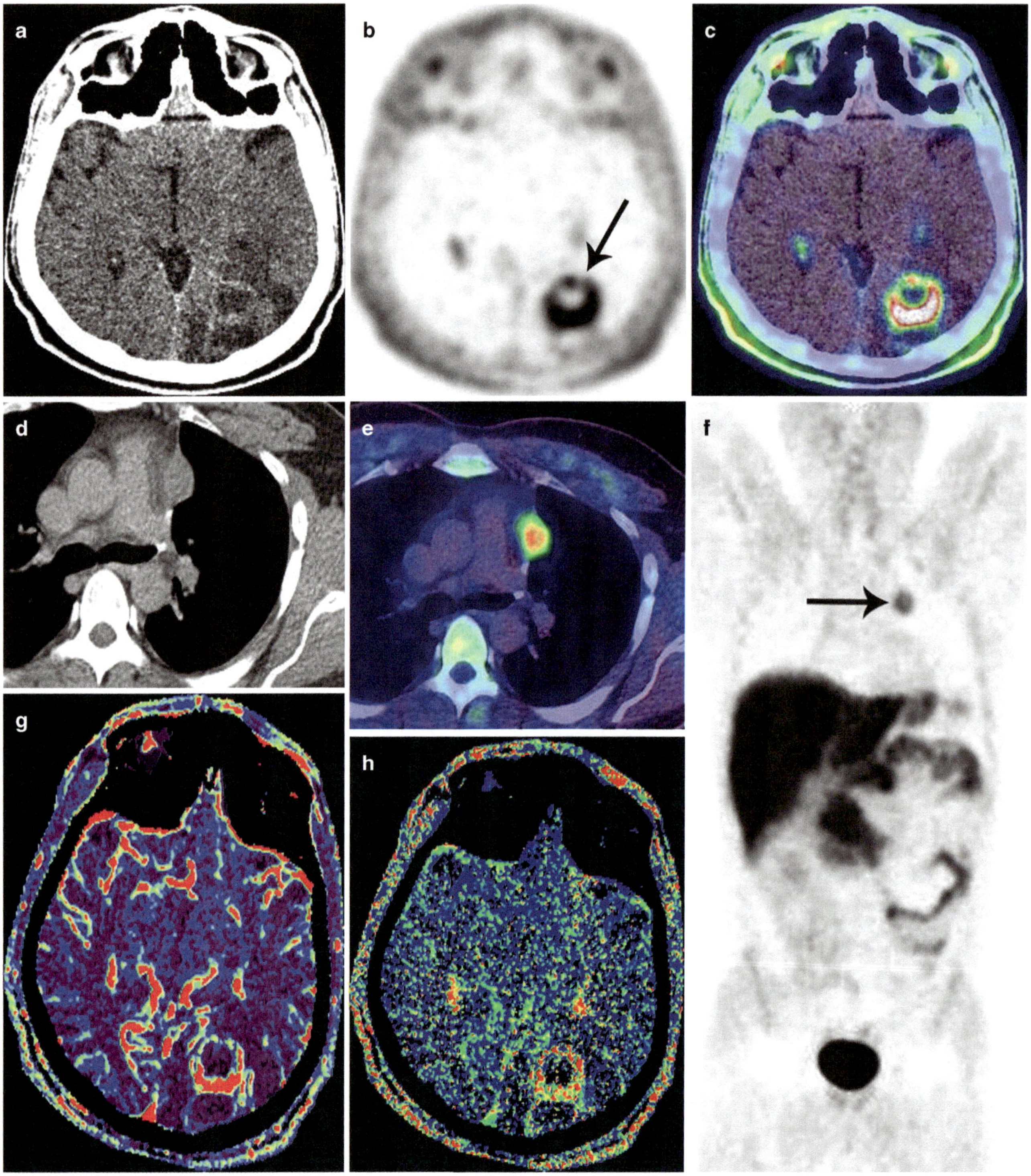

Fig. 12.43 A lung cancer metastasis in the brain. In the left occipital region, there is a solid-cystic lesion with a pronounced perifocal edema, moderately accumulating the contrast agent on CT (**a**). On PET with ^{18}F-choline, the lesion intensely accumulates RP (**b**, **c**) (the *arrow*). An additional body scanning showed a soft tissue lesion adjacent to the anterior mediastinum (**d**, **e**) in the upper lobe of the left lung, with similar RP accumulation values (the *arrow*); no other lesions with abnormal RP accumulation were identified (**f**). On CT perfusion maps, there is an increase in CBV (**g**) and MTT (**h**) values due to the solid structure of the tumor

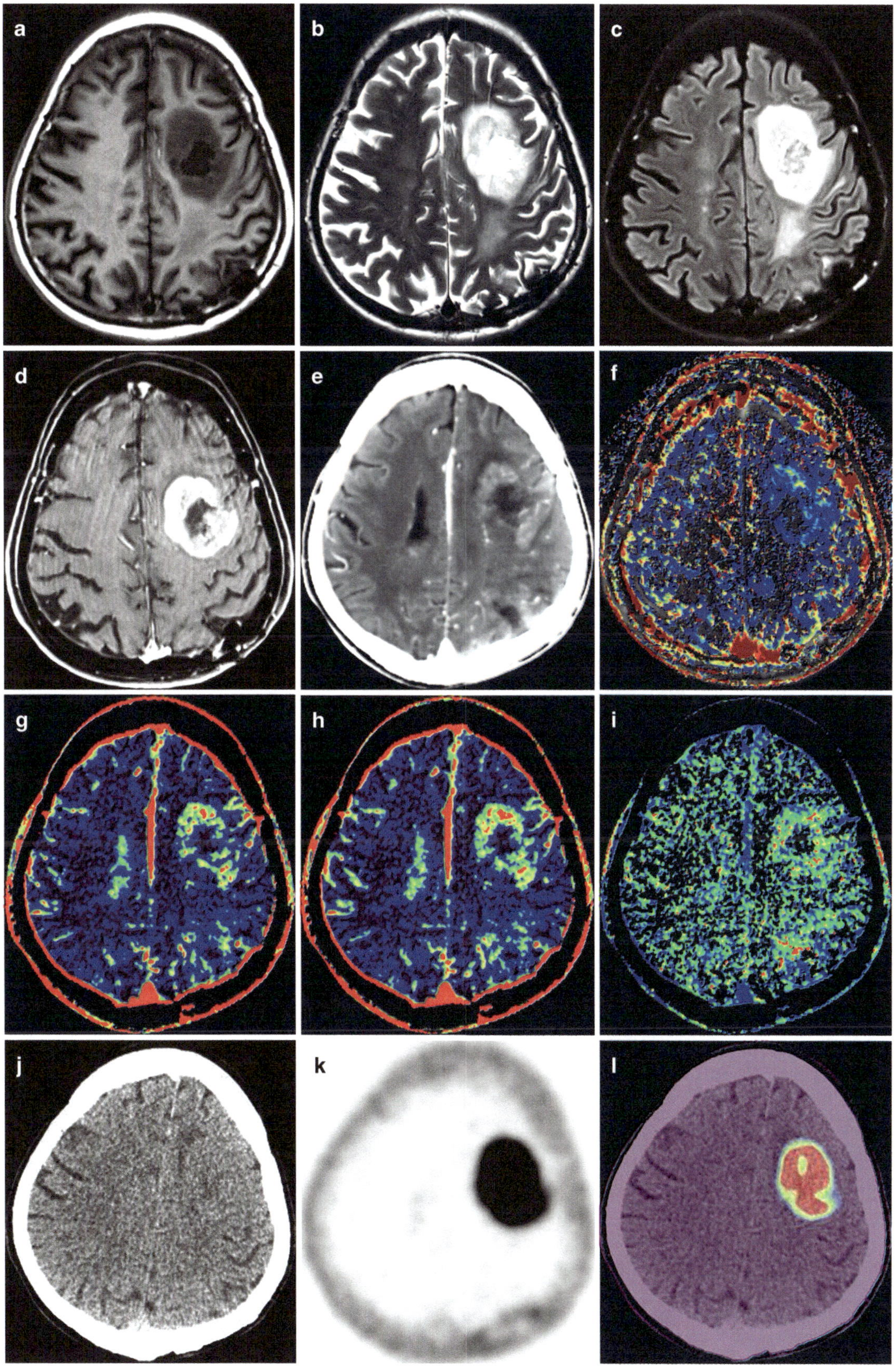

Fig. 12.44 A lung cancer metastasis in the brain. In the left frontal region, there is a large solid lesion with an isointense MR signal on T1-weighted MRI (**a**) and irregularly hyperintense on T2-weighted (**b**) and T2-FLAIR MRI (**c**). Following intravenous CA administration, its intense accumulation in the metastasis is observed both in an MRI and CT study (**d**, **e**). Dynamic MR contrast enhancement shows marked areas with increased blood-brain barrier permeability (**f**), as well as a marked increase in CT perfusion parameters CBV (**g**), CBF (**h**), and MTT (**i**). On PET/CT with ^{18}F-choline, the lesion is not visualized on routine CT scans (**j**) and intensely accumulates RP (**k**, **l**)

12.2 Post-radiation and Postoperative Changes

See Figs. 12.45, 12.46, 12.47, 12.48, and 12.49.

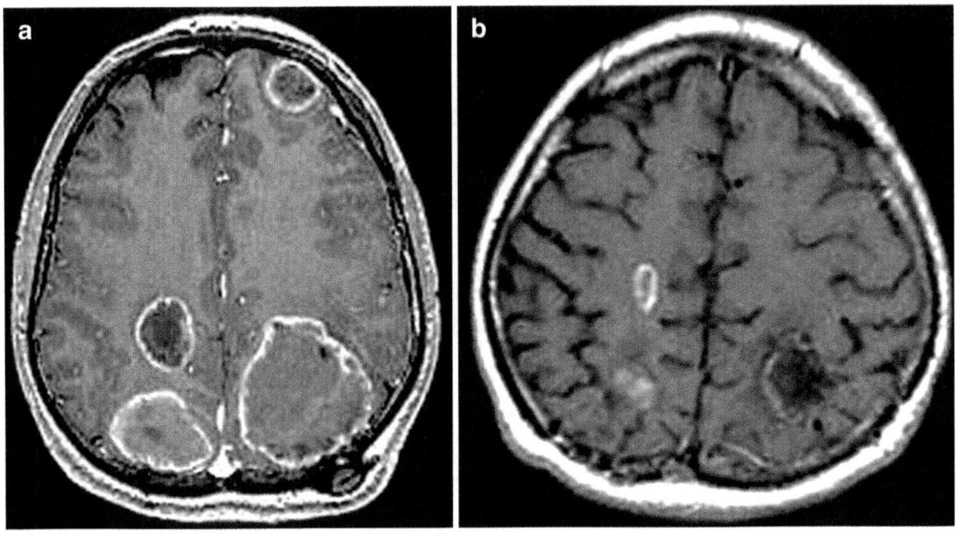

Fig. 12.45 Multiple lung cancer metastases in the brain. Condition before and after drug treatment. On T1-weighted MRI with contrast enhancement, multiple space-occupying lesions with different diameters and forms, with signs of intense accumulation of the contrast agent, mostly peripherally (**a**) are identified in the brain substance. The central parts of certain lesions have an increased signal due to hemorrhagic inclusions. After several courses of chemotherapy (**b**), there is a significant reduction in the size of metastases

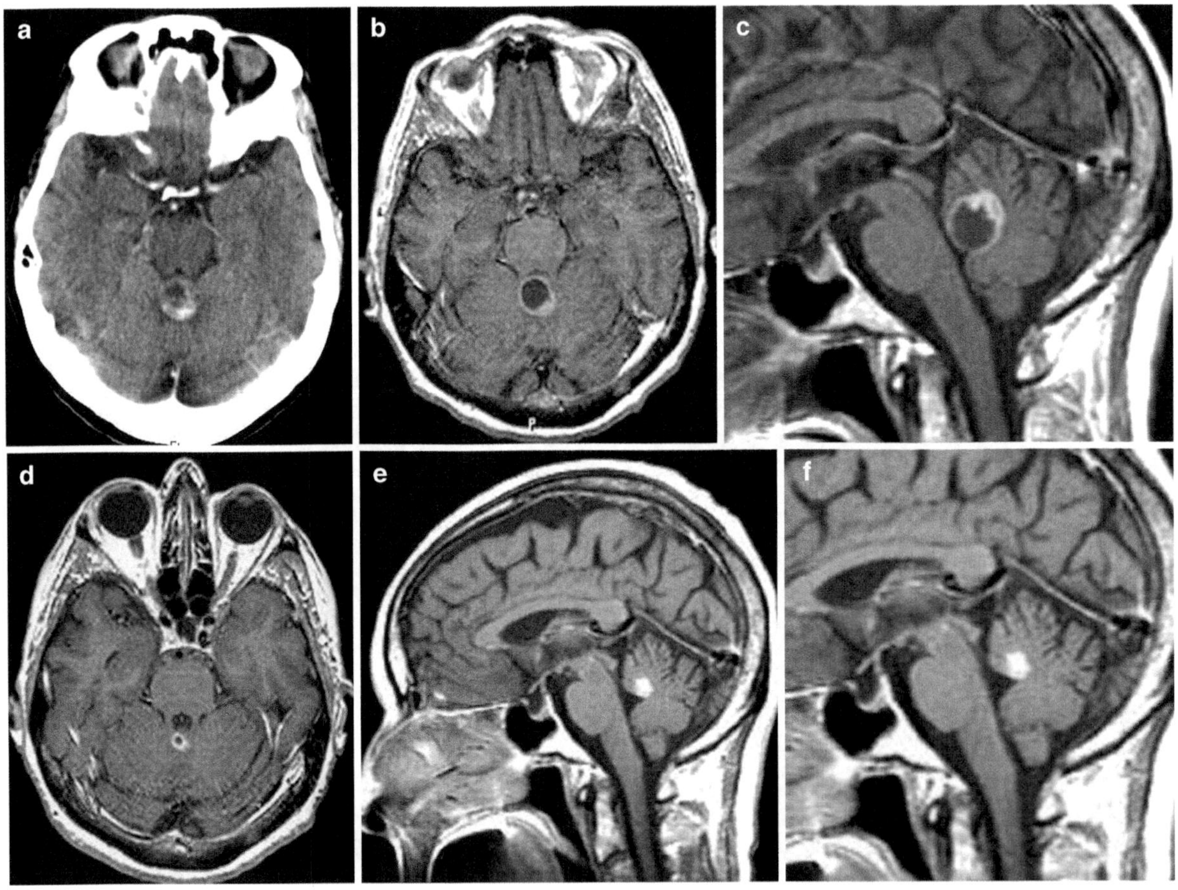

Fig. 12.46 A lung cancer metastasis in the brain. A follow-up during the treatment. Before the start of radiation therapy, a solid-cystic lesion that intensely accumulated CA was observed in the cerebellar vermis in CT (**a**) and MRI (**b**, **c**) studies. A follow-up during the radiation treatment showed a stable reduction in the tumor size at 3 months (**d**–**f**), at 6 months (**g**–**i**), and at 12 months after the treatment (**j**–**l**)—an incomplete response to the treatment

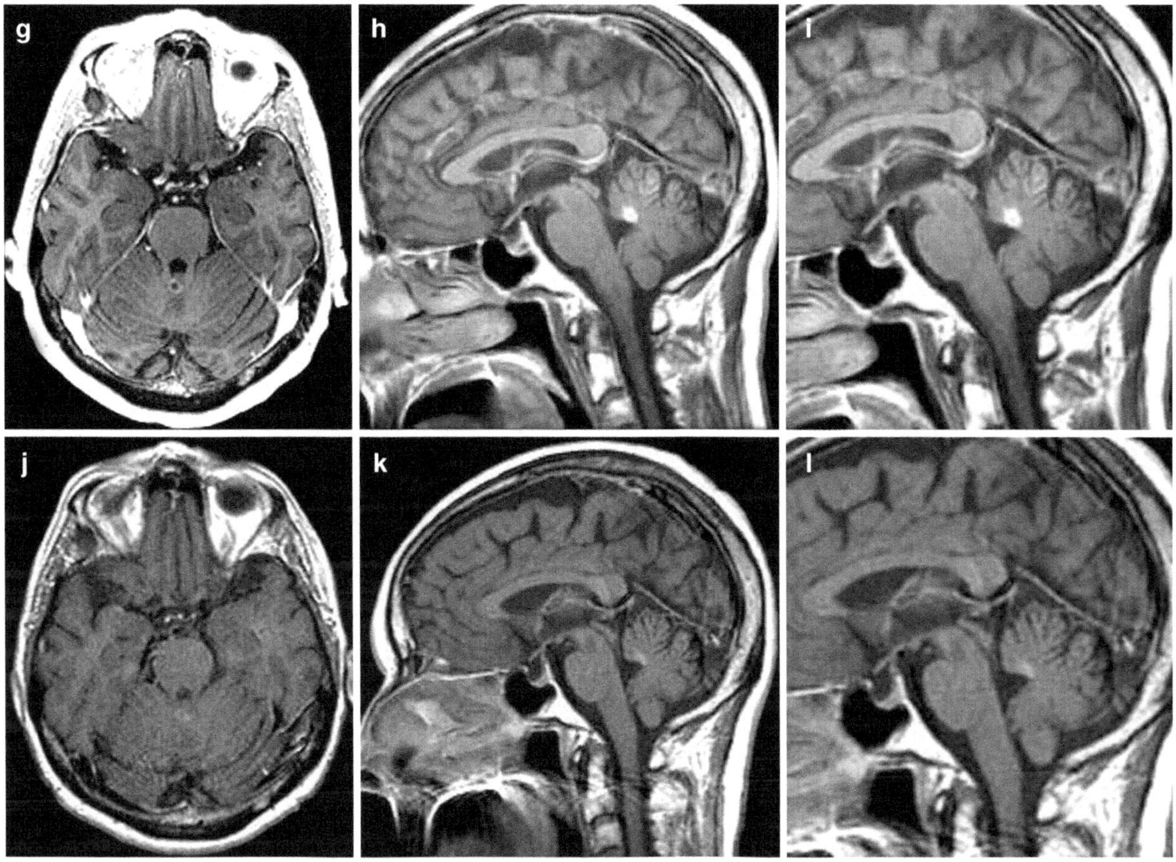

Fig. 12.46 (continued)

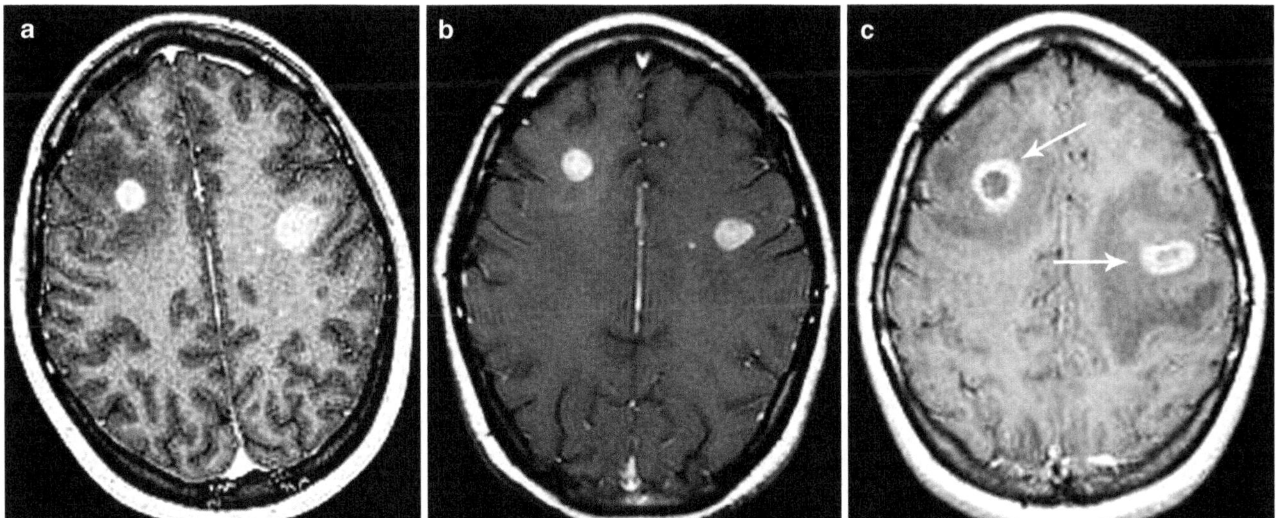

Fig. 12.47 Multiple lung cancer metastases in the brain. A follow-up study during the treatment. On T1-weighted contrast-enhanced MR images (**a**–**c**), there are multiple metastases in the frontal areas of the brain and an increase in the lesion size (the *arrows*) (**c**). On a CT scan before the treatment, these lesions initially also intensely accumulate CA (**d**, **e**), the perifocal edema zones are well visualized (hypodense areas), and there is poor CA accumulation with time (**f**). On CT perfusion before the radiosurgical treatment, an increase in the respective CBV, CBF, and MTT values (**g**, **j**, **m**) is observed, while 1 month after, a marked decrease in CBV and CBF (**h**, **k**) values and an increase in MTT values (**n**) are noted. CBV and CBF values were relatively reduced in relation to the brain substance (**i**, **l**), and MTT values (**o**) were increased 6 months after the radiosurgical treatment

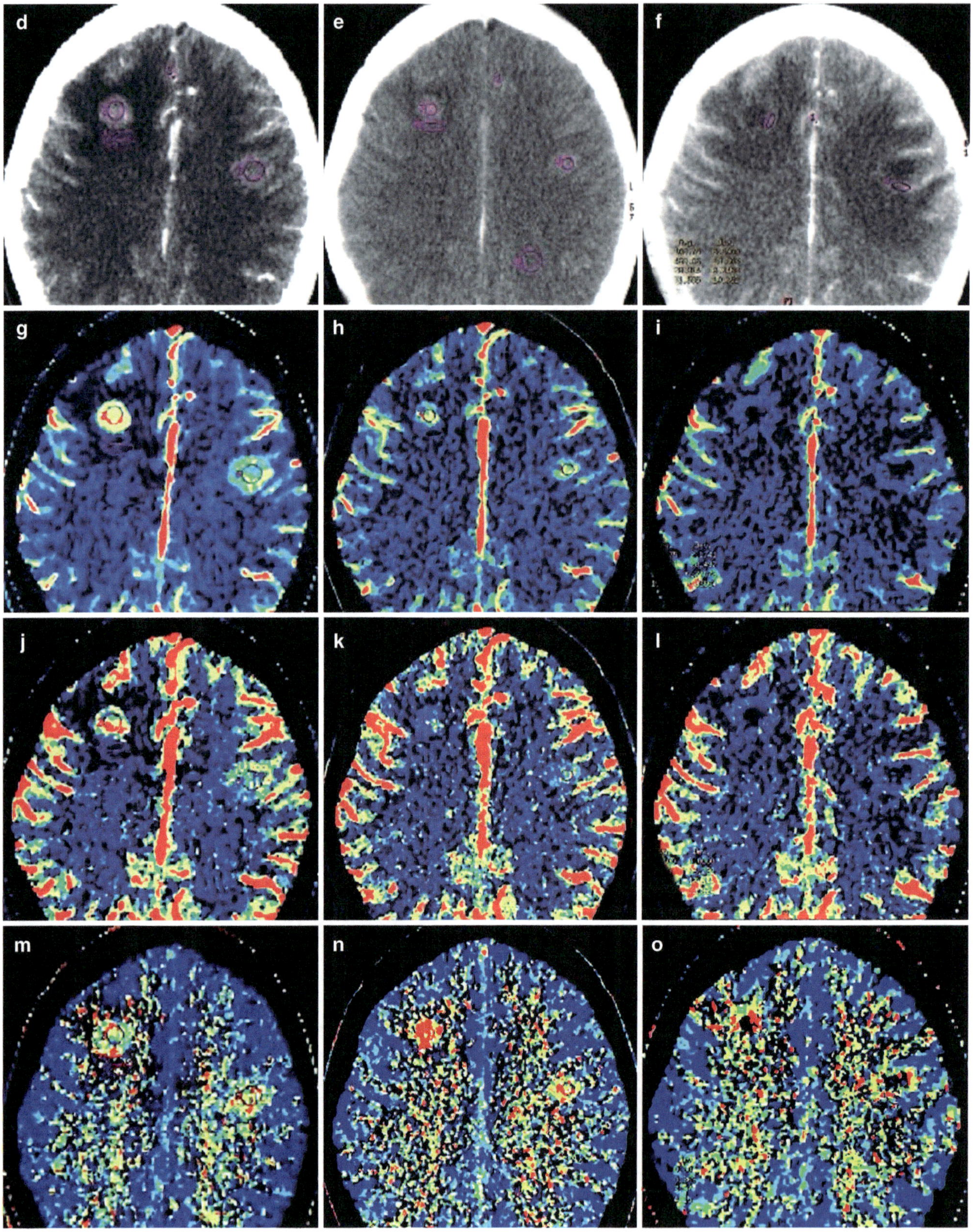

Fig. 12.47 (continued)

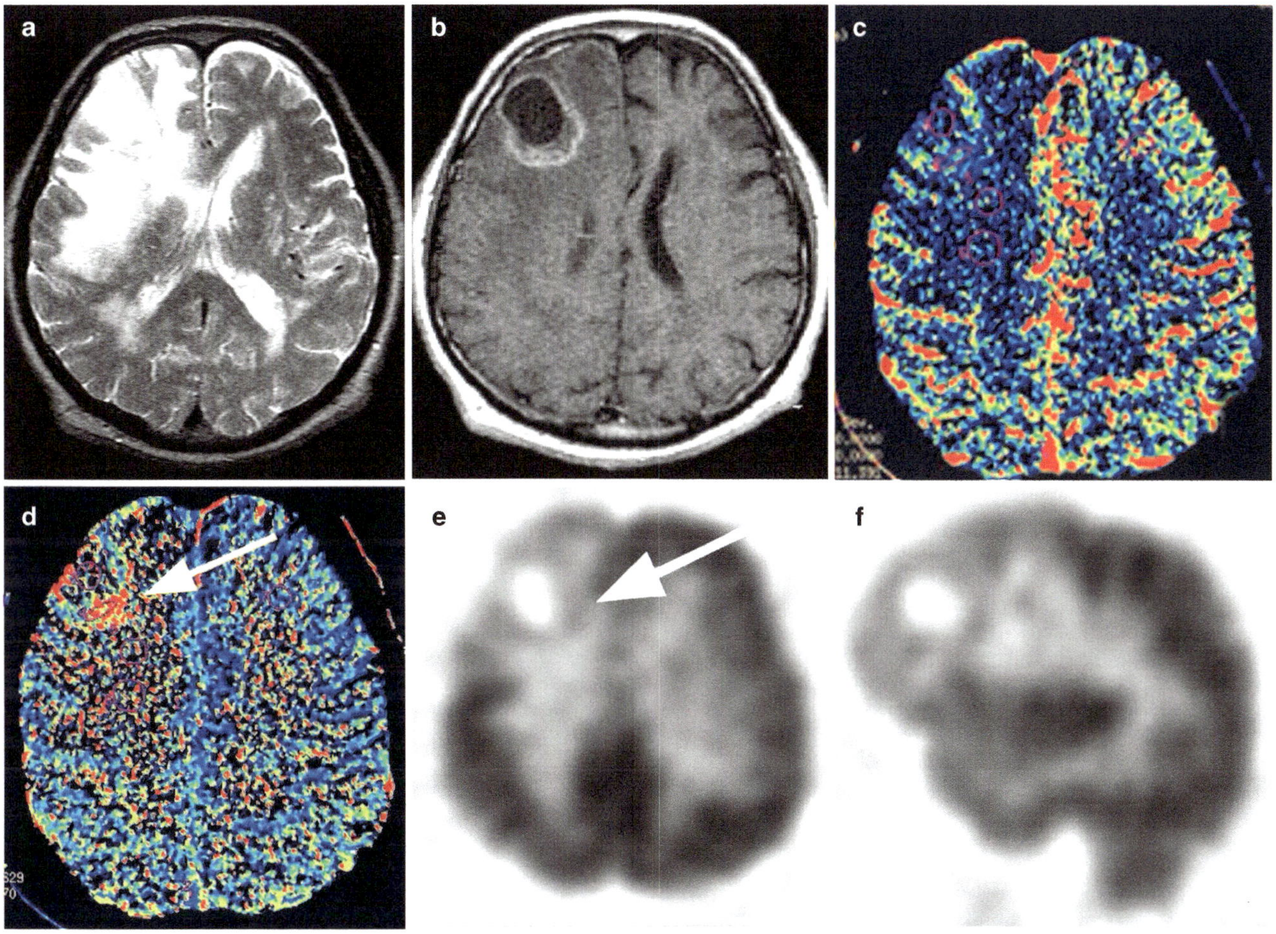

Fig. 12.48 A lung cancer metastasis in the brain 8 months after the radiosurgical treatment. On MRI in the right frontal area, there is a large cystic lesion with a pronounced perifocal edema (**a**) and non-uniform annular contrast enhancement (**b**). On perfusion maps, there are no signs of increased CBV values (**c**), with high MTT values (**d**) in the area of contrast agent accumulation along the posterior contour of the lesion. On PET with ^{18}F-FDG, there is no RP hyperfixation (**e**, **f**) (the *arrow*)

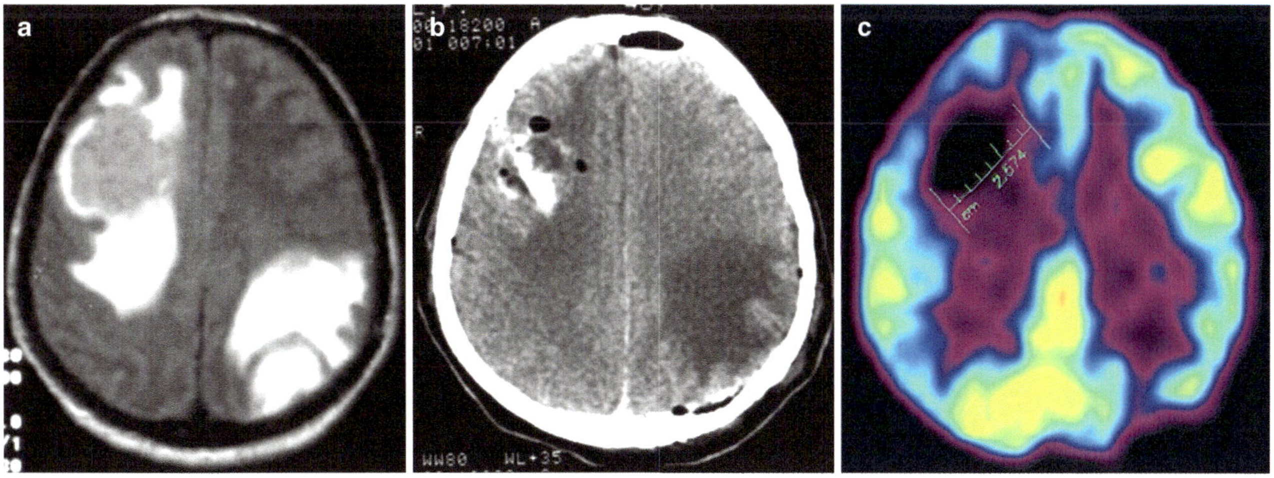

Fig. 12.49 Multiple intracranial lung cancer metastases. On T2-FLAIR MRI before surgical removal of tumors (**a**), large tumor lesions are identified in the right frontal and left parietal areas, with a pronounced perifocal edema. On a CT scan (**b**) after the simultaneous removal of two intracranial metastatic lesions, a hemorrhagic impregnation and pneumocephalus in the beds of the removed tumors are observed. There are no signs of RP hyperfixation on the follow-up PET with ^{18}F-FDG (**c**)

13 Breast Cancer (BC)

Breast cancer (BC) is the most common malignancy in women and occupies the first place in the structure of morbidity and mortality from malignant neoplasms in the female population of Russia: the absolute number of cases and deaths in 2013 has exceeded 57,000 and 25,000, respectively. According to Davydov and Axel (2014a, b) the incidence of malignant breast tumors tends to increase: from 42.8 per 100,000 in 2007 to 46.1 in 2012 among the female population of the Russian Federation. The growth rate was 7.7%, while mortality from malignant breast tumors tended to decrease from 17.1% in 2007 to 15.9% in 2012.

The risk of developing breast cancer increases with age: in 0.8% of cases, the disease manifests before the age of 30 years and in 6.5% at the age of 30–40 years, and more than 90% of breast cancer cases occur after 40 years of age.

The most common histological type of breast cancer is invasive ductal carcinoma, and lobular cancer is the second most common histological type of invasive breast cancer (Althuis et al. 2004). Less common are mucinous forms, tubular and cribriform cancer, and papillary, adenoid cystic, and secreting histological types of breast cancer characterized by low rates of metastasizing to the regional lymph nodes and a more favorable prognosis.

Breast cancer ranks second after lung cancer by frequency of brain metastases (Baker 1942; Baker et al. 1951; Lang and Slater 1964; Takakura et al. 1982; Lin et al. 2004; Stelzer 2013). According to several authors, MTS in the brain develops in 10–35% of all cases of breast cancer (Cifuentes and Pickren 1979; Le Chevalier et al. 1985; Lassman and DeAngelis 2003; Lin et al. 2004; Leone and Leone 2015) and 10% of patients in disseminated breast cancer (Boogerd et al. 1993; Fisher et al. 1997). According to our data, metastases of breast cancer accounted for 23% of cases.

Intracranial metastases of breast cancer are more common in case of massive extracranial metastasizing in 54% (Stark 2011). While lung cancer brain metastases are more common in men, in women breast cancer, metastases prevail. The incidence of breast cancer in men and women is estimated to be 1:100. Breast cancer metastases to the brain typically occur between 2 and 3 years from the time of diagnosis of the primary disease (van Eck et al. 1965; Nussbaum et al. 1996). According to Grigorov and Plotnikova (2012), the time interval from the detection of the primary tumor to the appearance of cerebral metastases depends on the initial stage of the disease and treatment of the primary lesion and, according to the authors, is 1 (at stage IV) to 4 years and 1 month (at stage IIA).

According to some authors, breast cancer metastases manifest in the brain as a single neoplasm (Zedeler et al. 1992; Flowers and Levin 1993; Yamada et al. 1997), according to other sources, these are often multiple lesions (Altundag et al. 2007).

In metastatic breast cancer, chemotherapy is effective in 70–80% of cases, while patients with treatment failure die from distant metastases. The average life expectancy in patients with stage IV breast cancer is 18–24 months, and this figure varies depending on the site of metastases. The 5-year survival rate of patients with breast cancer with distant metastases is 19%, with the disease having the worst prognosis in cases of visceral metastases (Zimm et al. 1981). However, Tevaarwerk et al. (2013) point out the apparent improvement in survival rates among patients with breast cancer over the last 30 years.

Breast cancer metastasizes to the cerebral hemispheres, cerebellum, brainstem, and spinal cord in 80–85%, 10–15%, 3–5%, and less than 1% of cases, respectively. Breast cancer metastases to the brain can spread through the bloodstream and lymphatic system. The presence of a lymphogenic metastasis determines an unfavorable outcome (Semiglazov et al. 2006).

In 5 to 20%, the meninges are involved (Grossman and Krabak 1999; Altundag et al. 2007; Kim et al. 2012; Scott and Kesari 2013), while in a percentage of cases, metastases in the spinal cord are detected in addition to brain lesions.

M. Dolgushin et al., *Brain Metastases*, DOI 10.1007/978-3-319-57760-9_13

According to Scott et al. (2016), the survival of patients with breast cancer leptomeningeal metastases is on average 4 months.

Given the frequent manifestation of breast cancer metastases in the form of cystic lesions, they have a decreased density and merge with the edema area on CT images. In cases of hemorrhagic inclusions or calcifications, breast cancer metastases have an increased density on CT before contrast enhancement. The deposition of calcium in the structures of metastases is more common during the treatment (chemotherapy or radiotherapy); therefore, the detection of calcifications in a long-term disease may indicate that they belong to the "old," not newly diagnosed metastases.

The majority of breast cancer metastases affecting the skull bones (47–85%) are characterized by an osteolytic form, although they can grow as osteoblastic metastases characterized by an increased density.

The contrast agent administration on CT allows to identify a solid part of breast cancer metastases in the brain. Small (<5 mm) metastatic lesions often accompanying the larger ones can remain undetected even with contrast enhancement.

On CT perfusion, a solid part of breast cancer metastases is characterized by an average blood volume CBV of 11.57 ± 5.79 ml/100 g with a large individual variation of the parameter values, close to the respective values of metastases of lung cancer, colorectal cancer, and uterine cancer. The parameter of blood flow velocity CBF has quite high values (92.04 ± 29.93 ml/100 g/min), also with a large dispersion of individual values. Average values of MTT parameter characterizing the blood transit through the capillary network of the metastasis were 7.6 ± 3.11 s. These perfusion parameters of metastatic breast cancer may provide important additional information required for the differential diagnosis of primary and secondary focal brain lesions, as well as metastatic lesions from primary tumors with various locations.

An MR study of suspected metastatic brain lesions in breast cancer is performed using the classical protocol. The nature of the CA accumulation by breast cancer metastases in our materials was diverse: along with homogeneous accumulation of the contrast agent by the solid part of the tumor, lesions with heterogeneous accumulation of the contrast agent were identified. In the majority of cases, after the contrast enhancement, a marked increase in the intensity of the MR signal from the tumor was noted, which facilitated the identification of sites and number of lesions.

The quality and reliability of visualization of metastases located in the posterior fossa, in the basal temporal region, and in convexital portions of the cerebral hemispheres are improving on T1-weighted MRI with fat signal suppression.

According to our observations, breast cancer is accompanied by significant involvement of the meninges (50% of cases), with the possible involvement of leptomeninges only. In cases of suspected metastases in the meninges, it is very important to use T1-weighted MRI with fat suppression and intravenous CA administration. Isolated metastases can spread through the dura mater and simulate meningioma, for example, if located at the base of the brain. Therefore, a differential diagnosis with the primary tumor or a non-tumor lesion must be carried out quite often for individual intracranial metastases of breast cancer.

Rarely breast cancer metastases in the brain can be detected at untypical sites, for example, in the sellar cavity. Metastases to the pituitary affect its posterior lobe and stalk more often than the anterior lobe, which can be associated with the direct blood supply to the neurohypophysis. About 35% of breast cancer metastases are located in the posterior cranial fossa, in the cerebellar peduncle, becoming multiple in some cases.

In our material, there are cases of patients with metastatic involvement of the orbit (6%), and, which is not typical for "untreated" metastases, tumor lesions contained small calcifications clearly detectable on CT. In metastatic involvement of the orbit, the uvea, the retrobulbar space, and its bony walls are often affected. Metastases of breast cancer in the orbit have diffuse and heterogeneous growth, whereas metastases of, for example, clear cell renal cell carcinoma and melanoma have clearly defined boundaries.

According to several authors, in adults, the primary source of metastases to the orbit is lung adenocarcinoma, breast cancer, prostate cancer, myeloma, lymphoma, and neuroblastoma (Lieb 2010). Malignant tumors of the orbit in 34% of cases are of metastatic origin or grow into the orbit from the adjacent areas. Women are almost two times more likely to get affected (Henderson et al. 1993).

On SWI (SWAN) MRI, breast cancer metastases in the brain have similar manifestations to those of lung cancer metastases, with a small number of hypointense inclusions in their structure. In the presence of hemorrhagic inclusions after radiotherapy, the use of standard MR protocols does not allow to reliably exclude the presence of a residual tumor. The combination of quantitative parameters of the coefficient of signal uniformity (CSU) on SWI (SWAN) maps and values of CT perfusion allows to obtain more accurate information about changes that reflect the "normal" course of post-radiation pathomorphism. After radiosurgical treatment, a pronounced accumulation of CA in the area of the irradiated metastasis can persist, which looks like a large hypointense area on SWI (SWAN) images, corresponding to the post-radiation changes (vasculitis).

On ASL maps in solid metastatic foci, even in the presence of pronounced hemorrhages, there is an increase in perfusion parameters. However, if the solid part is small (up to 1 cm), breast cancer metastases are difficult to differentiate on the background of the brain substance.

MR spectroscopy in breast cancer showed no reliable specificity. Changes similar to PMR spectra characteristic of metastatic lesions are also observed in glioblastoma and other tumors with necrotic decay.

The use of PET with ^{18}F-FDG for the primary diagnosis of breast cancer is not advisable. Today a series of activities is carried out aimed at finding specific radiopharmaceuticals to identify the "sentinel" lymph node. One of the most common drugs is ^{18}F-FES (fluoroestradiol): the drug is sensitive to ER+ receptors and can be used to assess the effectiveness of hormone therapy in breast cancer. A significant reduction in the accumulation of ^{18}F-FES in breast cancer metastases is noted following hormone therapy and, importantly, in the menopause period. Some patients may simultaneously have ER+ and ER− metastases, making it difficult to visualize tumor lesions (Vaalavirta et al. 2014).

Using whole-body PET as the first diagnostic step allowed in some cases to eliminate the need in ultrasound, CT, MRI, endoscopy, scintigraphy, and other study methods for a search of the primary tumor and, thereby, significantly reduce the time and costs of diagnostic activities. However, even upon identifying clear areas of abnormal CA accumulation on PET, the morphological verification of lesions is required.

13.1 Clinical Cases

See Figs. 13.1, 13.2, 13.3, 13.4, 13.5, 13.6, 13.7, 13.8, 13.9, 13.10, 13.11, 13.12, 13.13, 13.14, 13.15, 13.16, 13.17, 13.18, 13.19, 13.20, 13.21, 13.22, 13.23, 13.24, 13.25, 13.26, 13.27, 13.28, and 13.29.

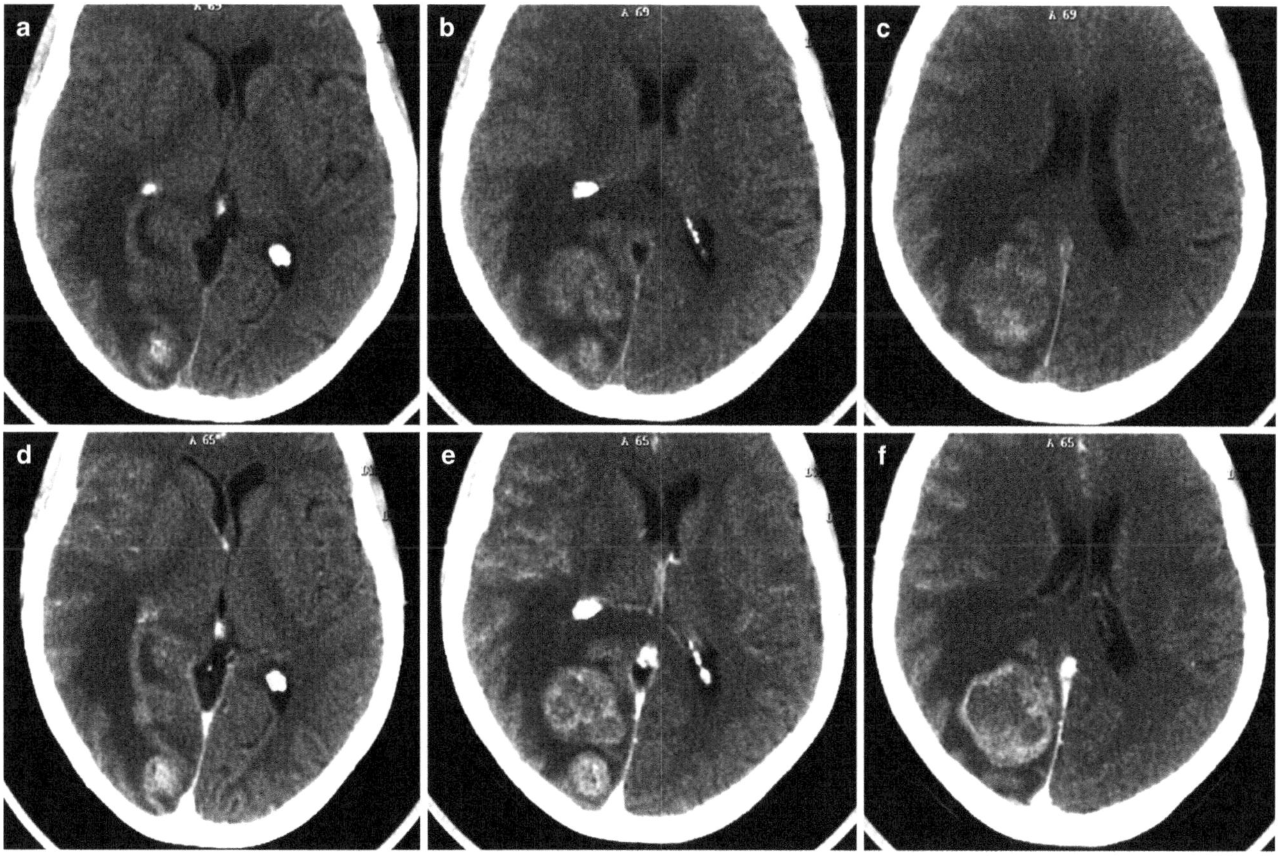

Fig. 13.1 Multiple breast cancer metastases in the brain. CT before (**a–c**) and after (**d–f**) intravenous contrast enhancement. On the background of edema, multiple tumor lesions with a solid structure and a marked contrast enhancement are determined. The ventricular system is deformed

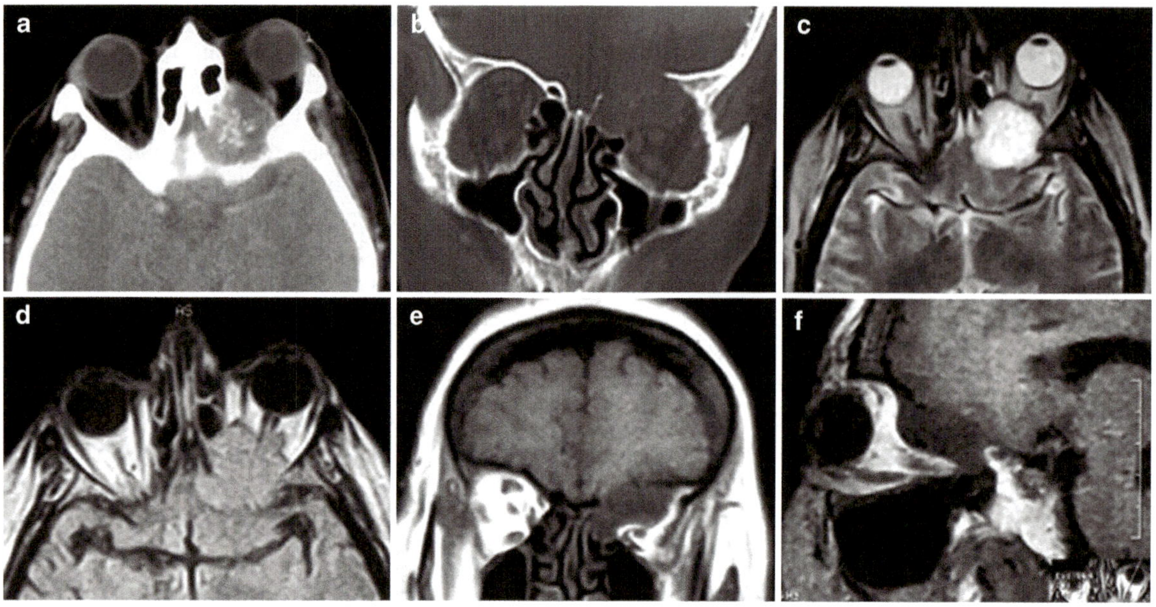

Fig. 13.2 A breast cancer metastasis. On CT in axial (**a**) and front (**b**) projections, an irregularly shaped tumor in the left orbital funnel is identified, causing the destruction of the orbital walls. There are small calcifications in the center of the tumor. On axial T2-weighted MRI (**c**) and T2-FLAIR (**d**) MRI, a quite homogeneous tumor is well defined. T1-weighted MR images in the frontal (**e**) and sagittal (**f**) views clearly show the destruction of the upper orbital wall and compression of the orbital fat and the optic nerve

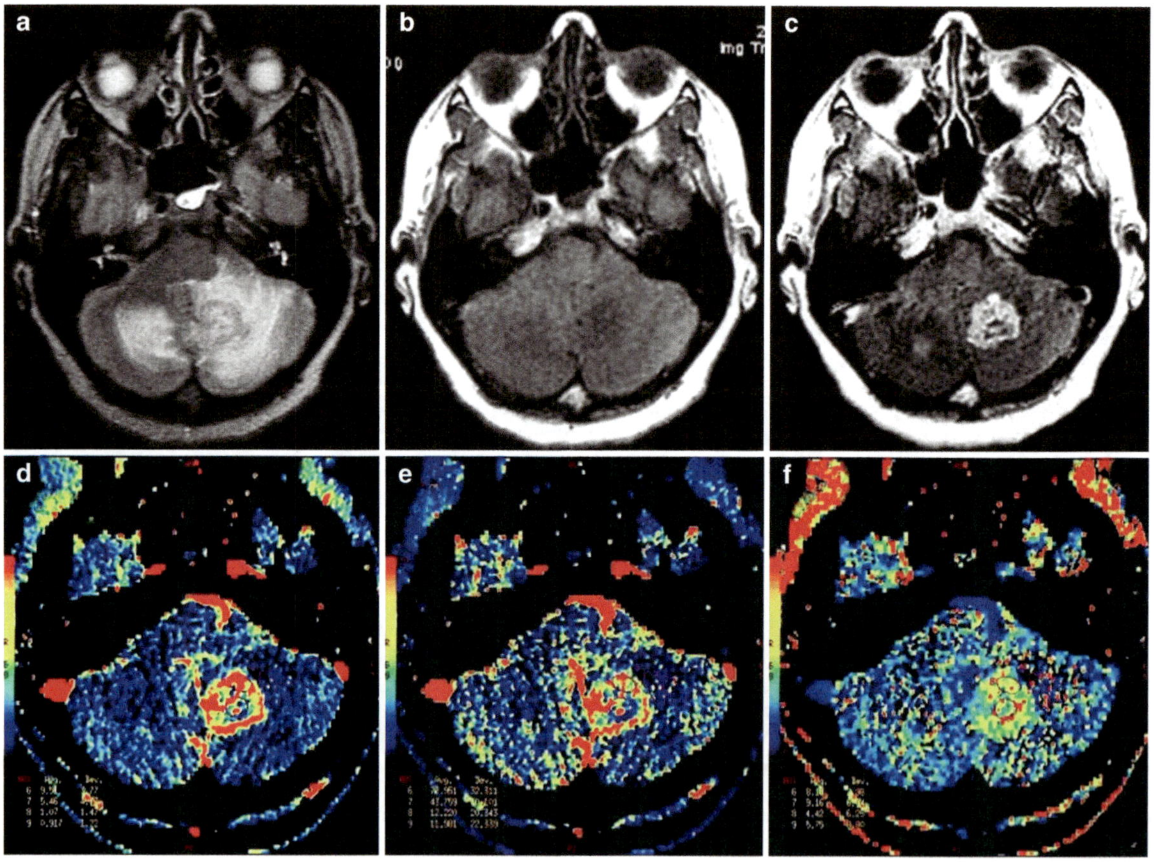

Fig. 13.3 Multiple breast cancer metastases in the brain. On MR images, in the left and right hemispheres of the cerebellum, there are areas with an iso-hyperintense signal on T2-FLAIR MRI (**a**) and a moderately hypointense signal on T1-weighted MRI (**b**). After the CA administration, its uneven intense accumulation is observed in a large lesion on the left and in a small lesion on the right (**c**). On CT perfusion maps, there is a marked increase in all perfusion parameters: CBF (**d**), CBV (**e**), and MTT (**f**)

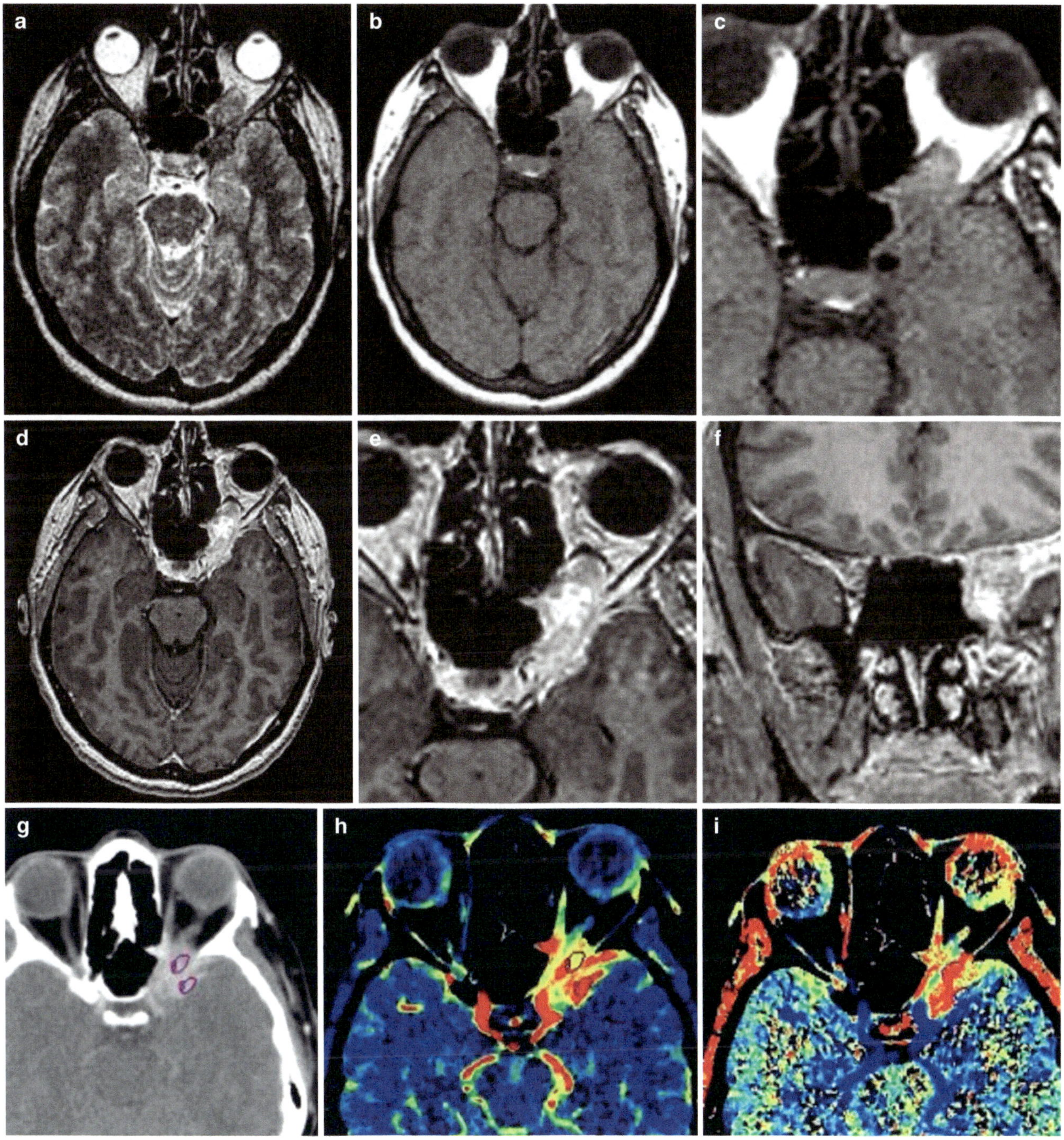

Fig. 13.4 A breast cancer metastasis. In the retrobulbar space on the left, there is a lesion with a low signal on T2-weighted MRI (**a**) and an isointense signal on T1-weighted MRI (**b**, **c**) with the spread to the orbital funnel. The lesion intensely accumulates CA (**d–f**), while the part of the tumor extending to the dura mater along the large wing of the sphenoid bone is well visualized. On contrast-enhanced CT (**g**), the tumor also intensely accumulates CA. On CT perfusion maps, the CBV (**h**) and MTT (**i**) values are increased both in the intraorbital portion of the tumor and along the meninges of the left temporal region

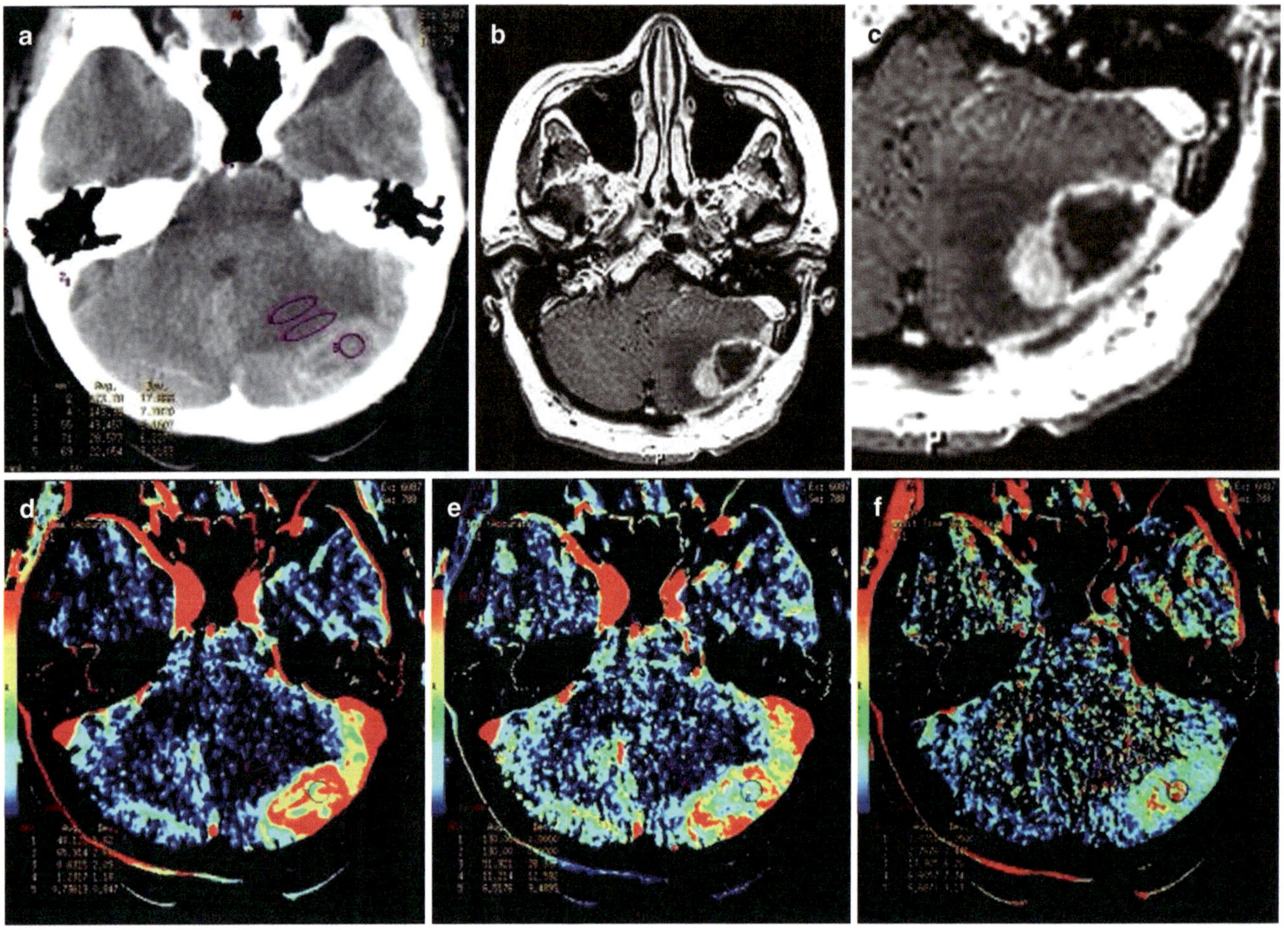

Fig. 13.5 A breast cancer metastasis in the brain. There is a solid-cystic lesion unevenly accumulating CA both on CT (**a**) and T1-weighted MRI (**b**, **c**) with signs of a moderate perifocal edema in the left hemisphere of the cerebellum. The fourth ventricle is compressed, and the brainstem is deformed. On CT perfusion, increased values of CBV (**d**), CBF (**e**), and MTT (**f**) are observed in the solid part of the metastasis

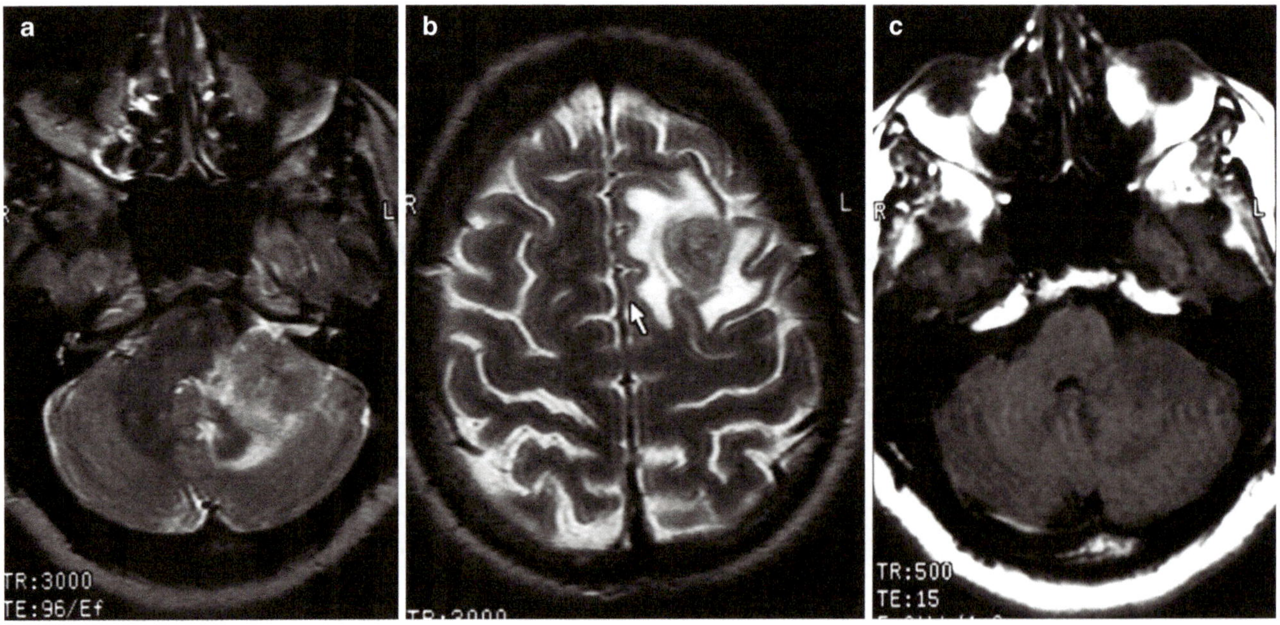

Fig. 13.6 Multiple breast cancer metastases in the brain. On T2-weighted (**a**, **b**) and T1-weighted (**c**, **d**) MRI, two solid tumor lesions are visualized supra- and subtentorially, which have low hyperintensity on T2 and low hypointensity on T1 signal intensity. The contrast enhancement is expressed and homogeneous (**e**)

Fig. 13.6 (continued)

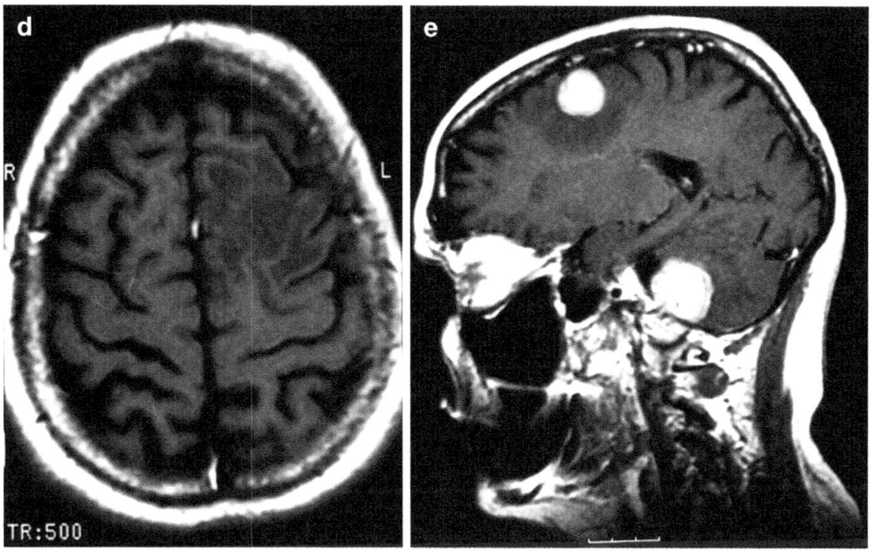

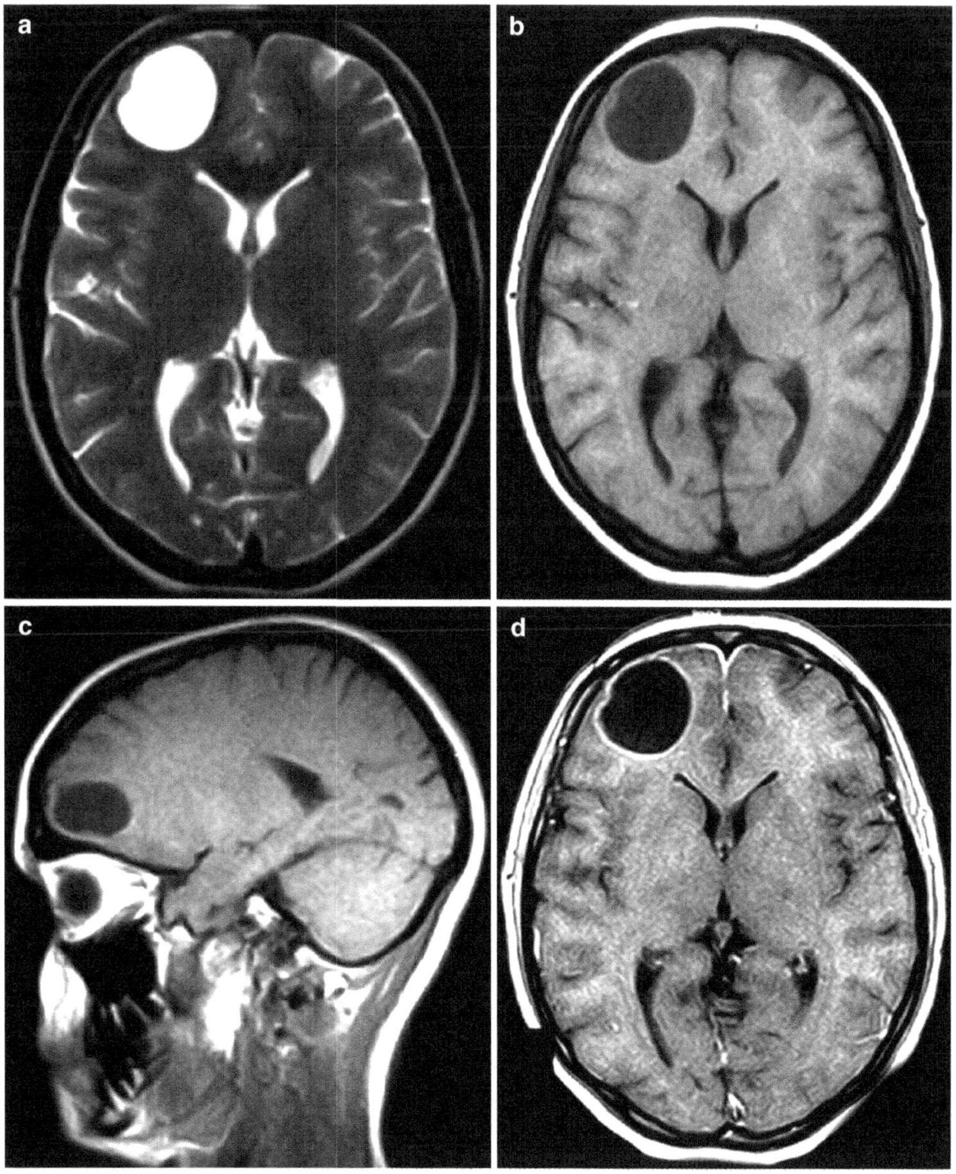

Fig. 13.7 A breast cancer metastasis in the brain. On MR images in the right frontal region, there is a large cystic lesion without a perifocal edema (**a–c**). After administration of the contrast agent, its intense accumulation is noted along the lesion contour in the form of a thin rim (**d**)

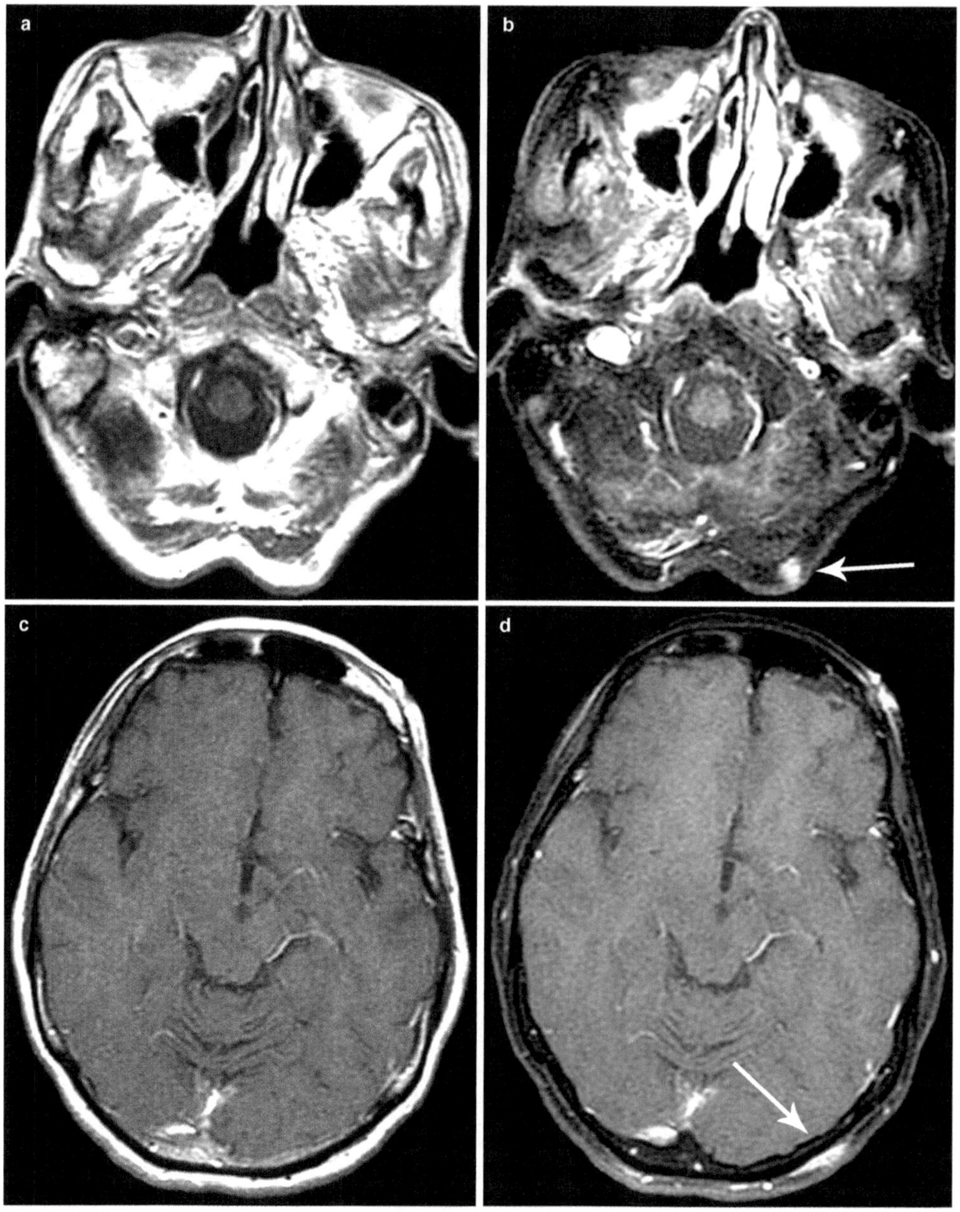

Fig. 13.8 Multiple breast cancer metastases in the brain. A two-level study. On T1-weighted MRI with contrast enhancement (**a**, **c**), no conclusive evidence of abnormalities have been detected. On T1-weighted MRI supplemented with fat suppression protocol (**b**, **d**), extracranially, in the soft tissue of the occipital region and the left occipital-parietal region, visualize lesions accumulating the contrast agent (the *arrows*)

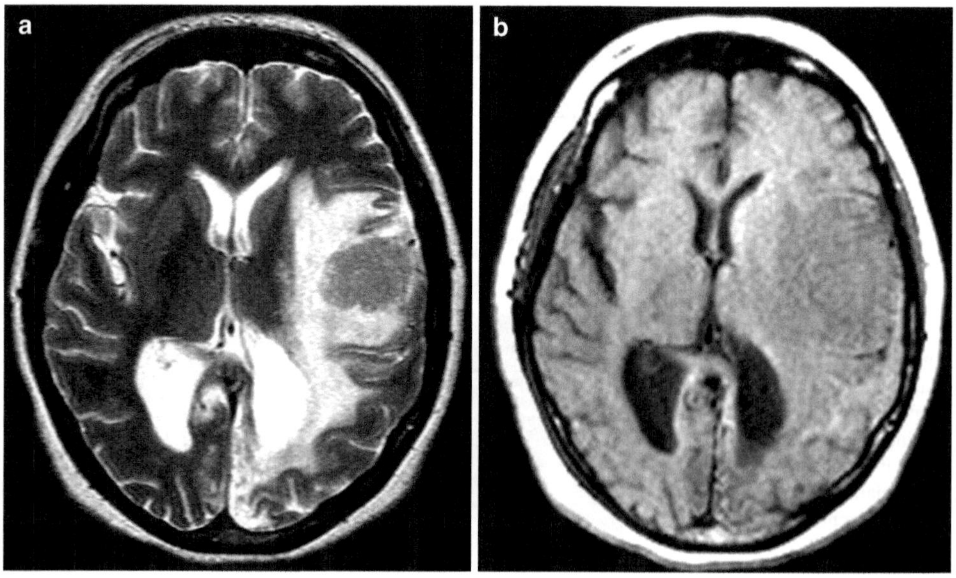

Fig. 13.9 A breast cancer metastasis in the brain. In the left frontotemporal region, there is a space-occupying solid lesion with an isointense MR signal on T2-weighted MRI (**a**) and moderately hypointense on T1-weighted MRI (**b**) with signs of a pronounced perifocal edema. The lesion intensely and uniformly accumulates the contrast agent (**c**, **d**). A pinpoint portion of accumulation medially to the main lesion is likely a blood vessel (**c**) (the *arrow*). There is displacement of the midline structures to the right and a moderate compression of the left lateral ventricle

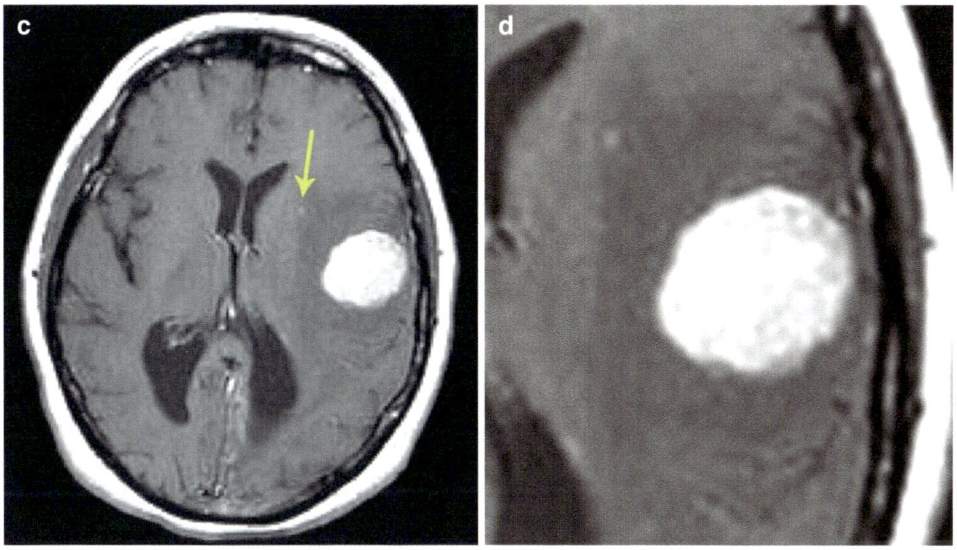

Fig. 13.9 (continued)

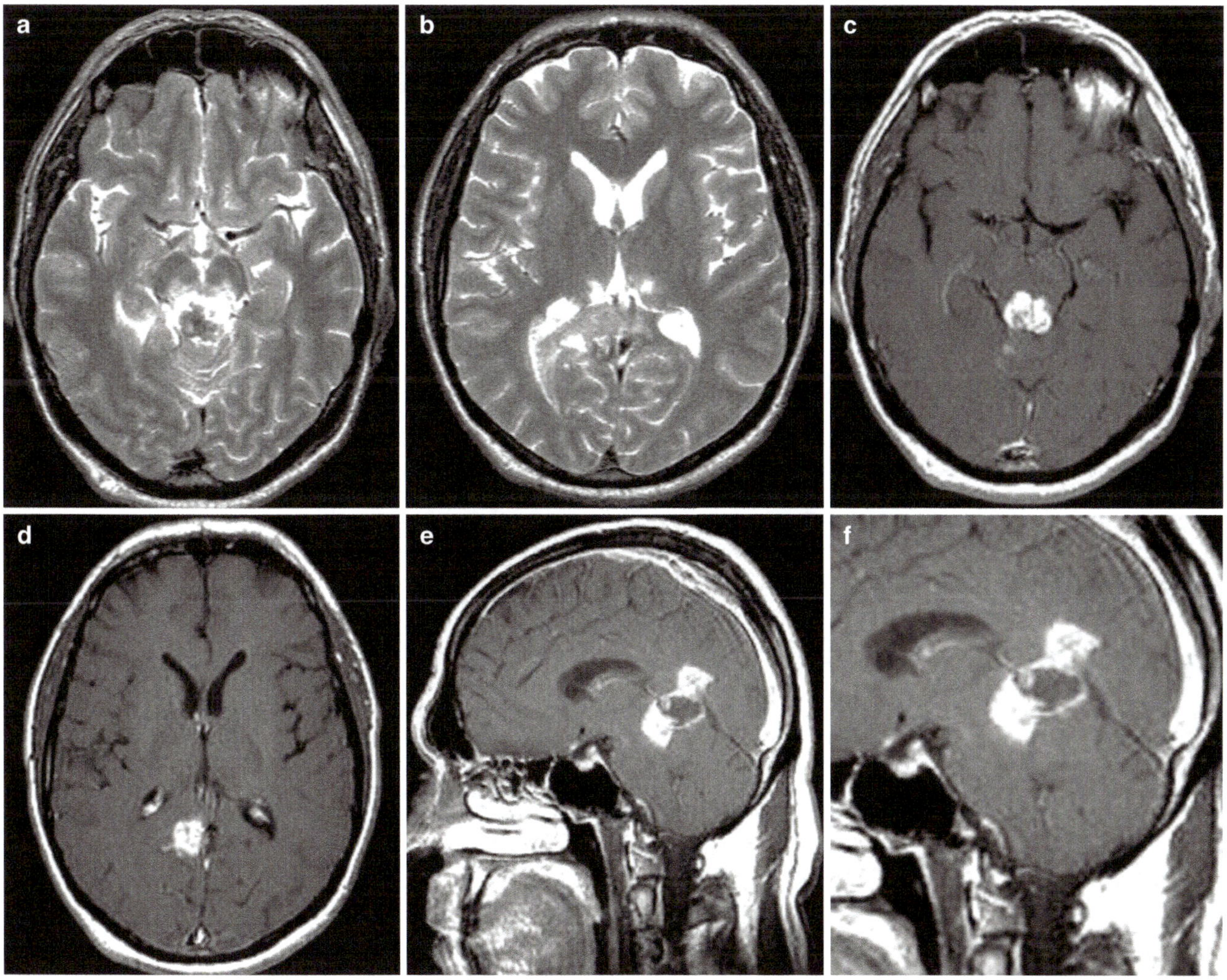

Fig. 13.10 A breast cancer metastasis. A two-level study. In the pineal region, there is an area with an iso-hyperintense MR signal on T2-weighted MRI without clear contours (**a**, **b**). After the CA administration, there is its intense uneven accumulation (**c**, **d**) in the specified area. In the sagittal projection, the upper and lower solid components of the tumor, as well as the central part of the cystic metastasis (**e**, **f**) are well visualized

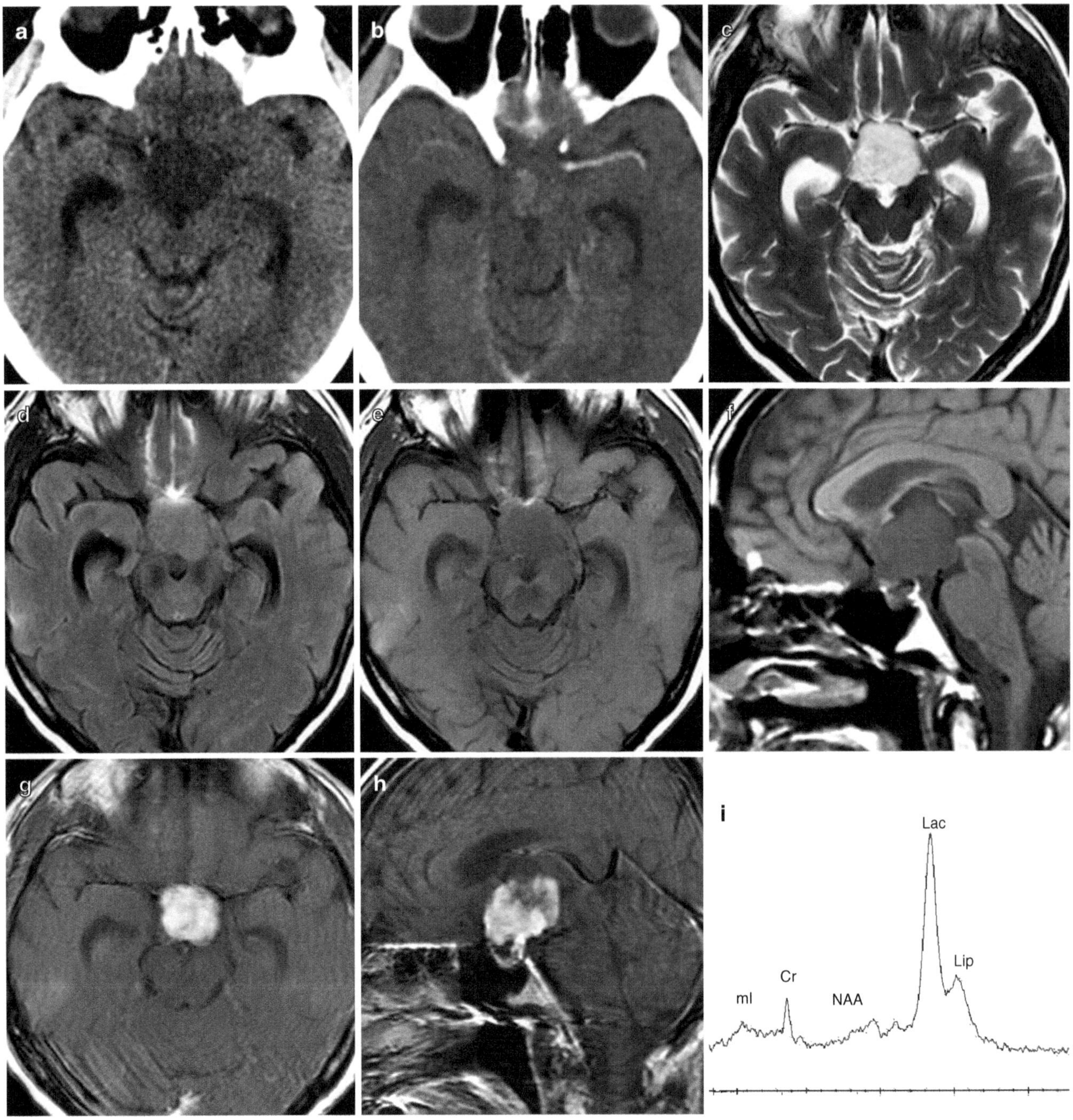

Fig. 13.11 A breast cancer metastasis in the brain. On axial spiral CT before (**a**) and after (**b**) contrast enhancement, there is a hypodense, rounded space-occupying lesion that moderately accumulates CA in the suprasellar region. The lesion has an increased signal on T2-weighted MRI (**c**) and an isointense signal on T2-FLAIR (**d**) and T1-weighted MRI (**e**, **f**). After contrast enhancement (**g**, **h**), the lesion has an unevenly increased signal, and the upper portions of the metastasis accumulate contrast agent in a lesser degree. On proton MR spectroscopy of the metastasis (**i**), a high peak of the Lip-Lac complex is determined

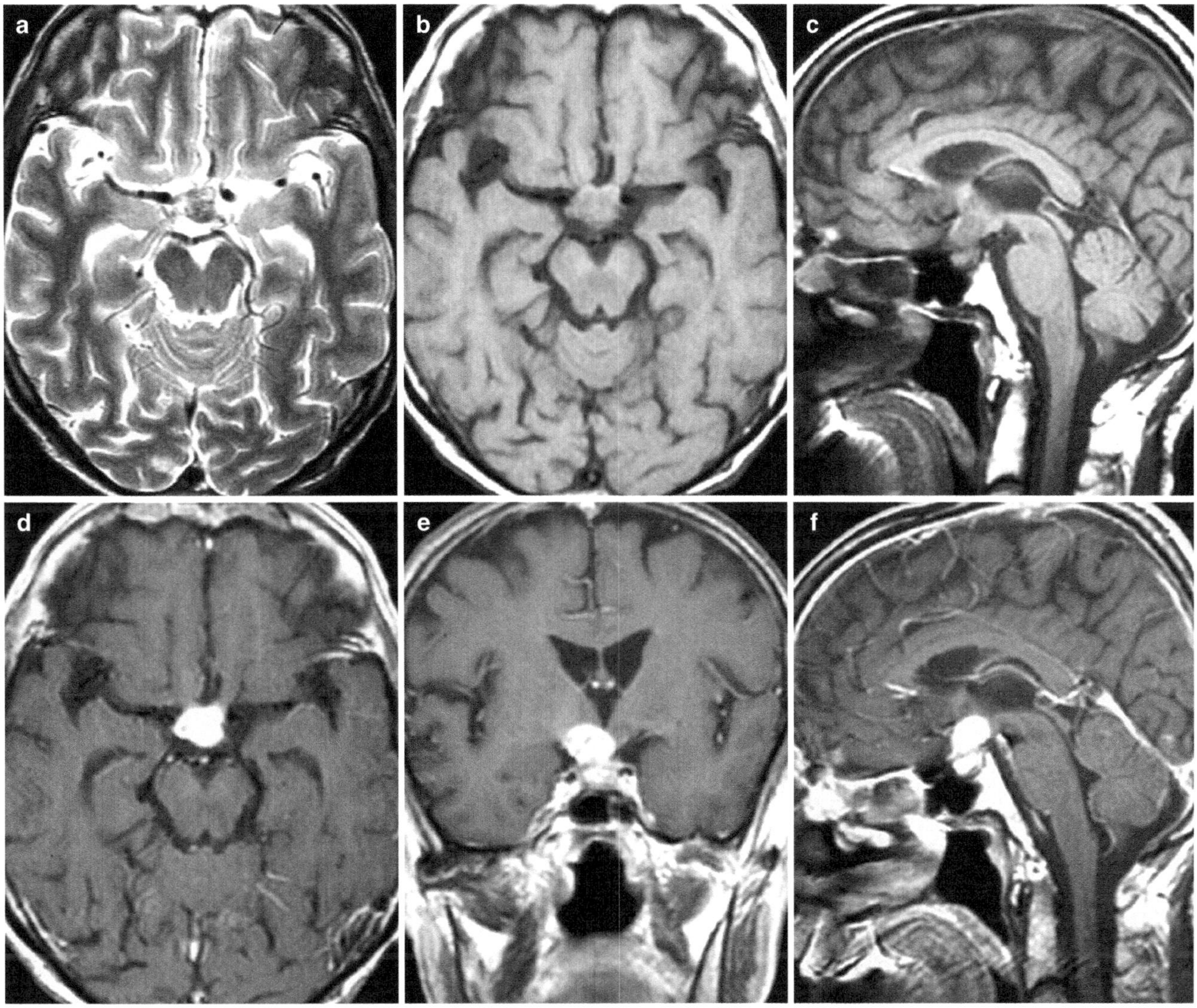

Fig. 13.12 A breast cancer metastasis in the brain. On T2-weighted MRI (**a**) and T1-weighted MRI (**b**, **c**), there is a small, isointense space-occupying lesion in the projection of the bottom of ventricle III. After intravenous administration of the contrast agent (**d**–**f**), the contours of the tumor with intense contrast enhancement, located over the Turkish saddle, are clearly identified

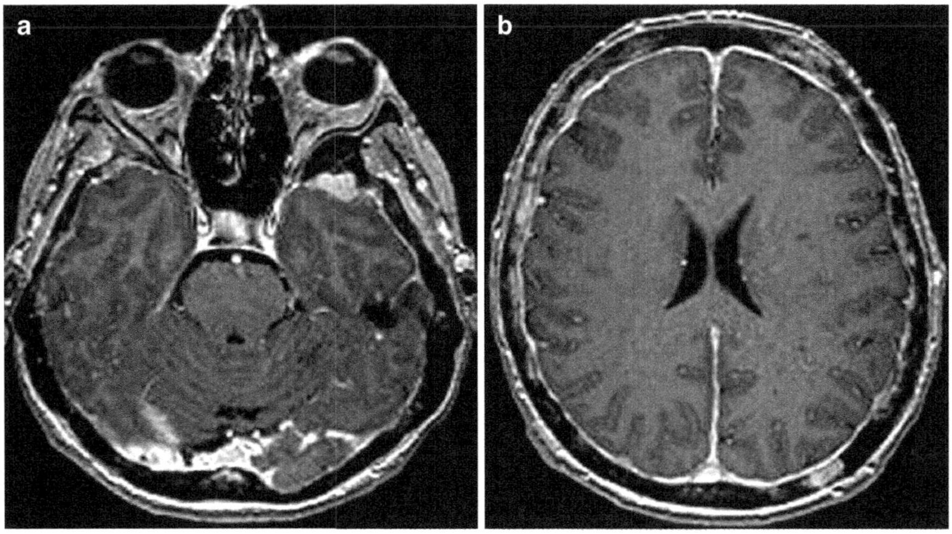

Fig. 13.13 Multiple breast cancer metastases in the brain. On T1-weighted fat sat MR images with contrast enhancement (**a**–**d**), there is a total thickening and accumulation of contrast agent along the dura mater of both hemispheres of the brain and multiple lesions of the bone structures of the cranial vault

Fig. 13.13 (conitinued)

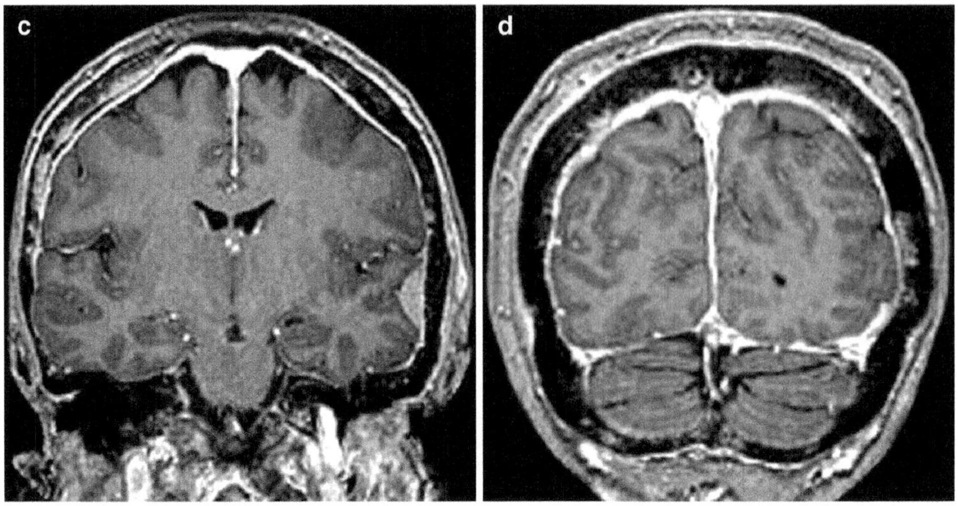

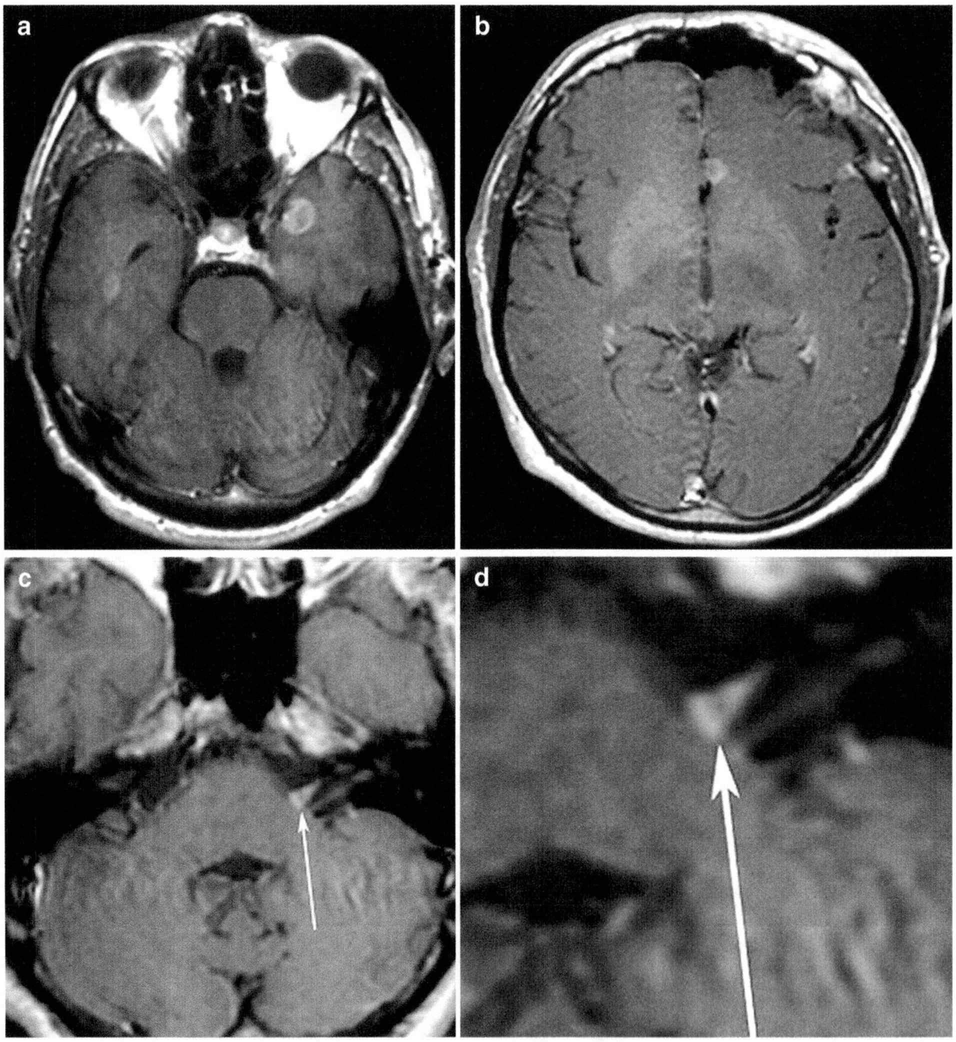

Fig. 13.14 Multiple breast cancer metastases in the brain. On MRI after administration of the contrast agent on T1-weighted images, there are multiple tumor lesions in the temporal and left frontal areas (**a**, **b**), and also abnormal CA accumulation is observed in the cisternal segment of nerve VII on the left (*arrow*) (**c**, **d**)

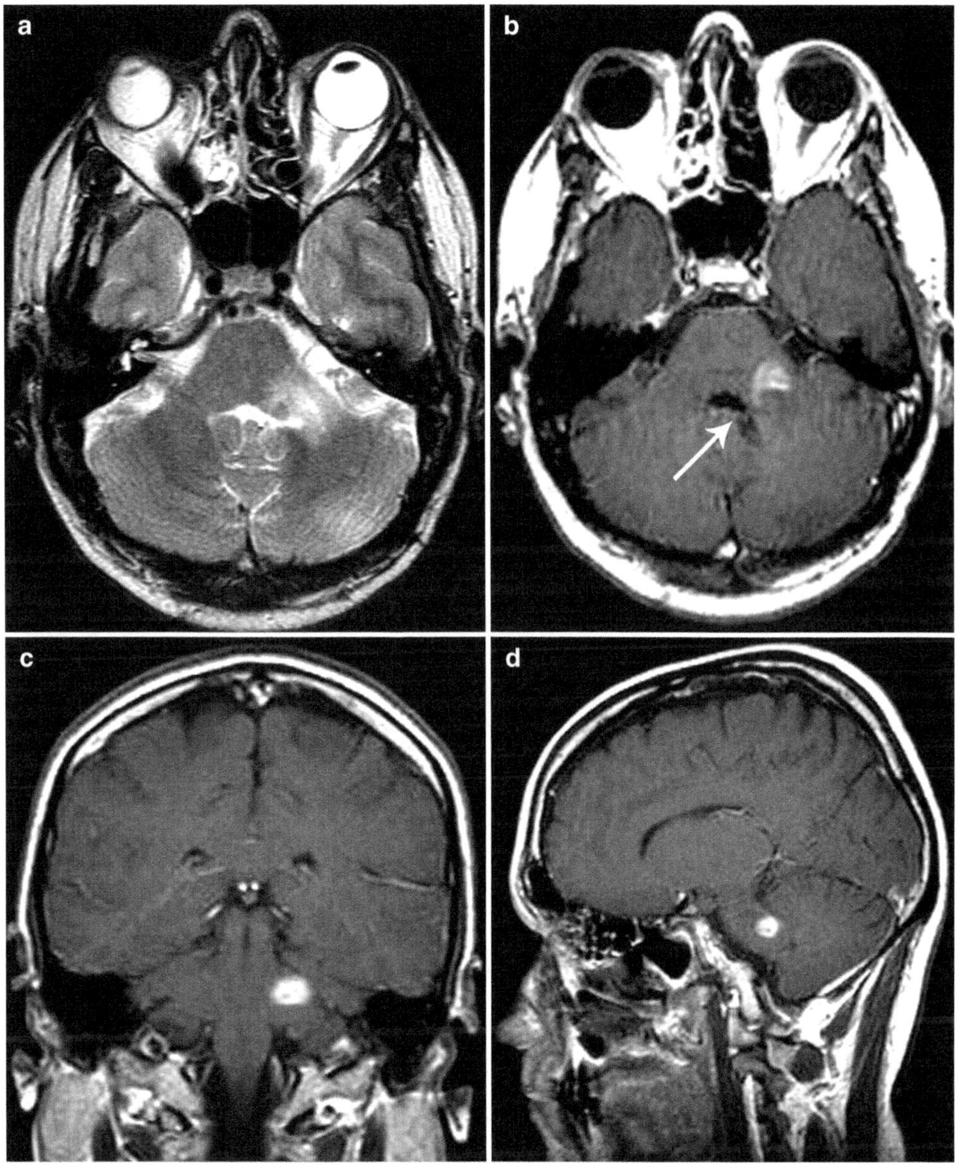

Fig. 13.15 A breast cancer metastasis in the brain. In the projection of the upper left cerebellar peduncle, there is a portion of a hyperintense T2-weighted MR signal (**a**). After CA administration, its intense accumulation in a small metastasis is observed: axial, coronal, and sagittal projections (**b**–**d**). Of note is the minimum compression of the fourth ventricle

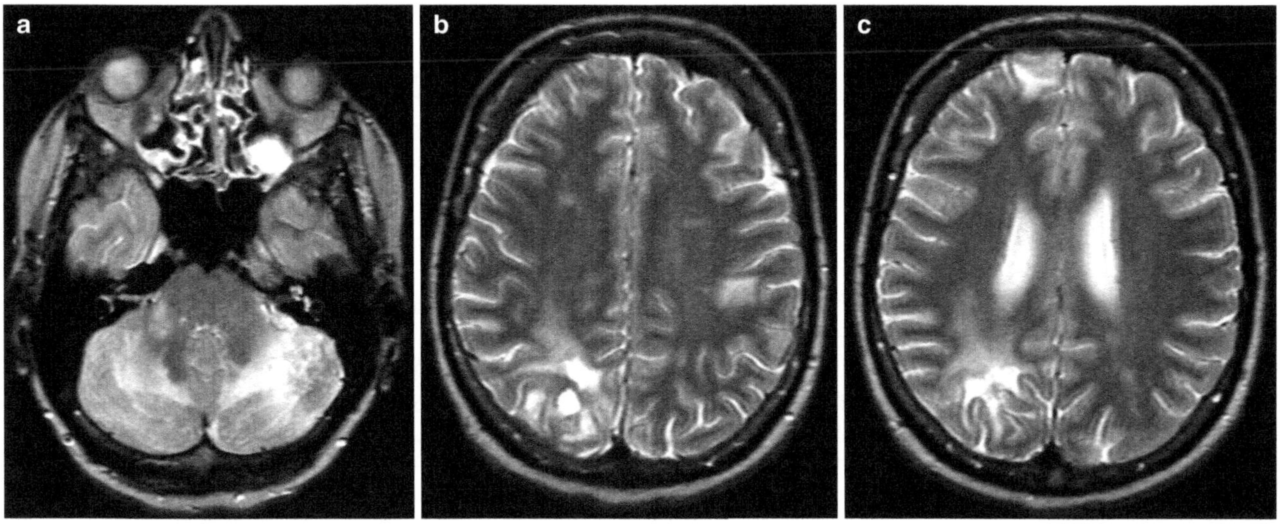

Fig. 13.16 Multiple breast cancer metastases in the brain. On T2-weighted (**a**, **b**, **c**) and T1-weighted (**d**, **e**, **f**) MRI following a double dosage of CA, multiple tumor lesions are identified sub- and supratentorially. Despite their small size, the lesions show signs of central necrosis

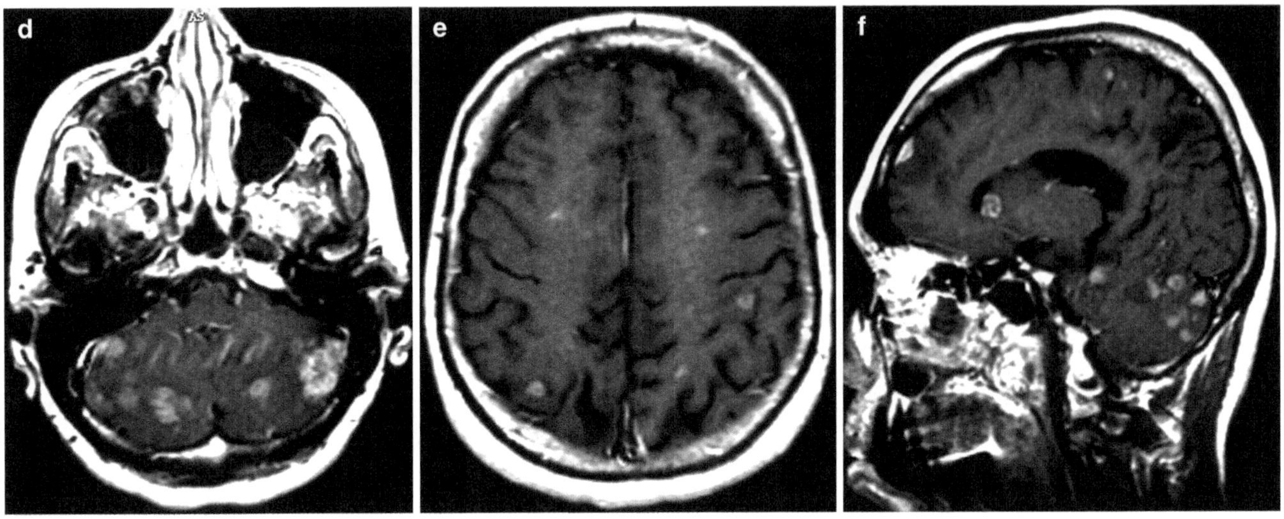

Fig. 13.16 (continued)

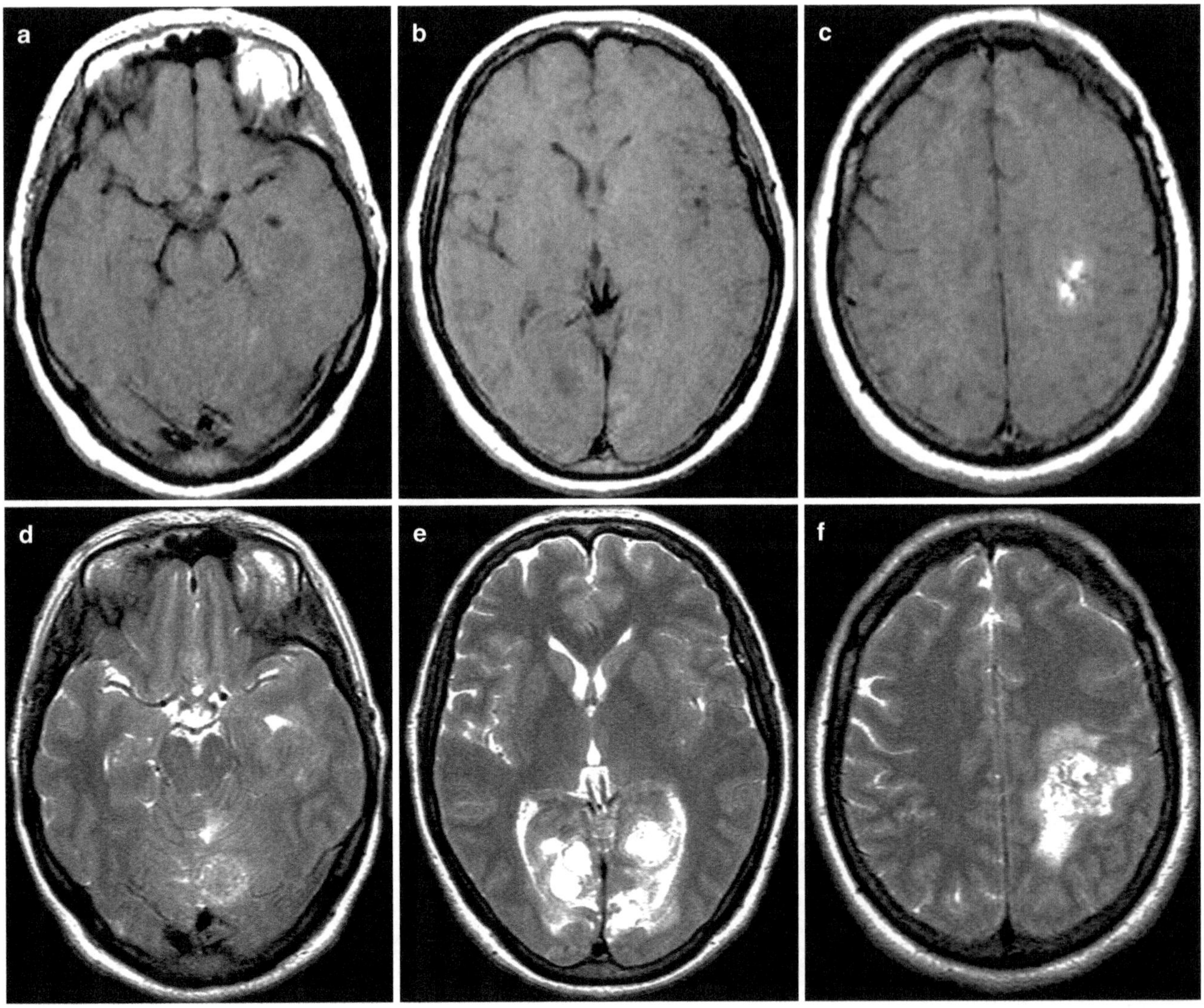

Fig. 13.17 Multiple breast cancer metastases in the brain. A three-level study. On T1-weighted MRI, there is a single site with an unevenly hyperintense signal on the border of the left frontal and parietal lobes (**a**–**c**). On T2-weighted MRI in both the occipital and left parietal regions, multiple areas of an iso-hyperintense signal are identified (**d**–**f**). After CA administration, on T1-weighted MRI, multiple metastatic lesions rapidly accumulating CA are observed in the axial (**g**–**i**), frontal (**j**), and sagittal (**k**, **l**) projections, in both cerebral and cerebellar hemispheres

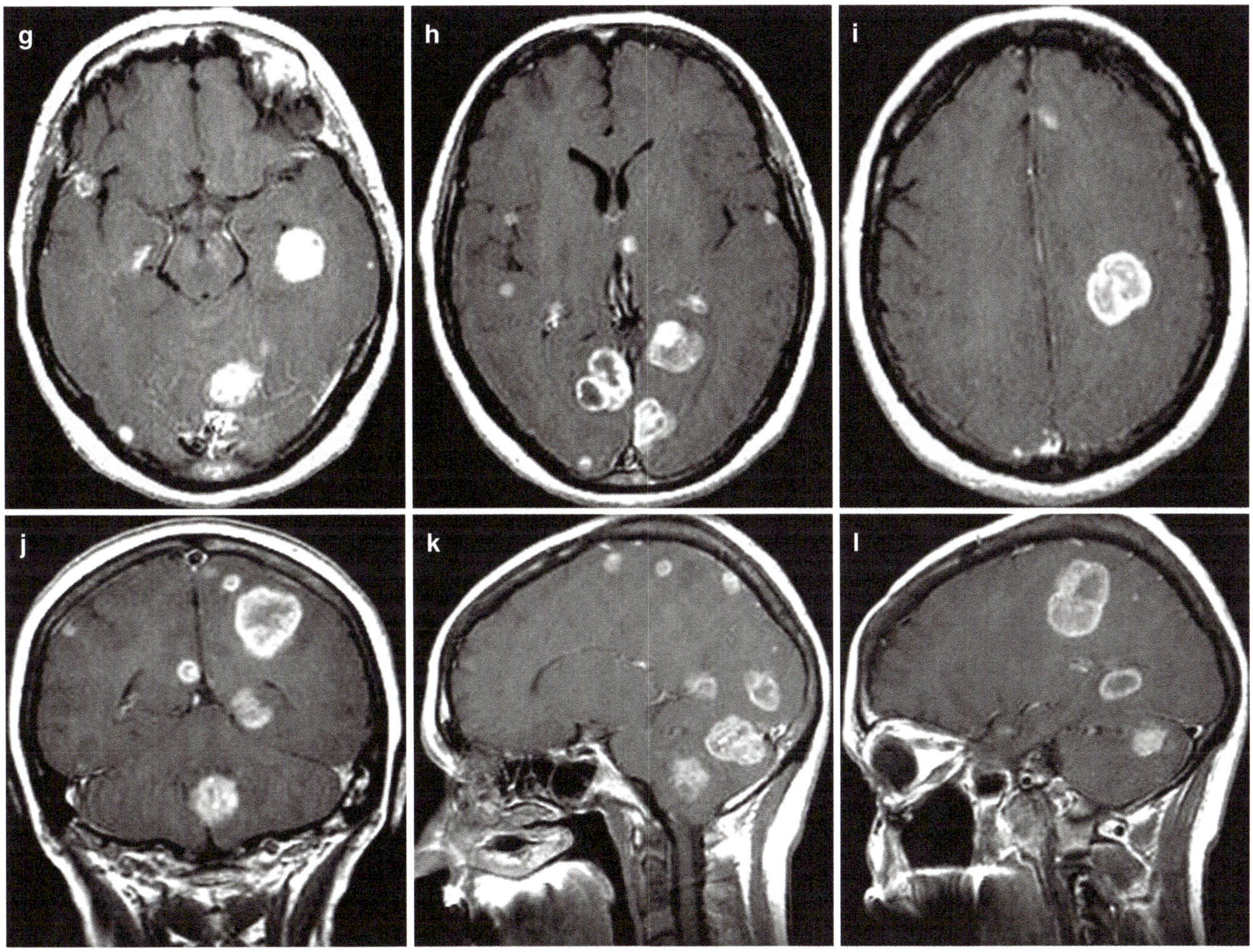

Fig. 13.17 (continued)

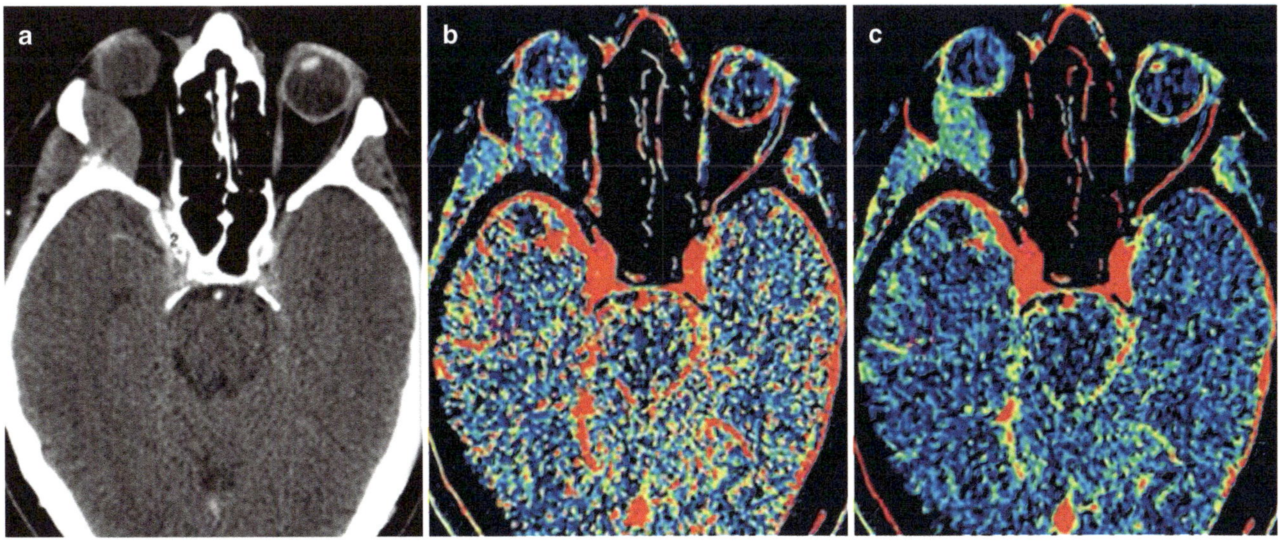

Fig. 13.18 A breast cancer metastasis in the right orbit. On a CT scan in the axial projection (**a**), there is a tumor located in the lateral parts of the right orbit, which causes the local bone destruction and significant exophthalmos. According to the CT perfusion study, an increase in CBF (**b**) and CBV (**c**) values and MTT prolongation (**d**) are observed. On T1-weighted MRI, at two levels (**e**, **f**), there are a homogeneous tumor, destruction of the lateral orbital wall, and spread of the metastasis in soft tissues of the orbit and infratemporal fossa

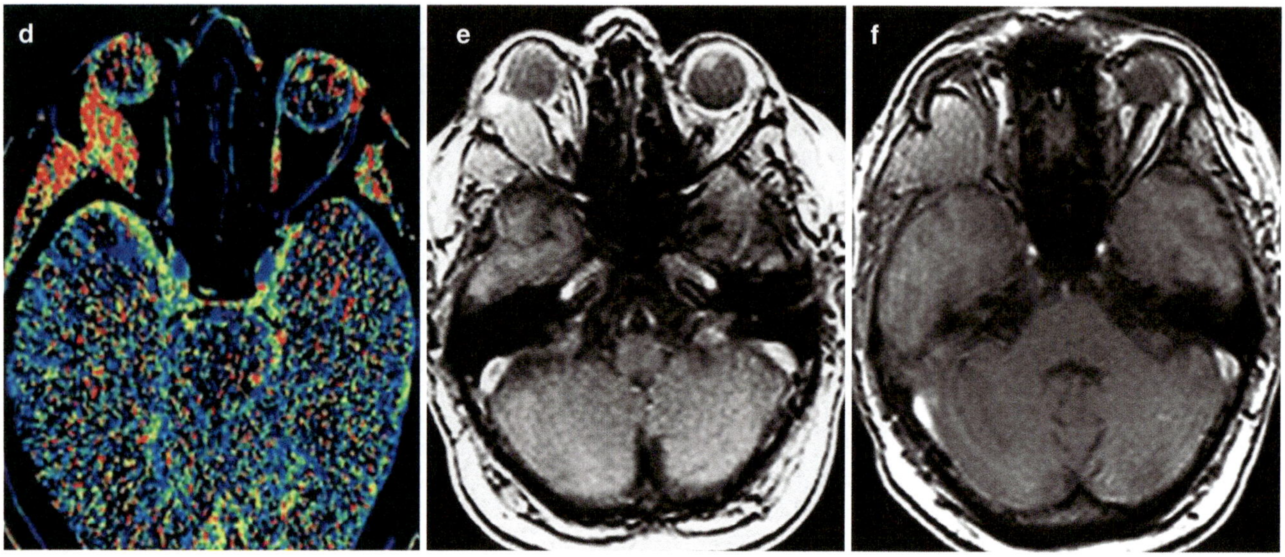

Fig. 13.18 (continued)

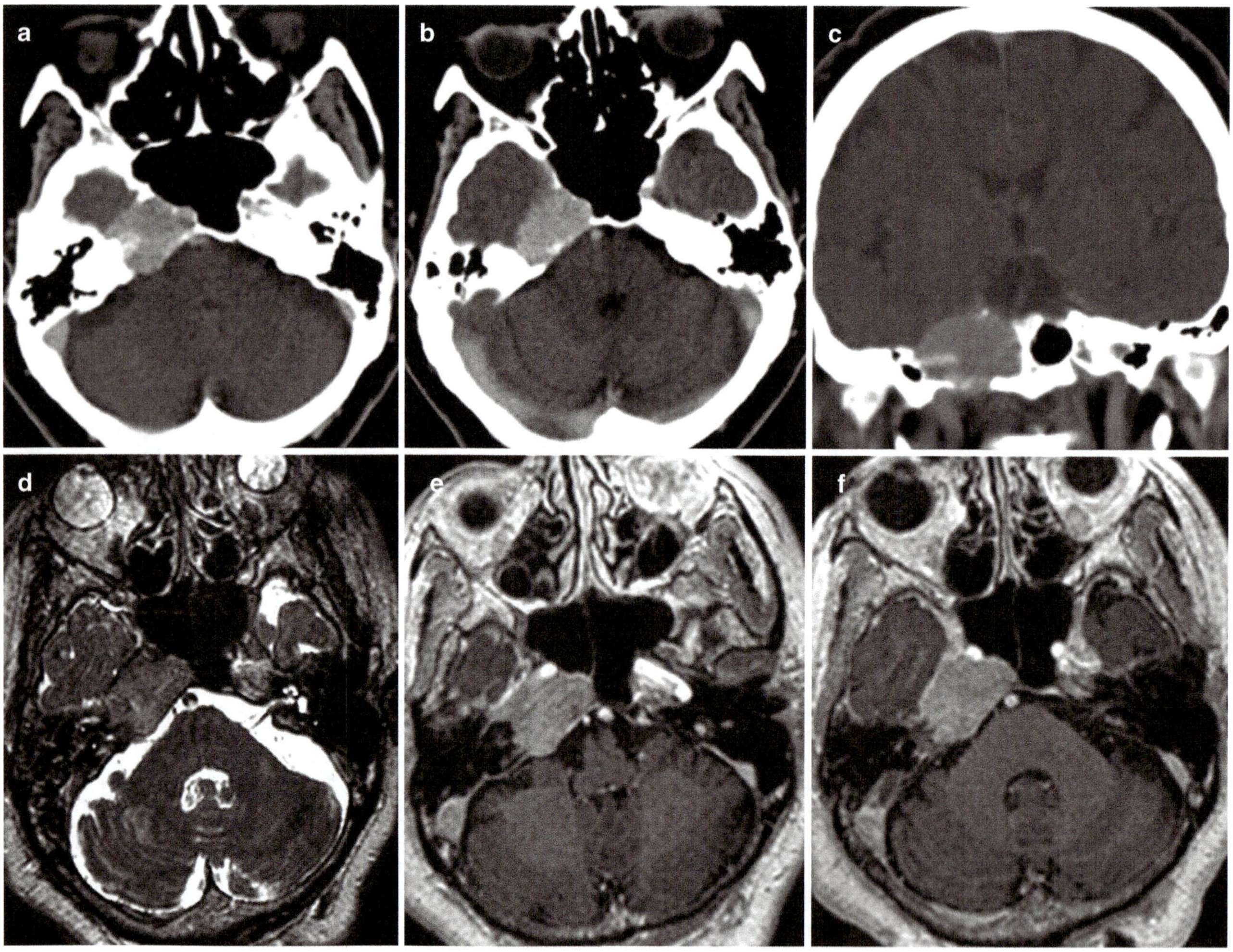

Fig. 13.19 A breast cancer metastasis. On CT (**a–c**) with contrast enhancement, a lesion is visualized in the projection of the apex of the petrous pyramid on the right and lateral sections of the sphenoid bone body, causing the destruction of surrounding bone structures. The tumor rapidly accumulates the contrast agent. On T2-weighted MRI (**d**), the metastasis has isointense characteristics relative to the brain. Contrast enhancement on T1-weighted MRI is homogeneous and pronounced (**e, f**)

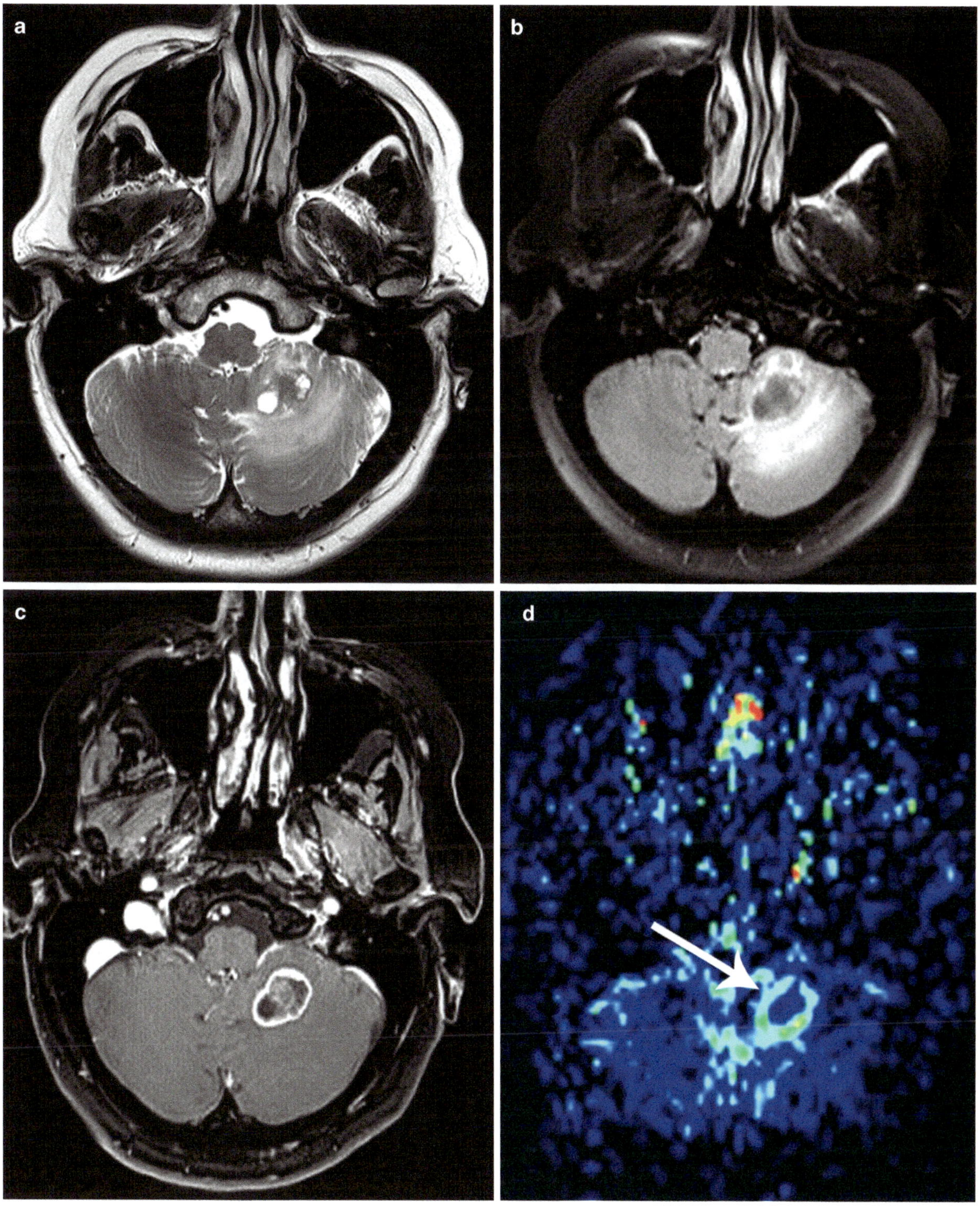

Fig. 13.20 A breast cancer metastasis in the brain. In the depth of the left cerebellar hemisphere, there is a solid-cystic lesion with a hypo-hyperintense signal on T2-weighted MRI (**a**) and a predominantly hypointense signal on T2-FLAIR MRI (**b**) with signs of a pronounced perifocal edema. After CA administration, the lesion unevenly accumulates CA mainly along the contour (**c**). On ASL MRI, there is an increase in CBF values on the periphery of the metastasis (d) (the *arrow*)

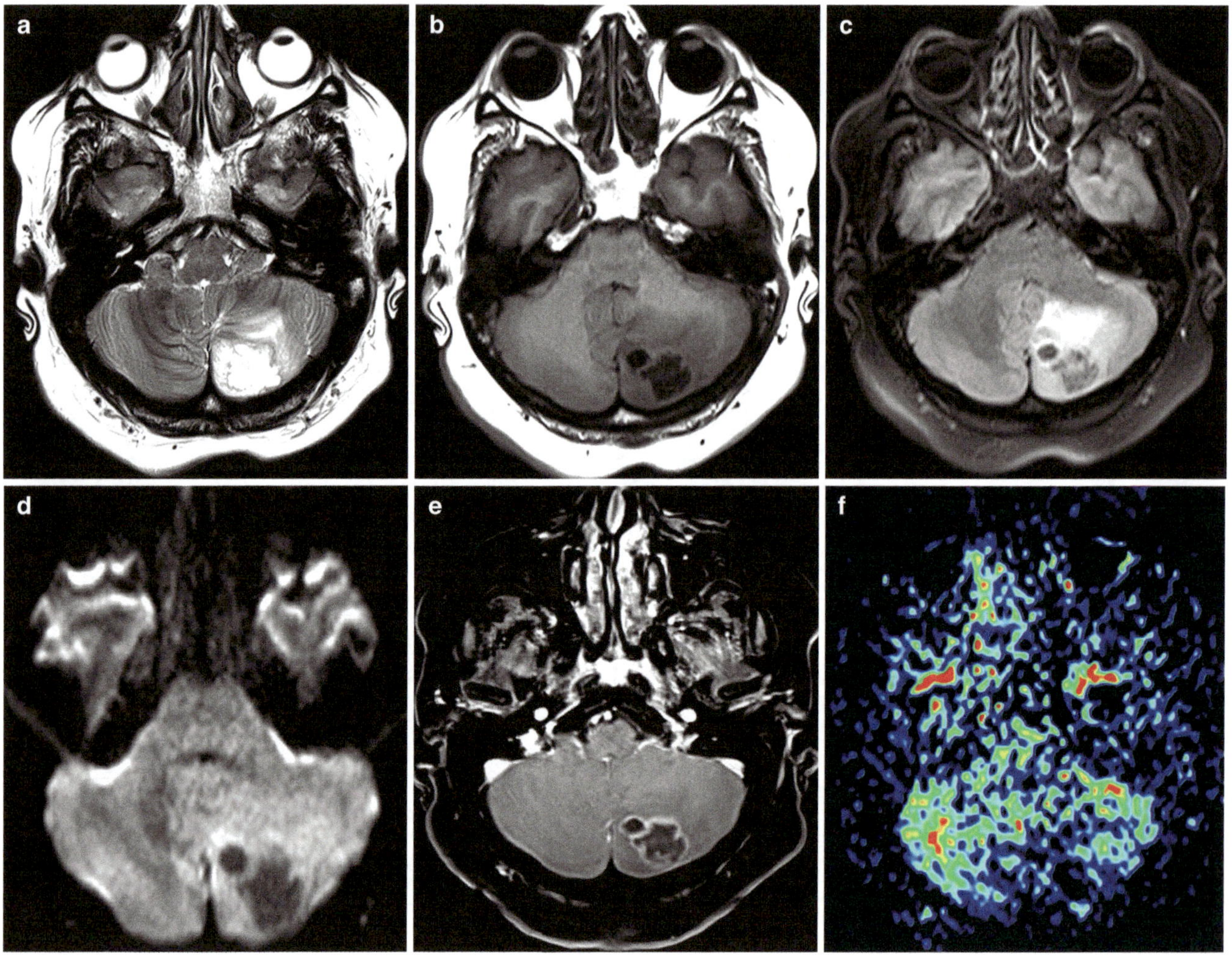

Fig. 13.21 A breast cancer metastasis in the brain during drug therapy. In the left cerebellar hemisphere, there is a cystic lesion with an increased signal on T2-weighted MRI (**a**), a hypointense signal on T1-weighted MRI (**b**) and DWI (**d**), and a heterogeneous signal on T2-FLAIR MRI (**c**). After CA administration, its intense accumulation along the contour of the metastasis (**e**) is observed, with well-visualized components of the multinodular lesion. On ASL MRI in the lesion area, there is a marked decrease in perfusion (**f**)

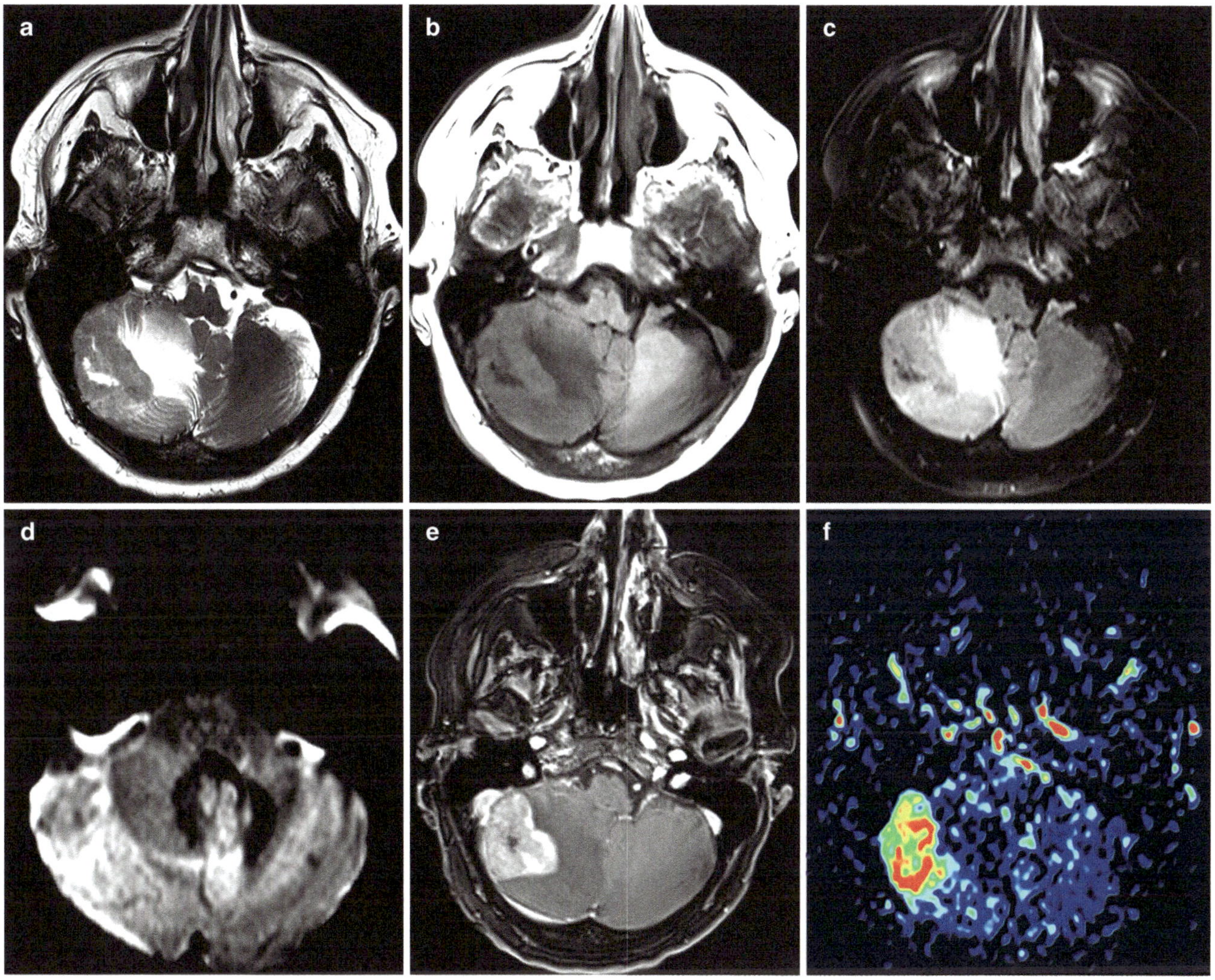

Fig. 13.22 A breast cancer metastasis. In the right cerebellar hemisphere, there is a lesion with a small area of decay in the central portion of a heterogeneously hyperintense signal on T2-weighted (**a**) and T2-FLAIR (**c**) MRI, an iso-hypointense signal on T1-weighted MRI (**b**), and a hyperintense signal on DWI MRI (**d**). There is intensive CA accumulation in the solid part of the metastasis (**e**). On ASL MRI (**f**), there is a pronounced uneven increase in CBF values. The lesion is surrounded by an area of perifocal edema, which causes the displacement of the adjacent brainstem structures and compression of the fourth ventricle. The tumor is closely adjacent to the transverse sinus

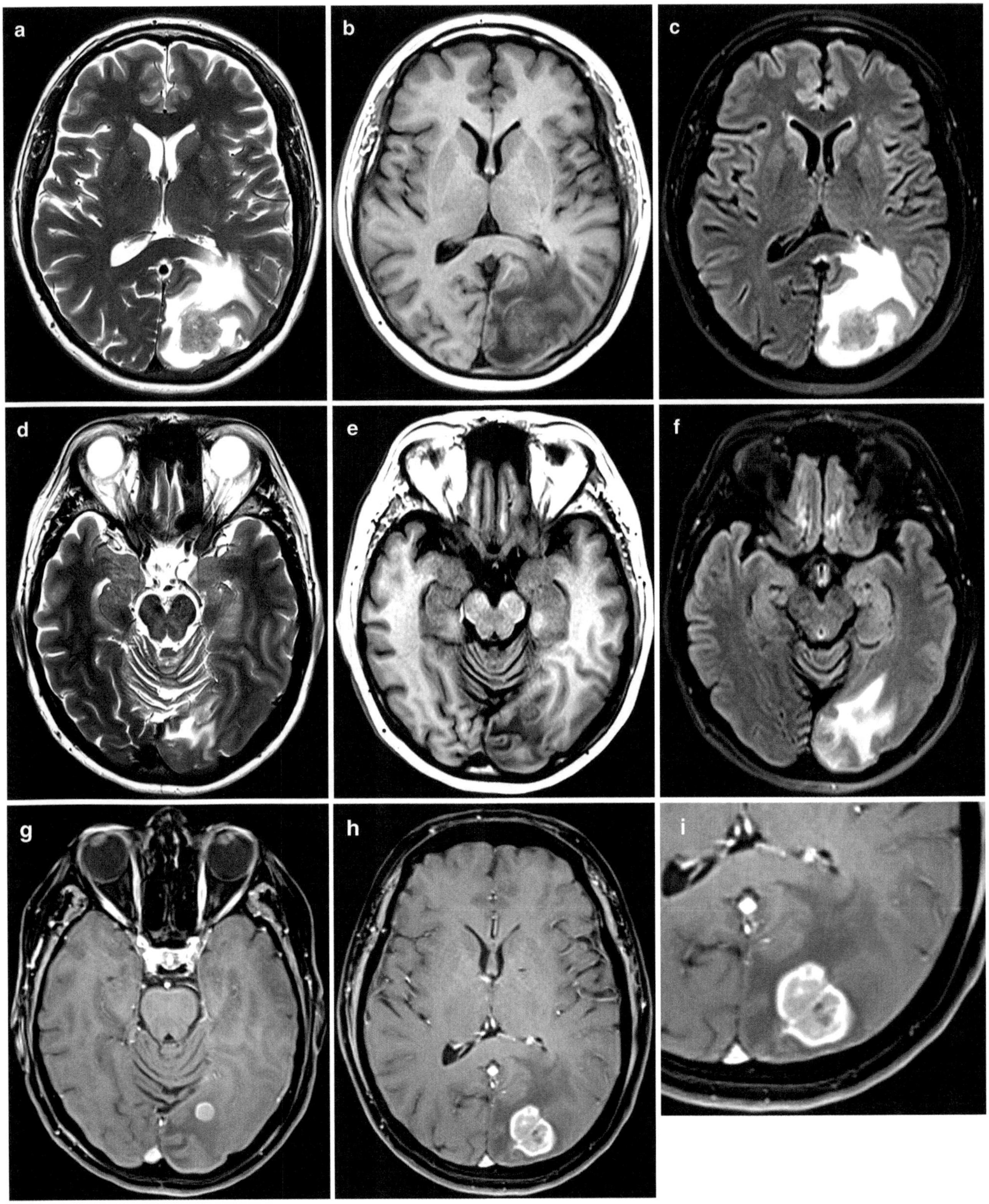

Fig. 13.23 Multiple breast cancer metastases in the brain. A two-level study. In the left occipital region, there are superimposed metastatic lesions with an iso-hyperintense signal on T2-weighted MRI (**a**, **d**), a hypointense signal on T1-weighted MRI (**b**, **e**), and an isointense signal on T2-FLAIR MRI (**c**, **f**) with signs of a pronounced perifocal edema. The lesions intensely accumulate the contrast agent (**g**–**i**). On ASL MRI, CBF values are high in both metastatic lesions (**j**–**l**)

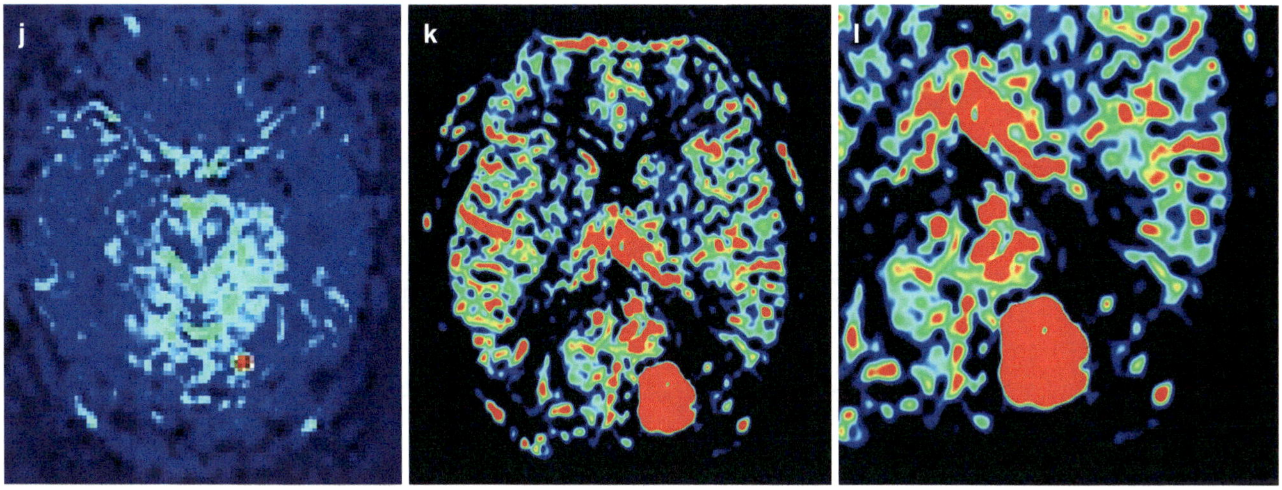

Fig. 13.23 (continued)

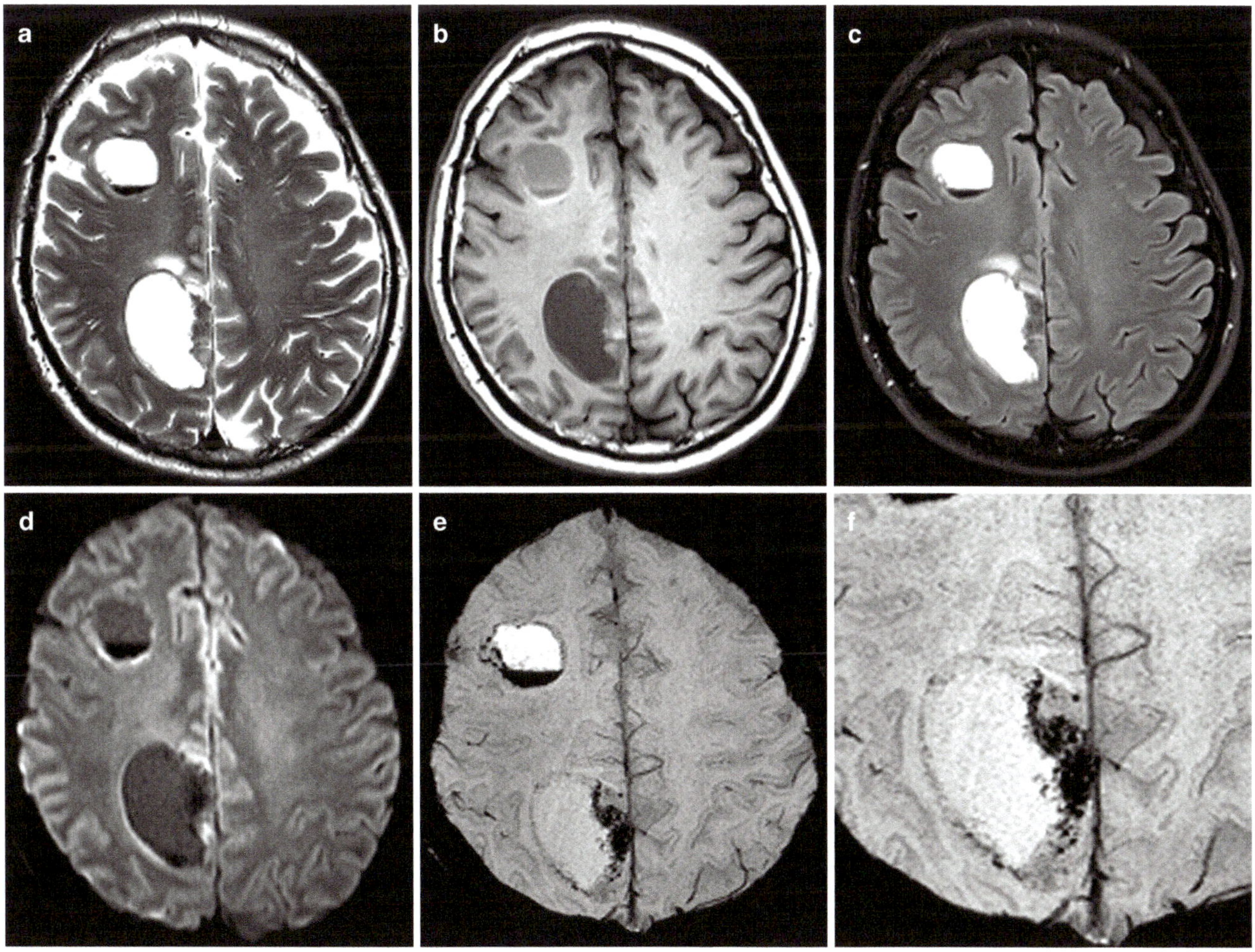

Fig. 13.24 Multiple breast cancer metastases in the brain. A follow-up study before and after chemoradiotherapy. In the right hemisphere of the brain, there are multiple lesions with the solid-cystic structure and a hyper-hypointense MR signal on T2-weighted MRI (**a**), hyper-hypointense signal on T1-weighted MRI (**b**), and hyper-hypointense signal on T2-FLAIR MRI (**c**). In the cystic portion of the lesion, in right frontal area, the "level" of hemorrhagic content is well visualized. The signal from the cystic content is increased on T1-weighted MRI due to blood. On DWI MRI, there are areas of a hyperintense signal on the periphery of the lesions (**d**). On SWI (SWAN) MRI, in the solid structure of the metastases, multiple pinpoint areas of hypointense signal (**e**, **f**) are observed. Following chemoradiotherapy, a significant decrease in the size of the lesions and change in their structure are noted (**g**–**i**). An increased signal from the white matter on T2-weighted (**g**) and T2-FLAIR (**h**) MRI represents post-radiation changes (leukoencephalopathy)

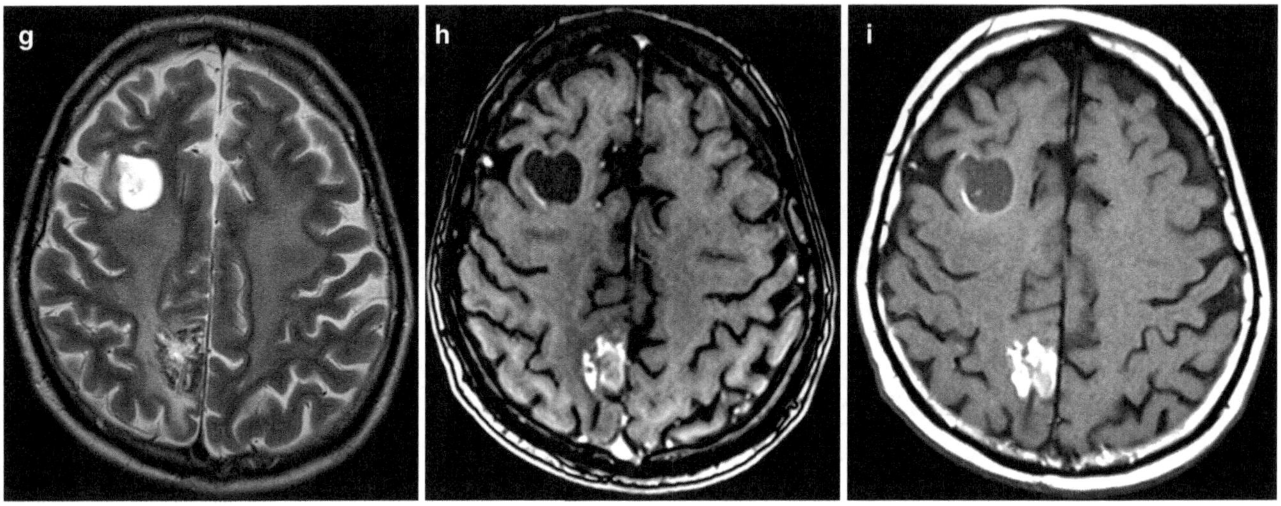

Fig. 13.24 (continued)

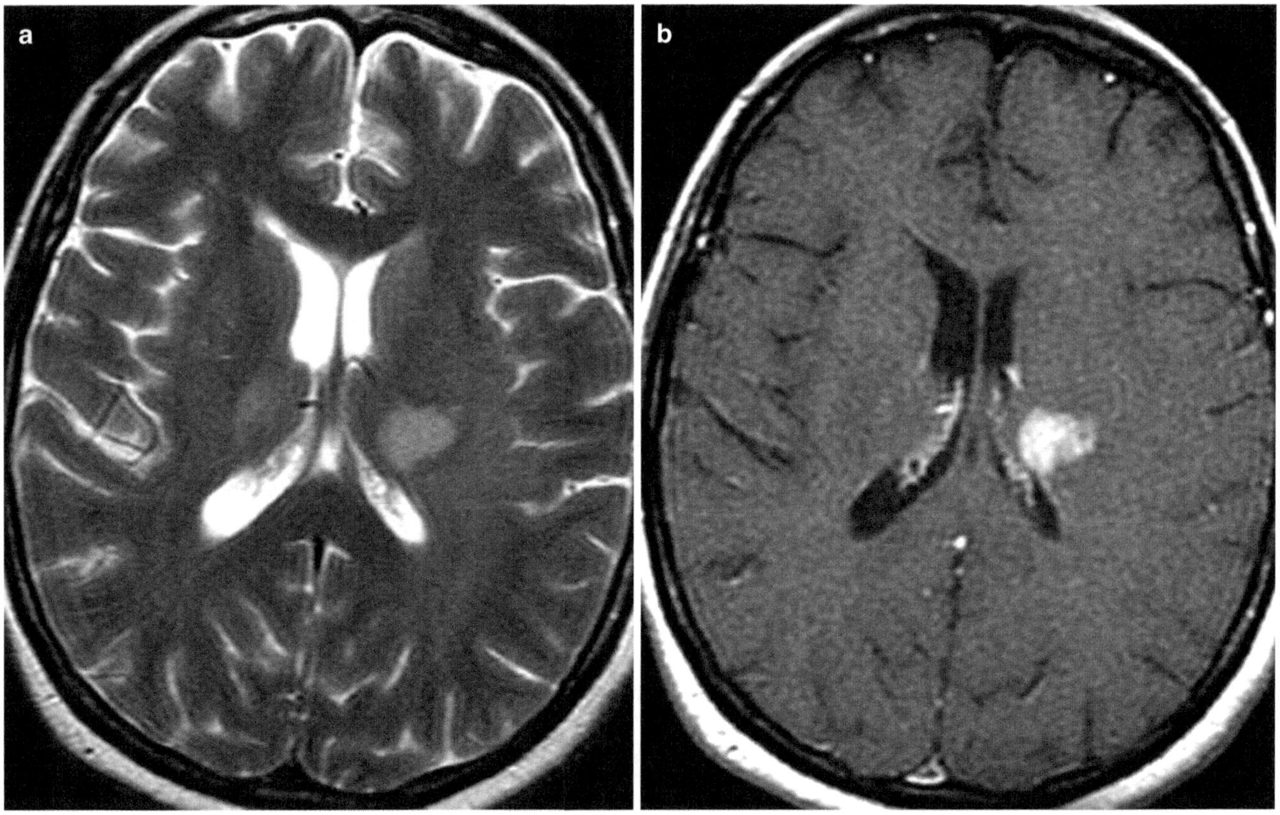

Fig. 13.25 A breast cancer metastasis in the brain. In the posterior thalamic region on the left, there is an area with a moderately hyperintense signal on T2-weighted MRI (**a**), intensely accumulating the contrast agent, without clear contours along the lateral pole (**b**). On MR tractography (**c**, **d**), there is a deformation of the conductive pathways medially and laterally with respect to the metastasis

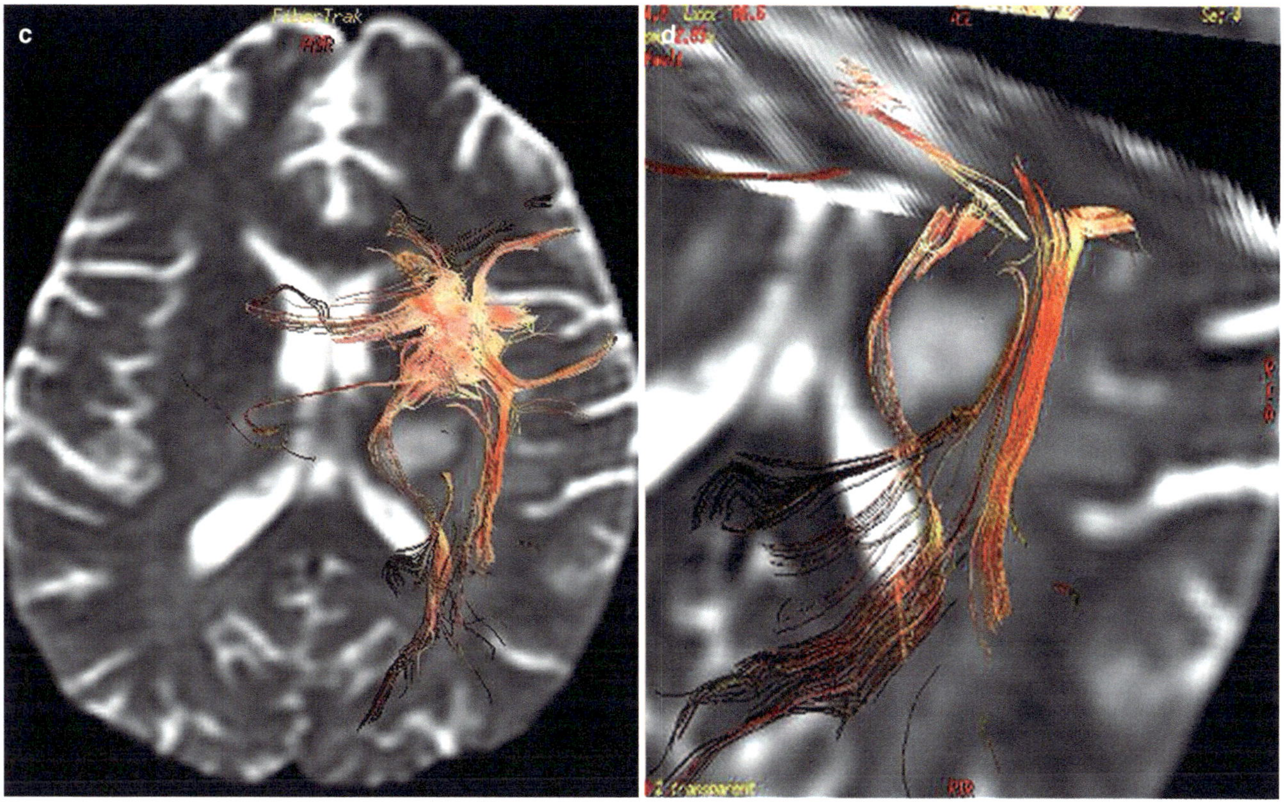

Fig. 13.25 (continued)

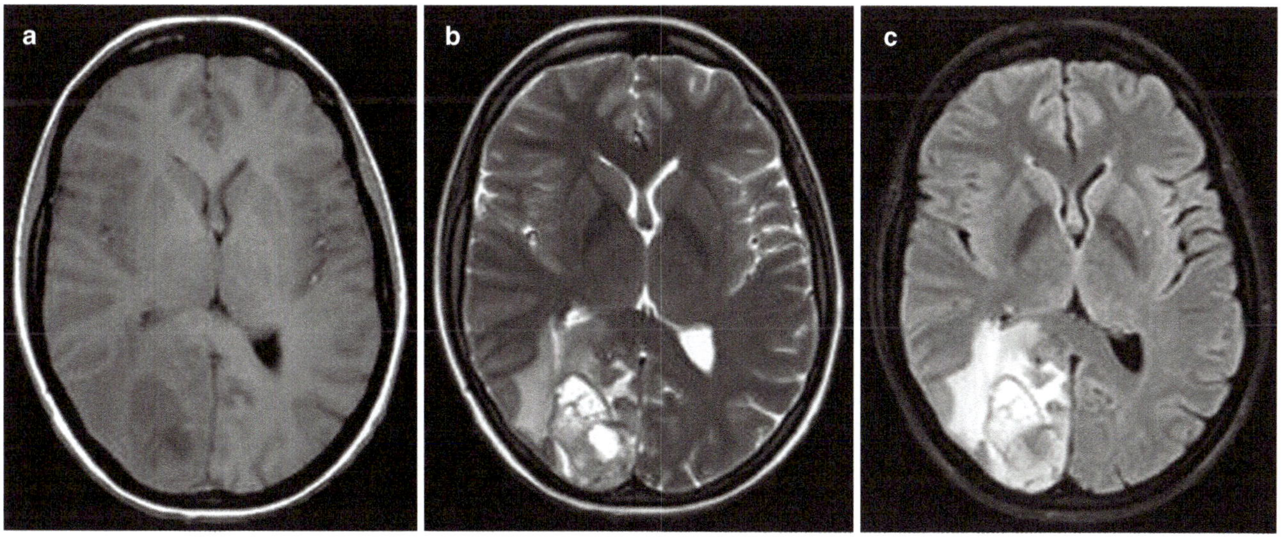

Fig. 13.26 A breast cancer metastasis. Metachronous cancer. In the right occipital region, there is a space-occupying lesion with an iso-hypointense signal on T1-weighted MRI (**a**) and a heterogeneously increased signal on T2-weighted MRI and T2-FLAIR MRI (**b**, **c**) with signs of a moderate perifocal edema. On DWI MRI (**d**), the signal from the metastasis is increased. After CA administration, its intense, uneven accumulation in the solid part of the tumor (**e**, **f**) is noted, and there is a marked hypointense portion along the front contour of the tumor. On whole-body DWI MRI (**g**–**j**), there are high-signal areas in the mammary glands, in the axillary regions, in the right adrenal gland, and in the head and body of the pancreas, corresponding to multiple tumor sites identified by T2-weighted MRI (**k**–**m**)

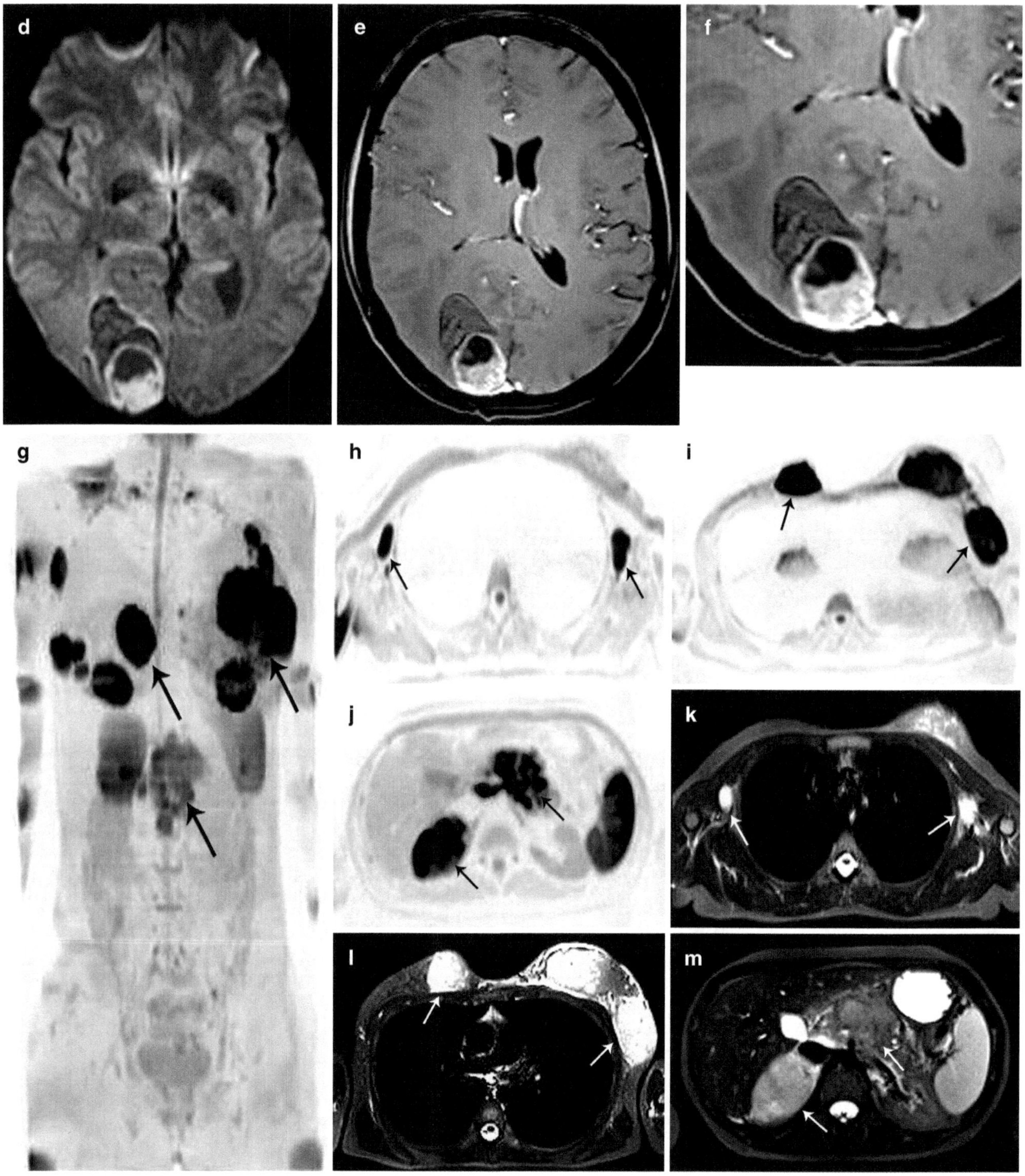

Fig. 13.26 (continued)

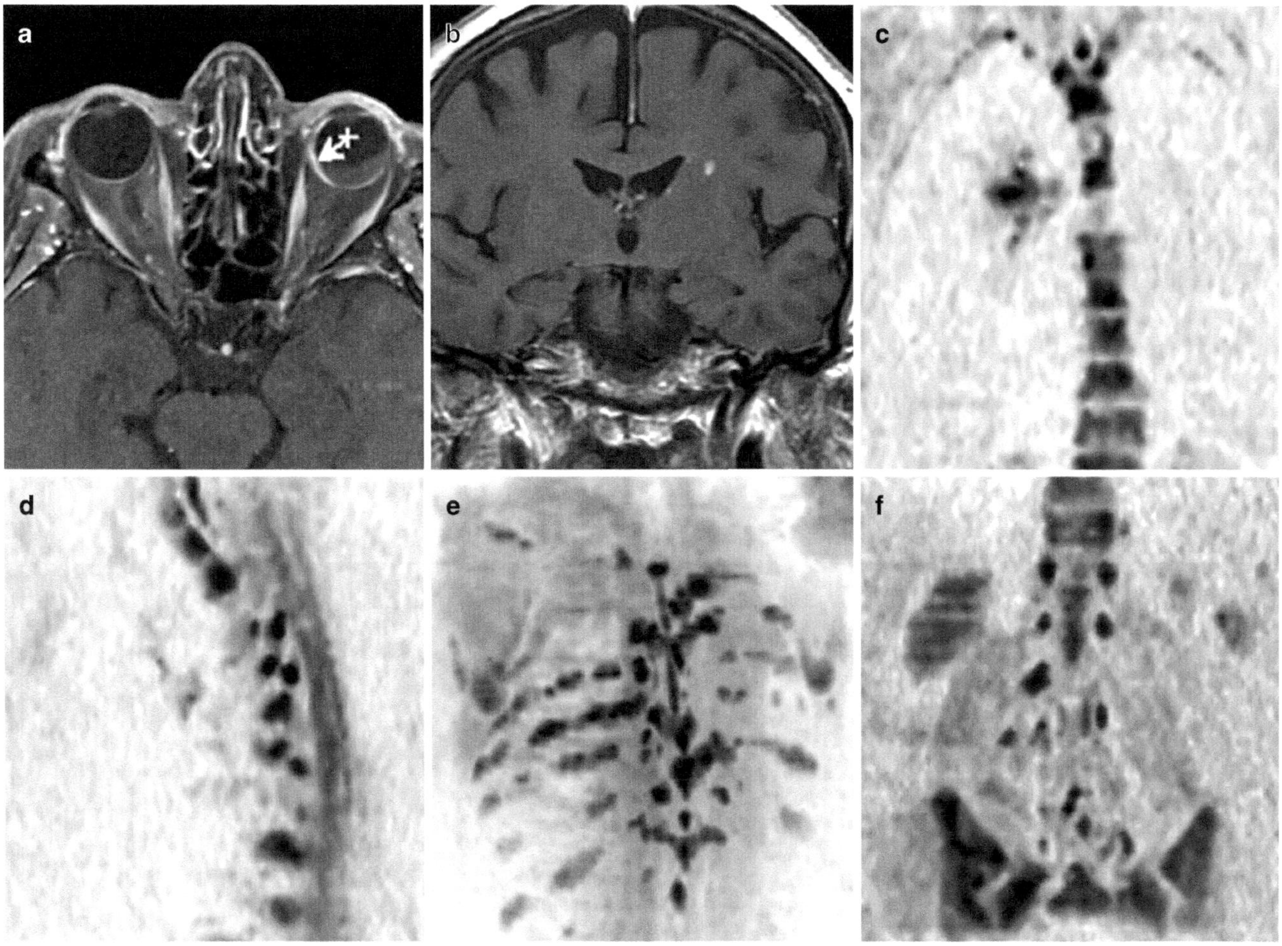

Fig. 13.27 Multiple breast cancer metastases. T1-weighted MRI after intravenous contrast enhancement which demonstrates metastases in the left eyeball membranes (**a**) (*arrow*) and a micrometastasis in the left frontal region (**b**). On the diffusion-weighted images of the whole body, there is a tumor lesion in the right lung apex (**c**) and signs of disseminated involvement of the skeleton (vertebrae, ribs) (**d**, **e**, **f**)

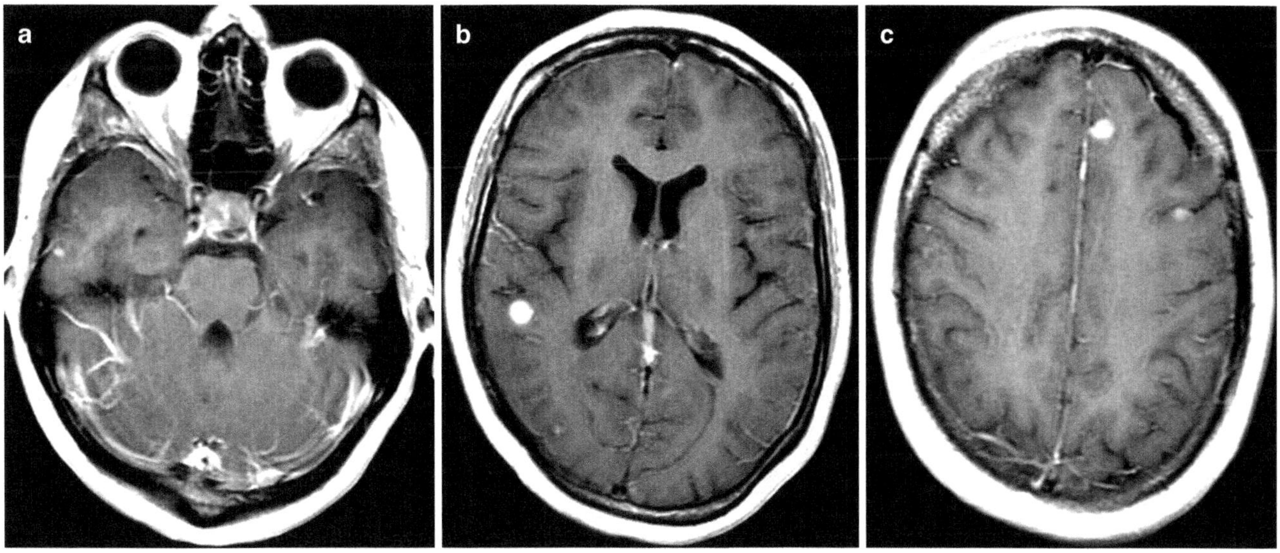

Fig. 13.28 Multiple breast cancer metastases in the brain. A three-level study. On T1-weighted MR images after CA administration (**a**–**c**), there are multiple metastases with various sizes, up to 1 cm in diameter. On PET images with ^{18}F-FDG, no signs of increased RP accumulation that would allow to differentiate the lesions on the background of physiological accumulation have been identified (**d**–**f**). Fusion PET/MR images (**g**–**i**)

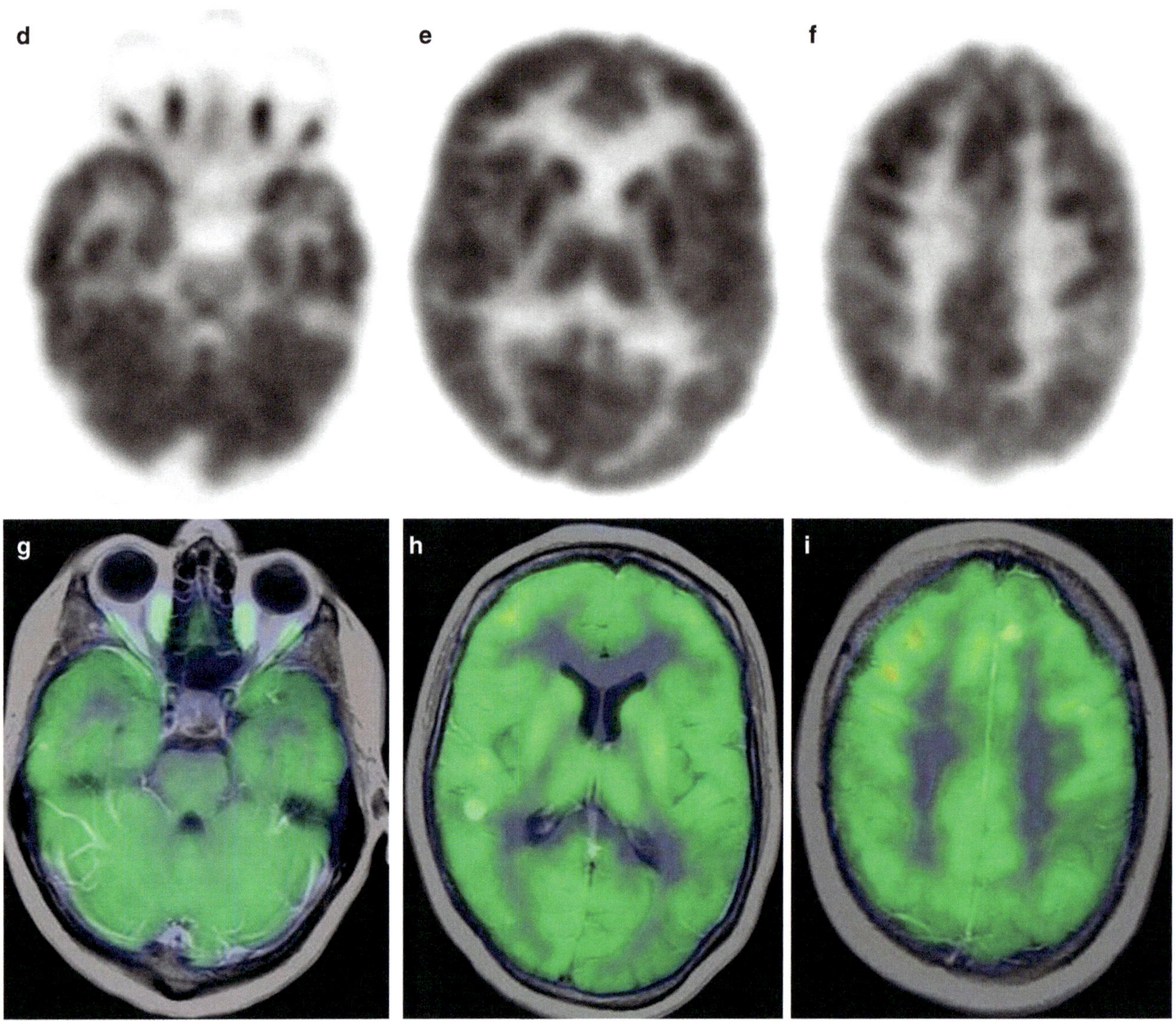

Fig. 13.28 (continued)

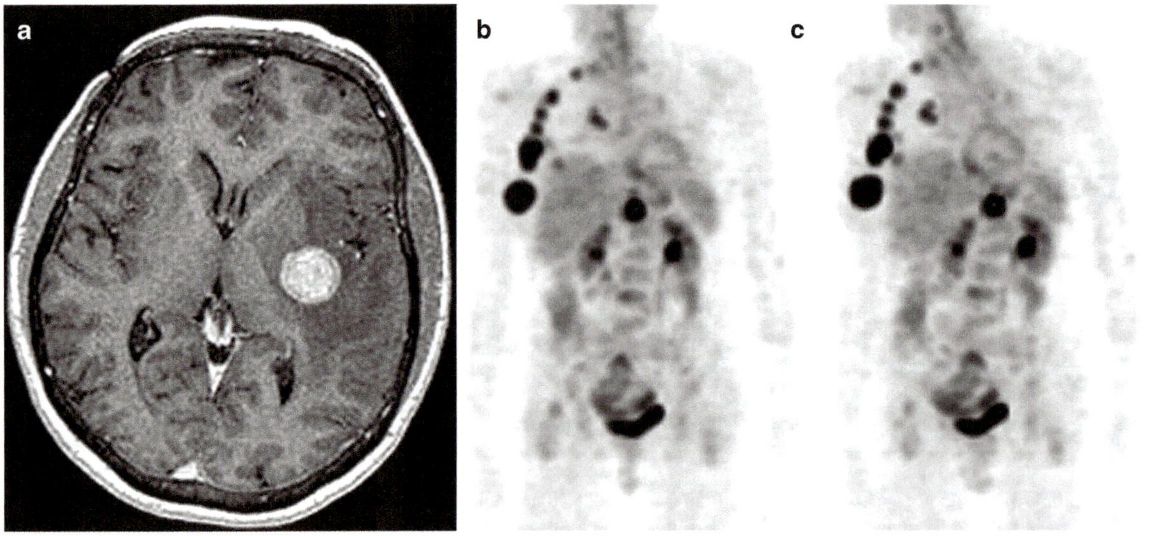

Fig. 13.29 A breast cancer metastasis in the brain. On T1-weighted brain MR images after intravenous CA administration (**a**), there is a solid tumor lesion intensely accumulating the contrast agent in the projections of basal ganglia on the left. Multiple areas of abnormal RP accumulation on whole-body PET (in the projection of the right breast and regional lymph nodes (**b**, **c**); there is an additional rounded lesion with abnormal RP accumulation in the projection of the aortic hiatus (lymph node)

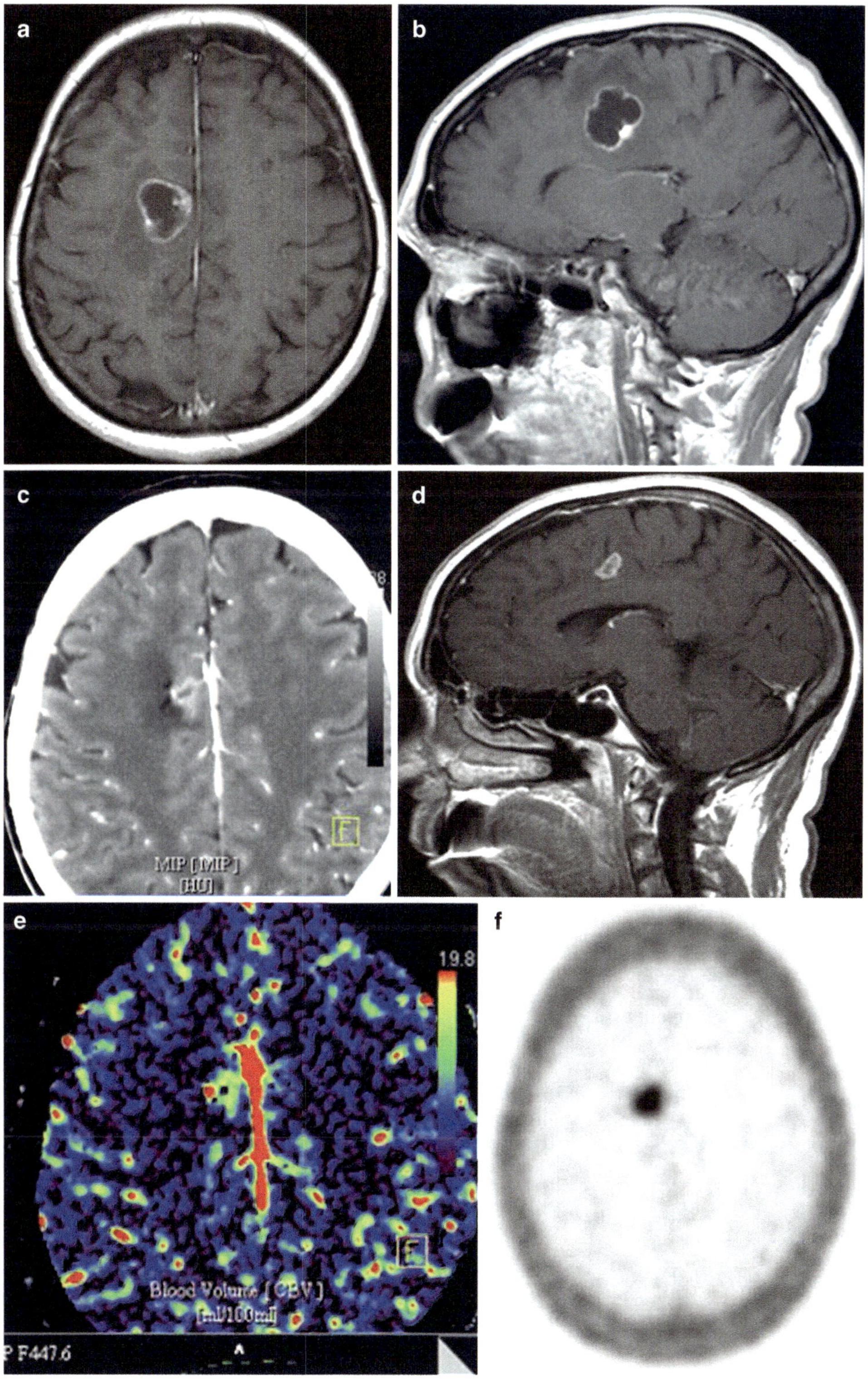

Fig. 13.30 A breast cancer metastasis in the brain before and after radiosurgical treatment, a residual tumor. In the right postfrontal region (before radiosurgery), there is a cystic lesion with signs of intense CA accumulation along the contour and with a small solid portion along the posteromedial contour—the axial and sagittal projections on T1-weighted MRI after the administration of the contrast agent (**a**, **b**). After radiosurgery, there is a small area accumulating CA parasagittally on CT (**c**) and MRI (**d**) images. On CT perfusion maps (CBV), there is an increase in blood flow values in the specified region (**e**). On PET with ^{18}F-choline (**f**), there is an intense RP accumulation in the residual tumor

13.2 Post-radiation Changes

See Figs. 13.31, 13.32, 13.33, 13.34, 13.5, 13.6, 13.7, and 13.8.

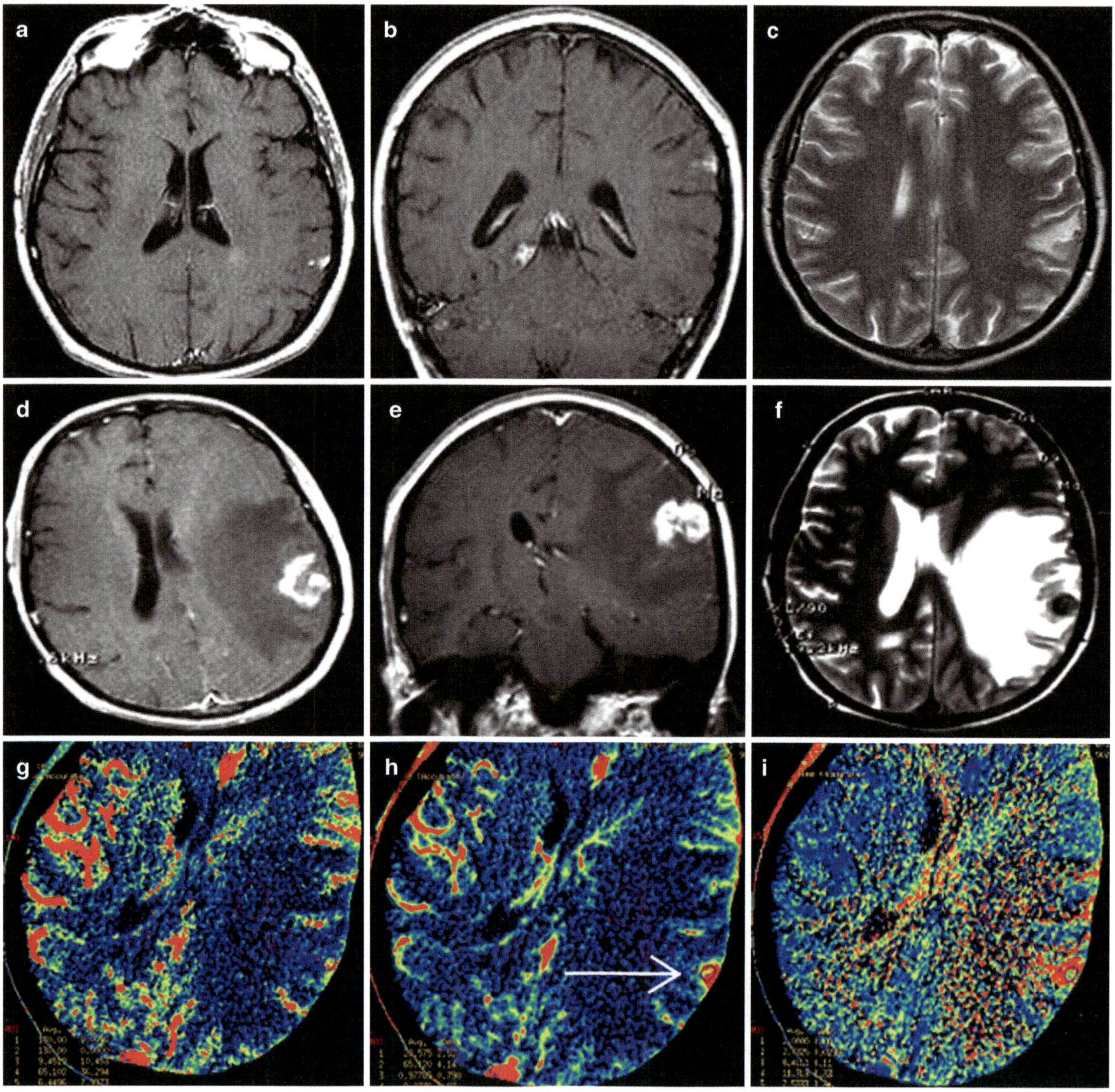

Fig. 13.31 A breast cancer metastasis in the brain. On T1-weighted MRI with contrast enhancement (**a**, **b**) and T2-weighted MRI (c) 3 months after the irradiation, there is a small region of abnormal CA accumulation in the convexital departments of the left parietal region. There is a significant increase in the size of the site with abnormal CA accumulation and an increase in edema 5 months after (**d**, **e** and **f**). On CT perfusion, a large part of this area is characterized by low perfusion values, with the exception of a small area with high CBF (**g**) and CBV (**h**) along the convex (arrow)—a residual tumor. MTT values (**i**) are increased throughout the area—post-radiation changes

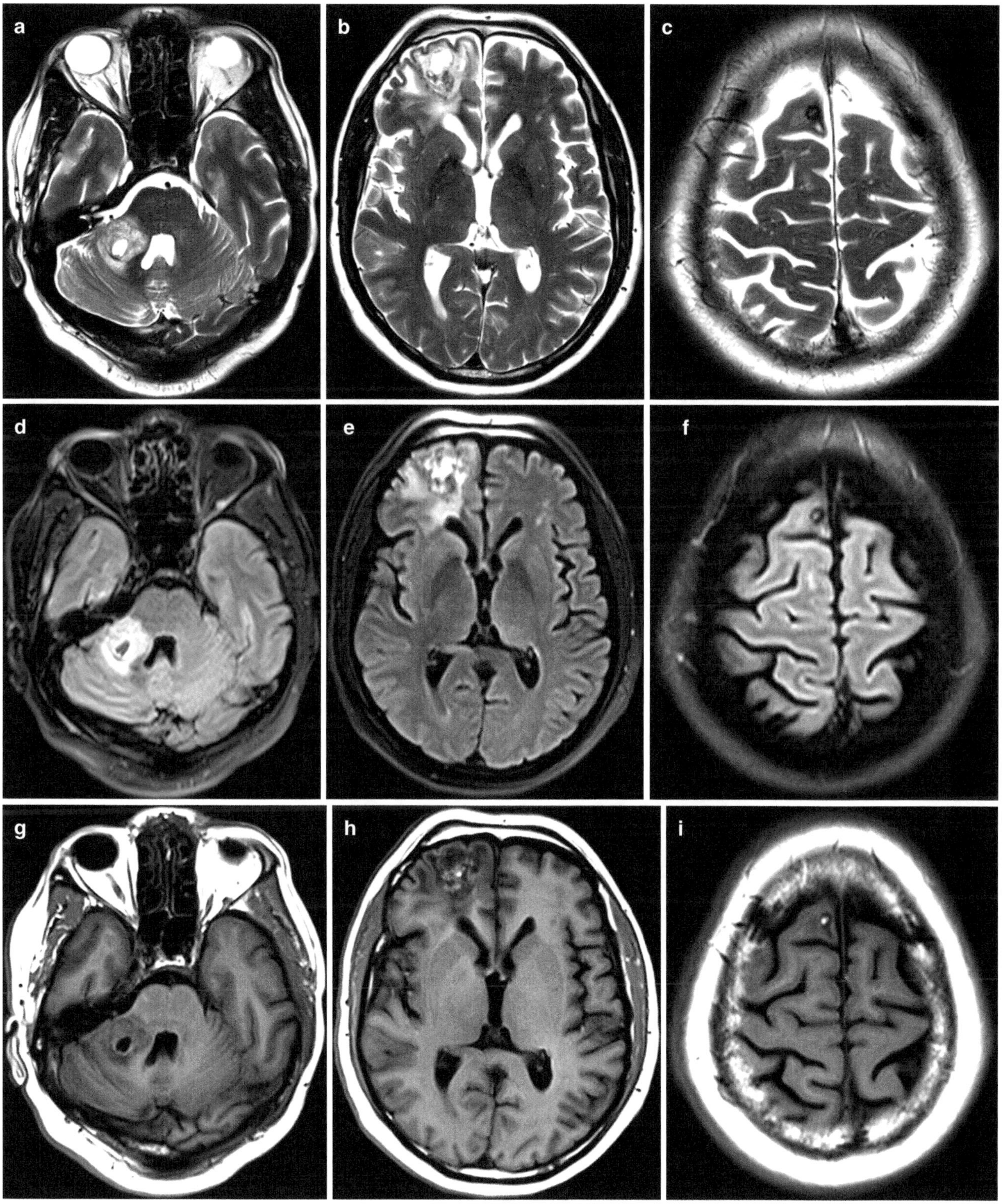

Fig. 13.32 Multiple breast cancer metastases in the brain during complex treatment. A three-level study. In the left cerebellar hemisphere, there is a space-occupying lesion with a hyperintense signal on T2-weighted MRI (**a**), a heterogeneous signal on T2-FLAIR MRI (**d**), and a hypointense signal on T1-weighted MRI (**g**). In the right frontal lobe, there is a lesion with a signal similar to that on T2-weighted MRI (**b**) and a heterogeneously increased signal on T2-FLAIR and T1-weighted MRI (**e**, **h**). In the right upper frontal region, there is a lesion with a hypointense signal on T2-weighted (**c**) and T2-FLAIR MRI (**f**)—hemorrhagic inclusions and an increased signal on T1-weighted MRI (**i**). After administration of the contrast agent, all lesions unevenly accumulate the contrast agent (**j**, **k**, **l**)

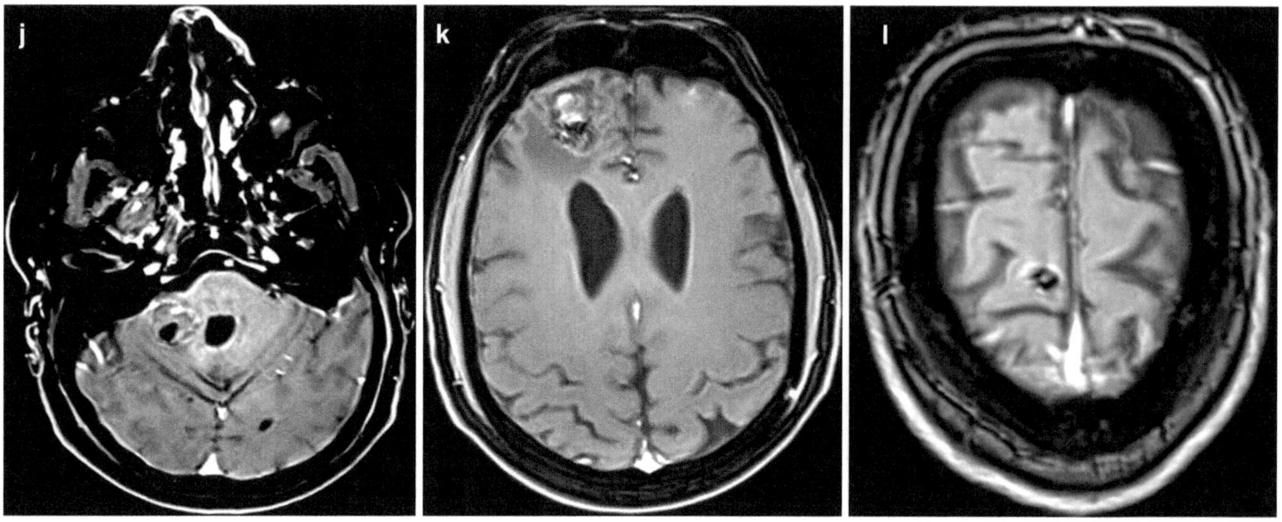

Fig. 13.32 (continued)

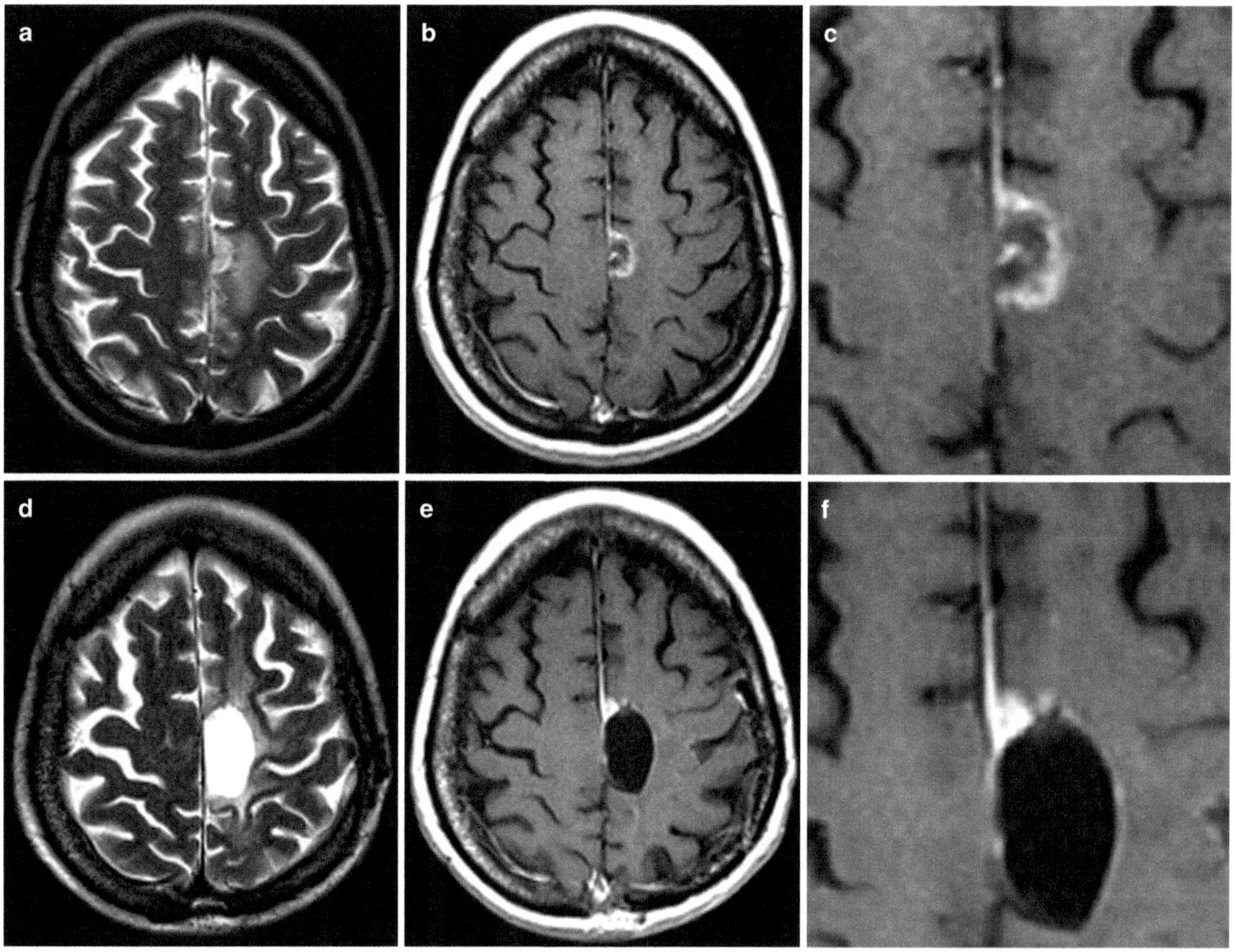

Fig. 13.33 A breast cancer metastasis in the brain before and after surgery, a residual tumor. In the parasagittal sections of the left frontal region after radiosurgery, there is an increased signal on T2-weighted MRI (**a**) with a moderate perifocal edema. After CA administration (**b**, **c**), its uneven, intense accumulation in the tumor is noted. On the MR images after surgical removal of the metastasis, there is a CSF cleft (**d**); along its front contour, a small portion of abnormal accumulation of the contrast agent, adjacent to the falx (**e**, **f**), is observed. On CT perfusion maps (**g**, **h**) and PET images with 18F-choline (**i**), along the front pole of the postoperative cyst, there is a small area with increased ^{18}F-choline accumulation and high perfusion parameters—a residual tumor

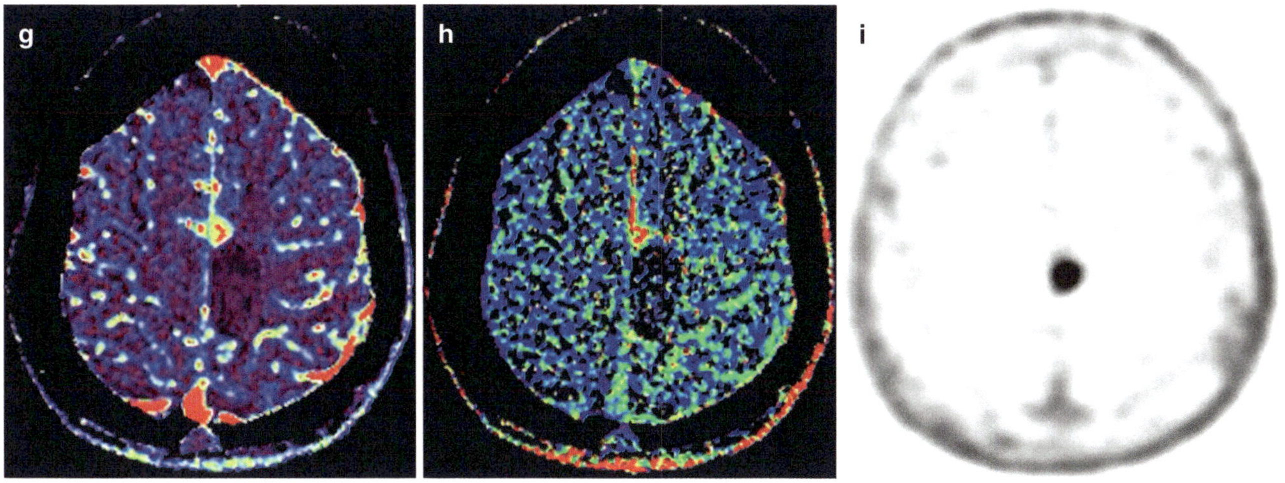

Fig. 13.33 (continued)

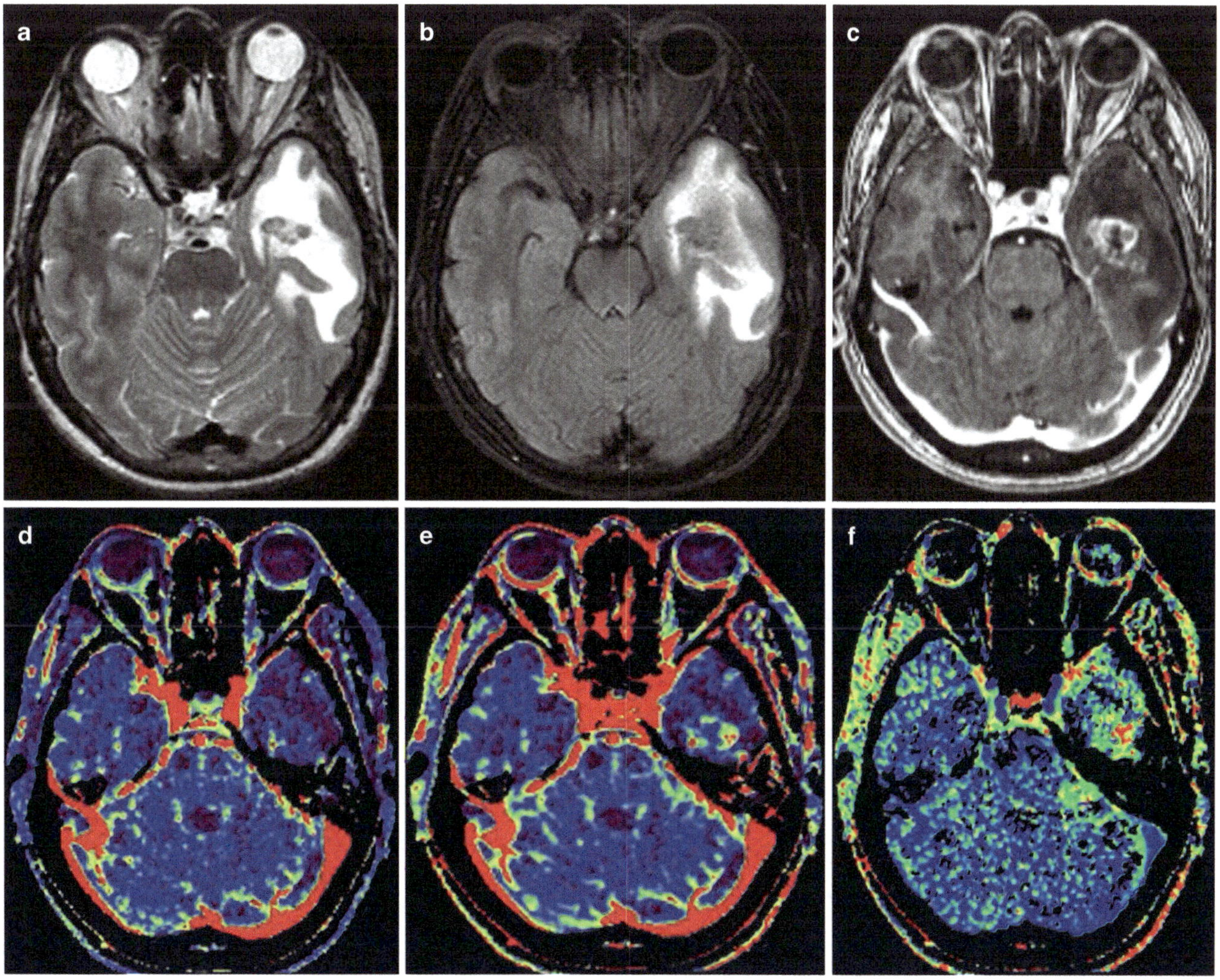

Fig. 13.34 A breast cancer metastasis in the brain. Condition after radiosurgical treatment (a residual tumor). On the MR images on the background of an expressed perifocal edema on T2-weighted and T2-FLAIR MRI (**a**, **b**), there is irregularly shaped abnormal CA accumulation (**c**) in the medial portion of the left temporal region on T1-weighted MRI. On CT perfusion maps in the specified area, there is a weak pinpoint increase in CBV values (**d**) (the *arrow*) and a marked increase in CBF (**e**) and MTT values (**f**). On CT in the left temporal region, there is a heterogeneous hypodense area (**g**). On PET with ^{18}F-FDG, there is moderate RP accumulation exceeding the background values (**h**) and expressed increased accumulation of ^{18}F-Tyrosine (**i**)

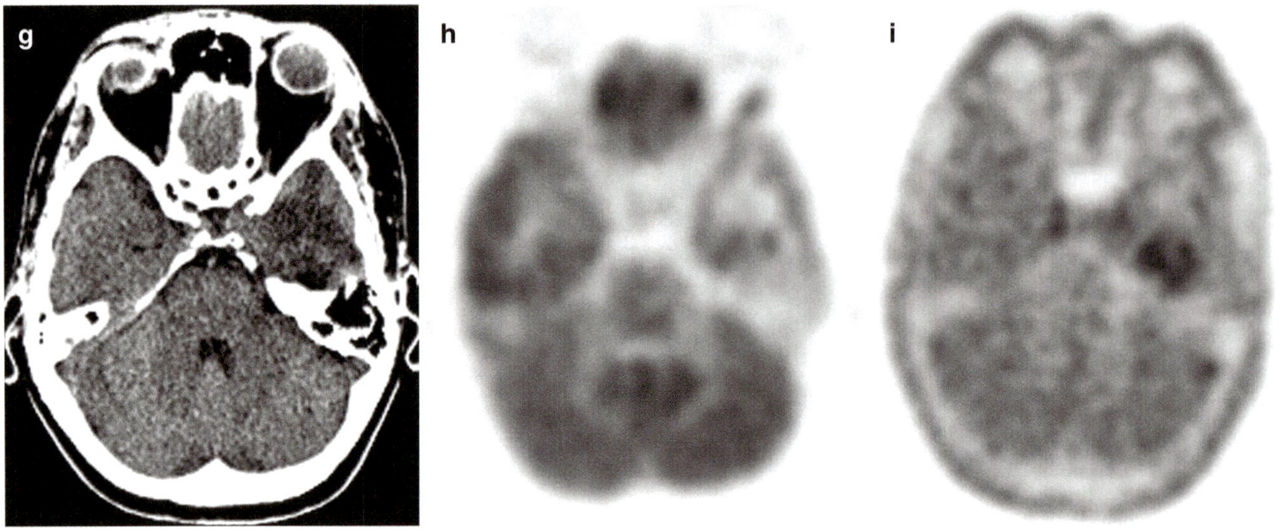

Fig. 13.34 (continued)

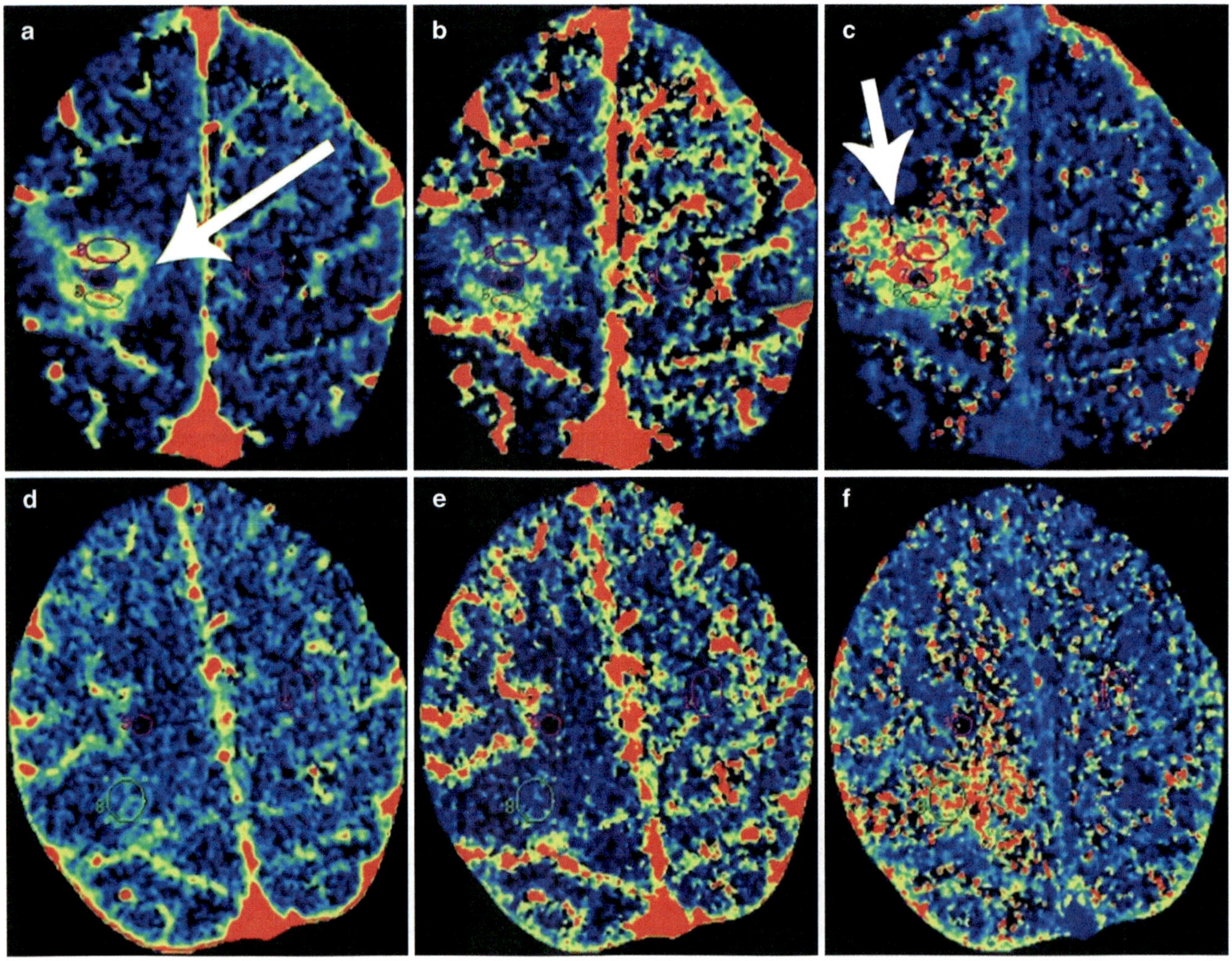

Fig. 13.35 A breast cancer metastasis in the brain. CT perfusion before the treatment (**a**–**c**): high rates of CBV, CBF, and MTT are observed in the lesion projection in the right frontal region. One year and 8 months after the treatment, a decrease in perfusion values CBV and CBF (**d**, **e**) and an increase in MTT (**f**) are observed; on T1-weighted MRI (**g**), intense CA accumulation persists; an edema zone is visualized on T2-weighted MRI (**h**); on SWI (SWAN) MRI (**i**), the lesion has a low MR signal—these are post-radiation changes with hemorrhagic inclusions

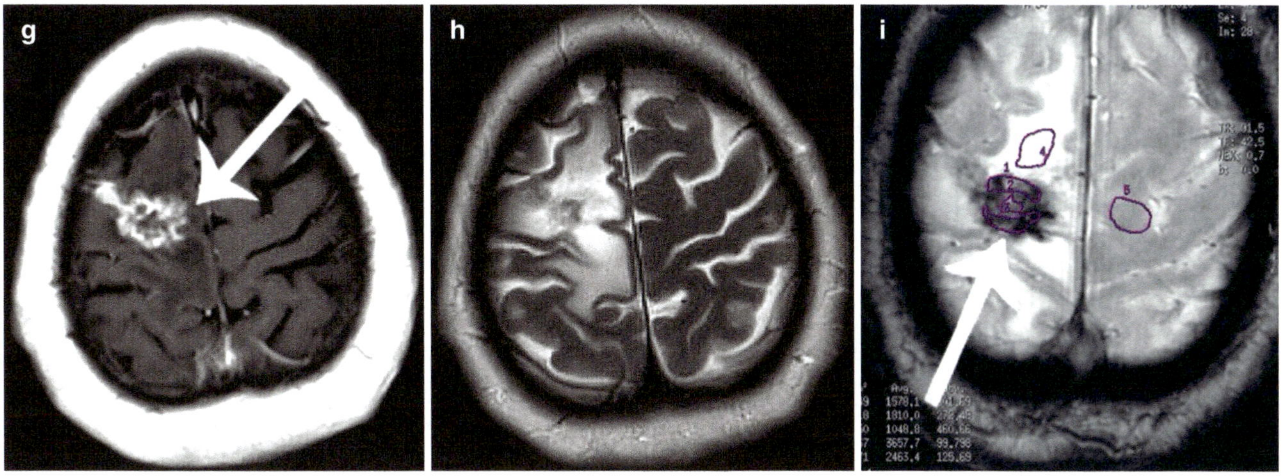

Fig. 13.35 (continued)

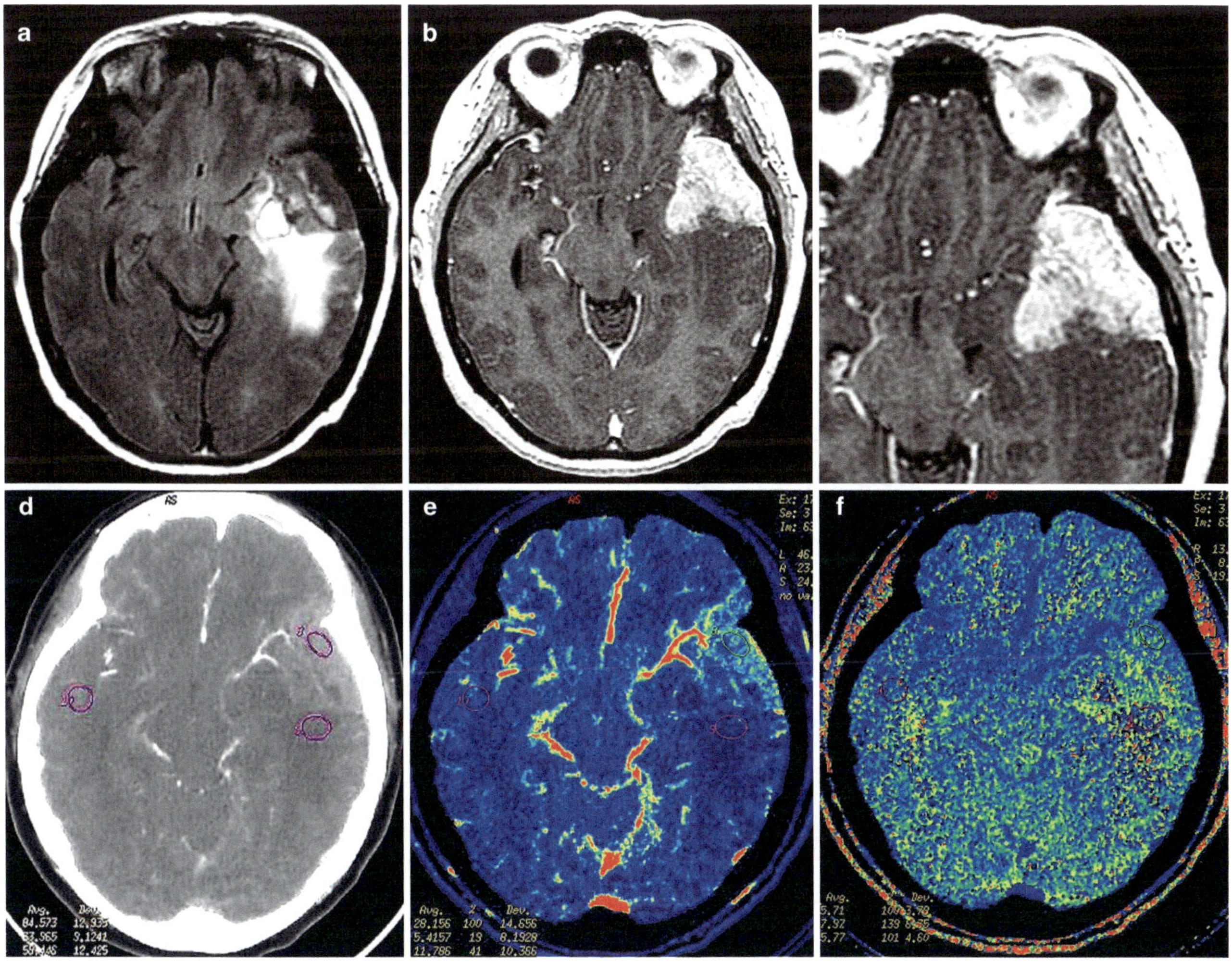

Fig. 13.36 A breast cancer metastasis in the brain. Follow-up studies during chemotherapy. In the left temporal region, there is an area with a hypo-hyperintense MR signal on T2-FLAIR MRI, without any precise contours (**a**) and with signs of a pronounced perifocal edema. After CA administration (**b**, **c**), its intense accumulation in the tumor is noted, with well-defined linear spread of the metastasis along the adjacent meninges with the formation of the “tail” effect. Of note is the displacement of the adjacent brain substance of the frontotemporal region, midline, and brainstem structures. On contrast-enhanced CT (**d**), the displacement of the middle cerebral artery anteriorly is well visualized. On CT perfusion, there is a moderate increase in CBF values (**e**) and insignificant MTT (**f**) in separate portions of the lesion. On T2-weighted MR images (**g**) and T1-weighted contrast-enhanced MR images (**h, i**) after chemotherapy, there is a marked reduction in the tumor size

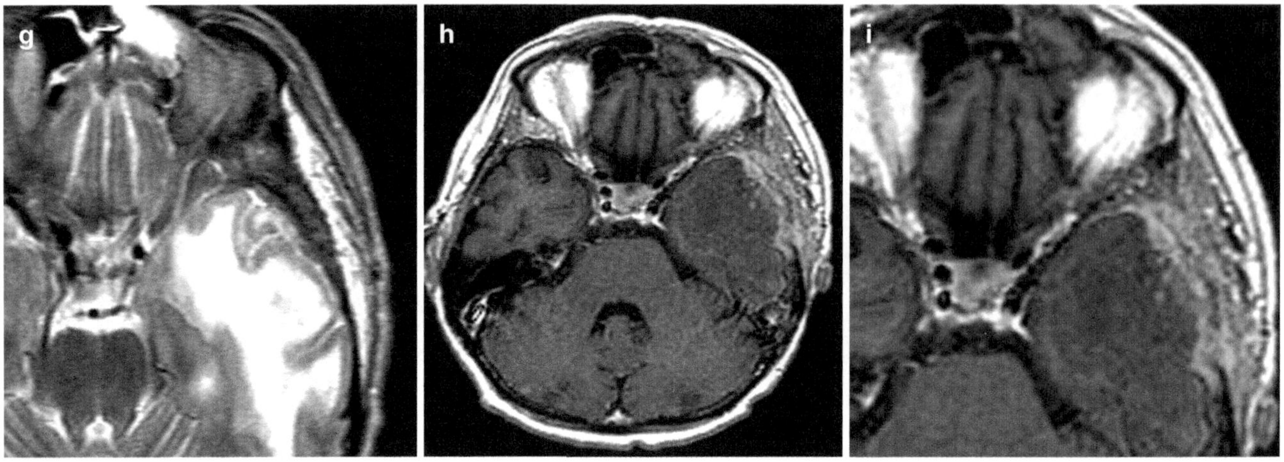

Fig. 13.36 (continued)

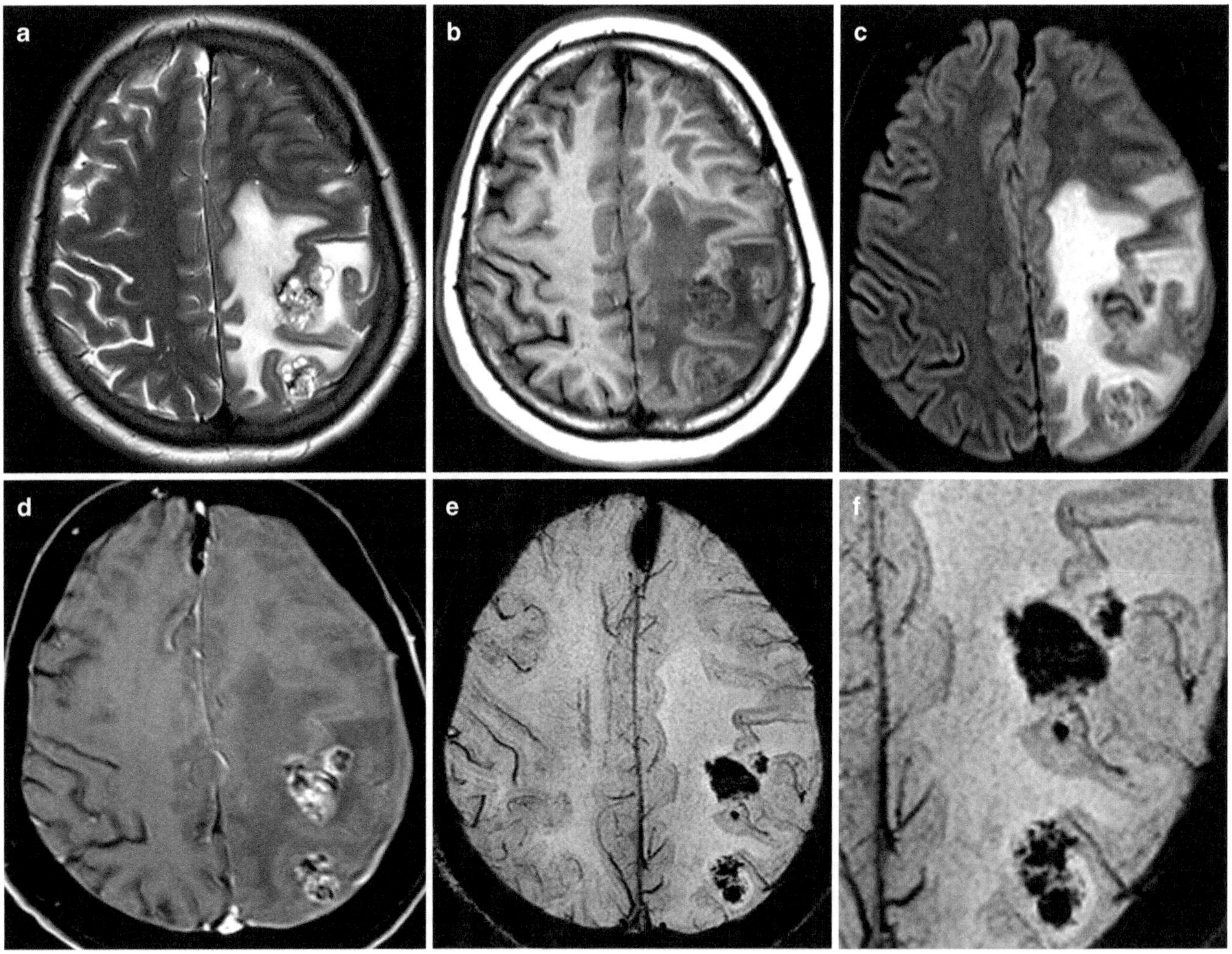

Fig. 13.37 Multiple breast cancer metastases in the brain during drug therapy. In the left parietal region, there are several merging lesions with a heterogeneously hyperintense signal on T2-weighted MRI (**a**), hypointense signal on T1-weighted MRI (**b**), and heterogeneous signal on T2-FLAIR MRI (**c**). After CA administration, its intense accumulation in metastases (**d**) is observed. On SWI (SWAN) MRI (**e**, **f**), there are signs of hemorrhagic transformation on the background of post-radiation changes (vasculitis with hemorrhagic impregnation)

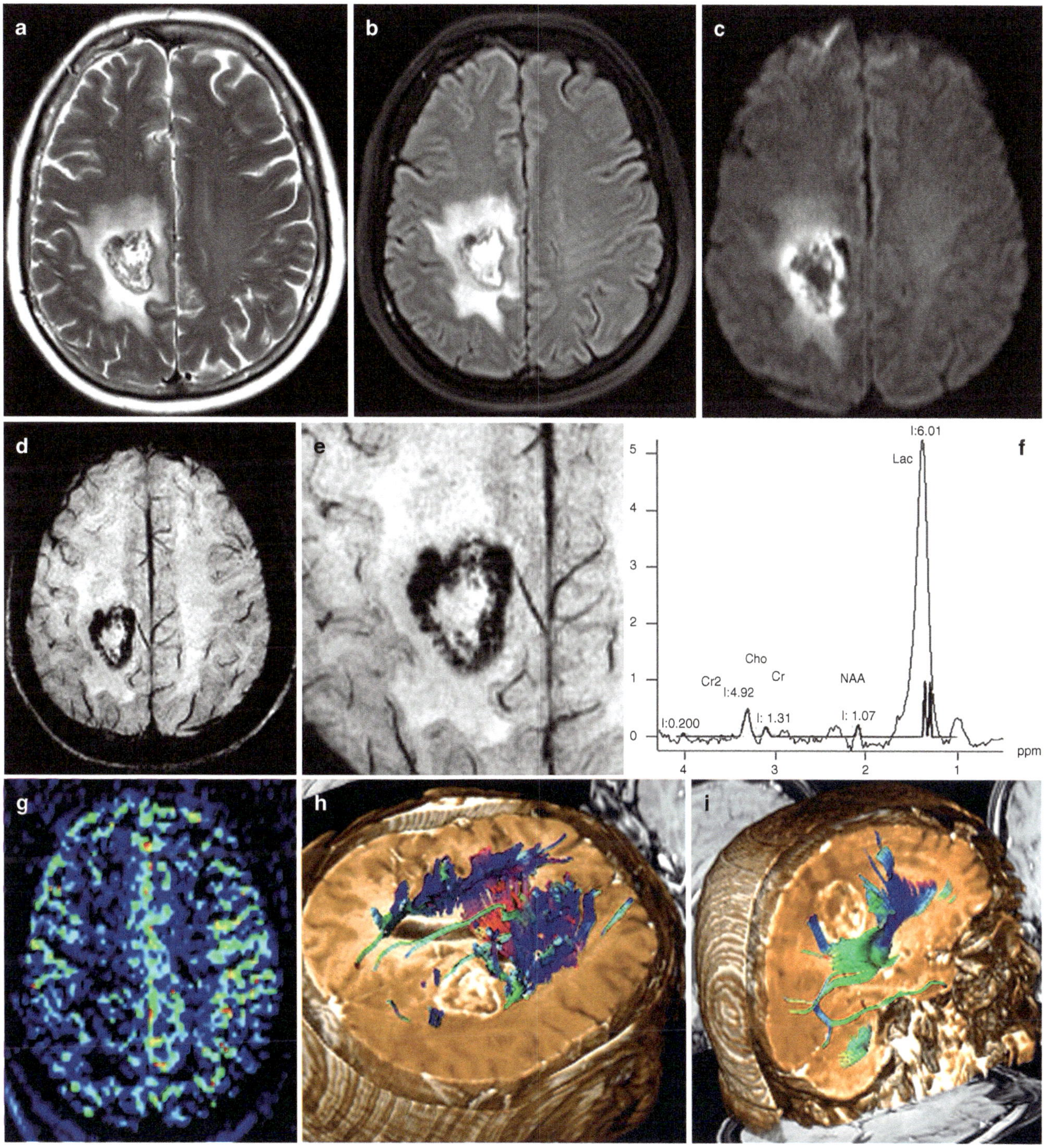

Fig. 13.38 A breast cancer metastasis in the brain. Post-radiation changes after radiosurgical treatment. In the deep parts of the right frontoparietal region, there is a lesion with a heterogeneous signal on T2-weighted MRI (**a**) and an increased signal on T2-FLAIR MRI (**b**) with a pronounced perifocal edema. On DWI MRI, in the central parts of the lesion, there is a reduced signal and a rim of a hyperintense signal on the periphery (**c**), significantly higher than the signal intensity from the perifocal edema. On SWI (SWAN) MRI, on the periphery of the lesion, there is a decreased signal (**d**, **e**), which is characteristic of hemorrhages. MR spectroscopy identified an increased peak of the Lip-Lac complex and a decrease in other peaks (**f**) and a decrease in blood flow in non-contrasted perfusion (**g**). When constructing the tracts, their marked deformation is observed (**h**, **i**). On PET images with ^{18}F-tyrosine, there is no increased CA accumulation (**j–l**), which confirms the post-radiation nature of changes

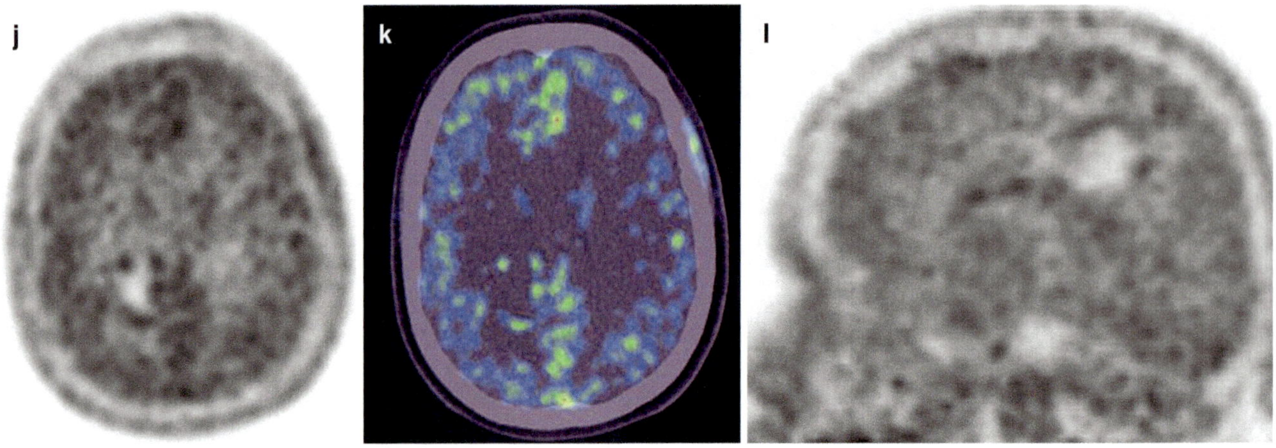

Fig. 13.38 (continued)

14 Melanoma

Melanoma is the most malignant tumor that develops as a result of malignant transformation of pigment cells—melanocytes located in various body tissues. The first mention of a "fatal black tumor with metastases and a black fluid in the body" appeared in European literature between 1651 and 1760. The term "melanoma" was first proposed by Carswell in 1838.

The incidence of melanoma in the world is more than 230,000 people annually. In the USA, more than 32,000 patients are diagnosed with melanoma each year, of whom 7200 annually die (Balch and Kirkwood 1997); in Russia this figure approaches 9000. In recent decades, a steady increase in the incidence of melanoma in all regions of the world is observed, with the tumor being more common in young people.

Melanoma is the third by frequency of metastases to the brain, although many authors put it on the second place, between lung cancer and breast cancer (Stehlin et al. 1965; Romodanov 1973; Hauward and Hayward 1976; Bullard and Cox 1981; Johnson and Smith 1995). According to Greenlee et al. (2001), melanoma metastases constitute 5–21% of the total cases of secondary brain malignancies, in spite of the fact that melanoma proportion in the structure of malignant tumors is only 4%. In our clinical material, melanoma metastases in the brain occurred three times less often (about 18.2%) than lung cancer metastases.

The mean interval between the diagnosis of melanoma and the development of MTSs in the brain is 1.2–3.5 years (Chason et al. 1963; Markesbery et al. 1978; Zimm et al. 1981; Damek 2003). When the size of brain tumor is <5 mm, survival of melanoma patients after surgery is 89–100%. When melanoma metastasizes in the internal organs, the 5-year survival rate is less than 10% (Rigel et al. 2000). The prognosis for patients with metastatic melanoma in the brain is the most unfavorable. The tumor volume, depth of invasion, ulceration, satellites, site, and radical treatment have a key prognostic value.

According to Rhodes et al. (1987), there is a definite relationship between the intensity of metastasizing and the age of melanoma patients. In children, melanoma metastases are rare. The authors noted the maximum intensity of metastasizing by 30–40 years of age; patients had metastases at various sites as early as after 3–4 months. A decrease in the tendency to metastasize was observed in elderly patients (Chao et al. 2004).

According to Akimov and Gershanowitch (2001), melanomas metastasize within the first months after the onset of the disease, while uncontrolled dissemination of the tumor was determined in many patients already at the time of diagnosis. According to McWilliams et al. (2008), metastases were detected at necropsy in 50–70% of patients diagnosed with melanoma, and only 60% of these cases of metastases in the brain were detected during their lifetime.

There are primary and metastatic melanomas in the brain. Primary melanoma in the central nervous system is very rare—1% of cases (Farrokh et al. 2001)—and is a surgical or necropsy finding. Primary melanoma usually develops in the choroidal plexus or the pial membrane of the fourth ventricle, or around the brainstem (especially in the ventral regions), as well as in the upper sections of the spinal cord, since these areas contain the greatest concentration of melanocytes (Gebarski and Blaivas 1996; Arbelaez et al. 1999). Primary melanoma usually metastasizes to the meninges, rarely affecting the parenchyma (Rubino et al. 1993; Arbelaez et al. 1999). Often primary melanoma spreads along the meninges after surgery. van der Ree et al. (1999) noted that, with the tumor located in the posterior fossa, 33% of patients experienced involvement of not only intracranial meninges but also of the spinal cord 2–13 months after the surgery.

In secondary metastatic brain lesions, primary melanoma is usually in the skin (97%), while in 2–3%, melanoma is detected in the vagina, anorectal area, choroid and iris, penis, and lungs. Melanoma metastases can also be found in the lymph nodes of the abdominal and thoracic cavities, lungs, gastrointestinal tract, adrenals, and heart. According Mogila (1979), melanoma metastases were found in the heart muscle in 9.4% of cases and in the adrenal tissue in 10.4%. The tumor lesions in the adrenal glands result in a decrease in the corticosteroid function up to the complete failure of this organ, which is often the cause of rapid deaths. According to

M. Dolgushin et al., *Brain Metastases*, DOI 10.1007/978-3-319-57760-9_14

the same author, the brain was the only place of melanoma metastases in 51.9% of patients.

Melanomas metastasize to the brain via both the hematogenous and lymphogenous routes Babchin et al. 1974a, b; Iconography et al. 1977). According to Martynov et al. (2002), melanoma cells enter the brain more often via the hematogenous route, through the arterial circle. Lymphogenous spread of melanoma metastases to the brain is possible, when the primary pigmented tumor is located in the skin of the head and neck. Zhuravlev et al. (1994) noted that metastases usually first appear in the regional lymph nodes, i.e., local lymphogenous spread of tumor cells occurs earlier than hematogenous one. However, other researchers believe, referring to the appearance of tumor cells in the regional lymph nodes and distant organs, that metastasizing occurs via a mixed route, i.e., both lymphogenically and hematogenically.

By their morphological structure, melanoma metastases in the brain, as compared with other metastases, most resemble the primary pigmented tumor. Just as in primary melanoma, metastases contain different histological variants of epithelium-like, spindle cell, and mixed structures. Metastases may differ from primary melanomas by the amount of melanin in the direction of both its increase and decrease (Ganina et al. 1978). In separate cases, amelanotic melanoma metastasized and became pigmented and vice versa.

Amelanotic (nonpigmented) forms of melanoma may still show some amount of melanin. However, according to Golbert (1975) and Tiraspolskaya (1975), a complete lack of melanin allows to suspect melanoma based on polymorphism of the tumor tissue, typical of this tumor, in combination with sarcomatoid or epithelioid cell structure. Both metastatic and primary CNS melanomas can be amelanotic. According to Ganina and Naleskina (1991), nonpigmented or weakly pigmented forms of melanomas have a pronounced tendency to metastasize and a poor prognosis. If primary melanomas remain undetected, according to Ikonopisov et al. (I977), the main reason for that is not only a microscopic tumor size but also its amelanotic form.

Metastases of melanoma in the brain are characterized by frequent hemorrhages(Hauward and Hayward 1976; Mogila 1979; Konovalov et al. 1997a, b, c; Karp et al. 2002). The main causes of hemorrhages in the tumor tissue are the degree of the tumor anaplasia and specifics of tumor vascularization. The clinical course of the disease in such cases drastically worsens.

On direct angiograms, manifestations of melanoma metastases in the brain are characterized by the "porous structure" with sharp edges and an abundant vascular pattern, and at the same time, an expressed dislocation of brain vessels is observed. It should be noted that, in some rare cases, pigmented tumors by their structure may resemble glioblastoma with formation of arteriovenous shunts on angiograms.

In contrast to metastases of other primary tumors to the brain, with iso- and/or hypodense characteristics, cerebral metastases of melanoma often have a heterogeneous density on CT due to frequent hemorrhages. In our experience, in 76% of cases of cerebral melanoma MTSs, the solid part of the tumor tissue was identified as a rounded site with moderately high density, and CA administration only enhanced its density characteristics. Our data correlate with data of other authors (Weisberg 1985; Patten et al. 1990; Ho Shon et al. 2008; Goulart et al. 2011). Thus, Weisberg (1985) noted using native CT in patients with metastatic melanoma that melanoma lesions were characterized by a hyperdense signal in 75%, while a hypo- and isodense signal was determined in 23% and 3%, respectively. It can be argued that CT manifestations of melanoma metastases in the brain are associated not only with the specifics of the tumor histogenesis but also with hemorrhages to its tissue, due to which the tumor density increases.

In case of detection in the brain of multiple tumor lesions with an increased density during a CT study, melanoma metastases should be suspected even if the primary tumor has not yet been detected. In terms of differential diagnosis in cases where there are hyperdense characteristics of the lesions on native CT, non-tumor hemorrhages should be first ruled out.

Even small metastatic melanomas are characterized by a pronounced perifocal edema.

As a result of CT perfusion studies, we noted that the tissue of melanoma metastases has one of the highest blood volume values—CBV = 15.03 ± 9.7 ml/100 g—only slightly inferior to that of kidney cancer metastases. Of note is a large dispersion of CBV values in melanoma, which is probably related to different degrees of tumor capillary network depending on its size and "age." These findings are supported by the fact that melanoma metastases are characterized by the highest values of the capillary blood flow in the tumor depth: CBF = 113.99 ± 24.25 ml/100 g/min. Melanoma metastases passed the blood through their parenchyma the fastest: they were characterized by the lowest MTT values (7.22 ± 2.1 s) in our group.

Our experience with CT perfusion techniques in the diagnosis of metastatic brain lesions allows to establish its high efficiency in the determination of perfusion characteristics of metastatic tumors, depending on the primary source and reliably differentiate melanoma metastases from metastatic lesions of other origin with similar CT manifestations during a native CT study ($p < 0.03$).

As noted earlier, a CT perfusion method was used not only in primary melanoma diagnosis but also in the monitoring of treatment effectiveness in radiation therapy, often revealing complications during the treatment. CT perfusion in some cases allowed us to unambiguously identify a residual tumor on the background of a hemorrhage, having similar manifestations on routine CT and MRI.

Similarly to other metastatic tumors, melanoma metastases tend to grow as nodular lesions without any signs of invasion of the surrounding brain substance, unlike primary malignant brain tumors that diffusely infiltrate adjacent tissues.

Melanoma metastasizes in any portion and structure of the brain and skull. The most common site is the brain. However, metastatic lesions may occur in the dura mater, choroid plexus, pituitary gland, and pineal gland. In our material, melanoma metastases were detected in the orbit.

Metastatic melanoma has a number of characteristic pathognomonic MRI manifestations that allow to assume the nature of the primary tumor with a greater probability, even based on routine MRI studies. It is known that melanin is characterized by the presence in its structure of unpaired electrons and has paramagnetic properties. This gives melanoma its characteristic signs in MR imaging, manifested as an enhanced MRI signal in T1-weighted MRI, even before the CA administration(Atlas et al. 1987a, b; Isiklaret al. 1995; Escott 2001; Breckwoldt et al. 2015). In our material, homogeneous metastatic melanomas (without signs of central necrosis) in T2-weighted images in 60% of cases had moderately hypointense or hypointense signals and in 31% of cases had iso-hypointense signals. In case of a tumor hemorrhage, the character of MR signal on T1-weighted MRI changed from hyperintense to hypointense depending on the "age" and the number of hemorrhages. Hemorrhages to the tumor tissue were detected in 60% of cases and were often identified both with single and multiple metastases of melanoma.

A decrease in the signal on T2-weighted MRI is typical not only for melanoma metastases (91%): colon cancer metastases were hypointense in 83% of our cases.

Often (about 9% of cases) melanoma metastases on T2-weighted MRI were visualized as hyperintense lesions, while on T1-weighted MRI as isointense ones, which may be indicative of amelanotic melanoma.

Complications in the form of a hemorrhage in the tumor tissue in our material were often observed in particular in melanoma metastases (34% of patients were operated due to an increase in the size of metastatic lesions in the brain). It should be noted that the cause to perform neurosurgery was often extensive hemorrhages, not further growth of the solid part of the tumor.

It should be noted that not only melanoma metastases may have an increased MR signal on T1-weighted MRI but also primary tumors, for example, protein-containing lesions (craniopharyngioma, atypical epidermoids, colloid cysts in the third ventricle), lipomas and lipomatous meningiomas, dural osteomas, as well as abnormal non-tumor lesions (multiple sclerosis, hamartomas, neurofibromatosis type I, intracranial forms of infections, etc.). Tumors with hemorrhages and hematomas in the early subacute stage may have MR characteristics similar to those in melanomas. In addition, according to many authors, the diagnostic range must also include pigmented meningioma, meningeal melanocytoma, melanotic schwannoma, and melanoblastosis—neoplasms containing melanin in their structure (Tatagiba et al. 1992; Faro et al. 1996; Painter et al. 2000; Doglietto et al. 2012). The next chapter will describe the differential diagnosis of metastases.

The need to identify additional small multiple lesions determines the requirement for mandatory contrast enhancement of intracranial melanomas. Characteristics of accumulation of the contrast agent by melanoma metastases allowed to identify various patterns occurring as a result of the contrast agent accumulation. The main pattern of CA accumulation by melanoma metastases corresponded to the "homogeneous" type of accumulation and reached 76% in our material. However, in the presence of necrotic areas in the central part of the tumor site, CA accumulation occurred along the periphery—a homogeneous ring-shaped accumulation with clear contours—a "target." Heterogeneous CA accumulation was also present but much less frequently. Perifocal edema was pronounced, which created, in turn, the picture of ring enhancement.

From our point of view, differences in the CA accumulation are due to, first of all, sizes, "age," intensity of growth, metabolic activity of the tumor tissue, presence or absence of necrosis areas, hemorrhages, etc.

Thus, it can be concluded that the standard MRI methods (T1, T2, T1 weighted + contrast enhancement, T2-FLAIR) in case of metastatic brain lesions in melanoma not only provide information about the synoptic features of the tumor lesion(s) and their numbers and structure but also allow to suspect the source of metastases based on particular characteristics (a signal change on T2-weighted MRI).

Melanoma metastases on SWI (SWAN) MRI are included in our study as a separate group and were studied in detail using other additional MRI techniques. Thus, a decrease in MR signal in SWI (SWAN) images, similar to that in T2-weighted MRI, is quite typical and is caused by the characteristics of the melanoma cellular structure. Paramagnetic melanin itself causes local inhomogeneity of the magnetic field not only on SWI (SWAN) MRI but also on standard T2-weighted images, except for a small number of cases with the cystic structure of this lesion (Gaviani et al. 2006).

As noted above, growth of melanoma—one of the most malignant tumors—is often accompanied by hemorrhages into the tumor stroma. On SWI (SWAN) images, due to higher sensitivity of the pulse sequence to the field inhomogeneity, the overall low signal from the neoplasm covers some features of the internal structure of melanoma.

During an MR spectroscopic study in patients with suspected melanoma metastases, it was noted that shimming frequency in melanoma metastases in cases of its solid type exceeds 7 Hz and sometimes reaches up to 14 Hz. In metastatic tumors with other histological structure, this phenomenon is not detected. Most likely, this difference is related to the paramagnetic properties of melanin and hemorrhages associated with melanoma metastases. In other cases, on the background of a significant decrease in NAA and Cr peaks, there was a sharp increase in the lipid-lactate complex and a moderate increase in the choline peak. It should be noted that these results were obtained only in the presence of tumor necrosis. In our material, increases in the peaks of choline, lactate, and lipids in the central part of metastases were noted in only 22% of cases.

On DWI images, in patients with melanoma metastases in the brain, no characteristic features were identified that could allow to differentiate melanoma metastases from other focal lesions with necrotic changes in the tumor tissue. However, the use of DWI allowed to obtain additional information on melanoma metastases with the solid structure: melanoma metastases in contrast to lymphomas and gliomas are characterized by higher ADC values, as degradation in the metastasis stroma starts earlier. Unlike glial tumors, melanoma metastases have a lower signal on DWI MRI in the edema area, which is most likely due to the lack of infiltration of the brain substance by the tumor cells and more free movement of water molecules in the extracellular space. The ADC values obtained in the solid parts of melanoma metastases were $0.9 \times 10^{-3} \pm 0.05 \times 10^{-3}$ s/mm^2; in the lesions with necrosis signs, they were $2.18 \times 10^{-3} \pm 0.05 \times 10^{-3}$ s/mm^2; in the edema area, they were $1.92 \times 10^{-3} \pm 0.07 \times 10^{-3}$ s/mm^2; in the white matter on the unaffected contralateral side, they were $0.7 \times 10^{-3} \pm 0.3 \times 10^{-3}$ s/mm^2.

Melanoma metastases and primary tumor are very well visualized on both DWI MRI and PET with ^{18}F-FDG. Since melanoma metastasizes to the soft tissues and bones, it is advisable to perform for diagnosis not scintigraphy, allowing to study only bone structures, but PET or MRI in order to investigate all tissues. ^{18}F-FDG PET is also highly sensitive to amelanotic melanoma cells. In our material, all patients with melanoma metastases in the brain had foci with increased accumulation of the radiopharmaceutical even on the background of hemorrhagic inclusions. More than in a half (57%) of the studies conducted, the PET picture corresponded to multifocal neoplastic lesions of the internal organs and lymph nodes. A histological examination of the biopsy material obtained allowed to prove the presence of a malignant melanoma.

For a search of the primary tumor, a whole-body PET study can be performed at different stages of the diagnosis. An absolute indication for PET is the presence of multiple tumor lesions in the brain on MRI, absence of history of cancer, and negative results of other diagnostic methods. PET is often performed in patients with a quite long history of cancer that received surgical therapy in the past for some tumor. In such cases, additional tumor lesions and lymph nodes affected with metastases are often found. Based on the whole-body PET study, we found abnormal RP accumulation in 88.6% of patients with melanoma in our material (n = 44). It should be noted that a PET/CT study should include the upper and lower extremities, which often allows to identify additional lesions. Given the difficulties of using DWI MRI with inclusion of extremities in the region of interest, PET is the method of choice.

14.1 Clinical Cases

See Figs. 14.1, 14.2, 14.3, 14.4, 14.5, 14.6, 14.7, 14.8, 14.9, 14.10, 14.11, 14.12, 14.13, 14.14, 14.15, 14.16, 14.17, 14.18, 14.19, 14.20, 14.21, 14.22, 14.23, 14.24, 14.25, 14.26, 14.27, 14.28, 14.29, 14.30, 14.31, 14.32, 14.33, 14.34, 14.35, 14.36, 14.37, and 14.38.

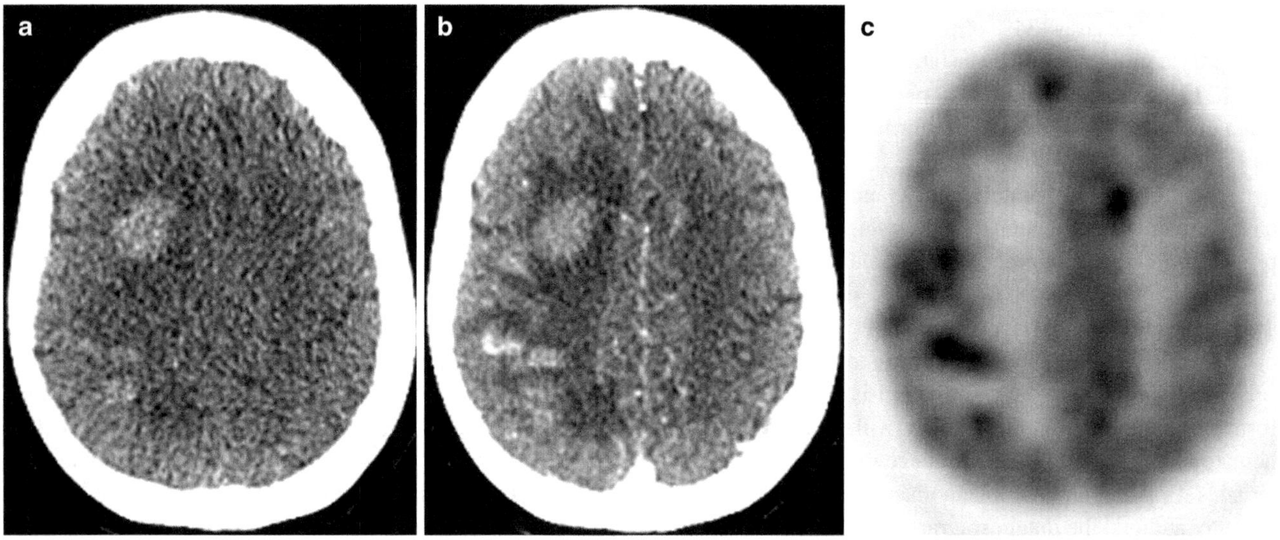

Fig. 14.1 Multiple melanoma metastases in the brain. On a CT scan before the administration of the contrast agent (**a**), there are multiple areas with an increased density in the right frontal and parietal regions. After the administration of the contrast agent (**b**), multiple metastases are additionally identified in both frontal regions, with the largest lesion with no apparent CA accumulation—blood. On PET with ^{18}F-FDG (**c**), lesions intensely accumulate RP, with the exception of the largest one, which is caused by a hemorrhage into its stroma

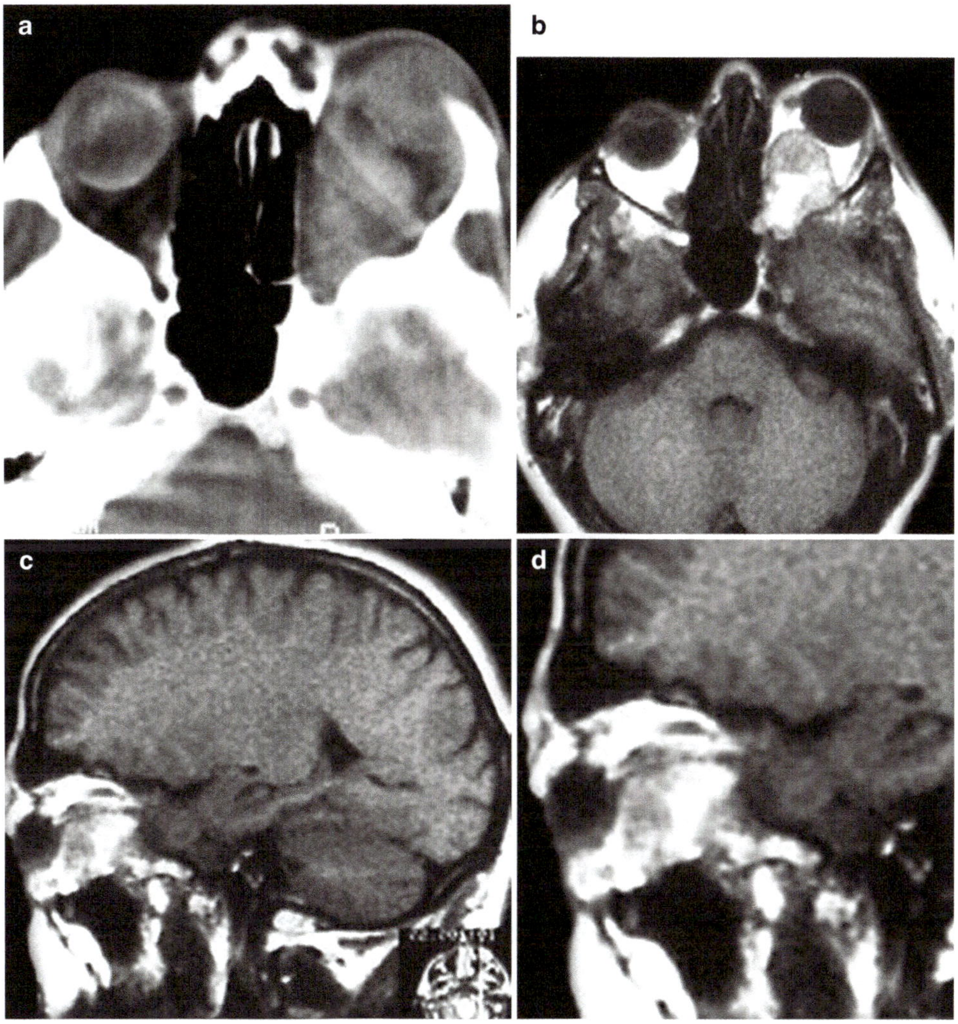

Fig. 14.2 A melanoma metastasis in the left orbit. On a CT scan in axial projection (**a**), there is a weakly hyperdense space-occupying lesion that causes destruction of the medial wall of the left orbit and exophthalmos. T1-weighted MRI with contrast enhancement in the axial (**b**) and sagittal (**c**, **d**) projections allows to visualize a tumor located in the retrobulbar region, with moderate and uneven contrast enhancement. The optic nerve is displaced upward

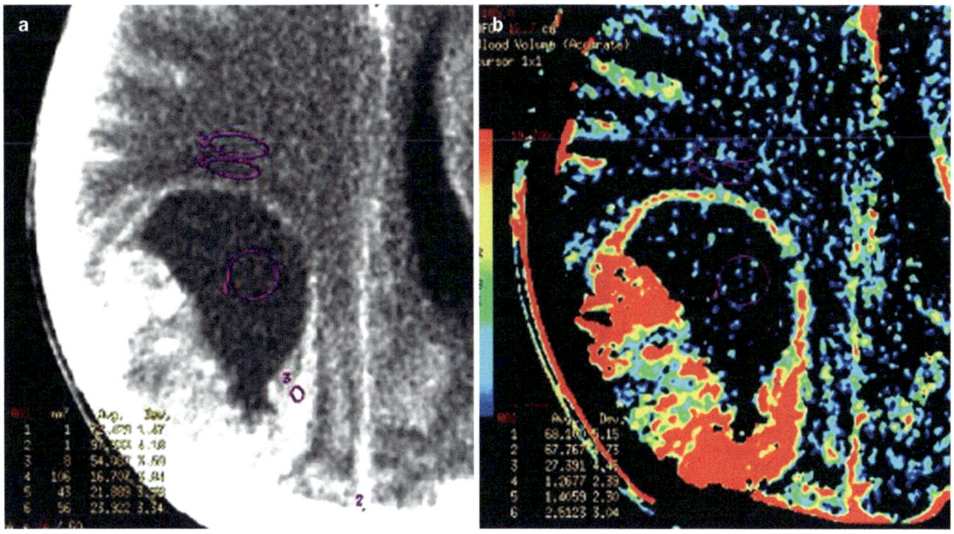

Fig. 14.3 A melanoma metastasis in the brain. CT and CT perfusion maps. In the right parietal lobe, solid-cystic space-occupying lesion is identified, whose solid component (along the lateral contour) intensely accumulates CA (**a**). On CT perfusion maps of CBV (**b**), CBF (**c**), and MTT (**d**), typical for melanoma, high CBV and CBF values and low MTT values are observed in the solid structure of tumors

Fig. 14.3 (continued)

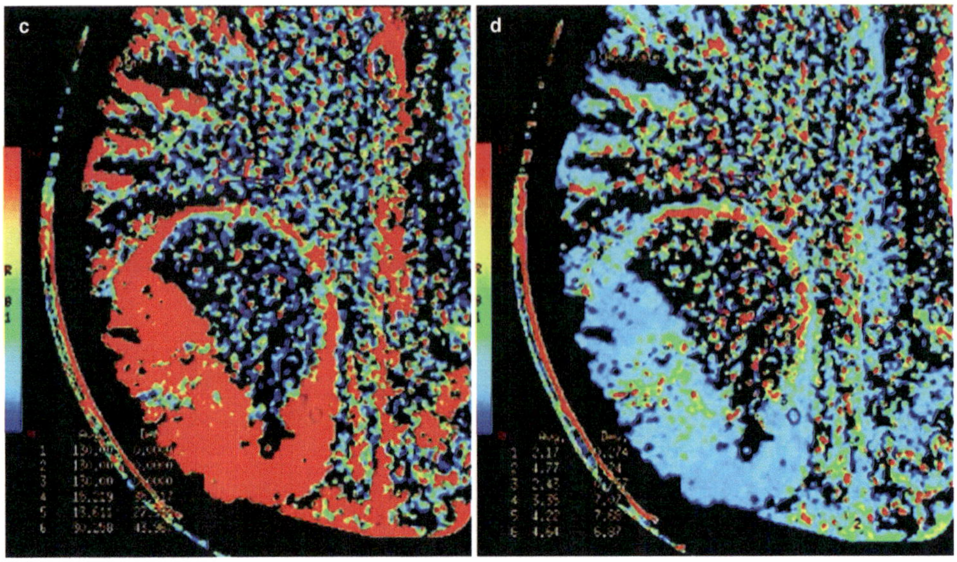

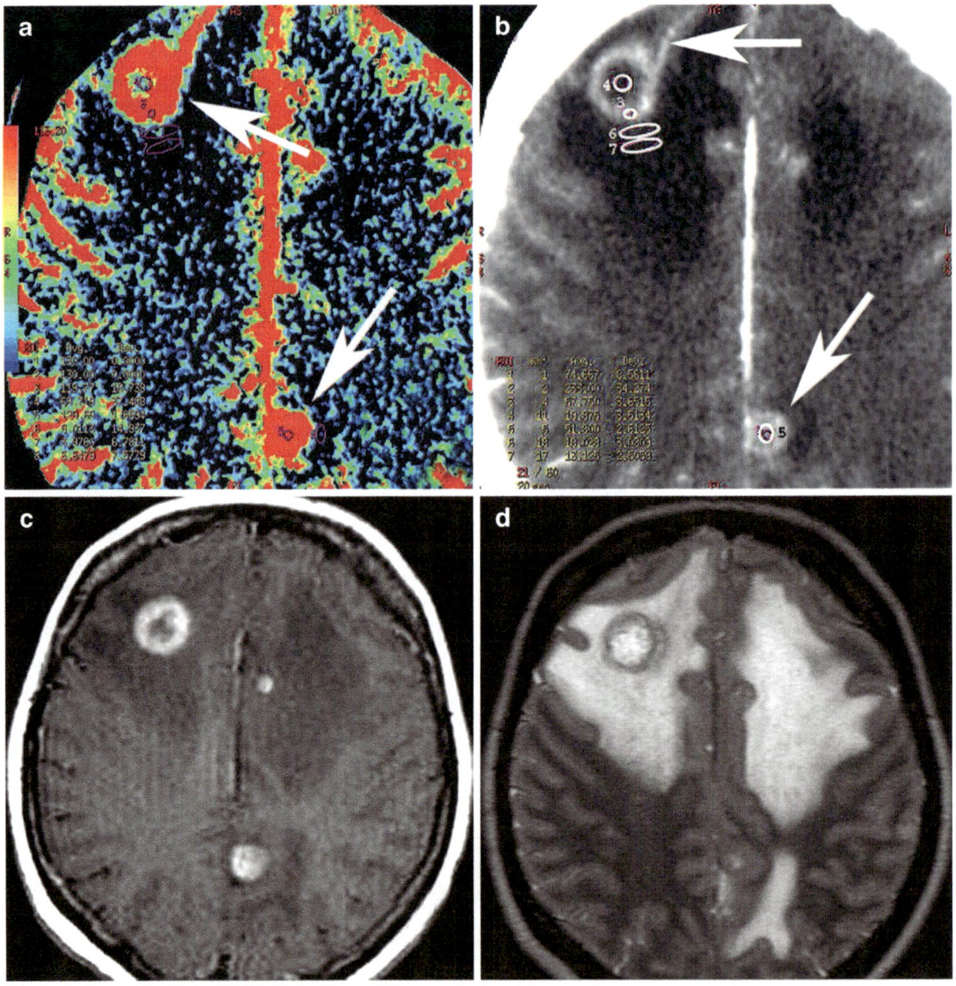

Fig. 14.4 Multiple metastases of melanoma. CBF map (**a**): melanoma metastases have elevated blood flow values (*arrow*). On CT with contrast enhancement (**b**), of note is a large artery approaching the front pole of the tumor (*upper arrow*) and an additional parasagittal tumor site (*lower arrow*). T1-weighted MRI with contrast enhancement (**c**) and T2-weighted MRI (**d**) allow to determine the true sizes of metastatic lesions and the severity of perifocal edema

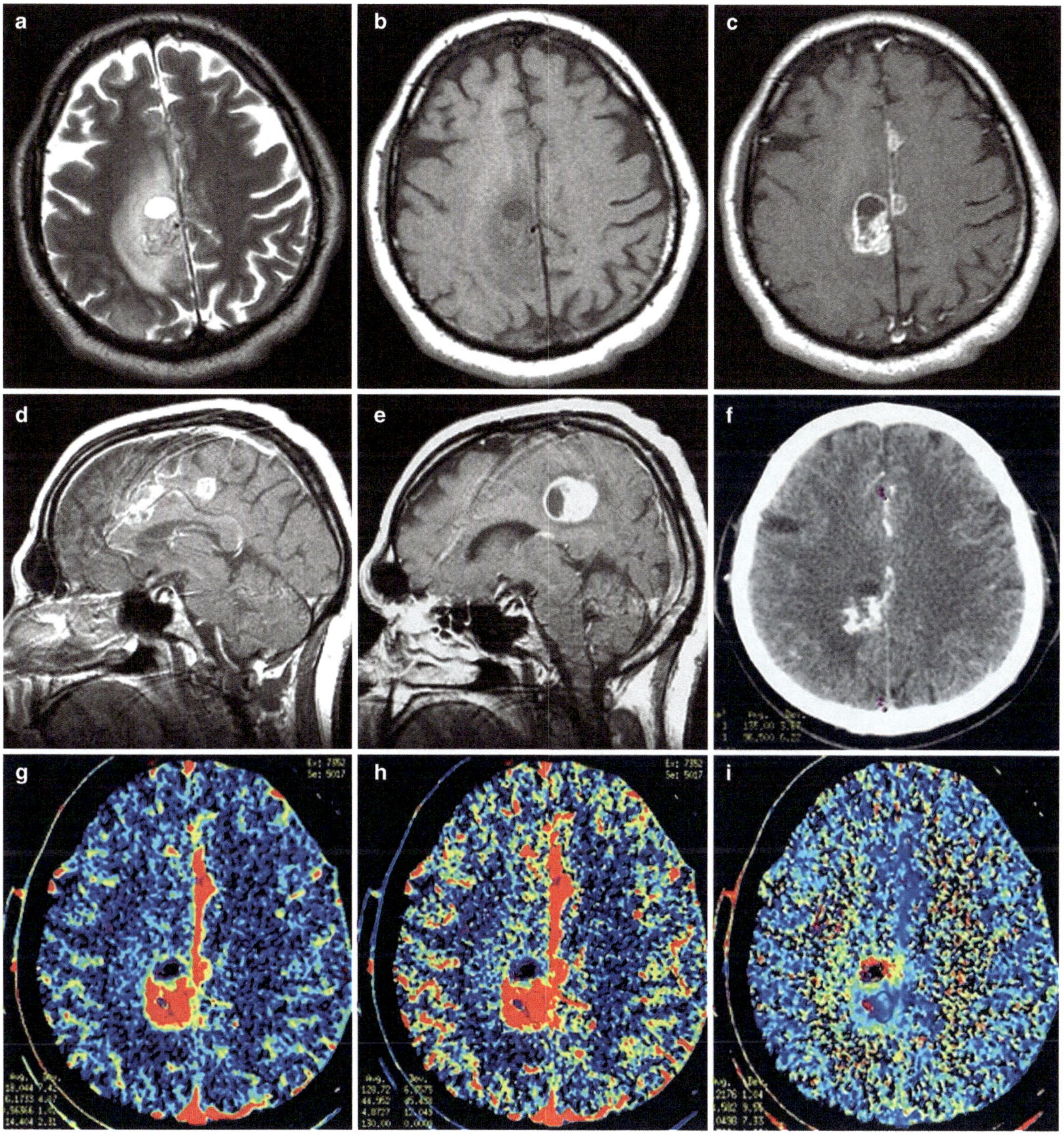

Fig. 14.5 Multiple metastases of melanoma. There are multiple lesions along the falx on both sides in the frontal and parietal regions. The largest lesion in the right frontoparietal region on T2-weighted MRI (**a**) has a heterogeneously hyperintense signal, and the brain substance along the periphery of the lesion is edematous. On T1-weighted MRI (**b**), lesions are weakly differentiated (no hemorrhages). After CA administration—axial (**c**) and sagittal (**d, e**) projections—there is its pronounced accumulation in the tumor lesions, while the well-visualized cystic fragment is well visualized along the anterior pole of the largest metastasis. On CT (**f**), the lesion also intensely accumulates the contrast agent. On CT perfusion maps of CBV (**g**), CBF (**h**), and MTT (**i**), typical for melanoma, high CBV and CBF values and low MTT values are observed in the solid structure of tumors

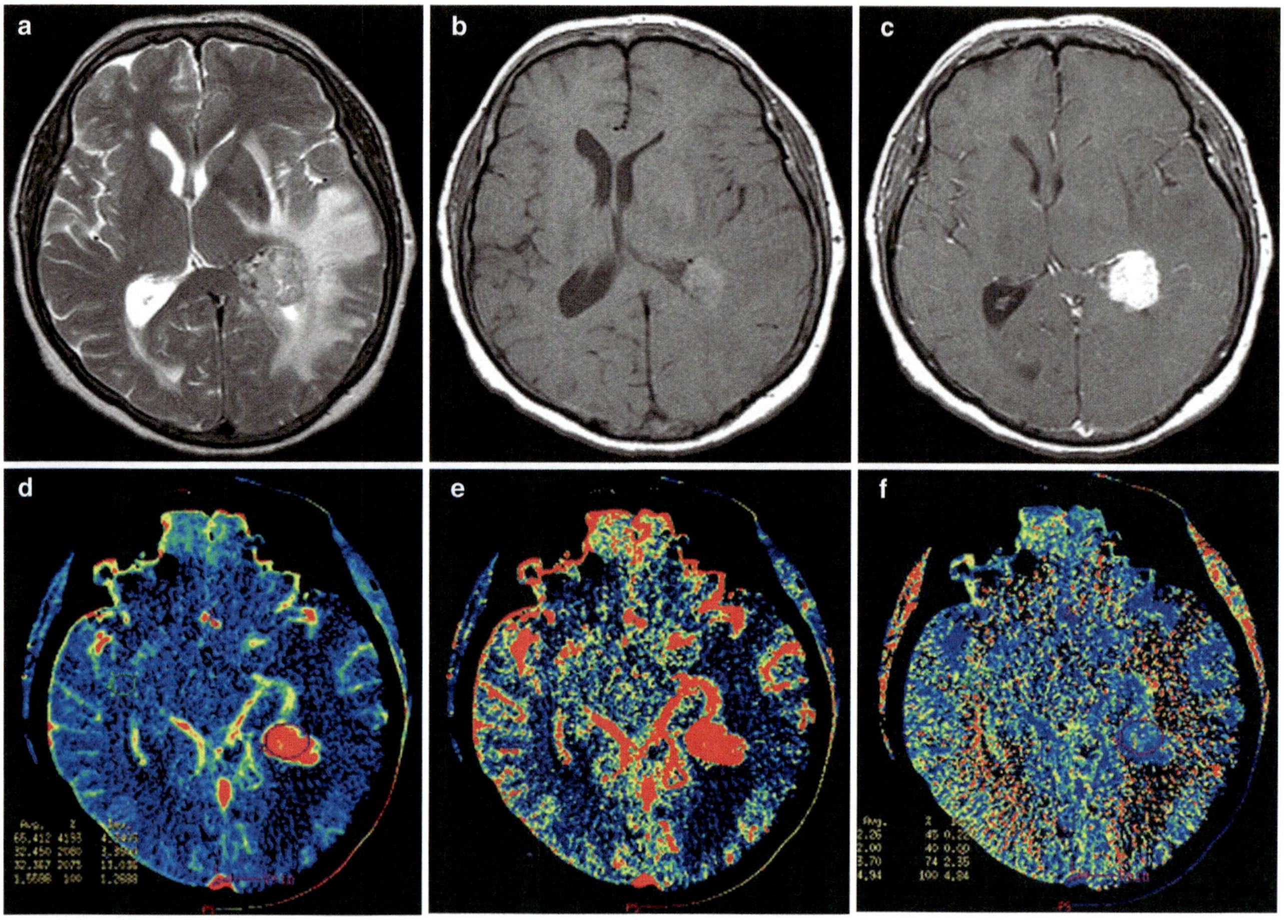

Fig. 14.6 A melanoma metastasis in the brain. In the posterior horn of the left lateral ventricle, there is a large solid metastasis with an increased signal on T2-weighted MRI (**a**) and a slightly increased signal on T1-weighted MRI (**b**). After the contrast agent administration (**c**), its accumulation is intense and uniform. Noteworthy is a pronounced perifocal edema with the displacement of the midline structures. On CT perfusion maps, the tumor lesion has sharply increased CBV (**d**) and CBF (**e**) values and low MTT values (**f**), which are characteristic of melanoma

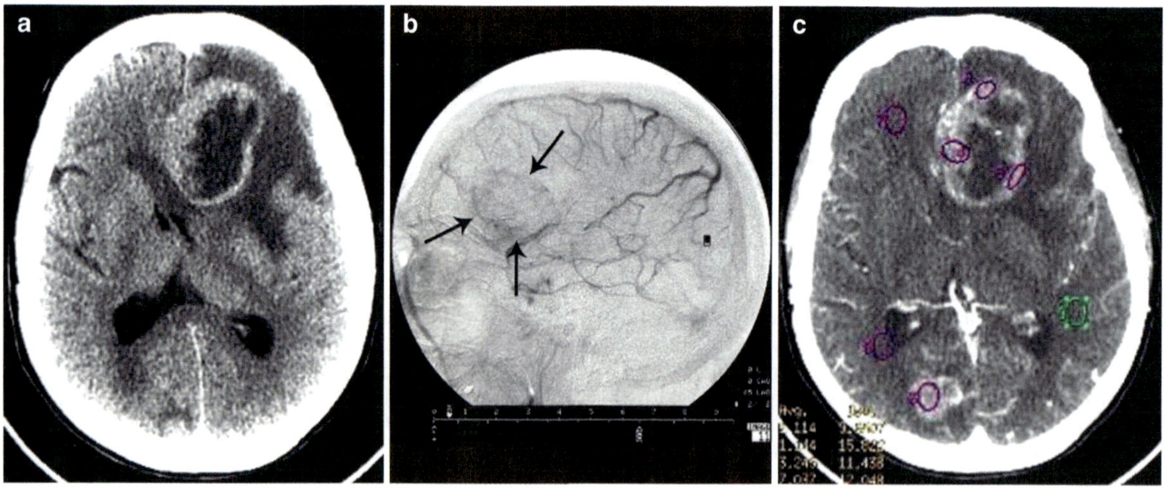

Fig. 14.7 A melanoma metastasis in the brain. In the left frontal and right occipital lobes, there are large, space-occupying heterogeneous lesions with areas of pronounced perifocal edema, intensely accumulating contrast agent in a CT study (**a**, **c**). On the lateral angiograms, there is a moderately expressed vascular network of the metastasis (**b**) (arrows). The largest lesion in the left frontal lobe extends to the falx. On CT perfusion maps of CBV (**d**), CBF (**e**), and MTT (**f**), there is a sharp, nonuniform increase in CBV and CBF values. MTT parameters are heterogeneous, and the most active part of the lesion (medial) is characterized by lower values. Perfusion parameters in the metastasis in the right occipital region are also significantly increased

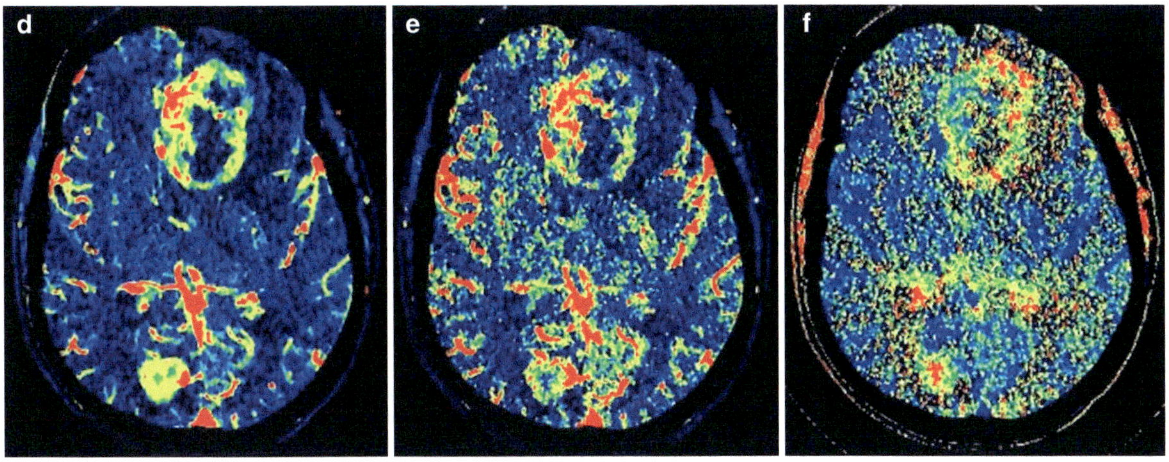

Fig. 14.7 (continued)

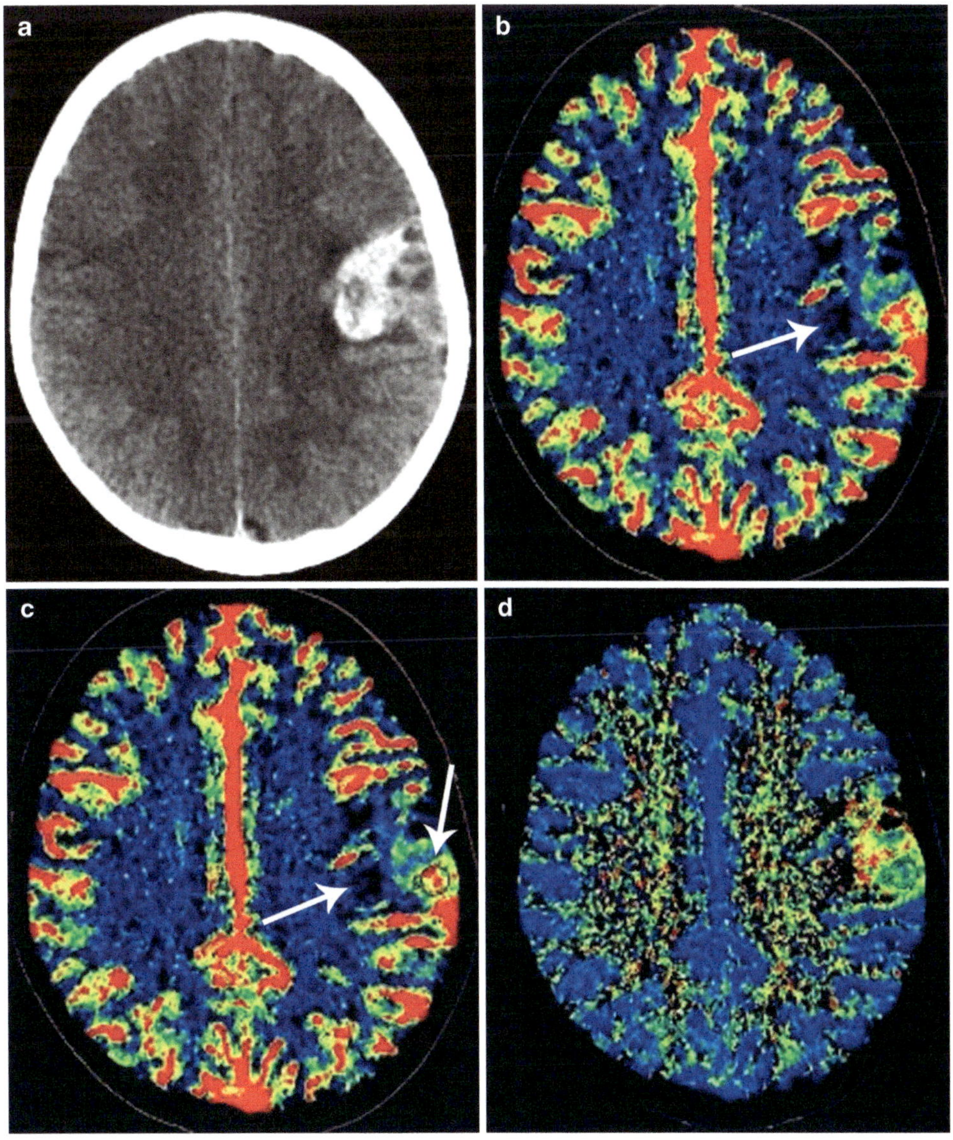

Fig. 14.8 A melanoma metastasis in the brain. Condition after radiosurgery. On CT in the left frontoparietal region, there is a lesion with a hemorrhage area with an increased density along the medial contour (**a**). On CT perfusion maps of CBV (**b**), CBF (**c**), and MTT (**d**) (*arrows*), there are dark regions in the hemorrhage areas—total absence of the blood flow. In the lesion residues, CBF values (**c**) (*arrow*) are increased and MTT values are high

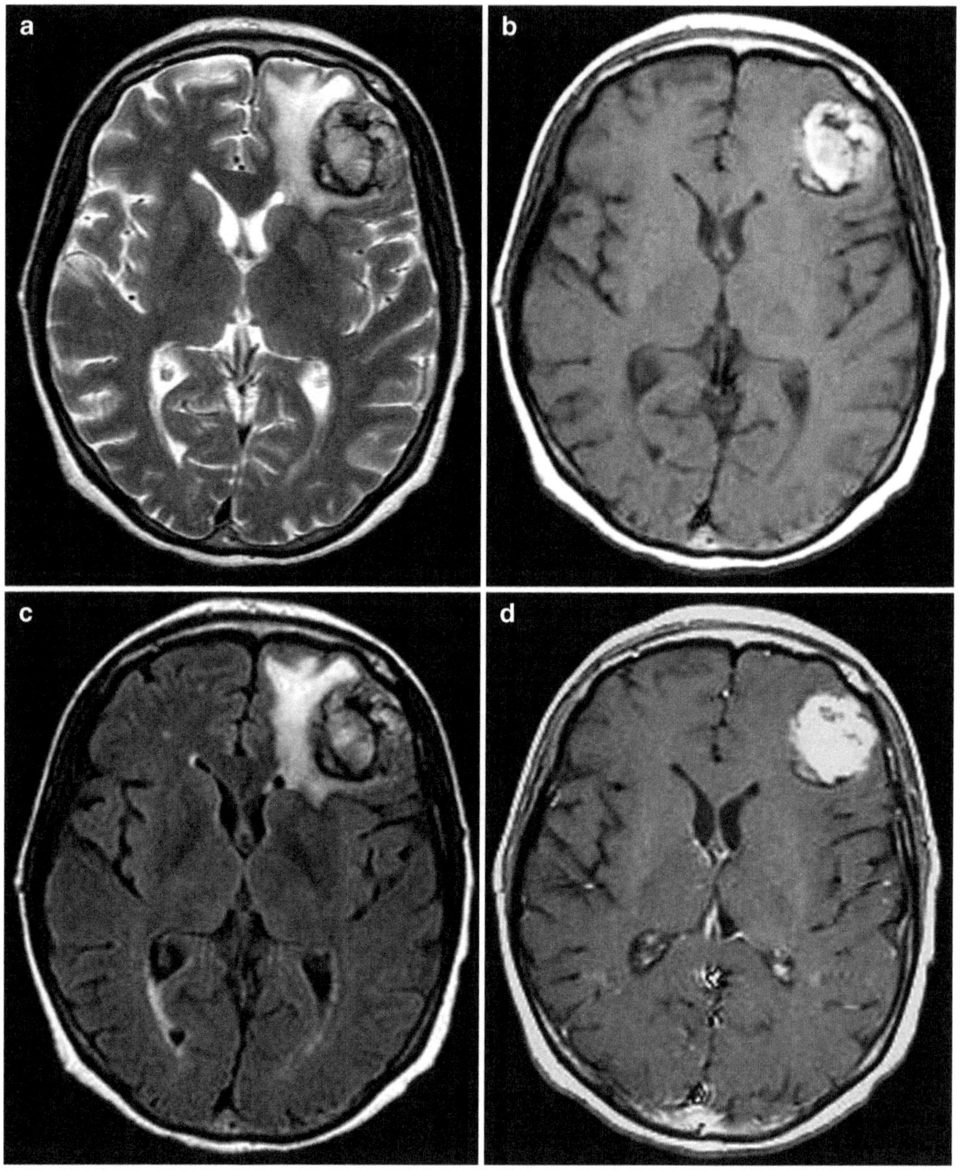

Fig. 14.9 A melanoma metastasis in the brain. In the left frontal region, there is a space-occupying lesion with a heterogeneous hypointense signal on T2-weighted MRI (**a**), hyperintense areas (hemorrhage) on T1-weighted MRI (**b**), and a moderately pronounced perifocal edema (a hyperintense area around the metastasis) on T2-FLAIR MRI (**c**). Following intravenous CA administration, its intensive accumulation in the tumor (**d**) is observed

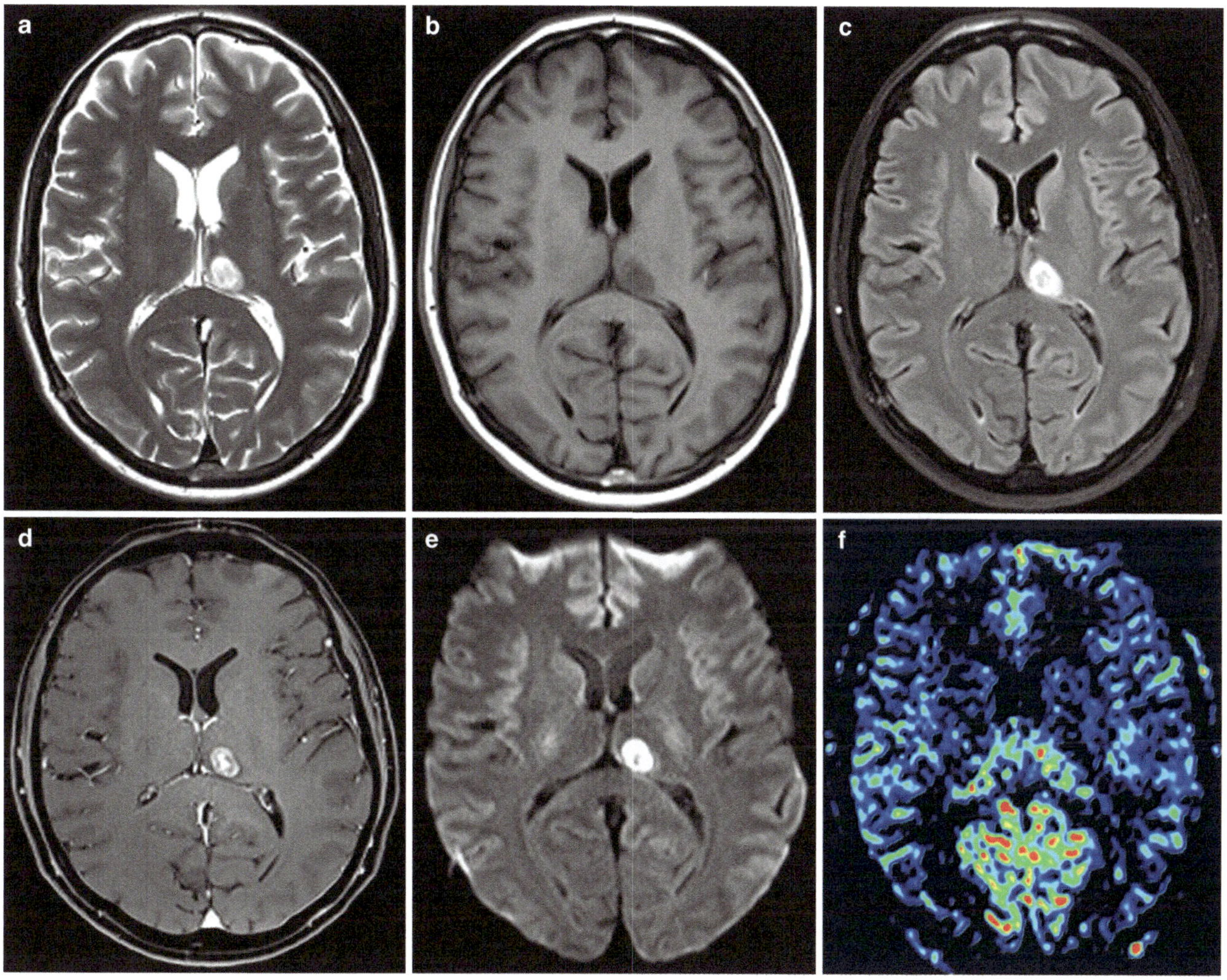

Fig. 14.10 A melanoma metastasis in the brain. In the left optic thalamus, there is a space-occupying lesion with an increased signal on T2-weighted, T2-FLAIR, and DWI MRI (**a**, **c**, **e**) and low signal on T1-weighted MRI (**b**), with signs of an increased blood flow on ASL MRI (**f**) and with no obvious signs of a perifocal edema. Following intravenous CA administration, its intense and uneven accumulation is noted in the tumor (D)

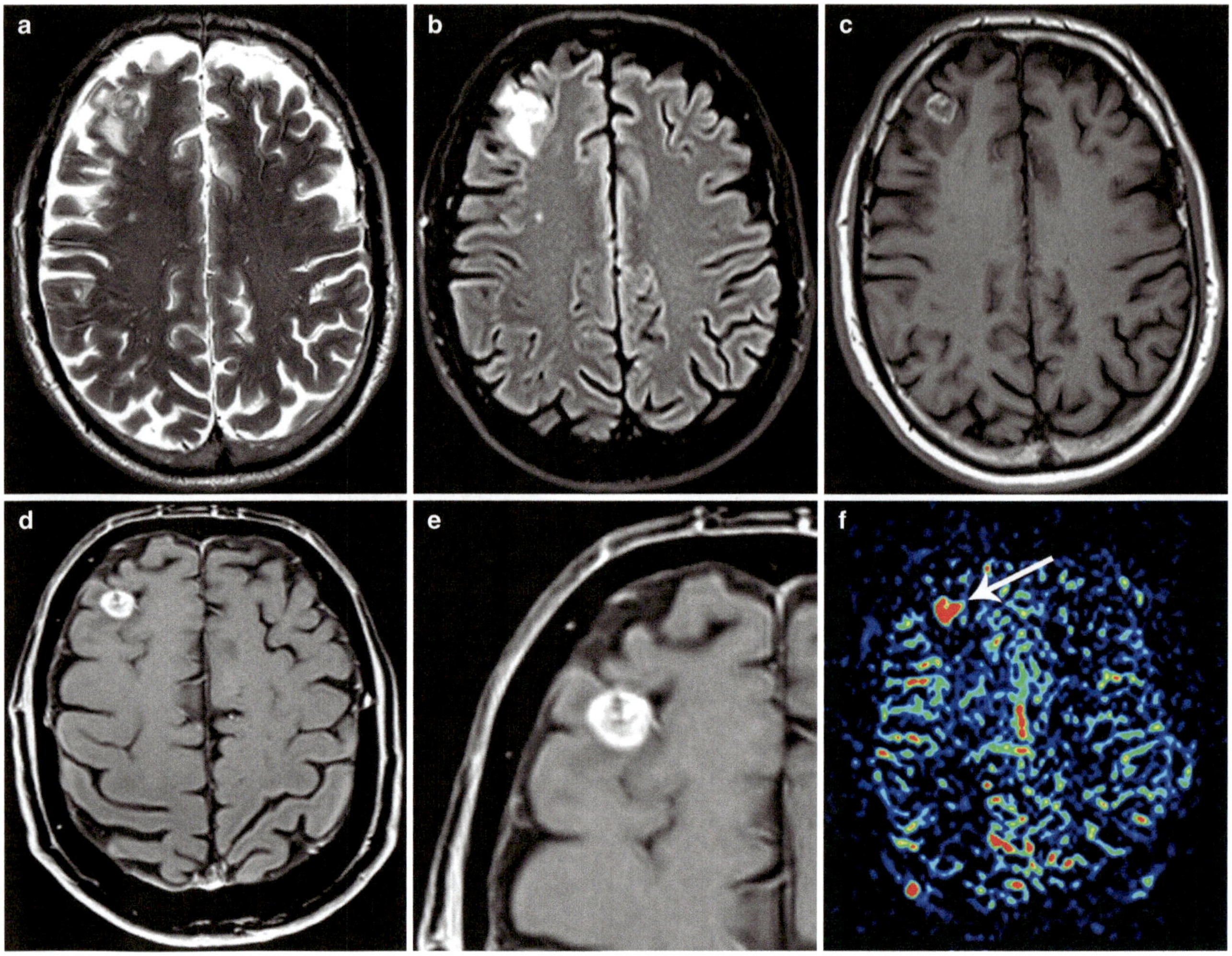

Fig. 14.11 A melanoma metastasis in the brain. In the right frontal lobe, there is a rounded space-occupying lesion with an iso-hyperintense signal on T2-weighted MRI (**a**) and an increased signal on T2-FLAIR MRI (**b**), with hyperintense areas (hemorrhage) on T1-weighted MRI (**c**) and with a moderate area of perifocal edema (**b**). After intravenous CA administration on T1 fat sat MRI (**d**, **e**), there is intense accumulation of the contrast agent in the tumor. The lesion is characterized by increased perfusion on ASL MRI (**f**)

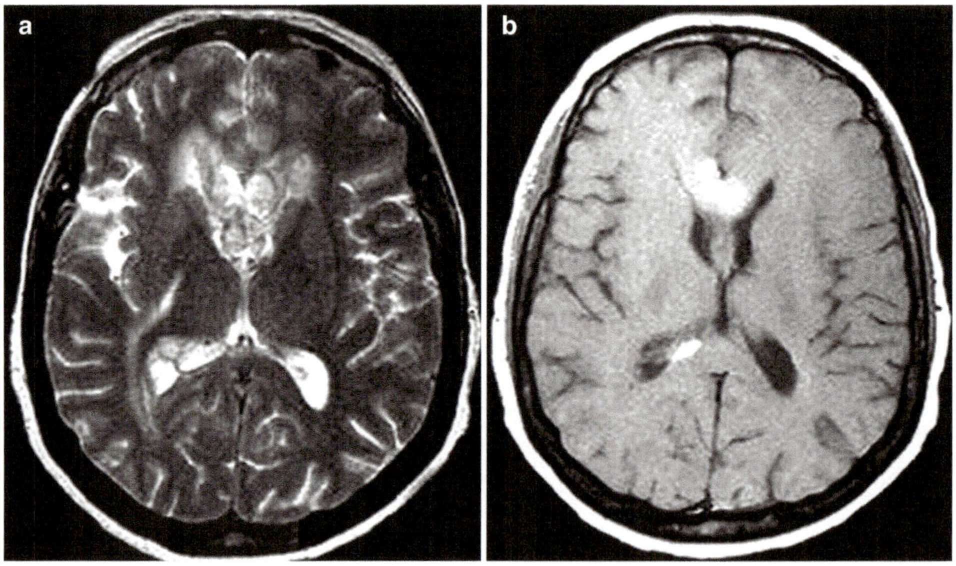

Fig. 14.12 Multiple metastases of melanoma. Along the meninges and ependyma of the lateral ventricles, there are multiple space-occupying lesions with an increased signal on T2-weighted (**a**) and T1-weighted MRI (**b**). After CA administration, there is its expressed accumulation in tumor lesions in the axial (**c**) and sagittal (**d**) projections

Fig. 14.12 (continued)

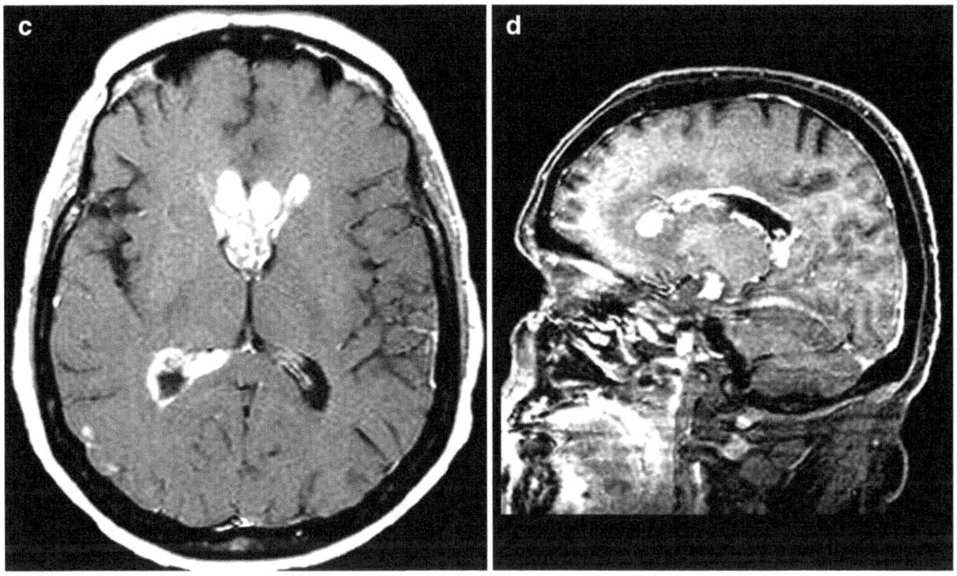

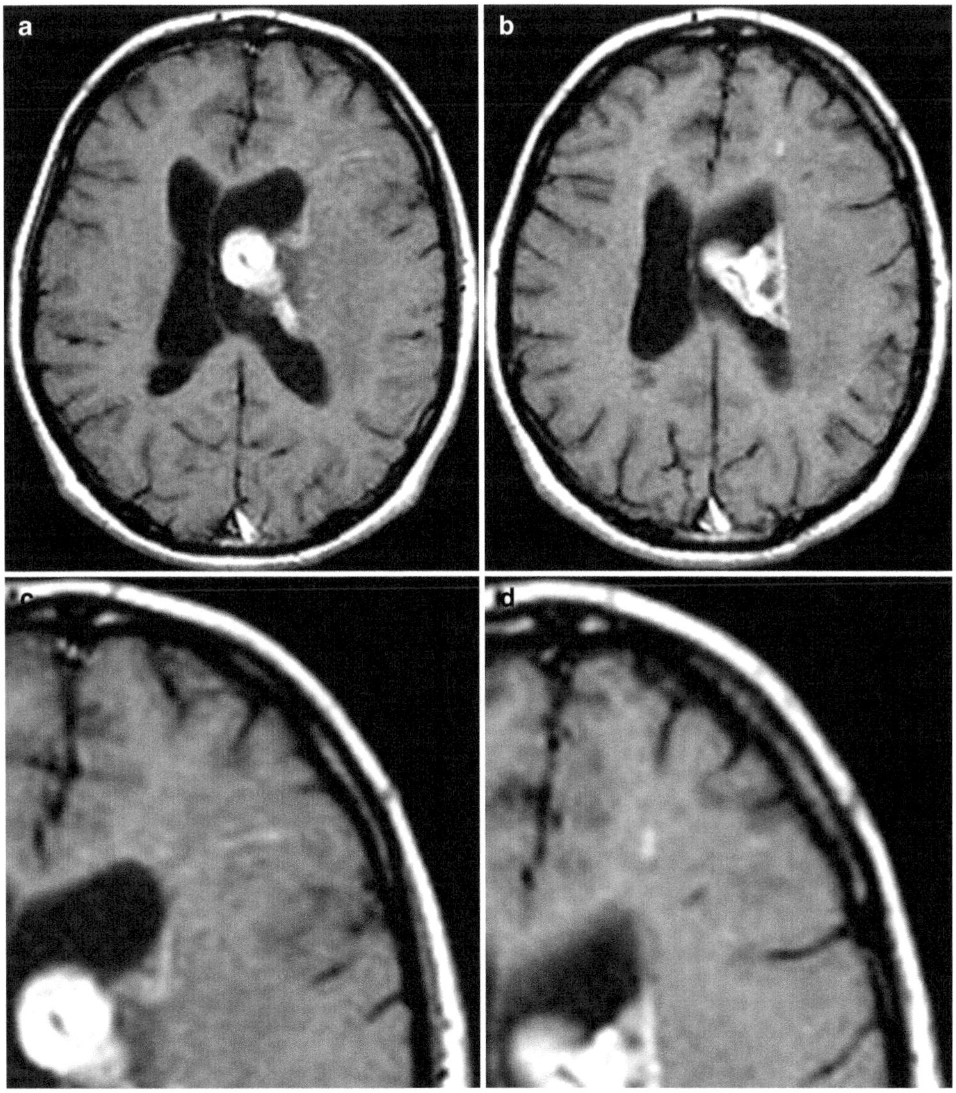

Fig. 14.13 Multiple melanoma metastases in the brain. On T1-weighted MRI with contrast enhancement in the projection of the left lateral ventricle, there are multiple confluent lesions (**a**, **b**) infiltrating the ependyma. Small inclusions with an increased signal in the substance of the left frontal region have vascular nature (venous angioma) (**c**, **d**)

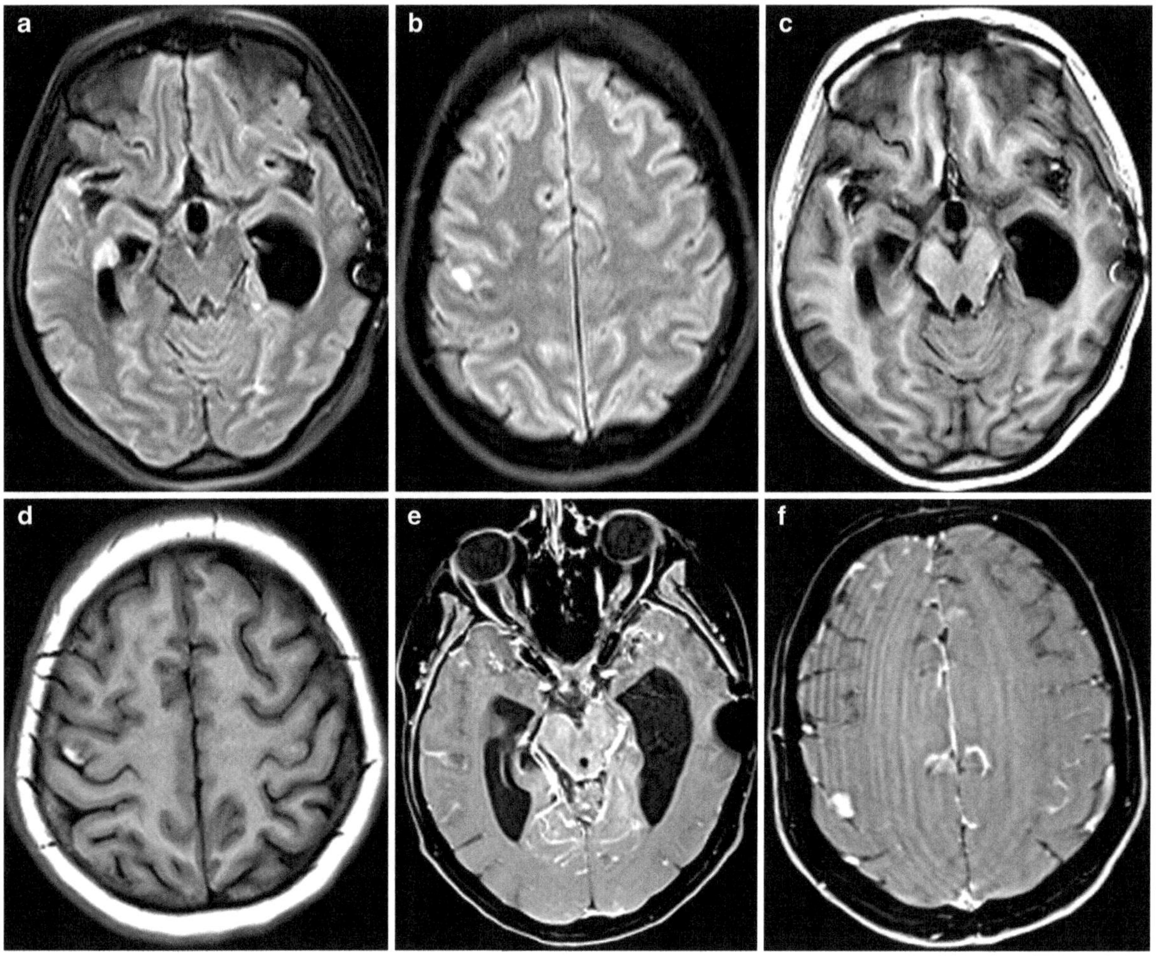

Fig. 14.14 Multiple melanoma metastases in the brain. A two-level study. Along subarachnoid meninges and ependyma of the temporal horn of the right lateral ventricle, there are multiple focal lesions with no obvious signs of a perifocal edema. Most of them are visualized only after intravenous CA administration on T1-weighted fat sat MRI (**e**, **f**). Some of the metastases in the right frontoparietal region have a hyper-intense portion (hemorrhage) on T1-weighted and T2-FLAIR MRI (**a**, **b**, **c**, **d**). The lesion in the ependyma of the right temporal horn is characterized by an increased signal on T2-FLAIR MRI (**a**) and a lower signal on T1-weighted MRI (**c**) without any clear signs of CA accumulation on T1-weighted fat sat MRI (**e**). In the left temporal area, there are artifacts from metal (**a**, **c**, **e**)

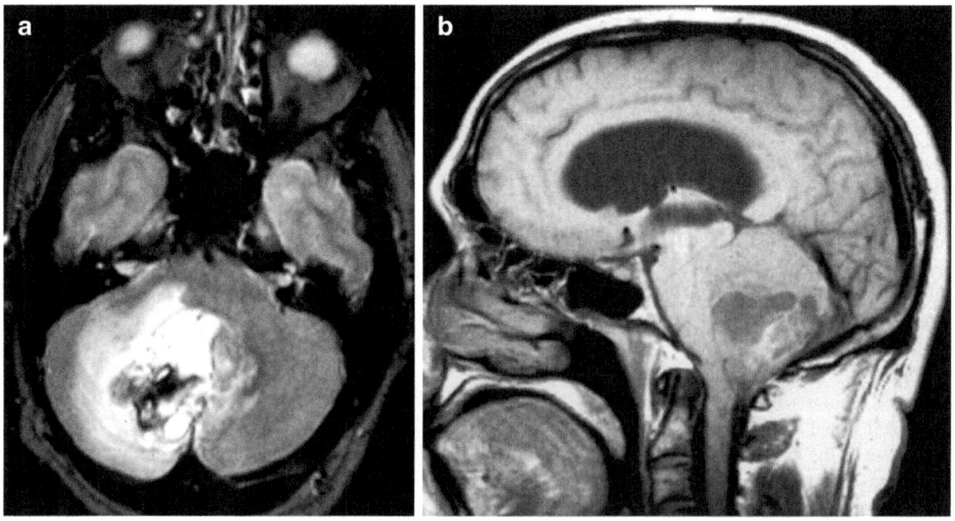

Fig. 14.15 A melanoma metastasis in the brain. In the right hemisphere of the cerebellum, there is a tumor lesion with a portion of a decreased signal in the central regions of the tumors on the T2-weighted MRI (**a**) and a high signal on T1-weighted MRI (**b**). On the periphery of the lesion, there are cysts and a significant perifocal edema. Obstructive hydrocephalus

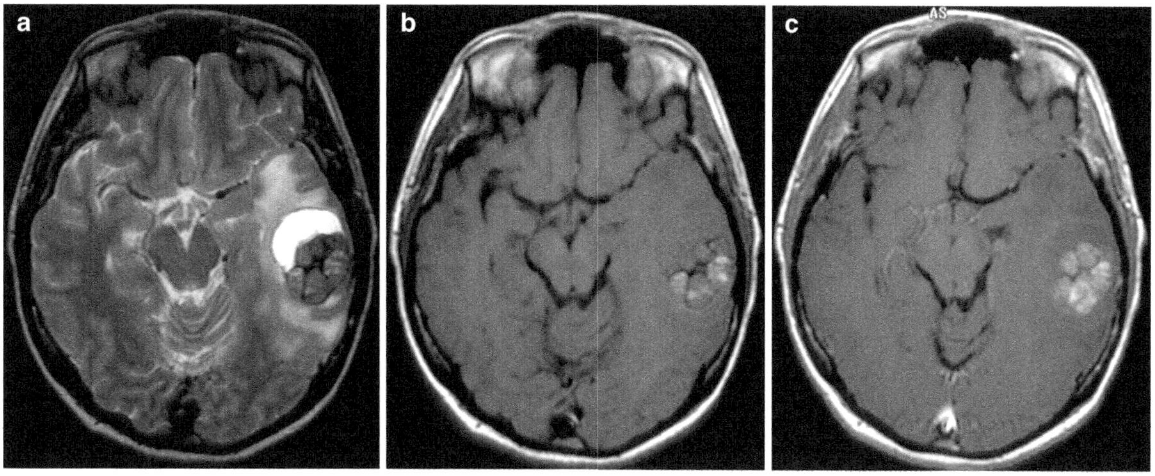

Fig. 14.16 A melanoma metastasis in the brain. On T2-weighted (**a**) and T1-weighted MRI before (**b**) and after (**c**) contrast enhancement: in the left temporal region, there is a tumor lesion with foci of subacute hemorrhages and melanin deposits (a hyperintensive MR signal on T1-weighted MRI). There is a hyperintense hemorrhagic cyst along the anterior contour of the lesion on T2-weighted MRI, with a solid part of the tumor having a decreased MR signal on T2-weighted MRI

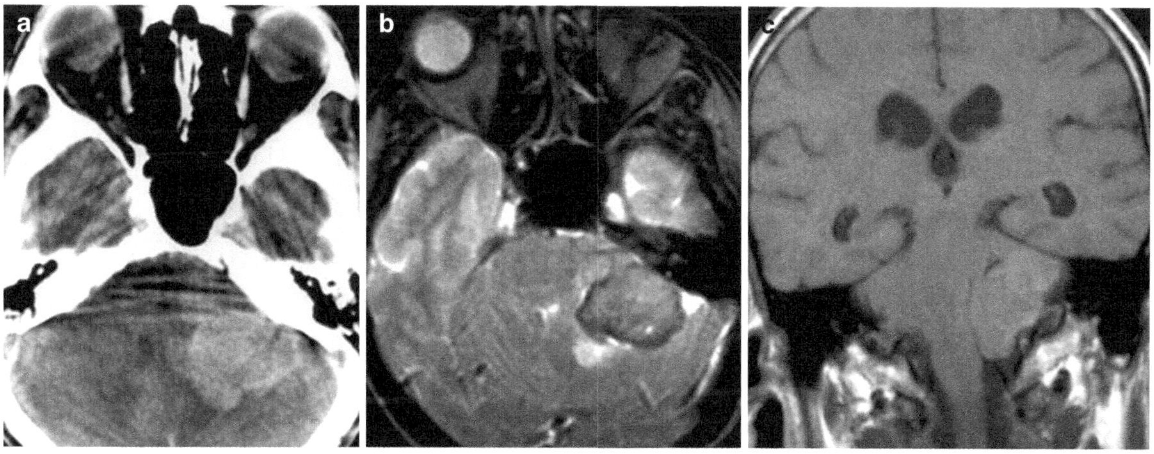

Fig. 14.17 A melanoma metastasis in the brain. On contrast-enhanced CT (**a**), in the projection of the left cerebellopontine angle, a tumor mass is visualized with a high density and a homogeneous structure. On T2-weighted MRI (**b**), the tumor is hypointense, and on T1-weighted MRI (**c**), it has the signal characteristics close to those of the brain substance

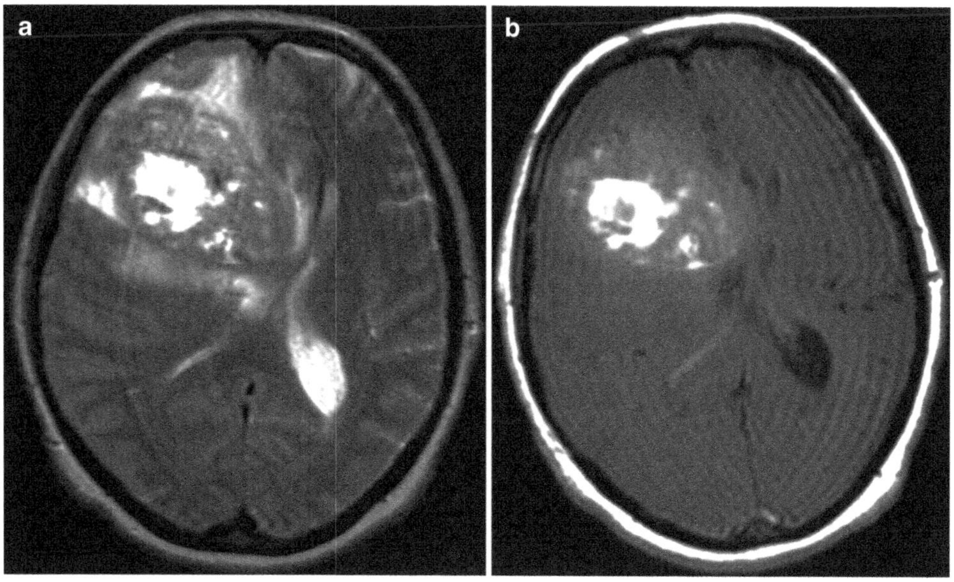

Fig. 14.18 A melanoma metastasis in the brain. On T2-weighted (**a**), T1-weighted (**b**), and T2*-weighted (**c**) MRI in the right frontal region, there is a huge tumor with foci of subacute hemorrhages (a hyperintensive MR signal in T2- and T1-weighted images), the perifocal edema is moderately expressed, and a sharp decrease in the MR signal on T2*-weighted MRI is caused by the presence of both melanin and subacute hemorrhages in the tumor

Fig. 14.18 (continued)

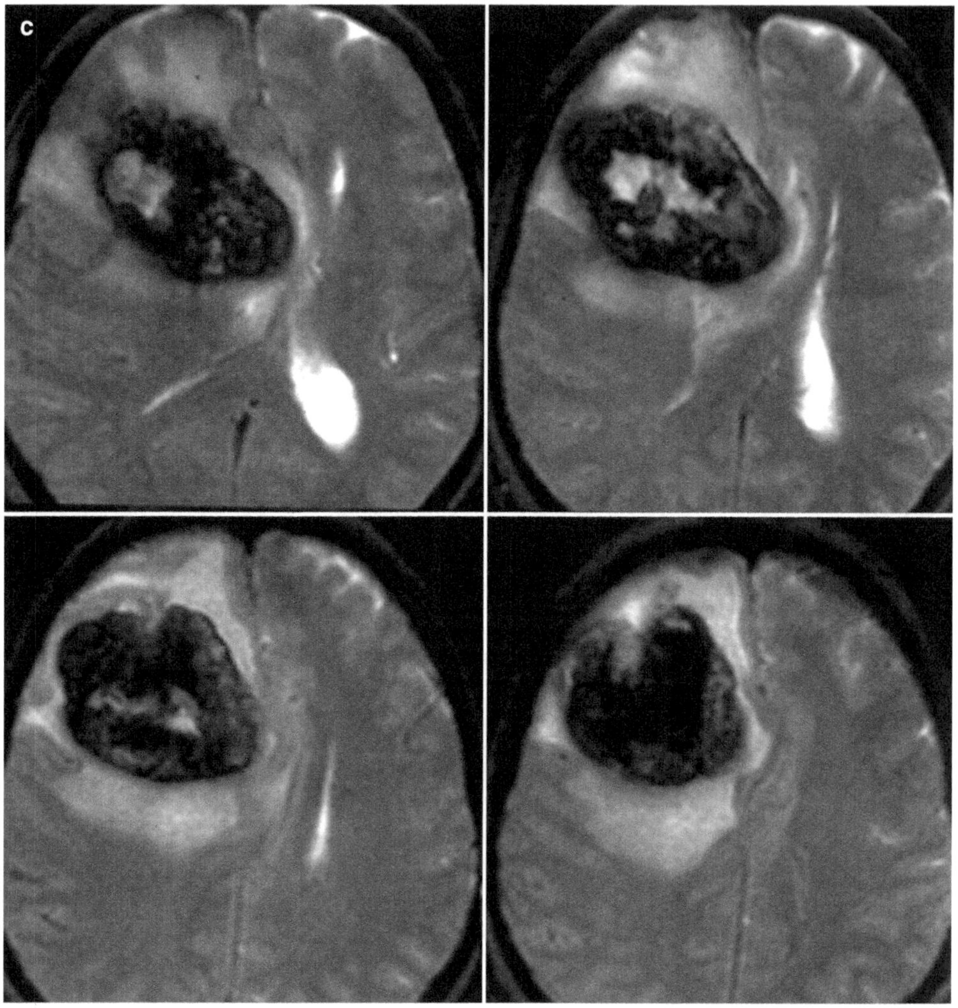

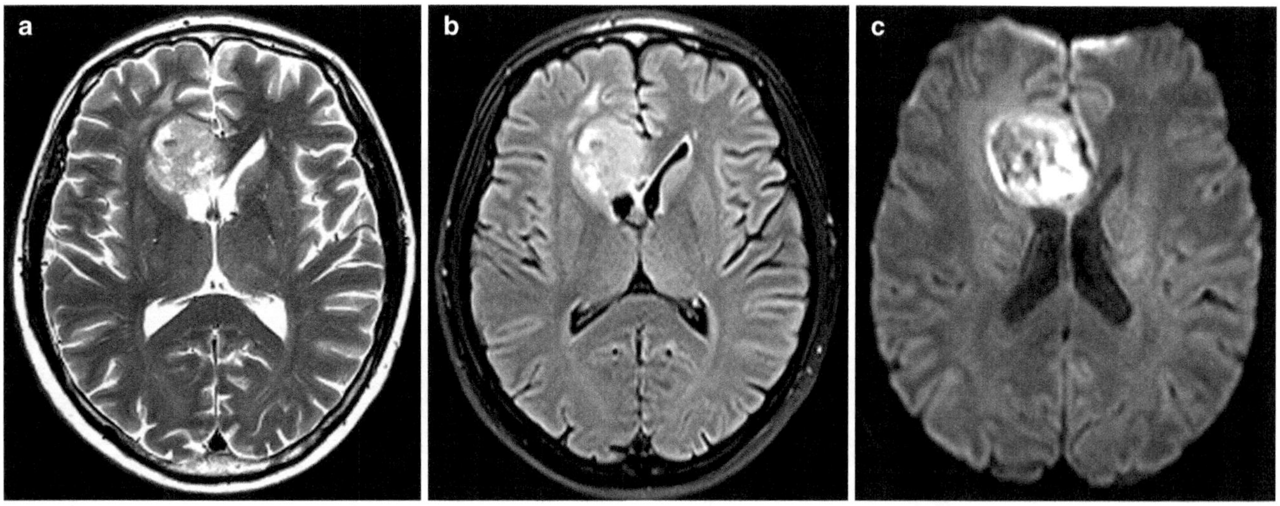

Fig. 14.19 A melanoma metastasis in the brain. In the area of the splenium of the corpus callosum, with the spread to the right hemisphere, there is a space-occupying lesion that deforms the falx and compresses the front horn of the right lateral ventricle. The metastasis is characterized by a heterogeneously hyperintense signal on T2-weighted (**a**) and T2-FLAIR (**b**) MRI, a sharply increased signal on DWI b-1000MRI (**c**), and a low signal onT1-weighted MRI (**d**). Following intravenous CA administration, its moderate and uneven accumulation is noted in the tumor (**d**). In the parasagittal sections, there is an area with increased perfusion on ASL MRI (F) (the *arrow*)

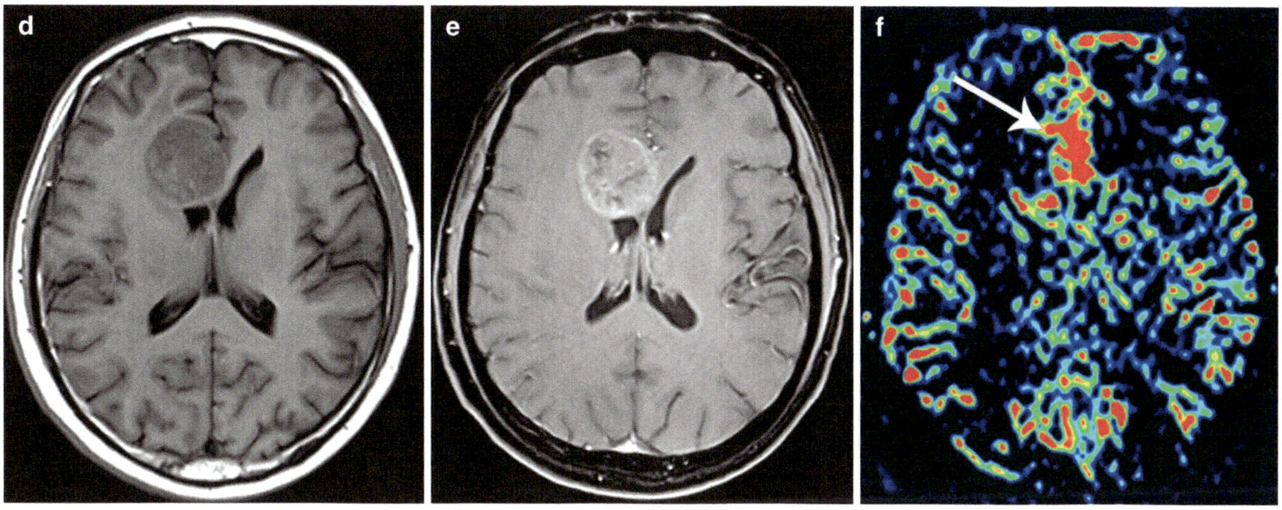

Fig. 14.19 (continued)

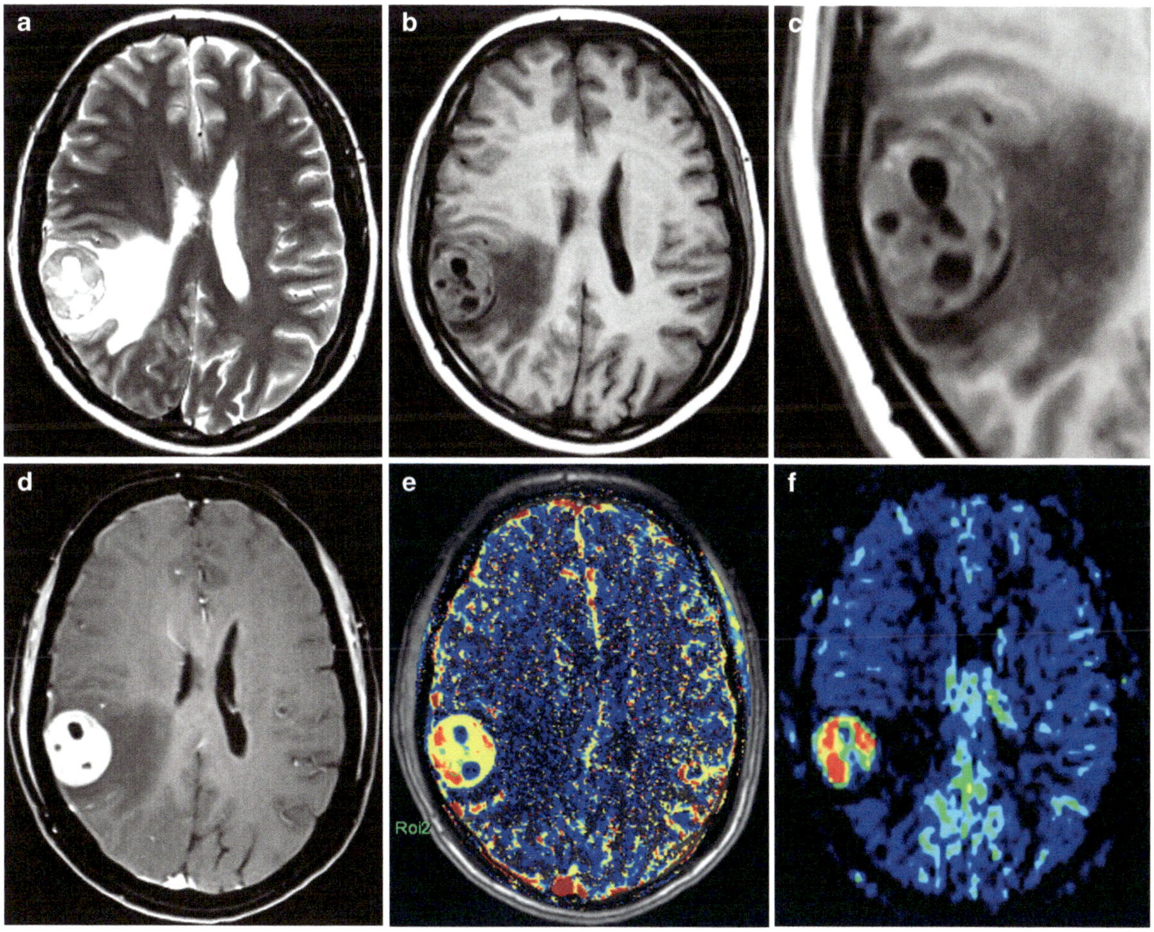

Fig. 14.20 Amelanotic melanoma metastasis in the brain. In convexital portions of the right frontotemporoparietal region, there is a heterogeneous space-occupying lesion with high signal on T2-weighted MRI (**a**), with areas of low MR signal on T1-weighted MRI (**b**, **c**). After CA administration (**d**), its intense accumulation in the solid part of the tumor is observed. With dynamic MRI contrast enhancement, Ktrans values (**e**) are increased, as there are increased perfusion areas on ASL MRI (**f**). On CT perfusion maps of CBV (**g**), CBF (**h**), and MTT (**i**), there are high CBV and CBF values and moderately elevated MTT values. On CT images (**j**), the lesion intensely accumulates the contrast agent. On PET/CT with 18F-tyrosine (**k**, **l**), there is an intense accumulation of the radiopharmaceutical in the structure of the lesion. A gross specimen of the removed metastasis of amelanotic melanoma (**m**, **n**)

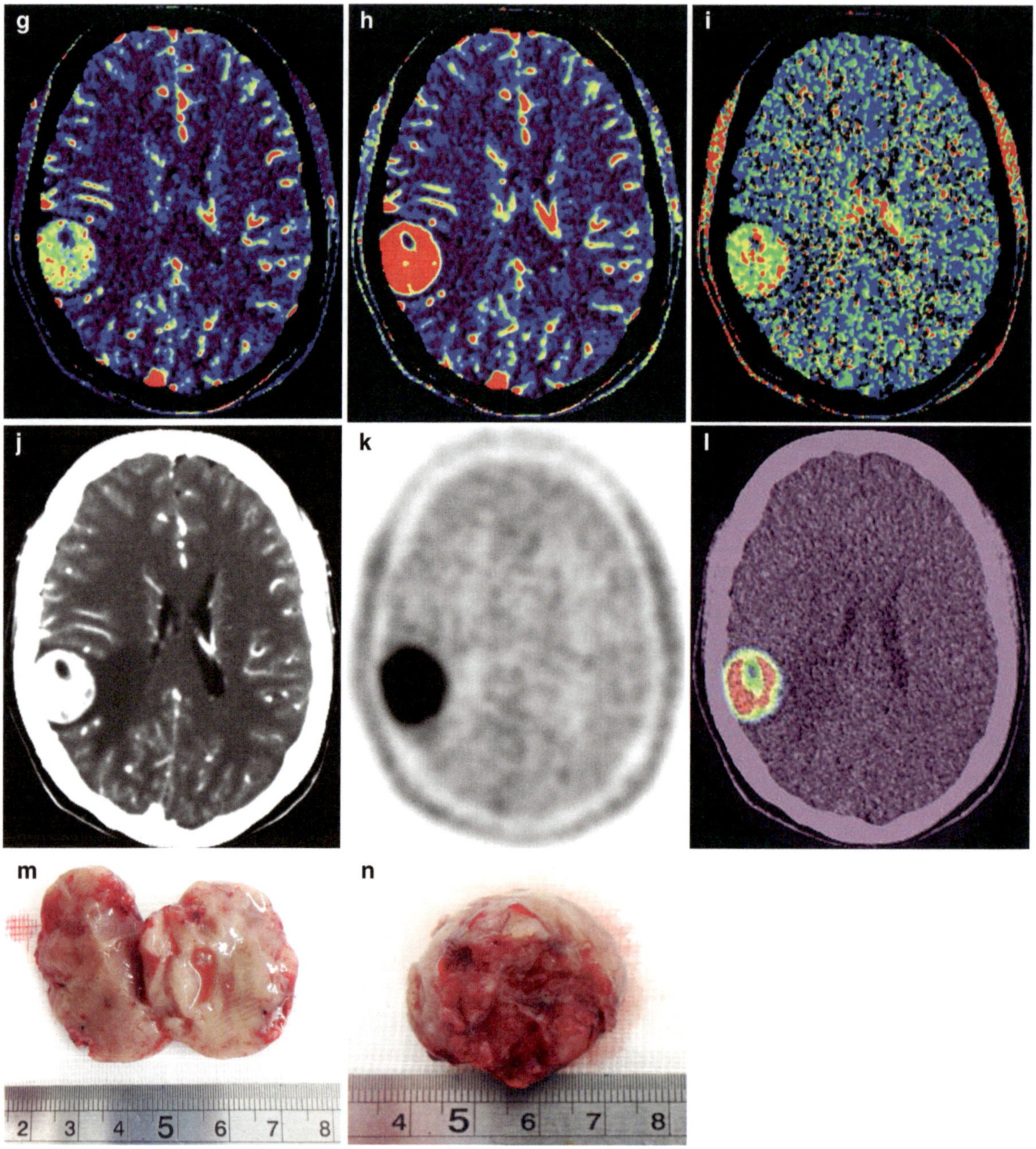

Fig. 14.20 (continued)

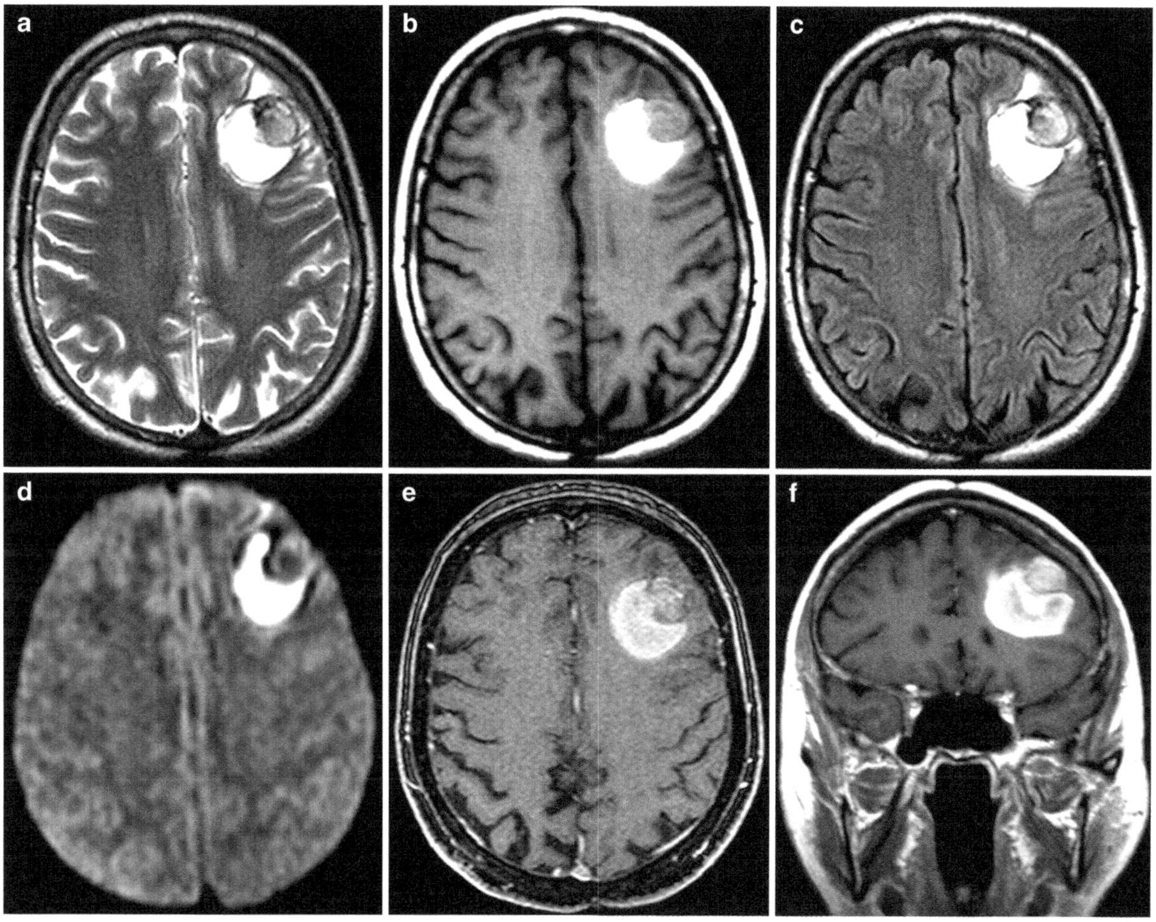

Fig. 14.21 A melanoma metastasis in the brain. In the left frontal region, there is a space-occupying lesion, whose solid part (anterior-lateral parts) has a heterogeneous hypointense signal on T2-weighted and T2-FLAIR MRI (**a**, **c**) and moderately increased signal on T1-weighted MRI (**b**), with an extensive hyperintense area (hemorrhage along the medial contour) with an increased signal in all sequences—T2-weighted, T1-weighted, T2-FLAIR, and DWI MRI (**a**, **b**, **c**, **d**). After intravenous CA administration on T1-weighted fat sat MRI in the axial (**e**) and frontal (**f**) projections, there is intense accumulation of the contrast agent by the solid component of the tumor

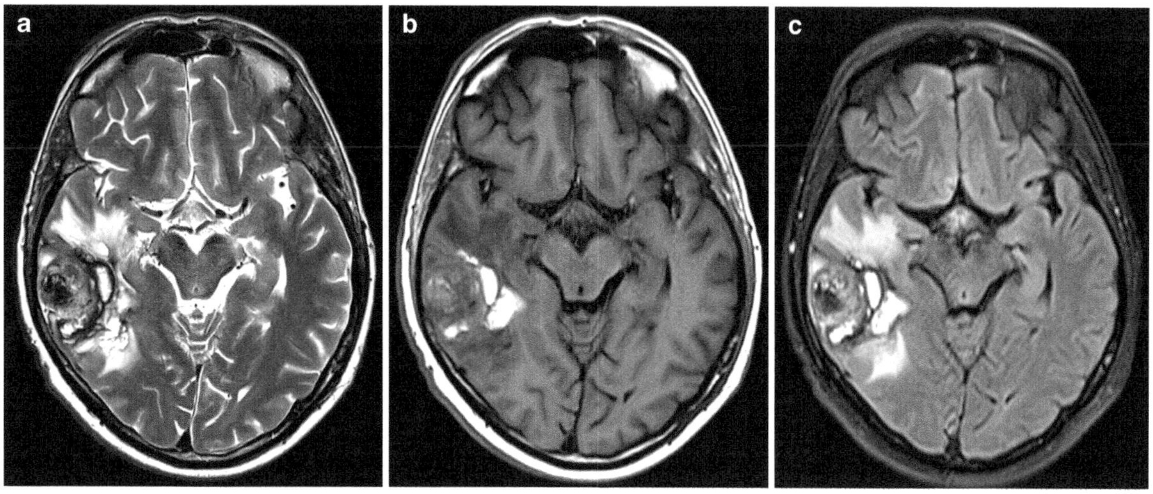

Fig. 14.22 Multiple melanoma metastases in the brain. A two-level study. The right temporal and parietal regions are identified as volumetric heterogeneous lesions with hypointense areas on T2-weighted MRI (**a**, **d**) and hyperintense (due to hemorrhages) areas on T1-weighted MRI (b, e). Perifocal edema is expressed only in the right temporal region on T2-FLAIR MRI (**c**, **f**). In the structure of the largest lesion in the right temporal region on ASL MRI (**i**), there is increased perfusion along the posterior contour, and the blood flow in the parietal region of the metastasis is also increased (**l**). Following intravenous CA administration on T1-weighted fat sat MRI, its uneven accumulation by the solid component of the tumor is observed (**g**, **h**, **j**, **k**)

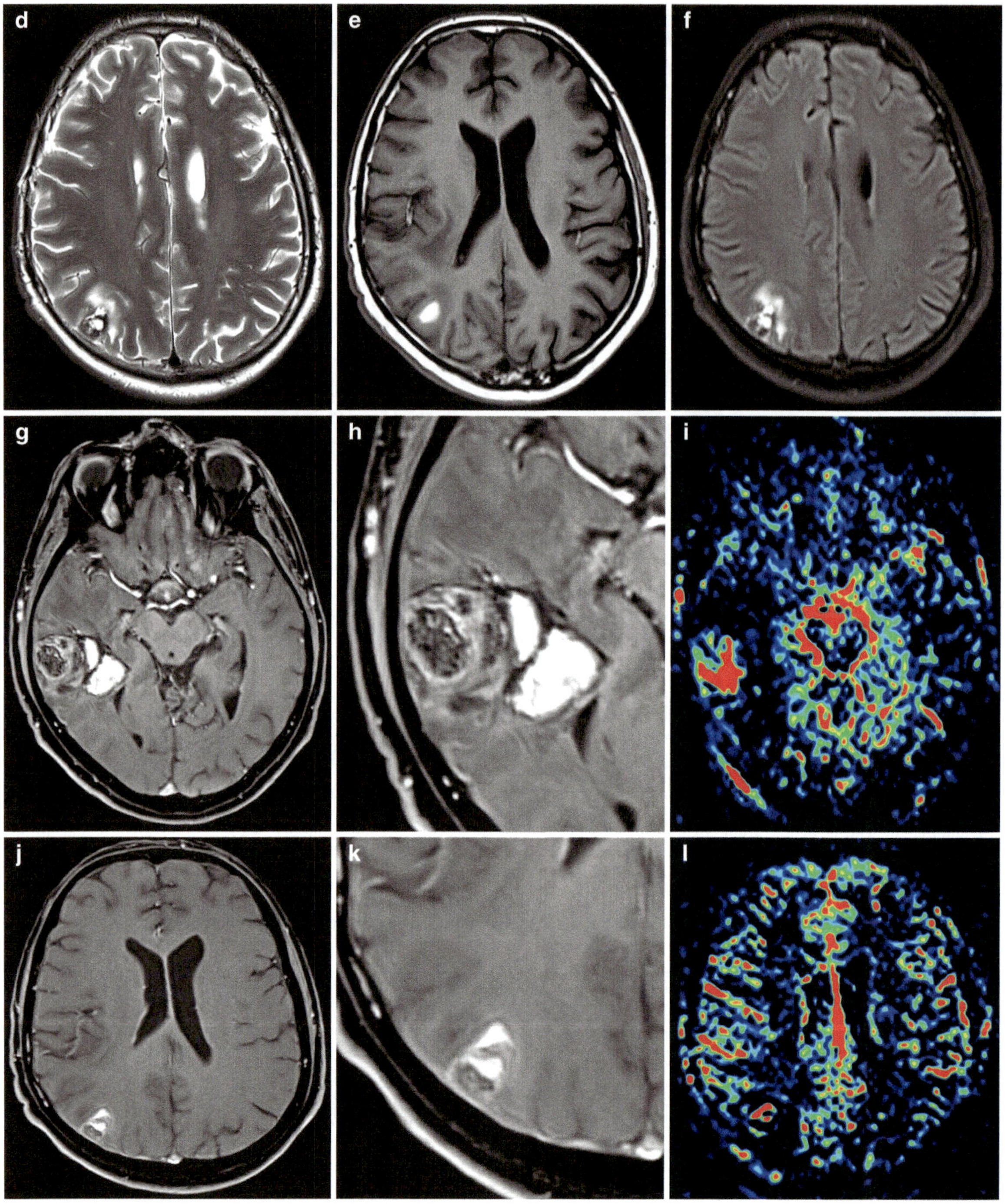

Fig. 14.22 (continued)

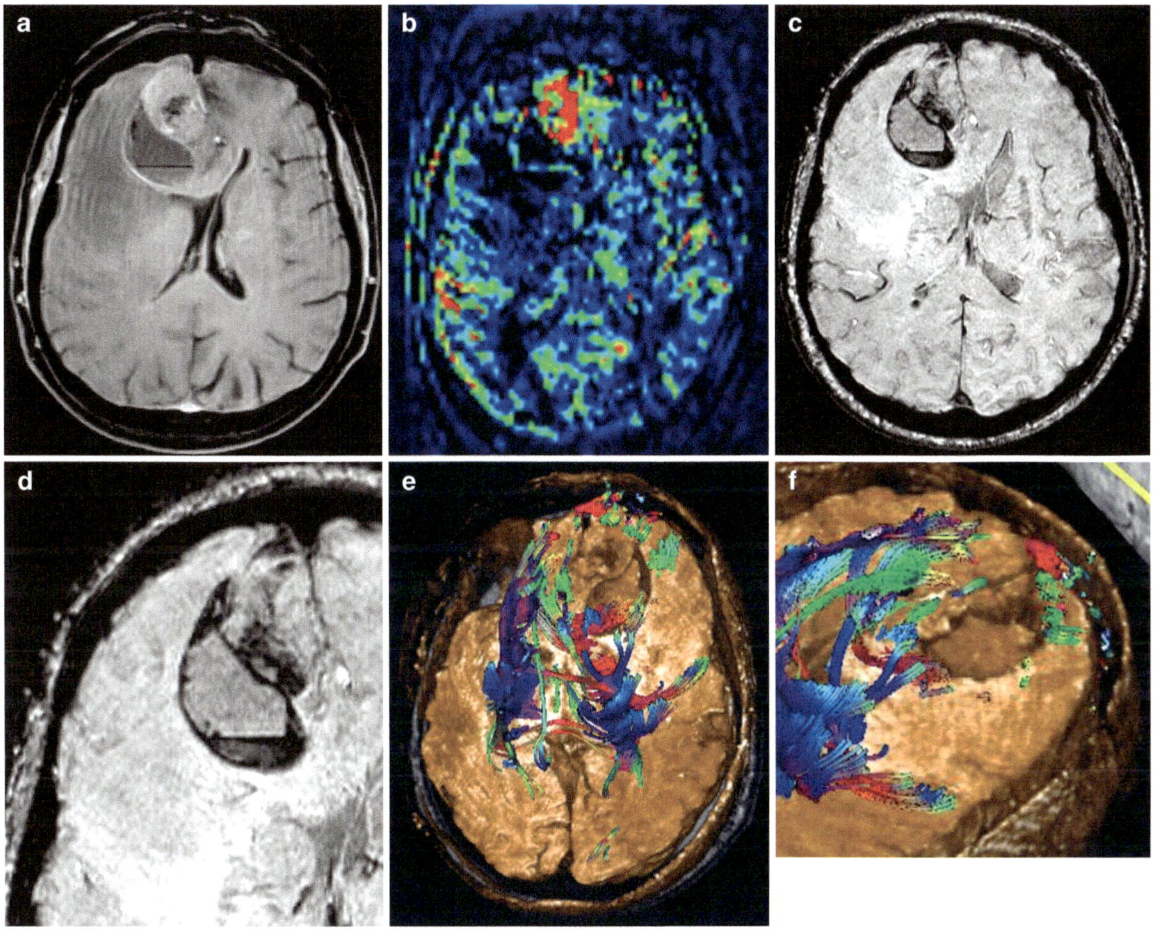

Fig. 14.23 A melanoma metastasis in the brain. In the right frontal lobe, there is a solid-cystic lesion intensely accumulating CA on T1-weighted MRI (**a**) that extends to the falx and compresses the front horn of the right lateral ventricle and the corpus callosum. In the cystic component, there is a horizontal level of hemorrhagic content with a moderately increased signal on T1-weighted MRI (**a**) and a decreased signal on SWI (SWAN) MRI (**c**, **d**), and the solid part of the lesion is also characterized by a low signal. On ASL MRI (**b**), there is increased perfusion in the anterior-medial tumor portions. On MR tractography (**e**, **f**) in this area, the conductive pathways are pushed aside and intact

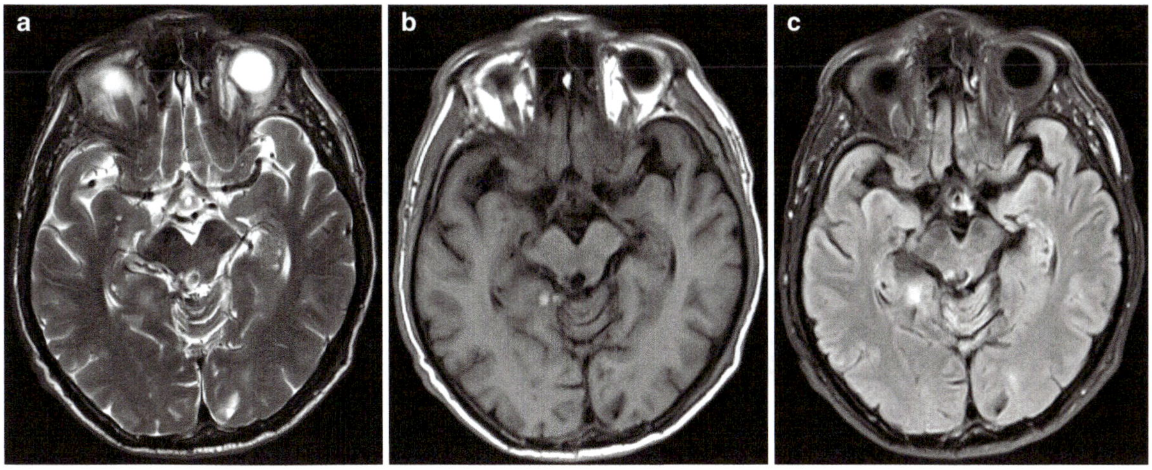

Fig. 14.24 Multiple melanoma metastases in the brain. Along the cerebellar tentorium on the right, there are areas with a moderately increased signal on T2-weighted (**a**), T1-weighted (**b**), and T2-FLAIR (**c**) MRI. On ASL MRI (**d**) on the background of increased perfusion in the cerebellum, perfusion in the tumor lesions is difficult to evaluate. Following intravenous CA administration, on T1-weighted fat sat MRI (**e**, **f**), there is its accumulation in the focal lesions spreading along the cerebellar tentorium on the right

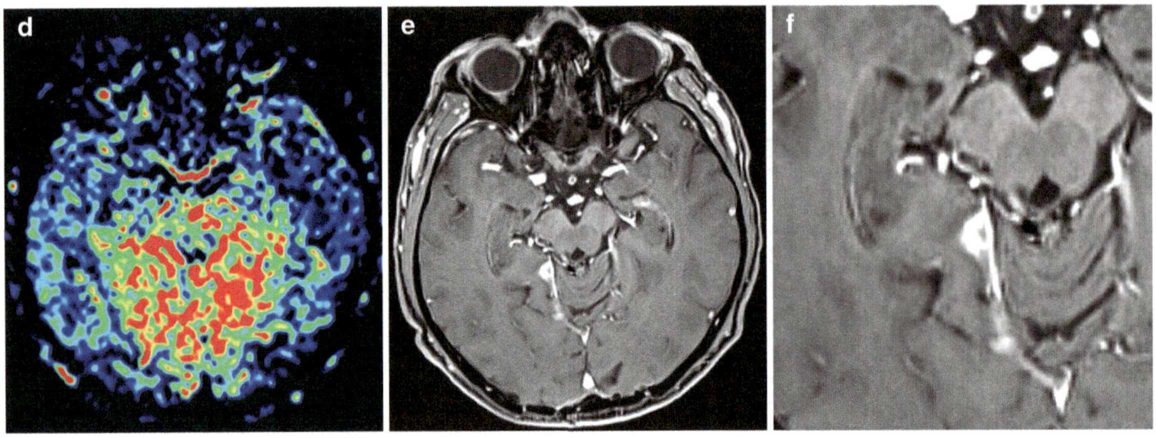

Fig. 14.24 (continued)

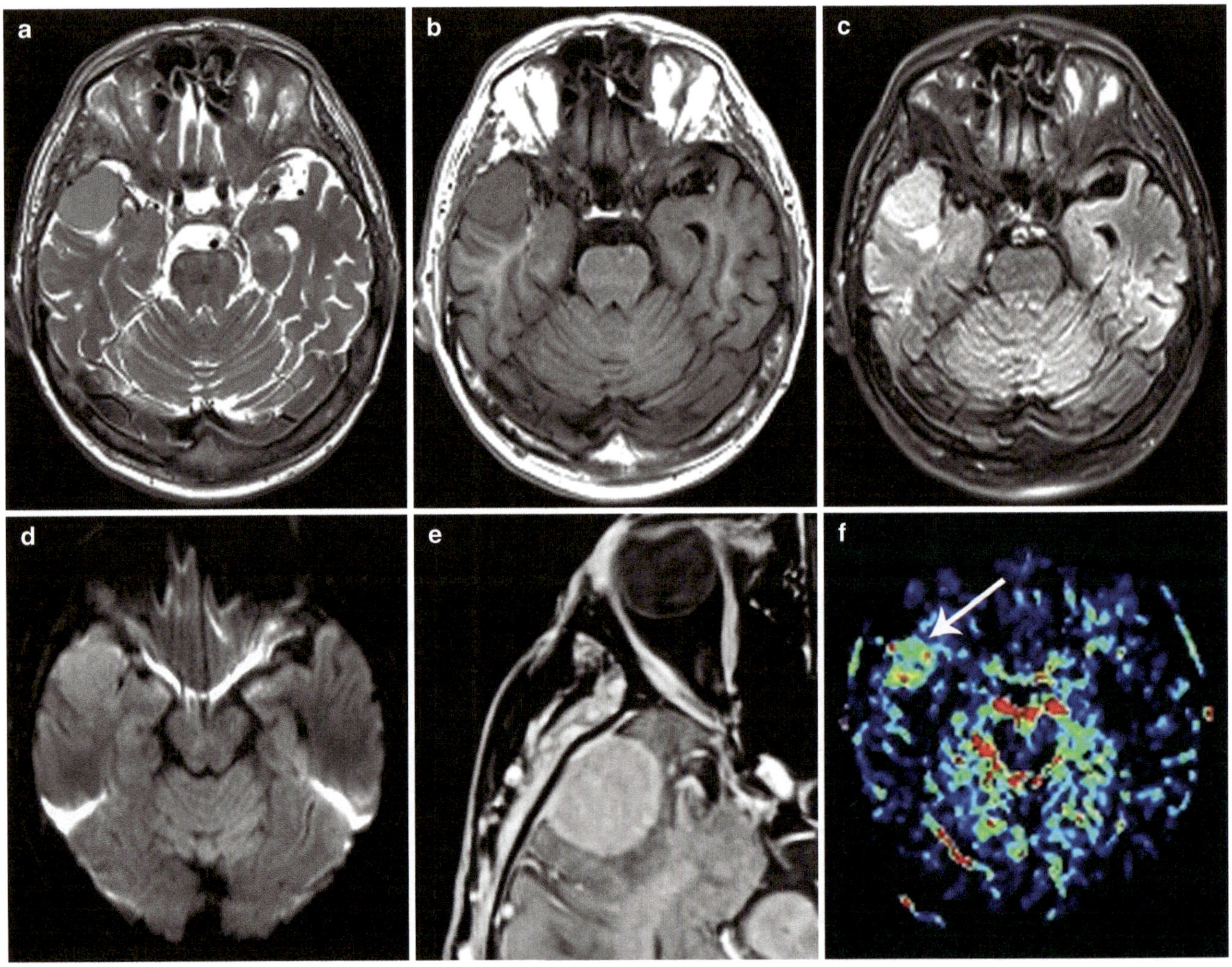

Fig. 14.25 A melanoma metastasis in the brain. In the right temporal lobe, there is a space-occupying lesion with an isointense signal on T2-weighted, T1-weighted, and DWI MRI (**a**, **b**, **d**) and a moderately increased signal on T2-FLAIR MRI (**c**) with an area of mild perifocal edema closely adjacent with its broad base to the meninges. Following intravenous CA administration on T1-weighted fat sat MRI (**e**), its intense and relatively uniform accumulation in the tumor is observed. Of note are the signs of the "tail" symptom—linear sections of abnormal accumulation of the contrast agent along the meninges adjacent to the tumor. On ASL MRI (**f**), there is an increased blood flow in the tumor (the *arrow*)

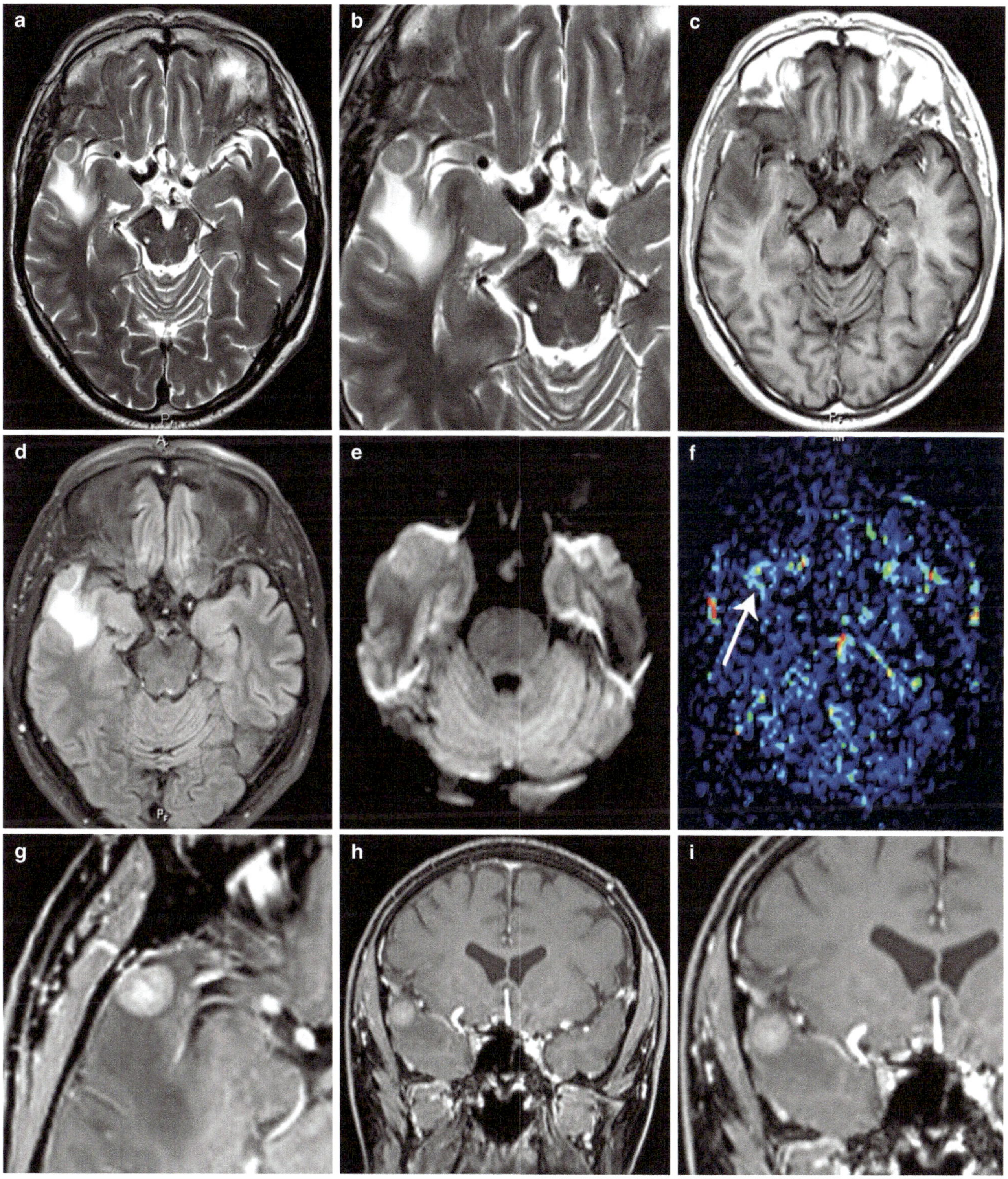

Fig. 14.26 A melanoma metastasis in the brain. In the convexital parts of the right temporal region, there is a small rounded space-occupying lesion with an intense signal on T2-weighted MRI (**a**, **b**) and T1-weighted MRI (**c**), increased on T2-FLAIR MRI (**d**) and slightly increased on DWI $b = 1000$ (**e**). The metastasis is characterized by moderately elevated blood flow rates on ASL MRI (**f**) (*arrow*). After intravenous CA administration in the axial (**g**) and frontal (**h**, **i**) projections, there is its intense and uneven accumulation in the tumor. The metastasis is partially adjacent to the meninges; however, there is no evidence of the "tail" symptom. The metastasis is characterized by a pronounced perifocal edema that simulates the CSF cleft in axial T2-weighted images

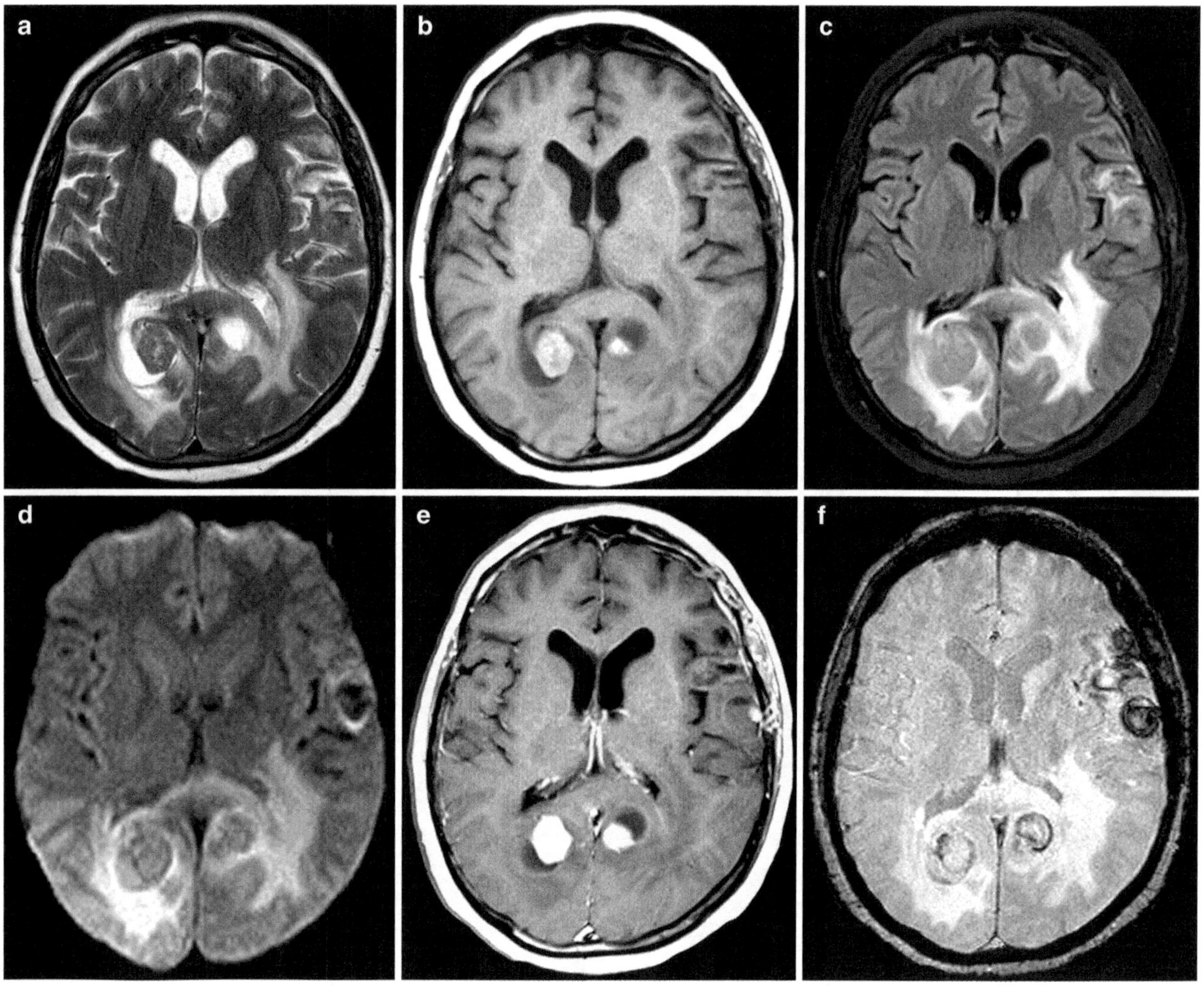

Fig. 14.27 Multiple metastases of melanoma. In the occipital region and cortical parts of the left frontotemporal region, there are multiple space-occupying lesions. The largest of them are accompanied by a severe perifocal edema (hyperintense area) on T2-weighted, T2-FLAIR, and DWI b-500 MRI (**a**, **c**, **d**). Hemorrhages are observed in the structure of metastases (hyperintense areas on T1-weighted MRI (**b**) and hypointense areas on SWI (SWAN) MRI (**f**)). Lesions in the left frontotemporal area are not differentiated on T1-weighted MRI (**b**); however, on SWI (SWAN) MRI (**f**), there are hypointense areas in its structure—more "fresh" hemorrhages. After intravenous CA administration, its accumulation is observed along the periphery (**e**) of the lesions and solid components of the metastases that have a boundary location

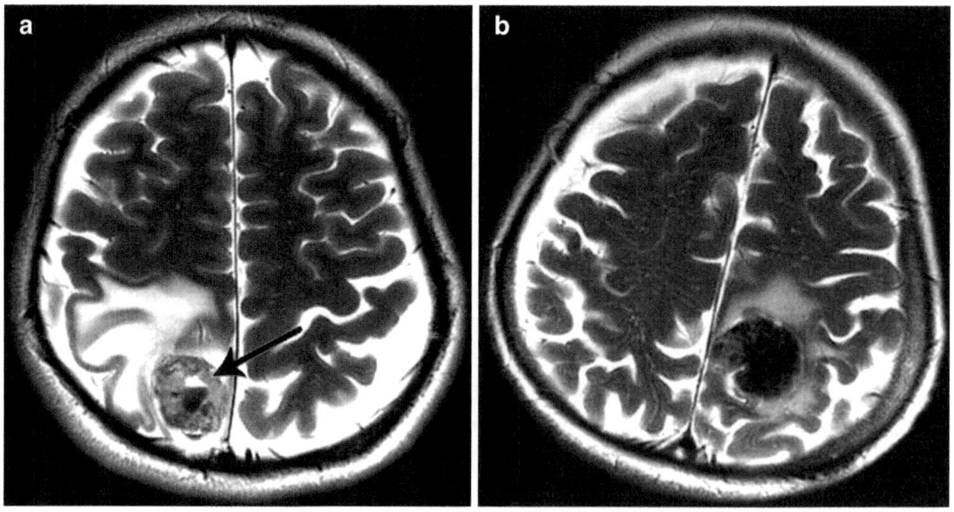

Fig. 14.28 Metastases of melanoma (**a**, **c**) and colon cancer (**b**, **d**). There is an expressed hypointense signal both on T2-weighted MRI (**a**, **b**) and SWI (SWAN) MRI (**c**, **d**) in both cases. In the melanoma metastasis, accumulation of free blood in the central parts of the tumor forms a hypointense "level" in the T2 image (**a**)—the *arrow*

Fig. 14.28 (continued)

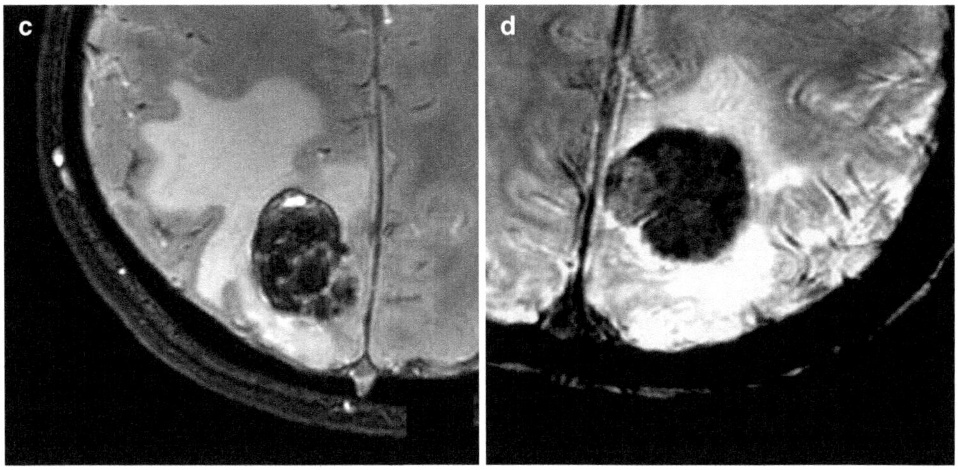

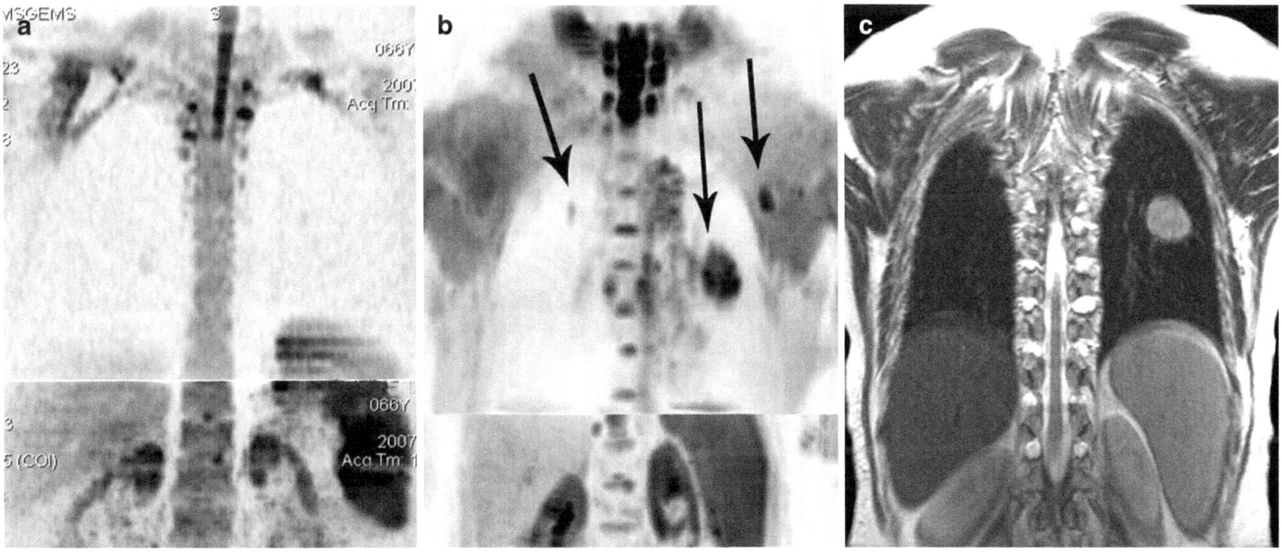

Fig. 14.29 A melanoma metastases in the left lung. The whole-body DWI MRI performed with 2-year intervals. On chest DWI MRI (**a**), no signs of abnormal changes have been identified. Two years after, a follow-up DWI MRI control (**b**) detected a large lesion with an increased signal in the left lung and lesions in the left axillary region (*arrows*) in the right lung. The study on T2-weighted MRI in the frontal projection (**c**) confirmed these diagnostic findings suggesting the disease progression

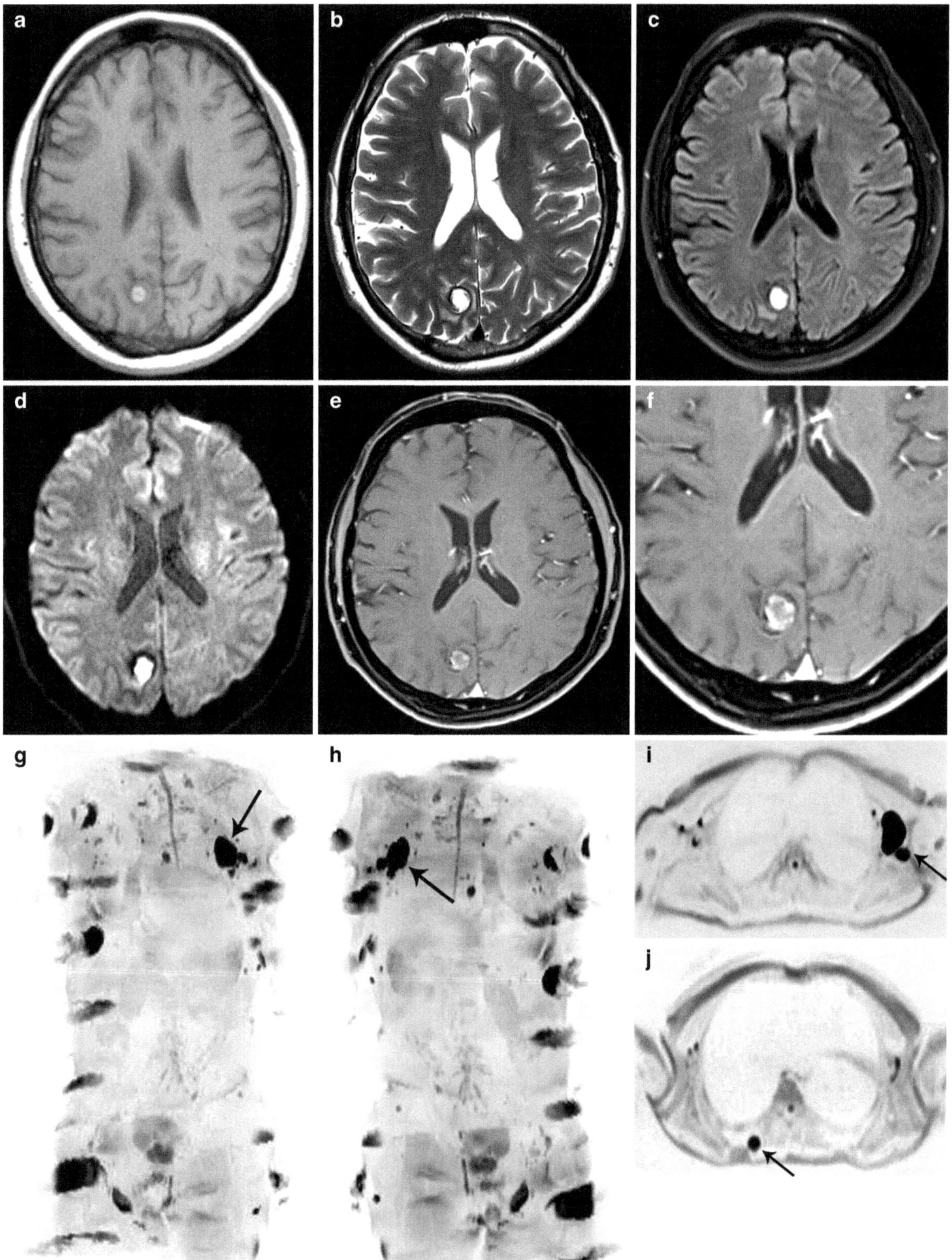

Fig. 14.30 Melanoma metastases. In the right occipital region of the brain, there is a solitary space-occupying lesion with a hyperintense signal on T1-weighted MRI (**a**), T2-weighted MRI (**b**), T2-FLAIR MRI (**c**), and DWI MRI (**d**), with signs of a minimal perifocal edema. The lesion moderately accumulates the contrast agent (**e**, **f**). In the whole-body DWI MRI study (**g**–**j**), there are areas with an increased signal in the right axilla on the left and in a small round-shaped area in the projection of the soft tissues of the middle third of the right side of the back: identified changes are consistent with metastatic lesions of the lymph nodes in the left axillary area and the primary tumor of soft tissues of the back at the said site (the *arrows*)

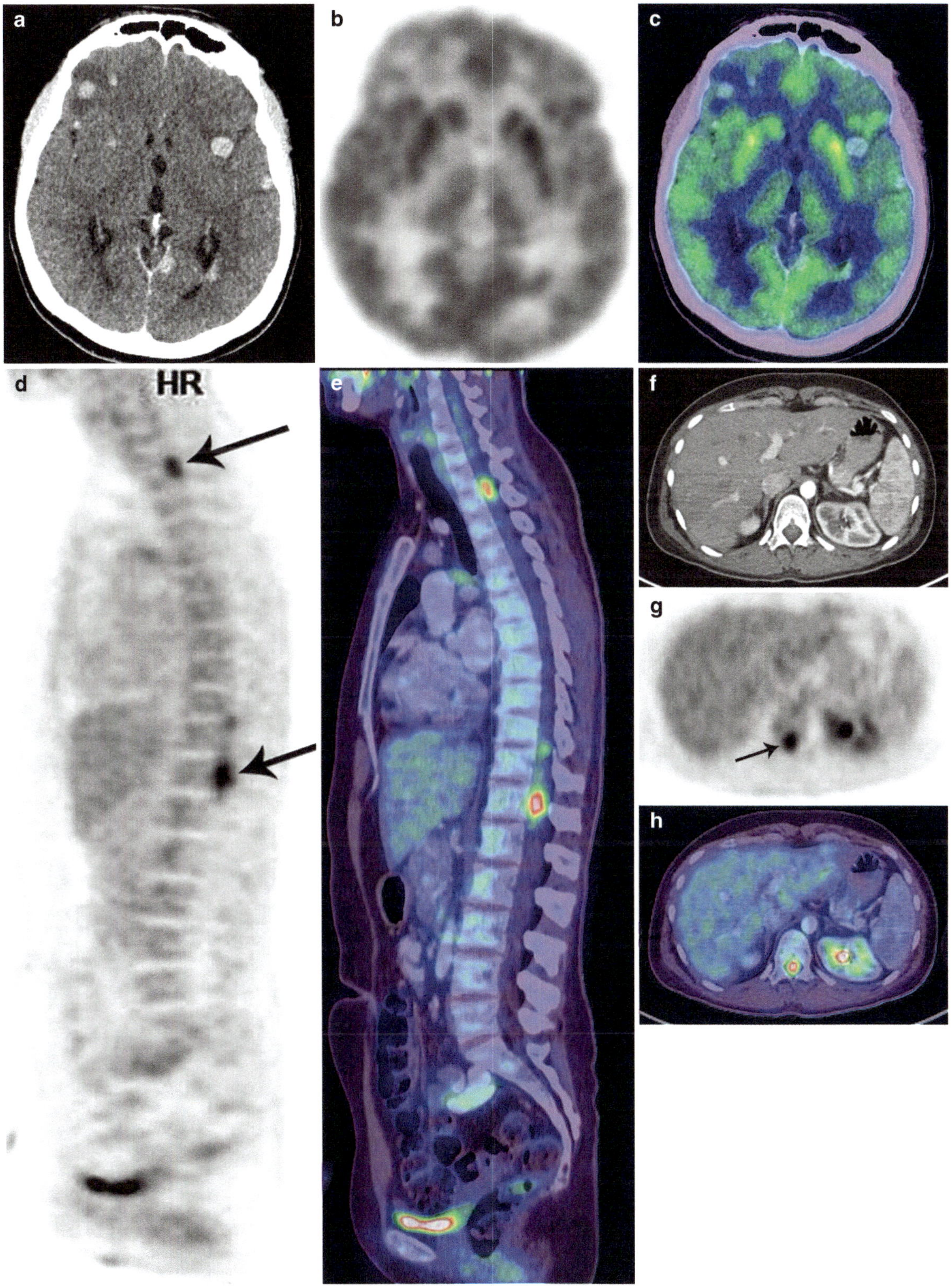

Fig. 14.31 Multiple melanoma metastases in the brain and spinal cord. On a CT image (**a**), there are multiple rounded lesions intensely accumulating the contrast agent with low perifocal edema. On brain PET/CT with ^{18}F-FDG (**b**, **c**), no signs of increased radiopharmaceutical accumulation are identified. The whole-body PET/CT scan shows marked multiple large lesions in the thoracic and cervical spinal canal: sagittal projection (**d**, **e**) and axial projection (**f**–**h**) (the *arrows*)

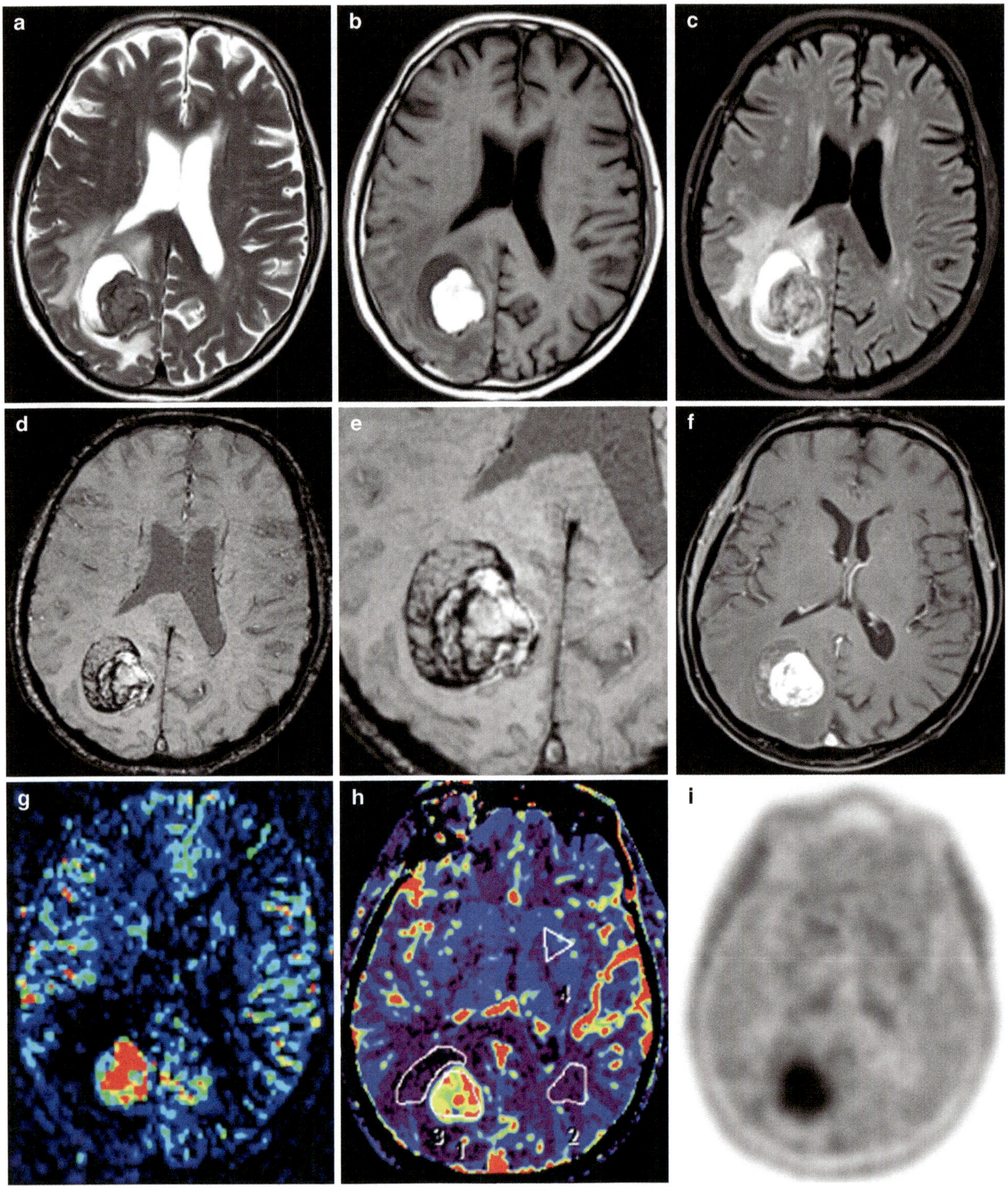

Fig. 14.32 A melanoma metastasis in the brain. In the right occipital lobe, there is a space-occupying heterogeneous lesion, whose solid component (along the medial contour) has a low signal on T2-weighted MRI (**a**), a drastically increased signal on T1-weighted MRI (**b**), and a heterogeneous signal on T2-FLAIR MRI (**c**). Both in the solid and in the cystic part of the metastasis on SWI (SWAN) MRI (**d**, **e**), there are marked multiple hypointense areas. After CA administration (**f**), there are separate portions of its accumulation in the solid part of the tumor fragments. On ASL MRI (**g**) and CBV maps of CT perfusion (**h**), there is a sharp increase in the blood flow. On PET with ^{18}F-Tyrosine (**i**), its intense accumulation in the lesion is observed

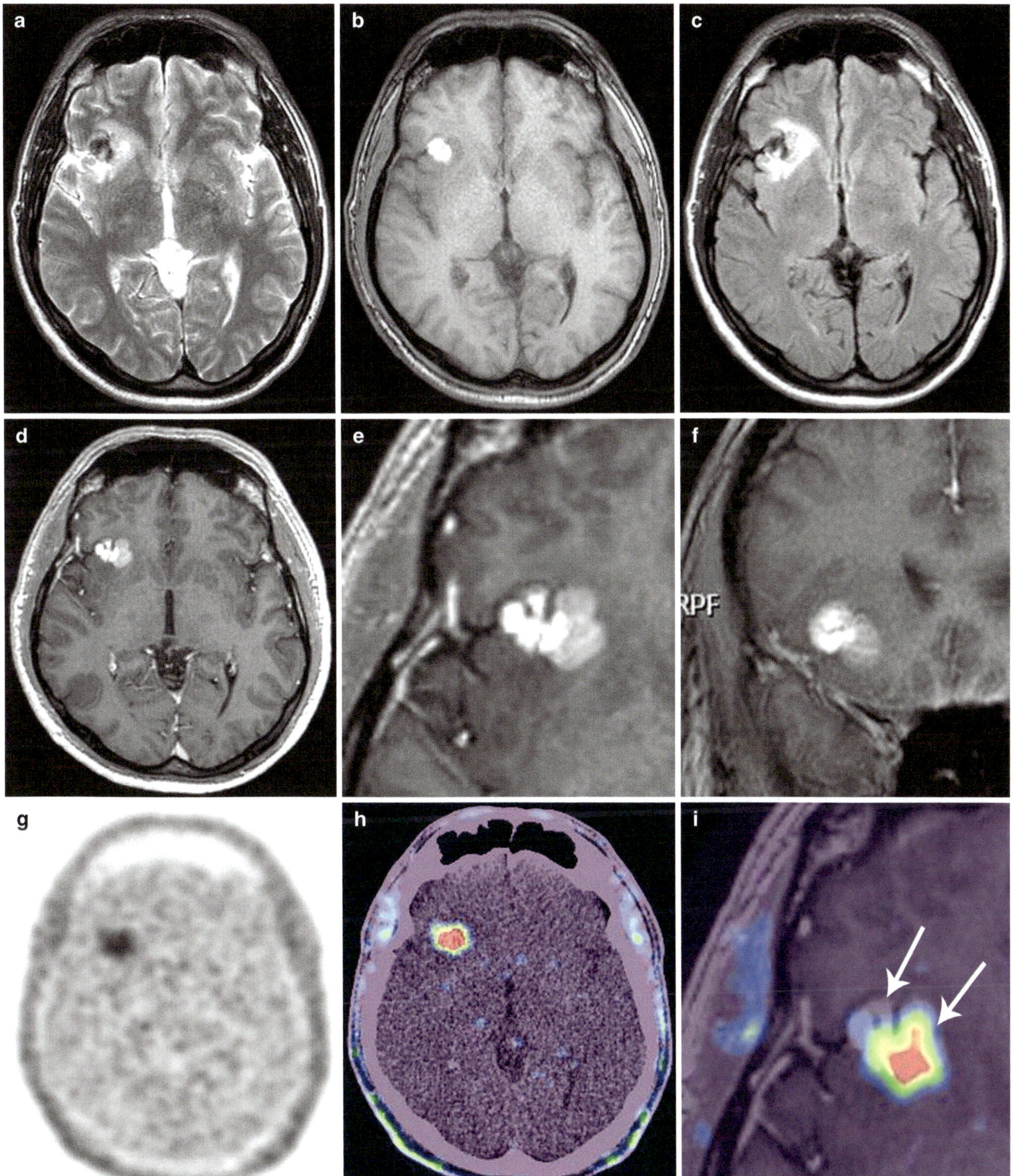

Fig. 14.33 A melanoma metastasis in the brain. In the right frontal lobe, there is a space-occupying lesion with a heterogeneously hypointense signal on T2-weighted MRI (**a**), a hyperintense signal on T1-weighted MRI (**b**), and a pronounced area of perifocal edema—an increased signal on T2-FLAIR MRI (**c**). After CA administration (**d–f**), its intense accumulation is determined along the medial contour of the lesion. On the PET/CT images with ^{18}F-tyrosine (**g**, **h**) and the PET-MR image (**i**), there is a clearly visualized intense RP accumulation in the solid part of the tumor and absence of RP accumulation in the hematoma (the *arrows*)

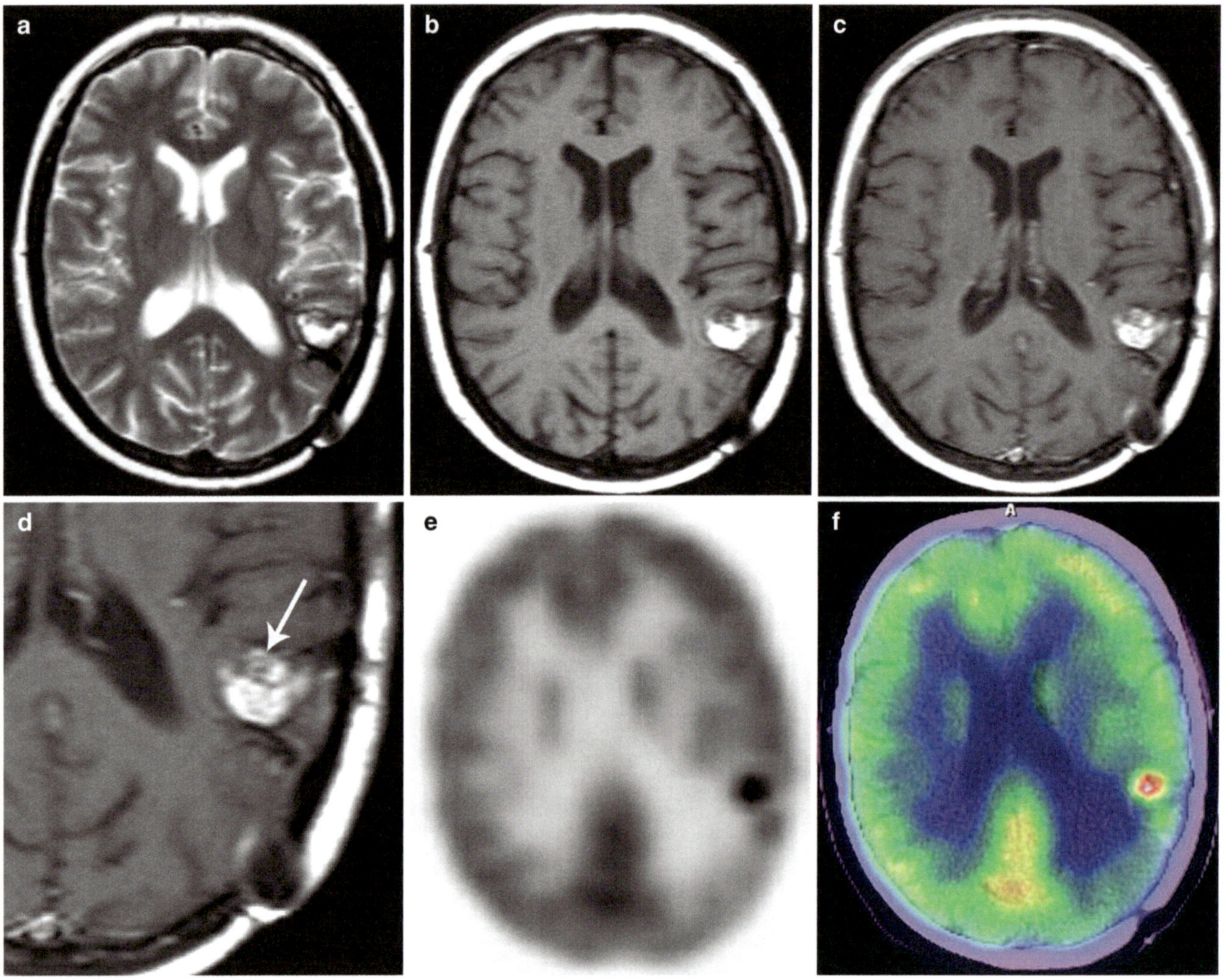

Fig. 14.34 A melanoma metastasis (a residual tumor after surgical removal). In the area of postoperative changes in the left temporal-occipital region, there is a heterogeneous signal on T2-weighted MRI (**a**) and an increased signal on T1-weighted MRI (**b**) representing blood. After CA administration, a small section of its accumulation is observed on the upper pole (**c**, **d**) (*arrow*). On PET/CT with ^{18}F-FDG (**e**, **f**), there is intense RP accumulation in the upper part of the lesion; no RP accumulation is observed in the hemorrhage area

Fig. 14.35 A large melanoma metastasis in the left frontal region. CT, CT perfusion, and MRI before and after radiotherapy. On CT with contrast enhancement, there is a space-occupying lesion in the anterior parasagittal sections of the left frontal region, and ROIs for perfusion measurements are indicated (**a**). On contrast-enhanced T1-weighted MRI (**b**) and T2-weighted MRI (**c**), the tumor weakly and heterogeneously accumulates the contrast agent; there are no symptoms of edema. On CT perfusion maps, there are high CBV (**d**) and CBF (**e**) values and low MTT (**f**) values, typical for melanoma. One month after the radiation treatment, the patient experienced an increase in cerebral symptoms. CT showed an increase in the tumor size (**g**). MRI (**h**, **i**) showed a significant increase in the abnormal site (an area with a heterogeneously increased signal on T1-weighted contrast-enhanced MRI) and deformation of the lateral ventricles, which was considered as continued growth of the tumor with a hemorrhage. On CT perfusion, posterior and central portions of the lesion had lower CBV (**j**) and CBF (**k**) values and high MTT (**l**) values. The anterior tumor pole retained parameters typical of melanoma. A life-saving surgery that confirmed the hematoma was performed

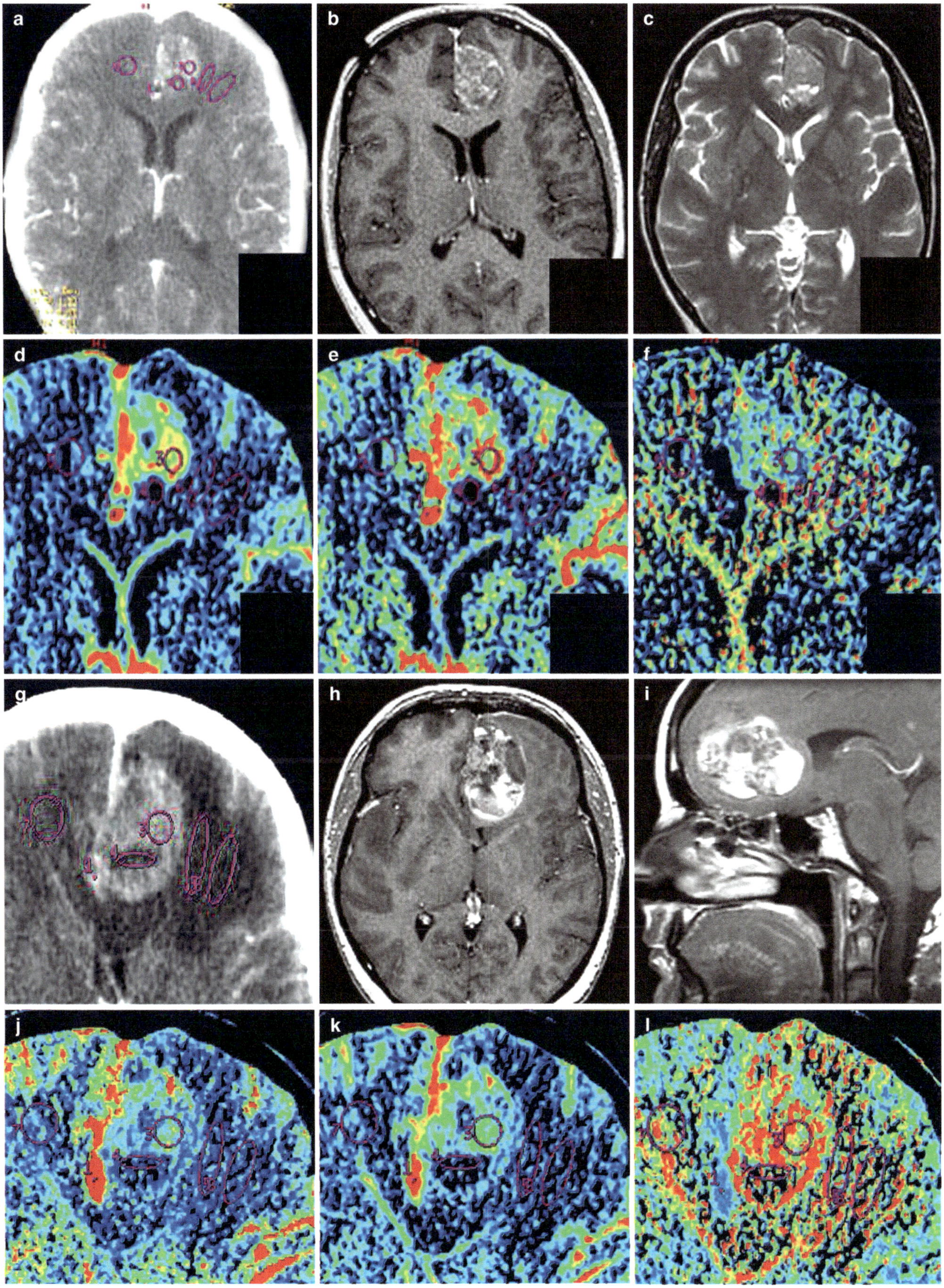
a
b
c
d
e
f
g
h
i
j
k
l

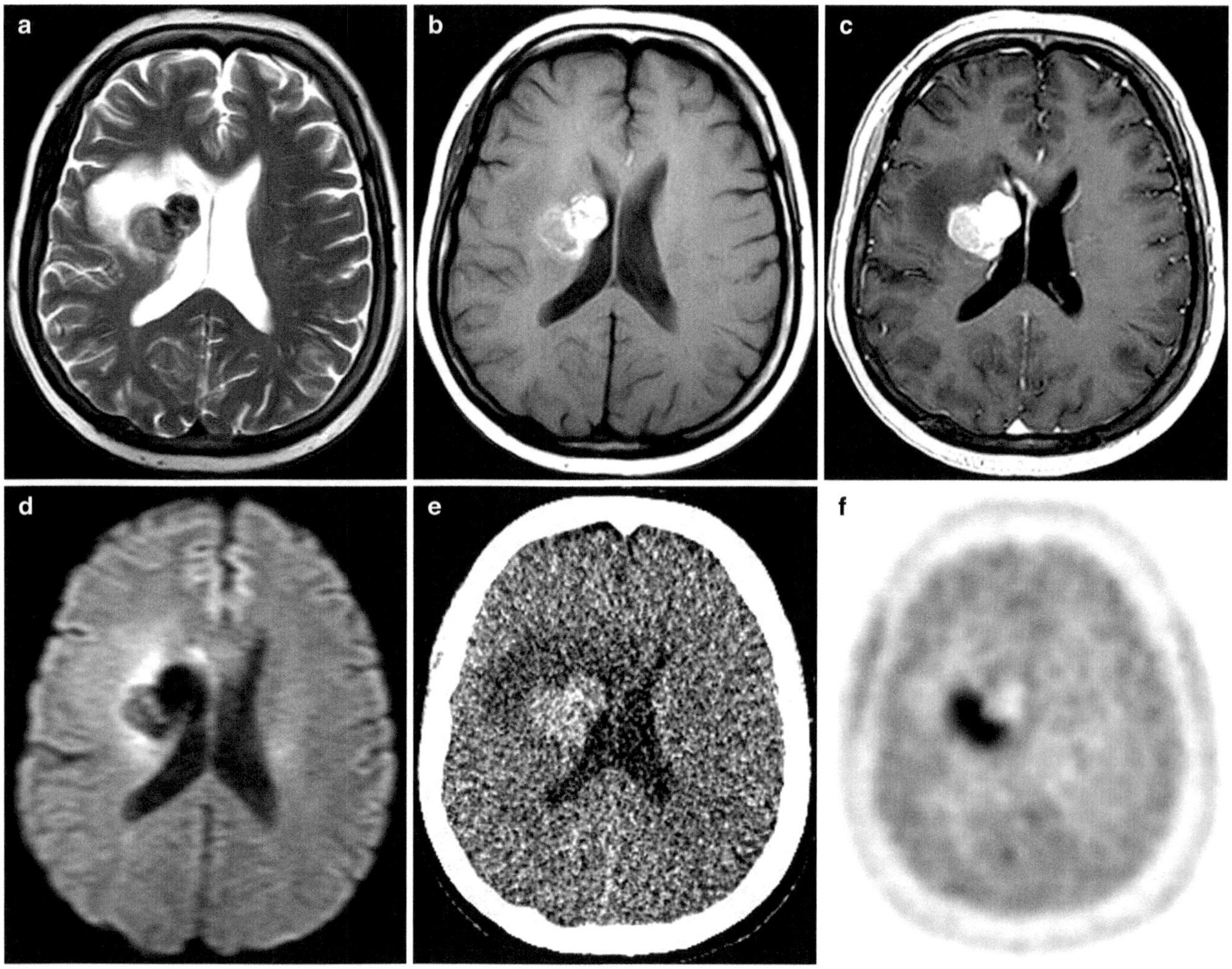

Fig. 14.36 A metastasis of melanoma in the brain after radiosurgery. In the deep portions of the right frontal region, there is a space-occupying lesion that extends to the ependyma of the right lateral ventricle, presses into the lumen of the latter, and causes a pronounced perifocal edema. The lesion has a heterogeneously reduced signal on T2-weighted MRI (**a**) and hyperintense signal on T1-weighted MRI (**b**). After CA administration (**c**), its intense accumulation in the posterior-lateral parts of the tumor is noted, and an increase in the signal from the anterior-medial parts of the lesion is much weaker. Also, linear portions of CA accumulation are observed along the medial contour of the anterior horn of the right lateral ventricle. On DWI MRI (**d**), the signal from the lesion is reduced. On CT images (**e**), there is a uniform moderate increase in the density. On PET with ^{18}F-tyrosine (**f**), its intense accumulation is observed in the posterior-lateral parts of the tumor, there is no intense RP accumulation in the anterior parts of the lesion (hematoma)

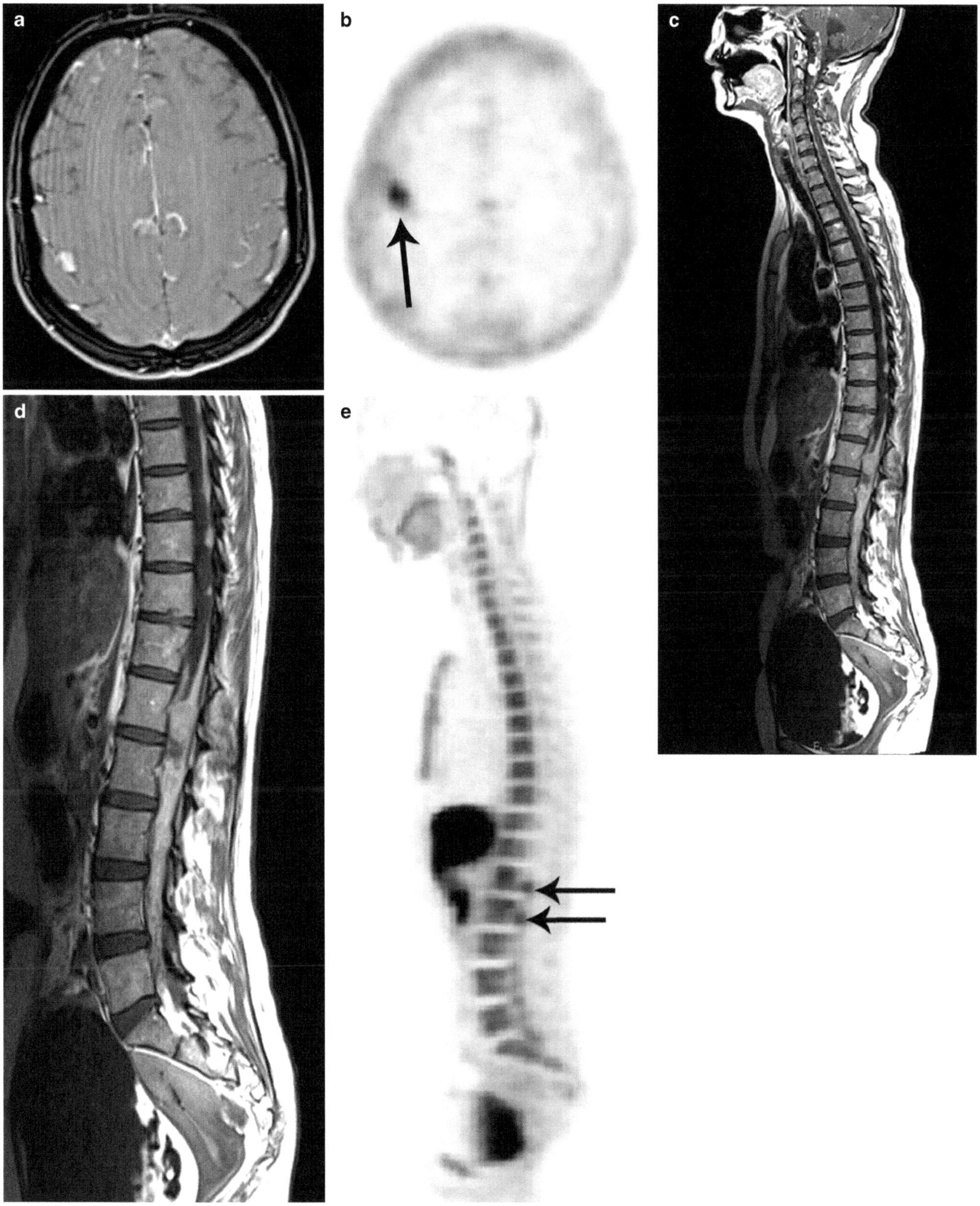

Fig. 14.37 Multiple metastases of melanoma: involvement of the brain and spinal cord. On T1-weighted MRI with contrast enhancement, there are metastases in the meninges of the brain (**a**), spinal cord, and roots of the spinal cord (**c**, **d**) with the formation of nodules in the convexital parts of the right parietal region and in the lumen of the spinal cord channel at the level of L1–L5 vertebral bodies. On PET with ^{18}F-choline, only nodules are well visualized both in the brain (**b**) and in the spinal canal (**e**) (the *arrows*)

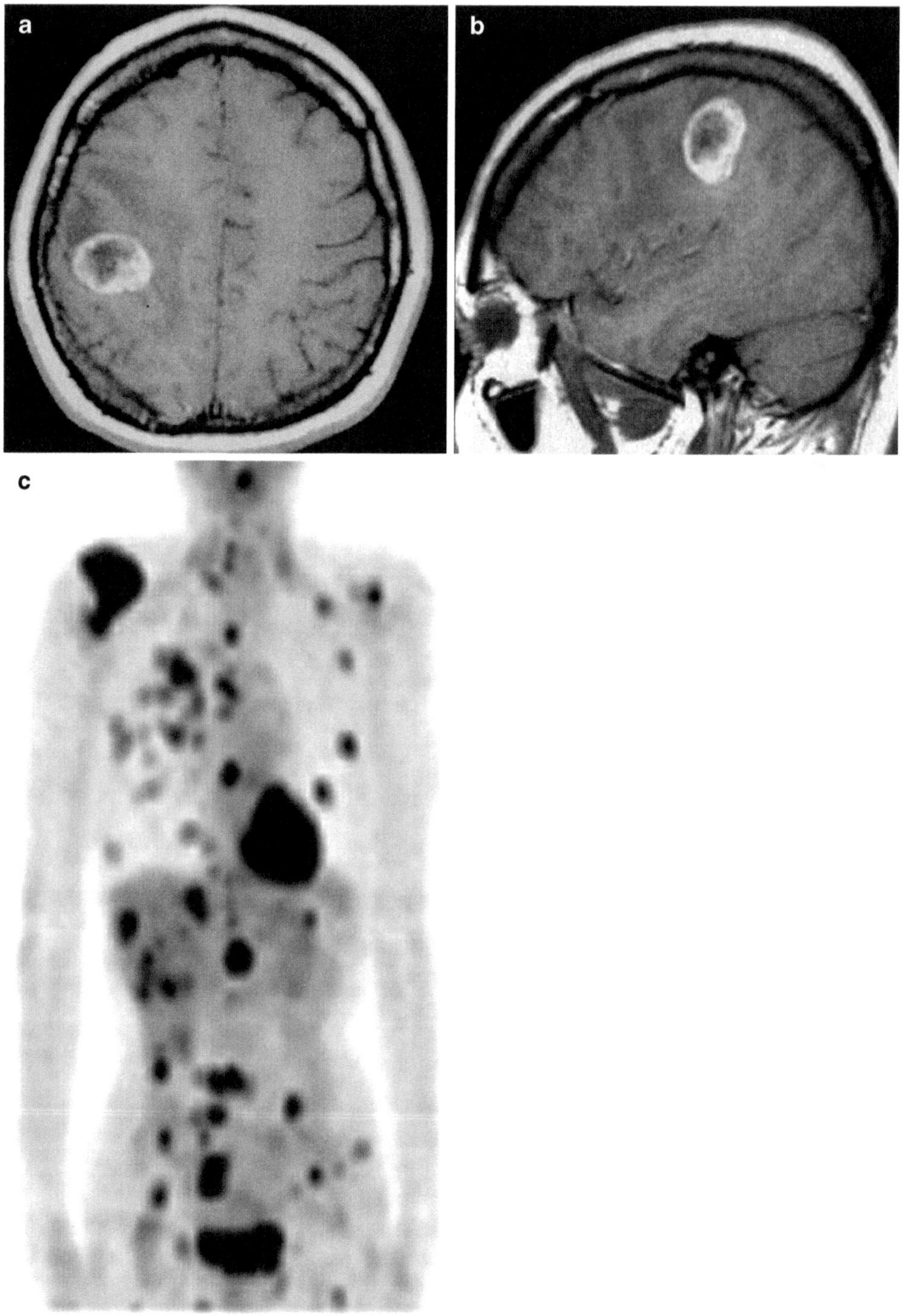

Fig. 14.38 A melanoma metastasis in the brain. On T1-weighted MRI with contrast enhancement (**a**, **b**) in the deep parts of the frontal region, there is an oval space-occupying lesion with signs of intense CA accumulation on the periphery. On PET with ^{18}F-FDG (**c**), there are multiple lesions in the bone and soft tissue structures. There is a large lesion with abnormal RP accumulation in the area of the right shoulder—primary melanoma

Renal Cell Carcinoma (RCC)

15

Renal cell carcinoma (RCC) is the most common malignant tumor of the kidney, accounting for about 80–90% of kidney tumors in adults and about 2–3% of all new cancer cases (Mori et al. 1998). RCC occurs twice as likely in men as in women, with the highest incidence in the age of 50–70 years (Muscat 2000). Each year, 30,000 and 20,000 new cases of kidney cancer are reported in the USA and in the European Union, respectively (Kirkali et al. 2001). In Russia, RCC occupies one of the first places among all forms of cancer in terms of the incidence rate: the number of cases in recent years approaches 20 thousand per year. Mortality rates from this disease in Russia are also high, 8000–9000 per year, accounting for 2–3% of all deaths of patients with malignant tumors. The 5-year survival in patients is 80–90% and 5–10% with localized and disseminated RCC forms, respectively (Motzer et al. 2004).

According to modern concepts, RCC is a multifactorial disease. A variety of factors can cause its development: genetic, hormonal, chemical, immunological, radiation, etc. (Ljungberg et al. 2011). Smoking, fatty and fried food, obesity, uncontrolled use of analgesics, diuretics, and hormone drugs significantly increase the risk of the disease (Lindblad et al. 1995; Coughlin et al. 1997; Godley and Stinchcombe 1999; Muscat 2000; Steliarova-Foucher and Parkin 2011). Thus, according to Parkin (2011), 42% of cases of RCC are caused by smoking and overweight. Men and women account for 47 and 34% among the cases, respectively. Vegetable diet and the use of vitamins with an antioxidant complex reduce the risk. Chronic renal failure and regular hemodialysis, polycystic kidney, nephrosclerosis often developing in diabetes mellitus, hypertension, and chronic pyelonephritis can also cause the development of kidney cancer.

Data from several meta-analyses indicate an increased risk of RCC up to fourfold in relatives of patients with renal cell carcinoma (Pfaffenroth and Linchan 2008; Karami et al. 2010). According to Clague et al. (2009), 4% of all RCC cases are due to hereditary factors. A family anamnesis of prostate cancer, melanoma, thyroid cancer, bladder cancer, as well as non-Hodgkin's lymphoma is associated with an increased risk of kidney cancer (Liu et al. 2011).

There are three forms of malignant kidney tumors: renal cell carcinoma, adenocarcinoma originating from the pelvis, and kidney sarcoma known as Wilms' tumor. Renal cell carcinoma has been described by Grawitz in 1883. This type of tumor is called hypernephroma; however, today the term renal cell carcinoma is used. The tumor develops from the epithelium of the proximal renal tubules.

Multifocality of RCC, characterized by the simultaneous presence of more than one lesion with the same histological tumor type in the kidney, is one of its morphological features. Many authors noted RCC multifocality in their studies (Gohji et al. 1998; Baltaci et al. 2000; Lang et al. 2004; Richstone et al. 2004; Crispen et al. 2008). For example, in the group of cases studied by Shus (2003), the incidence of multifocal renal cell carcinoma was 16.7%.

Renal cell carcinoma has various types of the histological structure. Clear cell cancer is the most common, which, according to WHO, is 70–75% of all RCC cases. Men more often have typical RCC forms—clear cell and papillary cancer—while women more often have rare forms, mucinous, medullary, chromophobe, unclassifiable, and benign kidney tumors(Jemal et al. 2007; Yurin 2007; Davydov and Axel 2014a, b).

Malignant kidney tumors metastasize via the hematogenous and lymphogenous routes. Metastases occur more than in a half of patients. Often a kidney cancer metastasis manifests clinically earlier than the primary tumor, but in some RCC cases, metastasizing may not occur for decades (Radley et al. 1993). The most common sites of metastases are the lungs, lymph nodes, bone, liver, adrenal glands, brain, contralateral kidney, and heart.

Thus, a series of autopsies in patients with kidney adenocarcinoma showed brain involvement in 11% of cases (Saitoh 1981). According to Harada et al. (1999), among 325 patients treated for kidney cancer at the Osaka University Hospital from 1957 to 1993, 5.5% of cases were with brain metasta-

M. Dolgushin et al., *Brain Metastases*, DOI 10.1007/978-3-319-57760-9_15

ses. Marshall et al. (1990) analyzed a series of cases of 106 patients with clinically localized renal adenocarcinoma, who underwent CT, and found metastases in the brain in 13% of cases. According to the authors, metastases to the brain most often occur in the later stages of kidney cancer, and the brain is likely to be the final site of the metastatic tumor. According to our data, kidney cancer metastases accounted for 13.9% of the total number of cases of metastatic brain lesions.

The interval between the detection of the primary kidney tumor and metastasizing to the brain ranges from 1 year to several years (Badalament et al. 1990; Nussbaum et al. 1996; Harada et al. 1999), and metastatic involvement of the meninges and skull bones in RCC occurs more frequently than in other histological forms of cancer. Multiple brain metastases of renal cancer are more typical for the young age ($p < 0.001$) (Bianchi et al. 2012). The most often metastasizing cancer is RCC (up to 50%), constituting 85% of all kidney cancers (Saitoh 1981).

Patients with renal cancer with distant metastases have a poor prognosis: their average life expectancy is 4.5–9 months. Kidney cancer patients with metastases to the brain have a poor prognosis as well: their average life expectancy is 5–9 months (Roser et al. 2002). Isolated cases of prolonged course of the disease with an identified kidney cancer metastasis were observed, which may be associated with low levels of mitosis, stability of the cell nucleus morphology, and, therefore, unexpressed chromosomal abnormalities. Treatment of these patients is complicated by the fact that kidney cancer belongs to radioresistant tumors, but radiosurgical treatment of metastases in the brain allows to reduce the tumor size. The effectiveness of chemotherapy in this form of cancer is low. Currently, the treatment of choice is surgery in combination with radiosurgery and immunotherapy(Patchell et al. 1990a, b; Coppic et al. 2000; Kleinberg 2009; Loudyi and Samlowski 2011; Nieder et al. 2011a, b; Blanco et al. 2011; Kusuda et al. 2011; Parashar et al. 2014; Raman and Vaena 2015).

A characteristic feature of intracranial metastatic RCC is intratumoral hemorrhages, often with the formation of an acute intracerebral hematoma requiring an urgent surgical intervention (Wronski et al. 1996). The author reports a series of cases of patients with renal cell carcinoma metastases, in which intratumoral hemorrhages were identified in 46% of cases and 4% of cases required emergency surgery. Our clinical cases are characterized by the relative homogeneity of renal cell carcinoma metastases: hemorrhages occurred not more than in 15% of cases.

Clinical symptoms of kidney cancer metastases in the brain are caused by a combination of cerebral and focal symptoms characteristic of metastases and primary tumors with other locations; it depends on the lesion site in the brain, size, and presence and severity of perifocal edema: headache, hemiparesis, cognitive impairment, seizures, and ataxia. Perifocal edema, often severe in kidney cancer metastases, results in an increase in the brain volume in a much greater degree than the metastasis per se. Intracranial pressure increases, which clinically can manifest by headache, often diffuse, dizziness, nausea and vomiting, and congested optic discs in the study of the fundus. In some cases, sleepiness, depression, diplopia, and transient episodes of visual impairment may occur.

On CT, RCC metastases in the brain are characterized by the presence of a solid lesion with a small area of degradation in the center. CA accumulation in the solid part of the tumor is homogeneous and expressed. Lesions most often have an annular shape with clear contours and hypodense content in the center. Perifocal edema on the background of the lesion is contrasted and strongly expressed, which creates, in turn, the picture of ring enhancement. Despite the relatively slow growth of metastases, often a very pronounced perifocal edema is observed, which by size considerably exceeds the size of the metastasis. CT is required in case of the involvement of bone structures of the cranial vault, characteristic for RCC, as well as for breast and prostate cancer. Involvement of the vertebral bodies is also often identified.

The analysis of CT perfusion data showed that, on average, the blood volume (CBV) for renal cancer metastases is characterized by high values (21.01 ± 6.21 ml/100 g), indicating the presence of rich tumor vasculature. Metastatic renal cell carcinoma has relatively low CBF values (73.93 ± 27.59 ml/100 g/min) and highest MTT values (18.38 ± 1.37 s). It should be remembered that the higher the MTT values obtained, the slower the blood passes through the metastasis structure per unit of time (second). The obtained perfusion parameters allow to establish, for example, that kidney cancer metastases pass larger volumes of blood through their tissue than, for example, melanoma (CBV = 15.03 ± 9.75 ml/100 g), but have lower blood flow velocity values (CBF) and high MTT values. Thus, CT perfusion in RCC metastases to the brain allowed to establish specific perfusion parameter values—the highest CBV and MTT values among metastases and average CBF values. These characteristics allow in some extent to differentiate this type of metastases from other metastatic lesions. Despite perfusion values, similar with those for metastatic melanoma, hemorrhages in the structures of kidney cancer metastases are much rarer.

On MRI, a standard set of sequences—T1 weighted, T2 weighted, T2-FLAIR, T1 weighted + Gd in three dimensions, as well as thin-sliced SPGR (VIBE) in multiple lesions—are mandatory sequences in MR diagnosis of metastatic brain lesions. In these sequences, metastases have tissue characteristics inherent in the majority of metastases with different histogeneses. Intracerebral RCC metastases often have a rounded shape and are usually distinguished from the brain substance. They are often presented by a solid tumor, homogeneously accumulate the contrast agent, and very rarely have central necrotic changes. However, if these changes exist, their contrast enhancement prevails over that of the solid part. The visual picture of kidney cancer metastases is very similar to that of colon cancer—a "thick" roll of the solid part and a small area of decay. In 75% of cases, metastases in renal cell carcinoma are multiple.

Single-voxel MR spectroscopy did not identify any significant specificity for RCC metastases in the brain. As with other metastatic brain lesions, a marked increase in peaks of lactate and lipids is noted. The NAA (N-acetylaspartate) peak in the central structure of RCC metastases is significantly reduced.

The solid part of metastatic RCC tumors on DW images is characterized by an isointense or hypo-isointense signal. Average ADC values of the metastatic lesion are, respectively, $1.15 \pm 0.9 \times 10^{-3}$ mm^2/s in the tumor stroma, $1.28 \pm 0.2 \times 10^{-3}$ mm^2/s in the near peritumoral area, and $1.56 \pm 0.2 \times 10^{-3}$ mm^2/s in the vasogenic edema area. ADC values in the tumor itself in our study were highly heterogeneous.

The use of PET with ^{18}F-FDG for the diagnosis of primary RCC does not make much sense due to the rapid physiological accumulation of the radiopharmaceutical in the urine, with an exception of large tumors extensively extending to perirenal fat. Kidney cancer metastases, according to our data, intensely accumulate ^{18}F-FDG in all structures of the body, including the brain. According to our data, ^{18}F-FDG in the primary diagnosis of brain lesions can be used in a single scanning. PET with ^{18}F-FDG showed its high sensitivity and specificity in the evaluation of the radicality of treatment; identification of a residual tumor, for example, in meningeal involvement; and differentiation of residual metastatic tumor in the brain from post-radiation changes.

15.1 Clinical Cases

See Figs. 15.1, 15.2, 15.3, 15.4, 15.5, 15.6, 15.7, 15.8, 15.9, 15.10, 15.11, 15.12, 15.13, and 15.14.

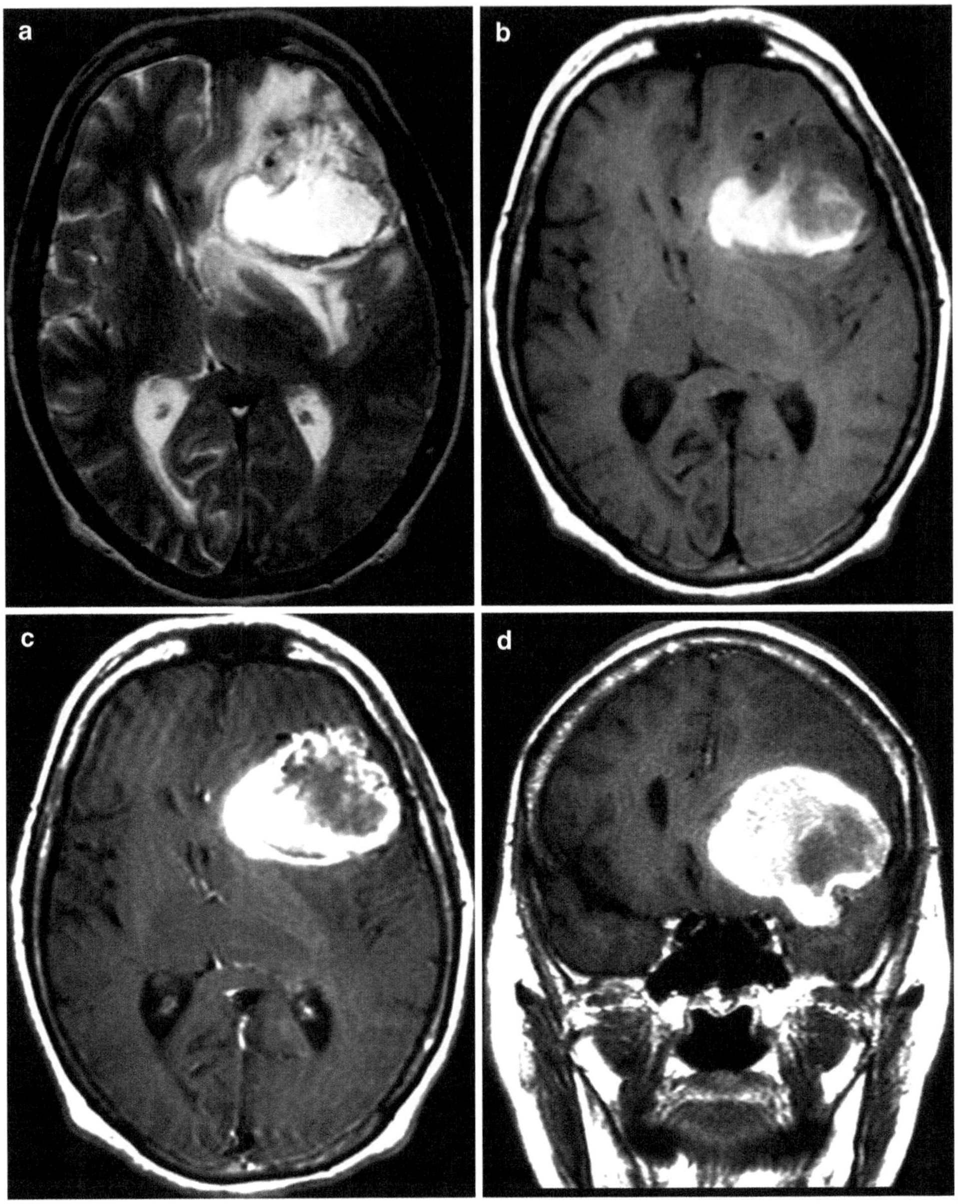

Fig. 15.1 A kidney cancer metastasis in the brain. MRI: in the left frontal area, there is a large tumor site with a pronounced perifocal edema (**a**) and with a hemorrhagic component—a high MR signal on T1-weighted MRI (**b**). After intravenous CA administration on T1-weighted MRI (**c**, **d**), an area of contrast enhancement is identified around the hemorrhage, in the solid part of the tumor. The ventricular system is deformed

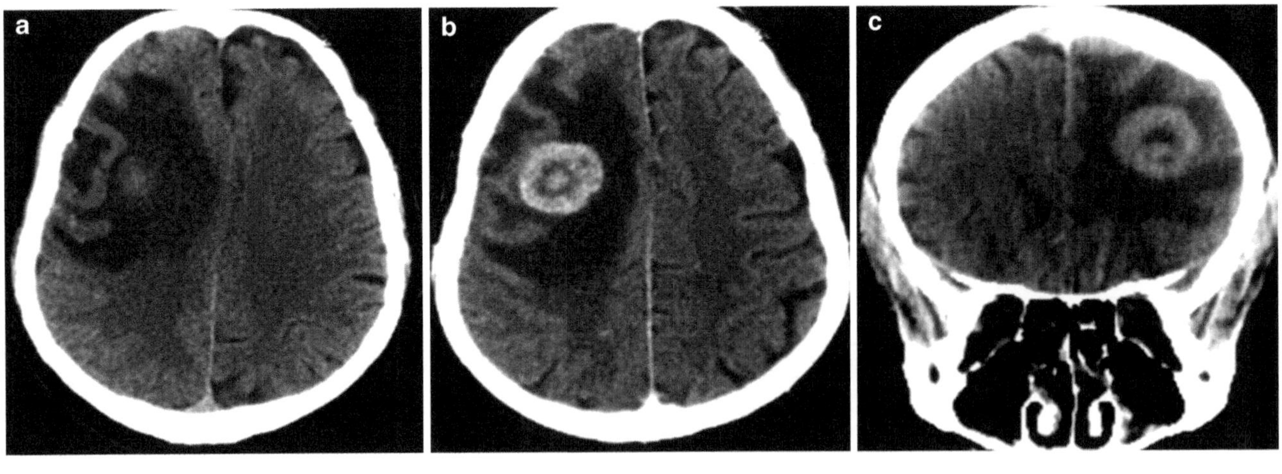

Fig. 15.2 A kidney cancer metastasis in the brain. In the right frontal region, there is an isodense lesion with a pronounced perifocal edema (**a**). Following intravenous CA administration, its pronounced accumulation in the solid part of the tumor (**b**, **c**) is observed; the typical picture of ring enhancement is observed on the background of the edema

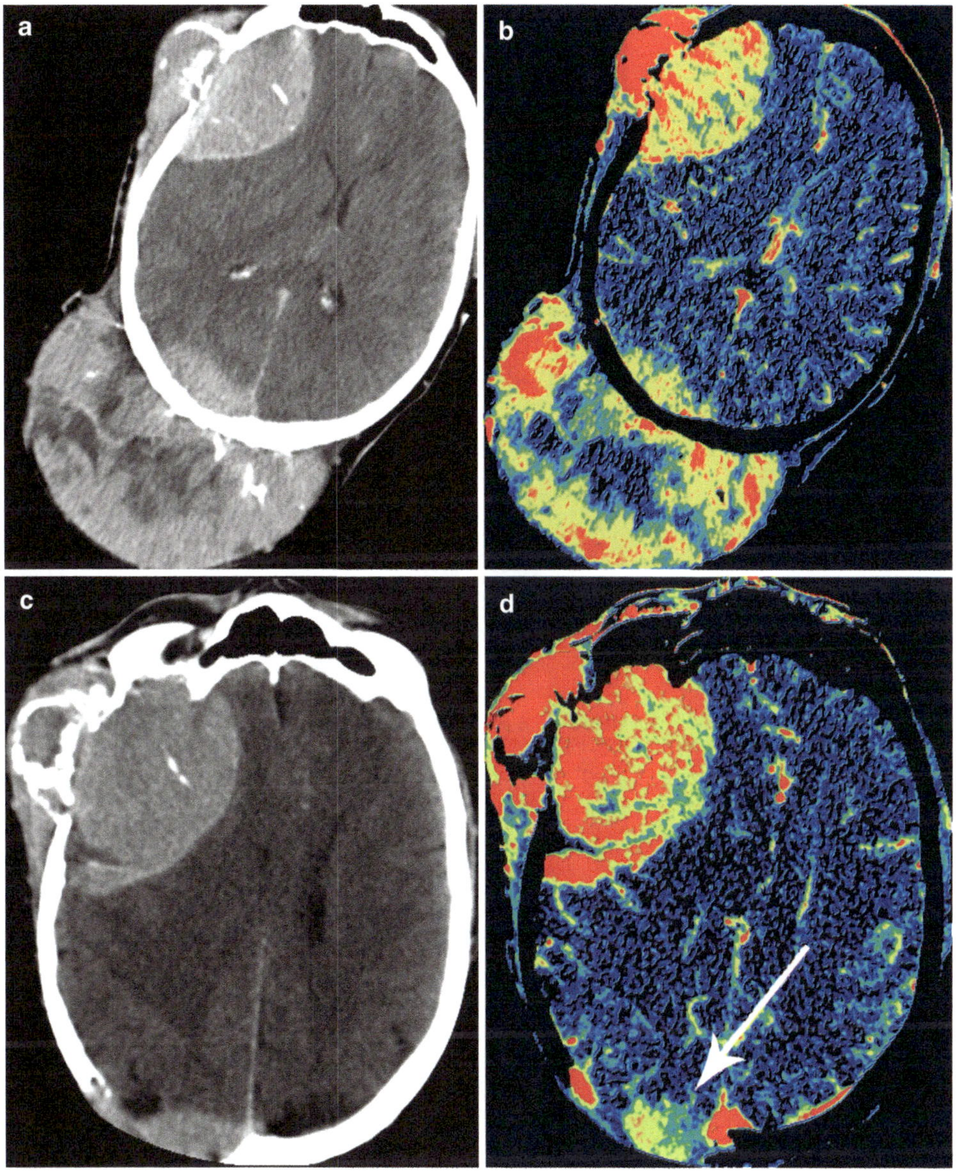

Fig. 15.3 Multiple kidney cancer metastases. A dynamic study before (**a**, **b**) and after (**c**, **d**) surgical removal. On CT images with contrast enhancement and CT perfusion maps, there are two large neoplasms with extra- and intracranial spread in the right frontal and parietal regions. The lesions are characterized by intense accumulation of the contrast agent and increased CBV values. After removal of the metastatic lesion in the right parietal region, there is a small residual tumor adjacent to the sagittal sinus (the *arrow*)

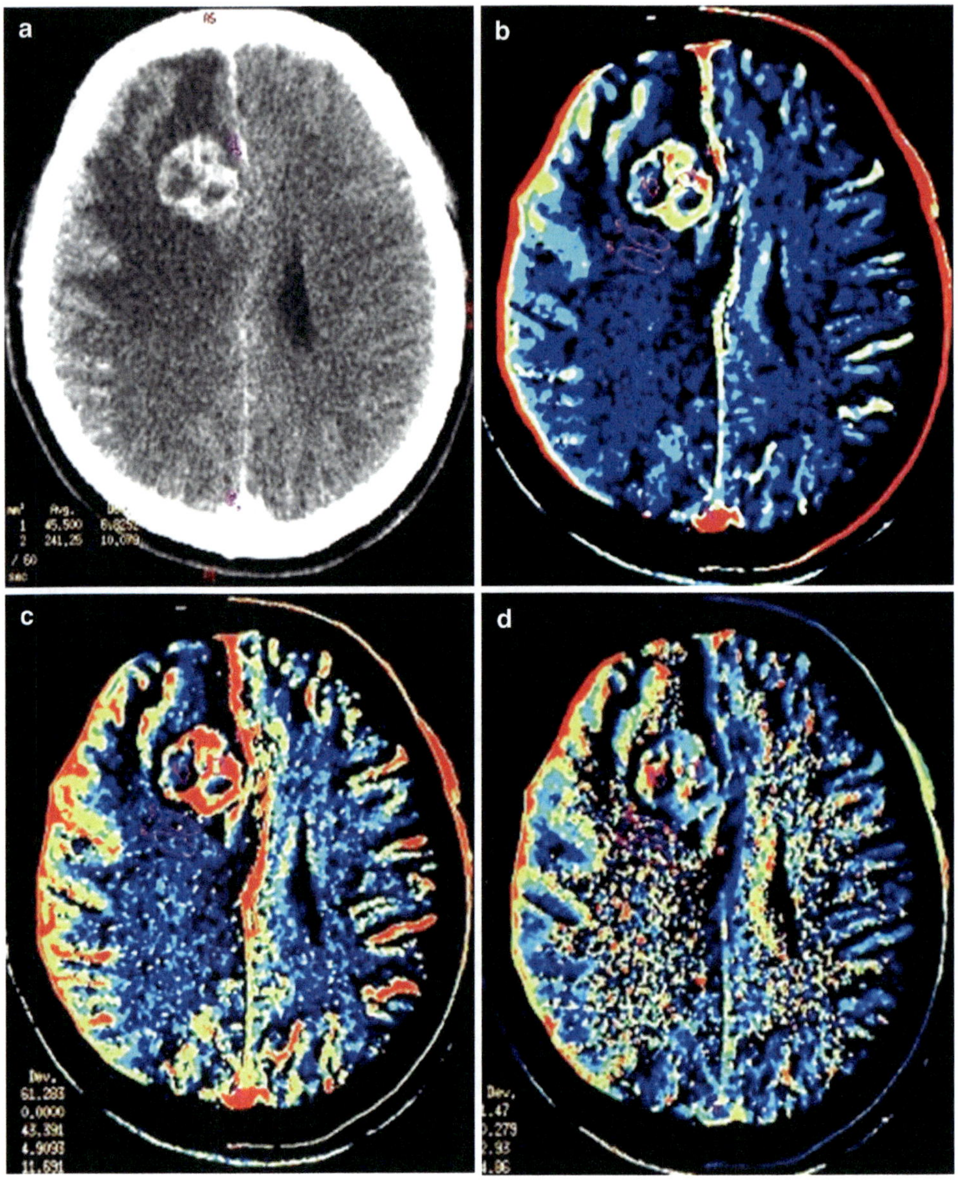

Fig. 15.4 A kidney cancer metastasis in the brain. On CT in the right frontal region, there is a solid-cystic lesion intensely accumulating the contrast agent (**a**) with a pronounced perifocal edema—ring enhancement. On CT perfusion, there is a significant increase in CBF (**b**), CBV (**c**), and MTT (**d**) values in the metastatic lesion

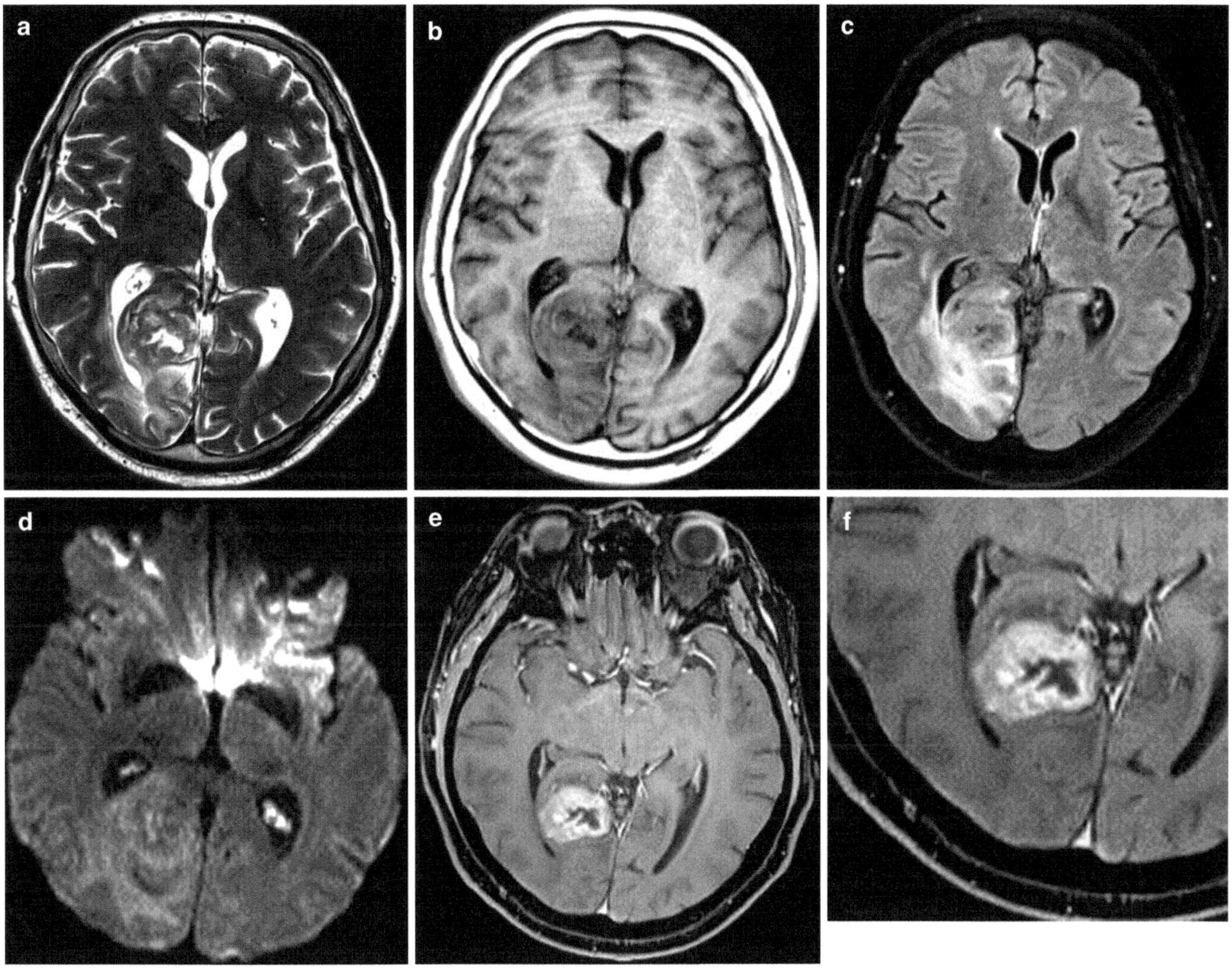

Fig. 15.5 A kidney cancer metastasis in the brain. In the right occipital region, there is a lesion iso-hyperintense on T2-weighted (**a**) and T2-FLAIR (**c**) MRI. On T1-weighted and DWI images, the tumor is predominantly isointense (**b**, **d**). After CA administration, its intense, inhomogeneous accumulation in the solid part of the metastasis is observed, with the well-visualized central necrotic portion (**e**, **f**)

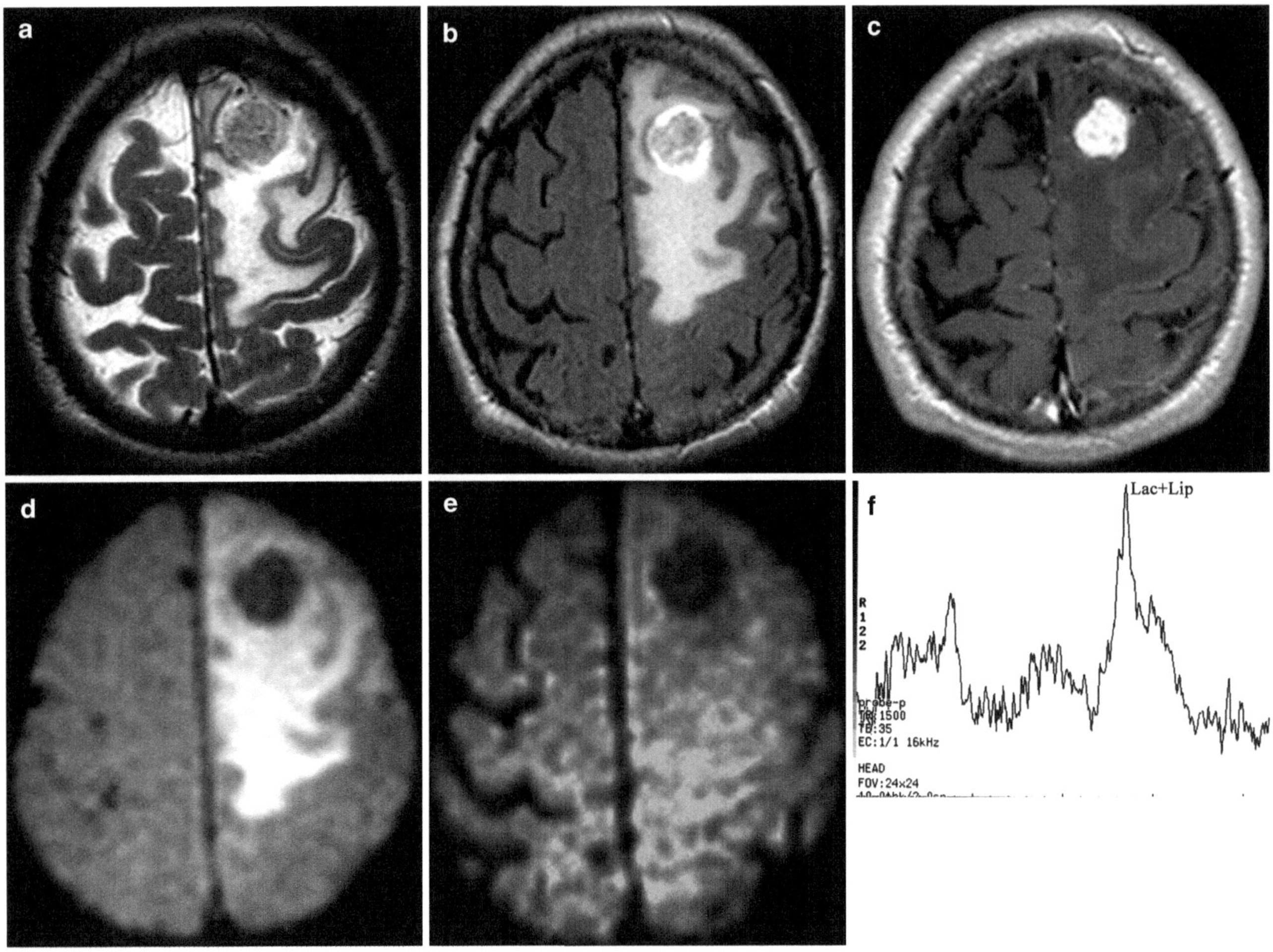

Fig. 15.6 A kidney cancer metastasis in the brain. On T2-weighted (**a**), T2-FLAIR (**b**), and T1-weighted MRI with contrast enhancement (**c**) in the left frontal region, there is a solid tumor lesion surrounded by a pronounced perifocal edema. Of note is a hyperintensive rim on T2-FLAIR images. On DWI with $b = 500$ (**d**) and $b = 1000$ (**e**), a perifocal edema is extracellular or vasogenic, while the metastasis is hypointense. On MR spectrogram, there is a high peak of the Lip-Lac complex (**f**)

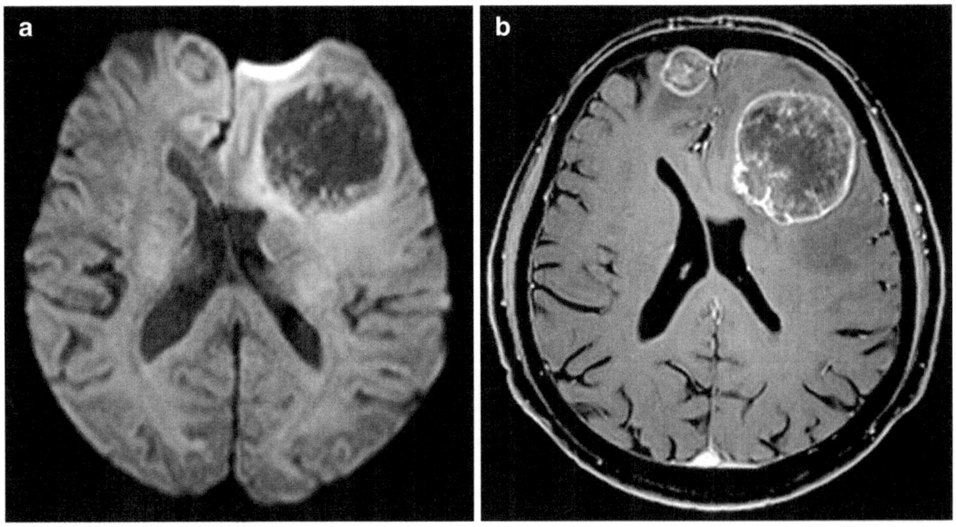

Fig. 15.7 Multiple kidney cancer metastases in the brain. On DWI MRI (**a**) and T1-weighted MRI after intravenous CA administration (**b**), there are space-occupying lesions in the left and right frontal areas. The lesions are characterized by a hypointense signal on DWI MRI, intense, inhomogeneous accumulation of the contrast agent, while the marginal sections of tumors most intensely accumulating the contrast agent on DWI MRI have the highest signal

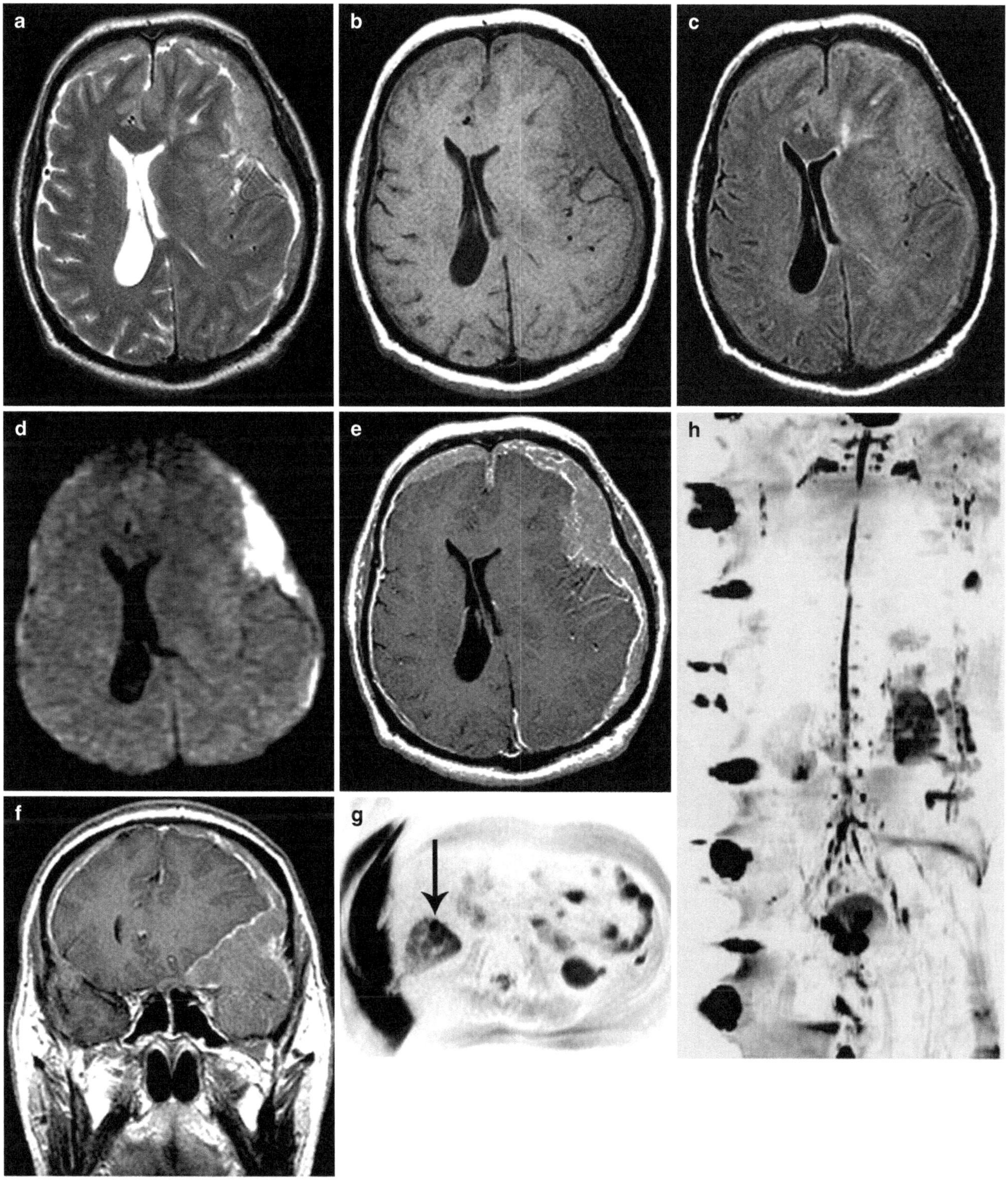

Fig. 15.8 Multiple kidney cancer metastases. Along the meninges of both hemispheres, there are multiple confluent space-occupying lesions with an iso-hyperintense signal on T2-weighted MRI (**a**) and an isointense signal on T1-weighted MRI (**b**) and T2-FLAIR MRI (**c**), without perifocal edema; the signal from the tumor is increased on DWI MRI (**d**). After CA administration, its intense accumulation in tumors is observed (**e**, **f**). In the whole-body MR-DWI study (**g**, **h**), there is a marked area with inhomogeneously high signal in the lower pole of the right kidney. Of note are a large number of artifacts on DWI MRI due to a significant fat tissue (**h**)

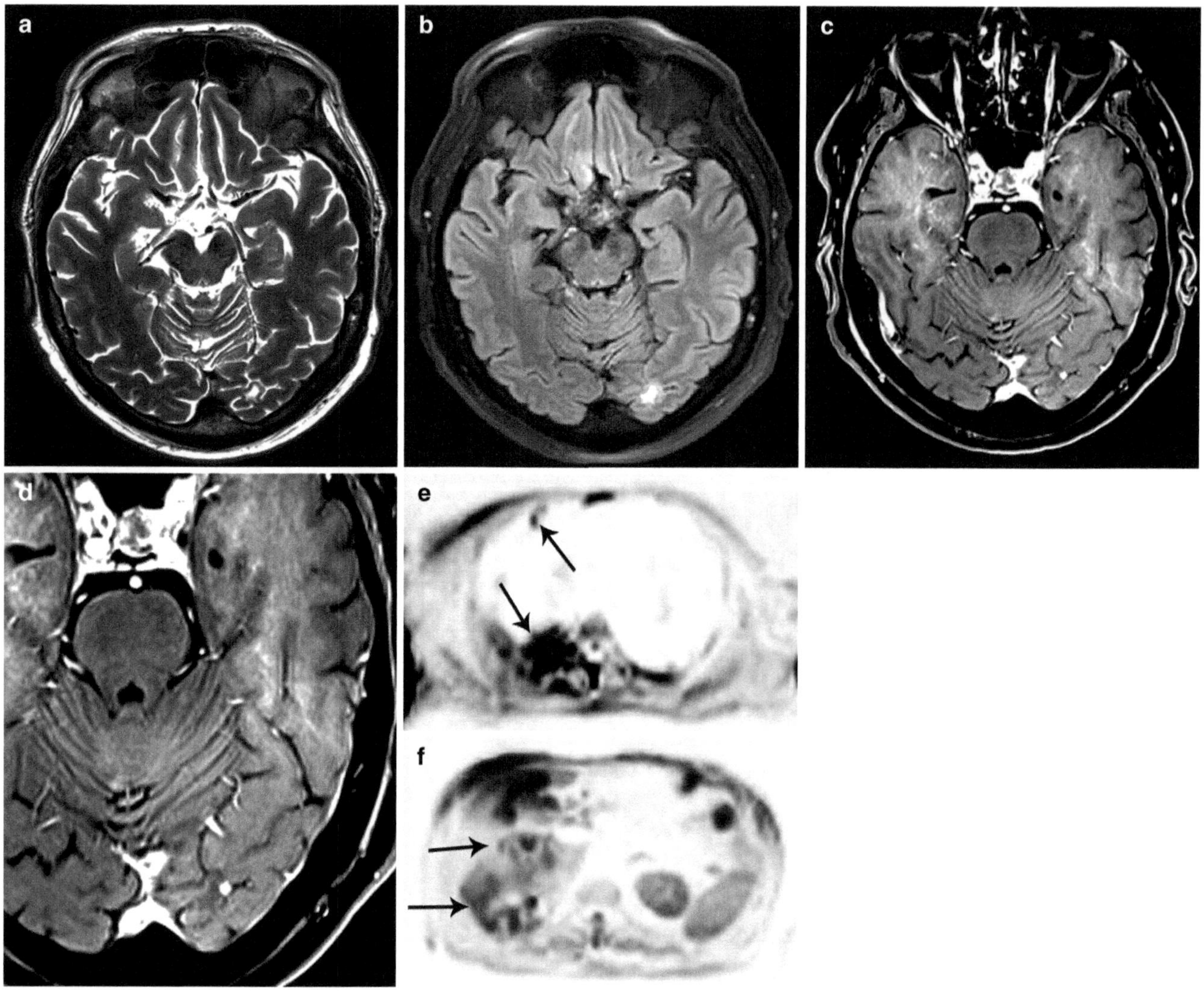

Fig. 15.9 A kidney cancer metastasis in the brain. In the left occipital region, there is a pinpoint lesion with signs of a perifocal edema and an increased signal on T2-weighted and T2-FLAIR MRI (**a**, **b**) that intensely accumulates contrast agent (**c**, **d**). In the whole-body MR-DWI study (**e**, **f**), there are areas with an increased signal in the upper pole of the right kidney, in the ribs on the right with a pronounced extraosseous component, in the sternum, and in the lung parenchyma, consistent with the tumor in the right kidney with metastatic involvement of bone structures and lungs

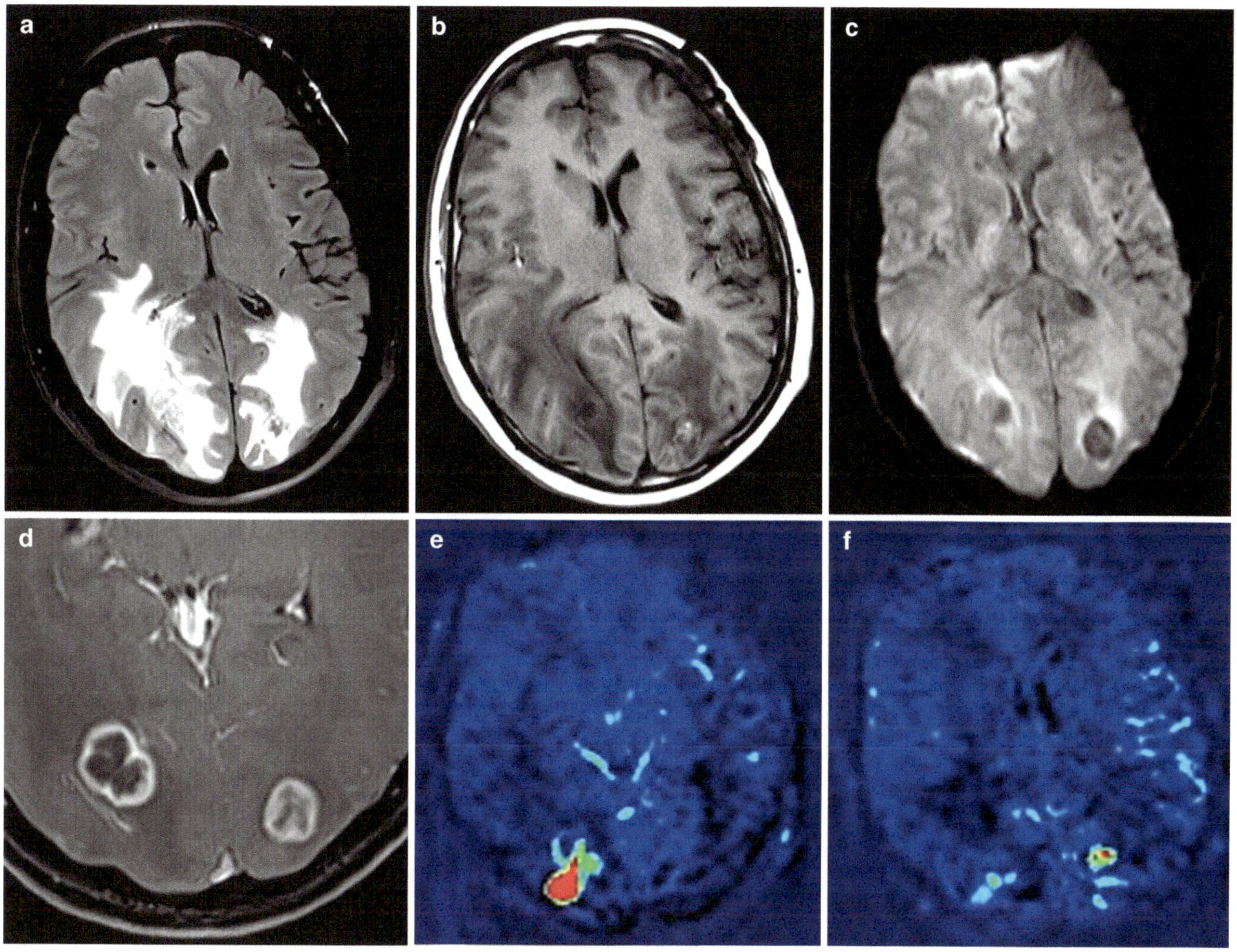

Fig. 15.10 Multiple kidney cancer metastases in the brain. In the occipital regions, solid-cystic lesions are identified with an increased signal on T2-FLAIR MRI (**a**), with a pronounced zone of perifocal edema and hemorrhagic changes hyperintense on T1-weighted MRI (**b**). On DWI MRI, lesions are characterized by a hypointense signal (**c**). CA accumulation in the lesions is intense, mainly on the periphery (**d**). All lesions have increased CBF values on non-contrasted perfusion (**e**, **f**)

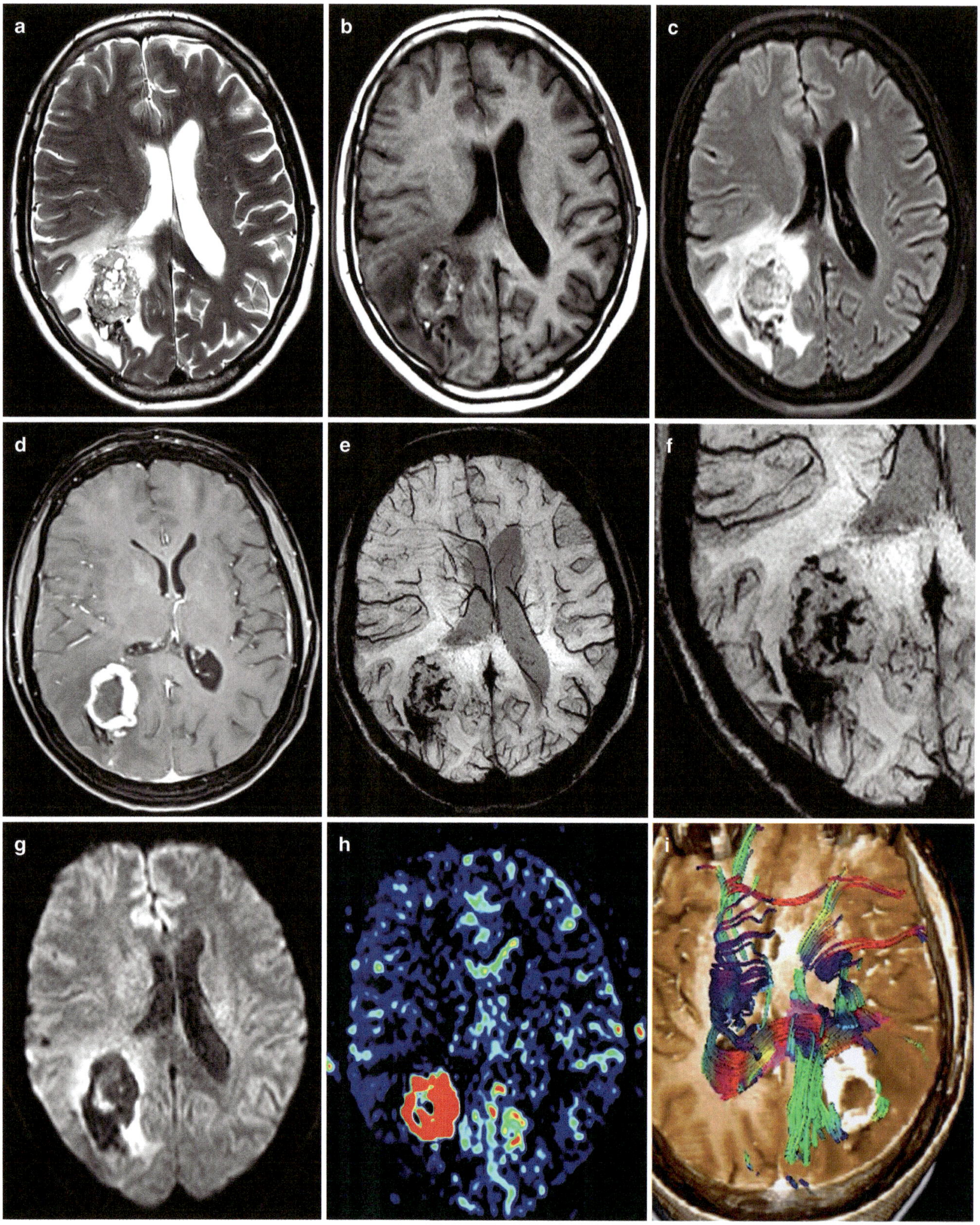

Fig. 15.11 A kidney cancer metastasis in the brain. In the right parietal-occipital region, there is a lesion with a heterogeneously high signal on T2-weighted MRI (**a**), with areas of hemorrhages—an increased signal on T1-weighted MRI (**b**) and a pronounced perifocal edema (**c**). After intravenous administration of the contrast agent, the lesion intensely accumulates the contrast agent on the periphery (**d**). There are multiple portions with a decreased signal in the lesion structure on SWI (SWAN) MRI (**e**, **f**). On DWI MRI (**g**), the lesion is characterized by a reduced signal. On ASL maps (**h**), a marked increase in the blood flow is observed. When constructing the tracts (**i**), the conductive pathways of the radiate crown are intact and deformed, and part of the beam is located along the outer contour of the tumor

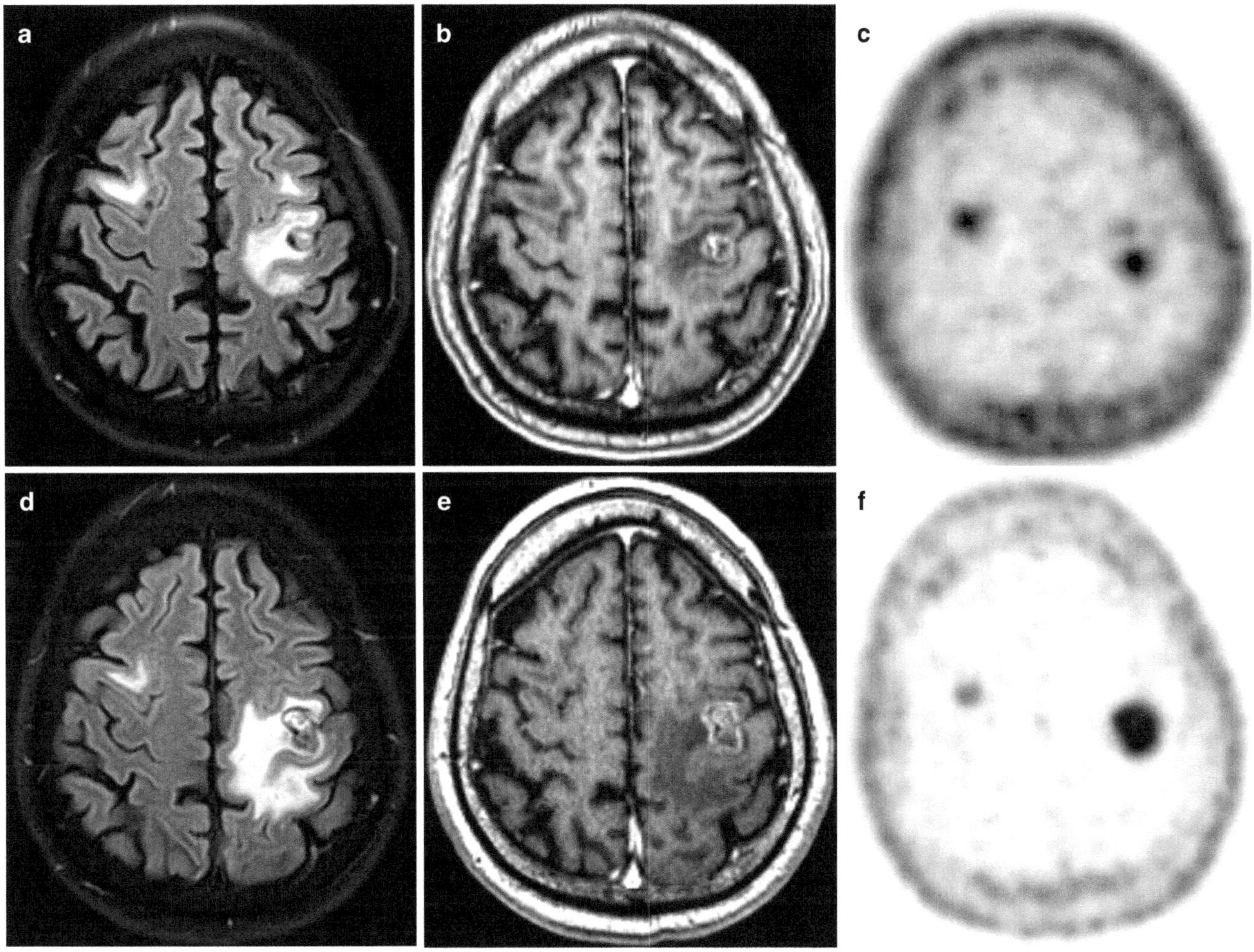

Fig. 15.12 Multiple kidney cancer metastases in the brain. Follow-up studies after the treatment by CyberKnife. On a series of MR tomograms on T2-FLAIR MRI (**a**, **d**) and T1-weighted MRI after CA administration (**b**, **e**) before and after radiosurgery (follow-up for 1 year), multiple metastases are identified heterogeneously accumulating the contrast agent. There is an increase in edema (**d**) and an enlargement of the area with abnormal CA accumulation of the lesion in the left post-frontal region (**e**), while no significant changes being observed in the lesion in the right frontal region. On PET images with ^{18}F-choline (**c**, **f**), there is also an increase in the area and intensity of RP accumulation on the left, indicative of the activity of the neoplastic process and stabilization of the process on the right

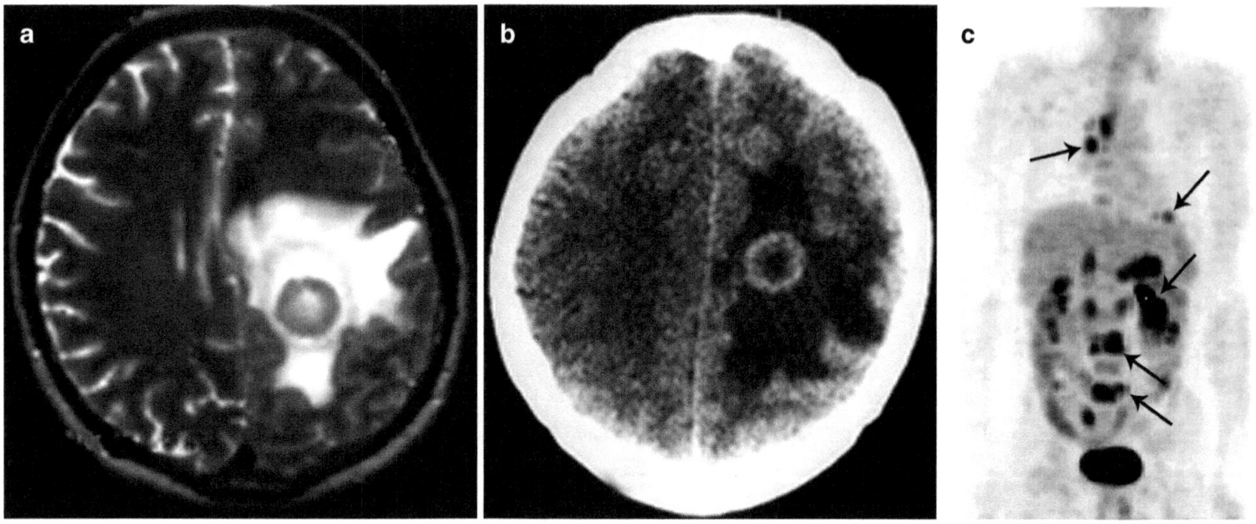

Fig. 15.13 A kidney cancer metastasis. In the left frontoparietal region, there is a rounded space-occupying lesion with a heterogeneously high signal on T2-weighted MRI (**a**) and high density on CT (**b**) with a pronounced perifocal edema—ring enhancement. On the PET image, in the frontal projection (**b**), there are a large tumor in the upper pole of the left kidney and multiple metastases in the bones, in the lower lobe of the left lung, and in the hilum of the right lung (the *arrows*)

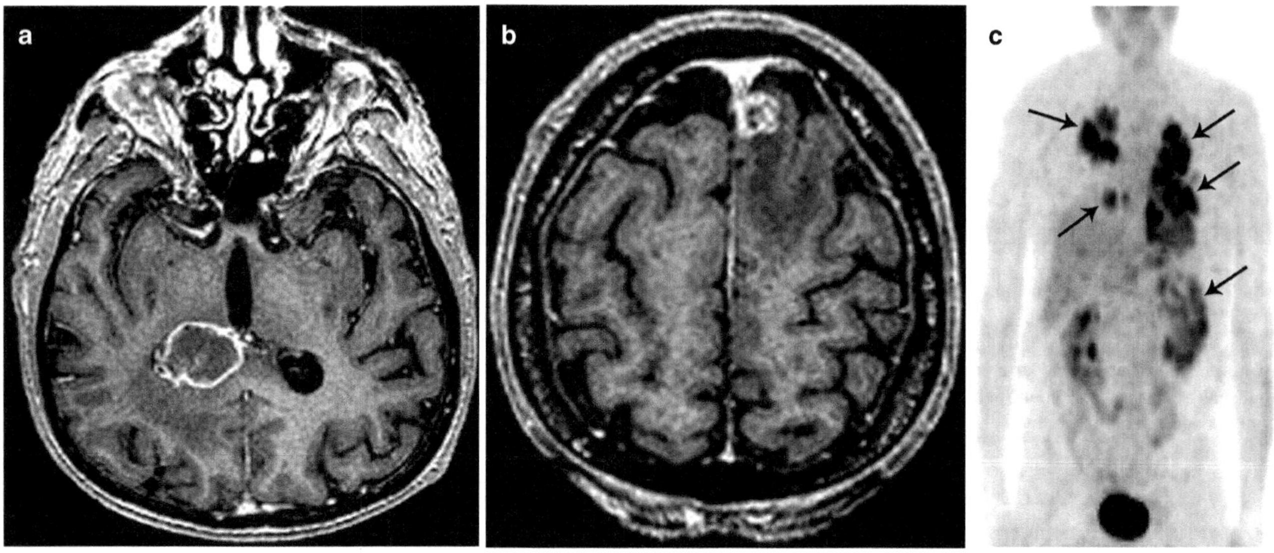

Fig. 15.14 Multiple kidney cancer metastases. On T1-weighted MRI with contrast enhancement (**a**, **b**), there are lesions with abnormal CA accumulation in the splenium of the corpus callosum on the right and in the convexital areas of the left frontal regions with signs of pronounced regional contrast enhancement. A PET study shows multifocal involvement of the lungs and a large tumor lesion in the upper left kidney with irregular RP accumulation (**c**) (the *arrows*)

15.2 Postoperative and Post-radiation Changes

See Figs. 15.15, 15.16, 15.17, and 15.8.

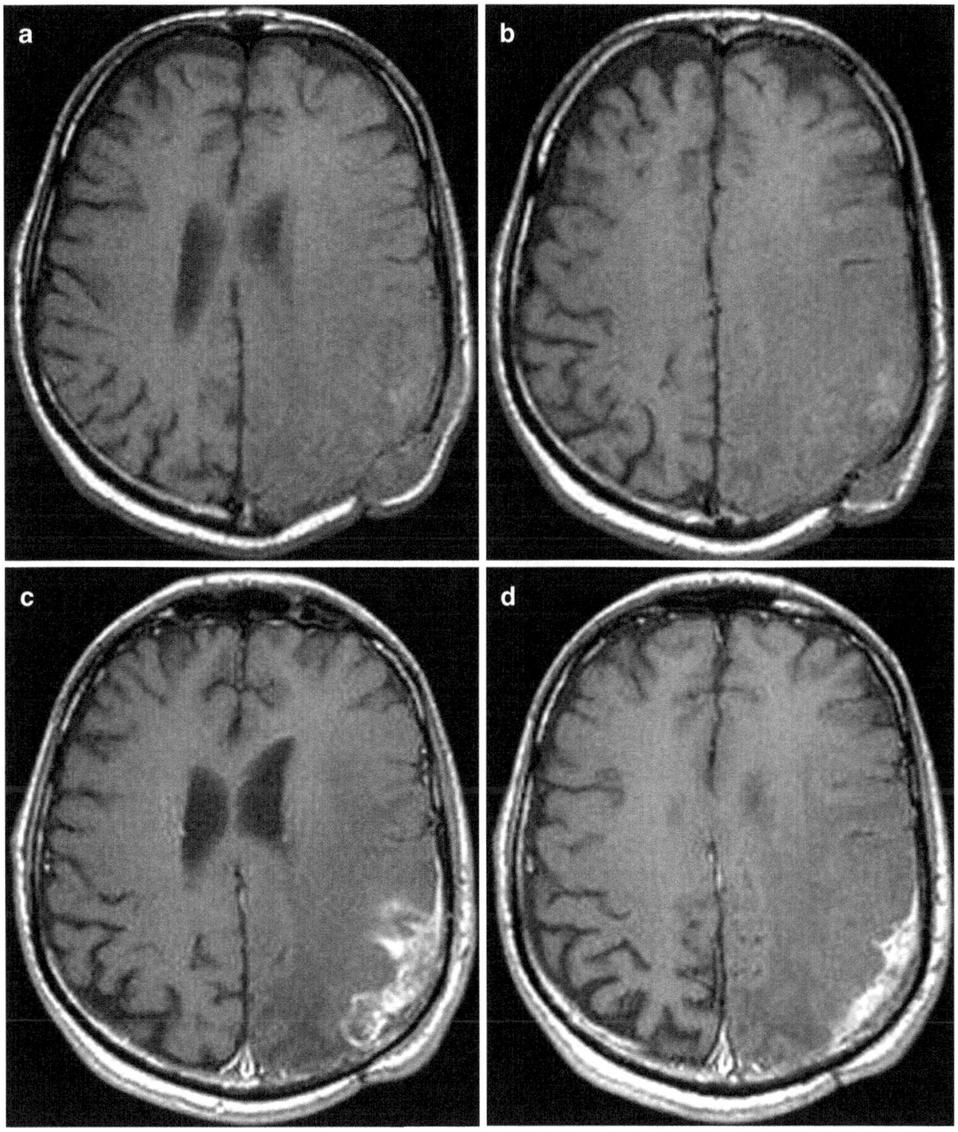

Fig. 15.15 A kidney cancer metastasis in the brain. Recurrence after surgical removal of the metastasis. In the frontoparietal region on the left, on the background of postoperative changes, there is a lesion with an isointense signal on T1-weighted MRI (**a**, **b**). Following intravenous CA administration (**c**, **d**), its intense, inhomogeneous accumulation is observed, and of note is the diffuse spread of the tumor into the brain parenchyma and lateral-spreading growth along the brain meninges

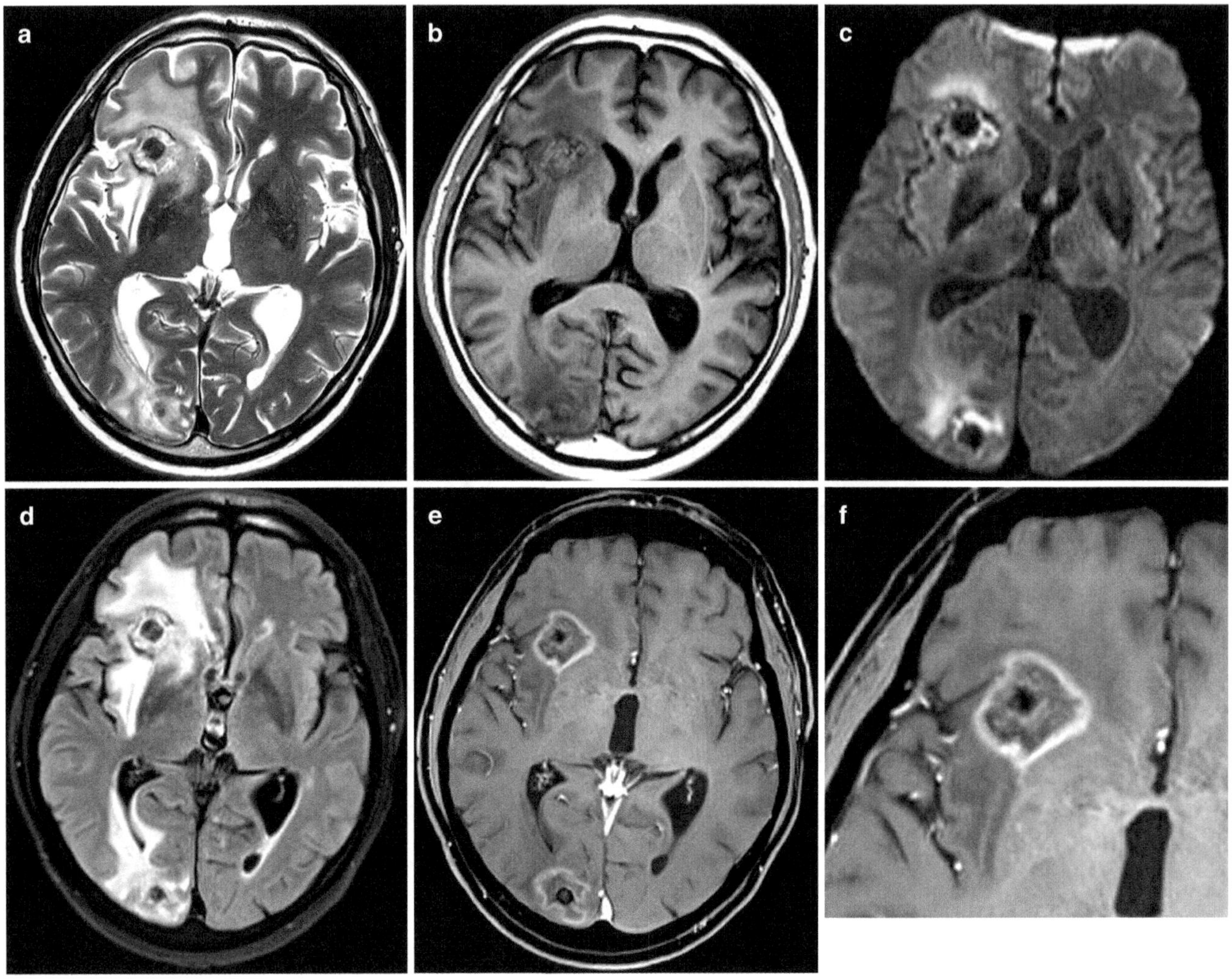

Fig. 15.16 Multiple kidney cancer metastases in the brain. Condition after radiosurgery—post-radiation changes. In the right frontal and occipital lobes, there are lesions with an iso-hypointense MR signal on T2-weighted (**a**) and T1-weighted MRI (**b**) and a heterogeneous signal on DWI (**c**) and T2-FLAIR MRI (**d**) with an area of a pronounced perifocal edema. After intravenous CA administration, the lesions accumulate it mostly along their contours (**e**, **f**). Central portions of the lesions are hypointense in all sequences due to the presence of a calcified component

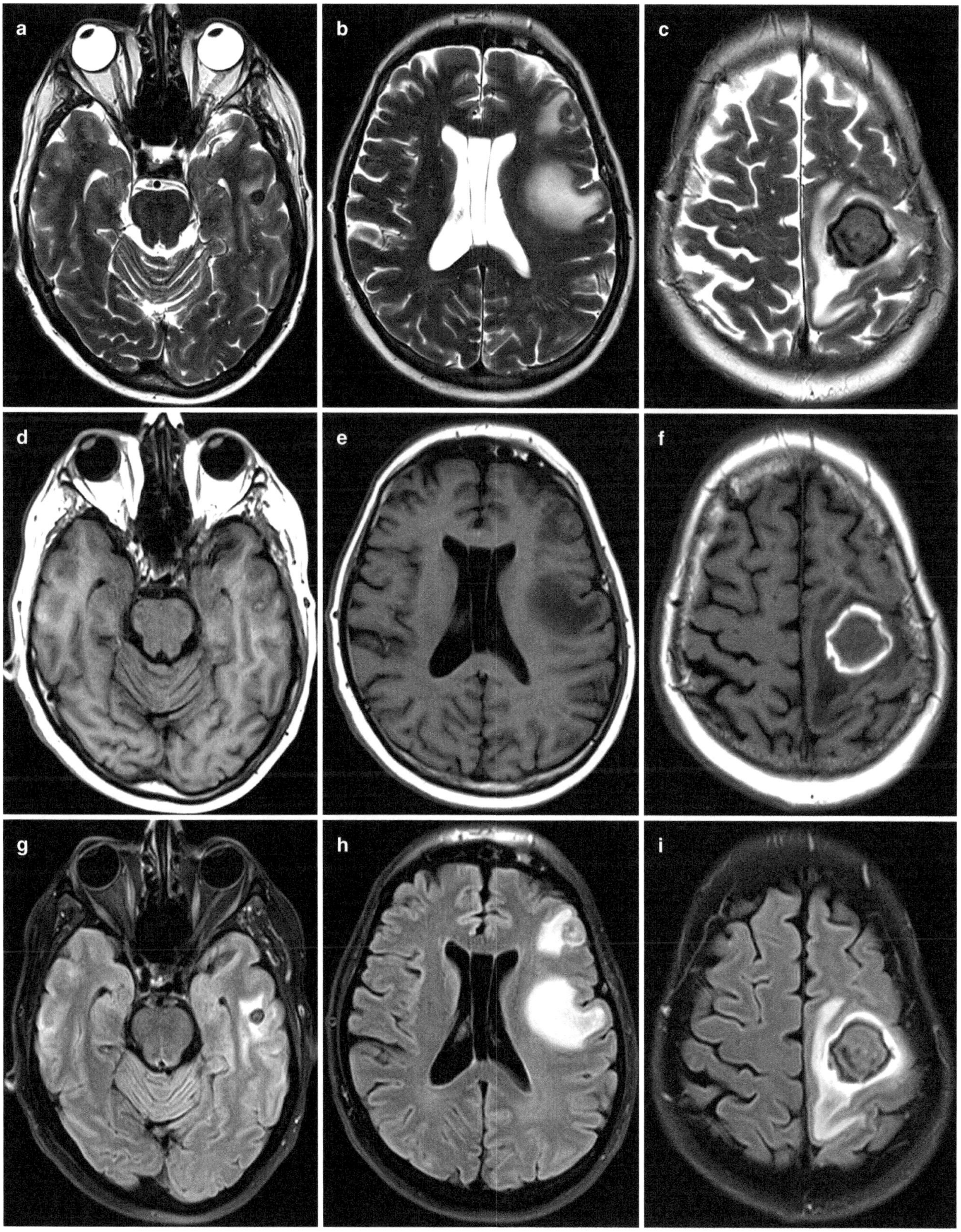

Fig. 15.17 Multiple kidney cancer metastases in the brain. A three-level study, condition after the radiosurgery—mixed changes with time. In the left temporal, frontal, and postfrontal areas, there are multiple lesions with a hypointense signal on T2-weighted MRI (**a**–**c**), a hypointense signal in the central part with a hyperintense rim on T1-weighted MRI (**d**–**f**), and a moderately high signal on T2-FLAIR MRI (**g**–**i**). On DWI MRI, the most prominent lesion has an increased MR signal along the periphery (**j**, **k**, **l**), and a small metastasis in the left frontal area has an increased signal. On ASL MRI, a small lesion is visualized in the left frontal area, with signs of an increased blood flow (**o**); the rest are not visualized (**m**, **n**). Following intravenous CA administration, the lesion inhomogeneously accumulates it (**p**–**r**)

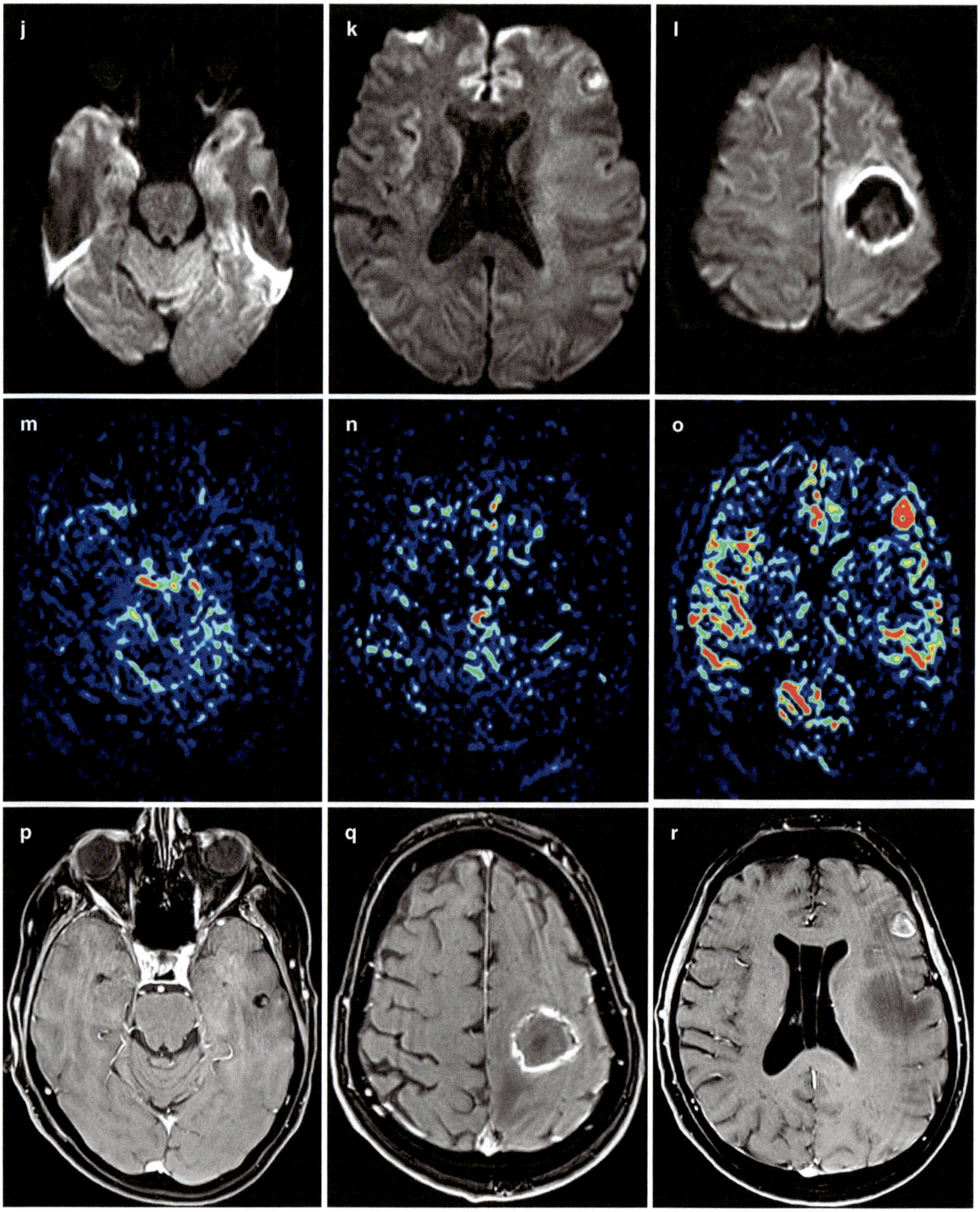

Fig. 15.17 (continued)

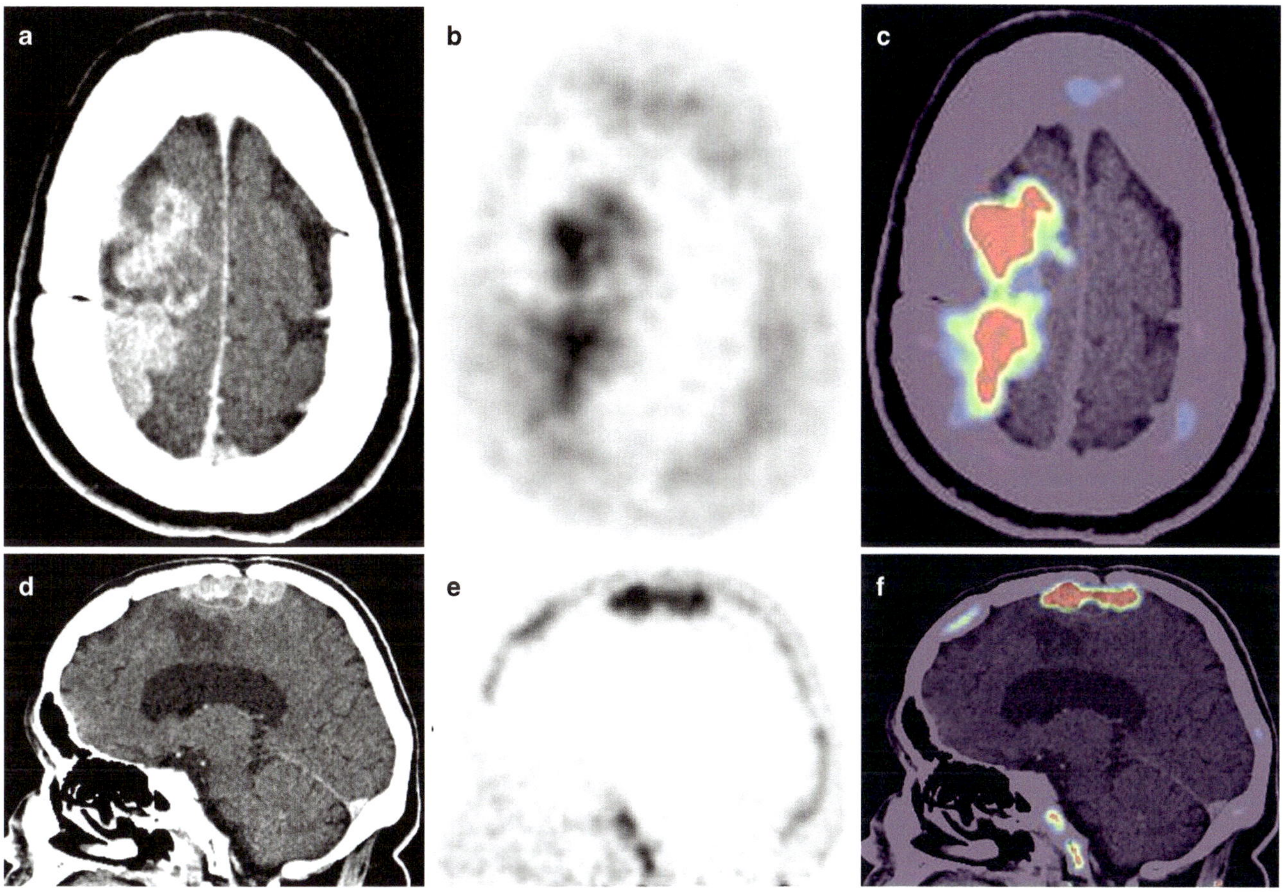

Fig. 15.18 Multiple kidney cancer metastases in the brain. Recurrence after surgical removal. In convexital parts of the right frontal region on CT in the axial view (**a**) and sagittal constructs (**d**), there are several confluent space-occupying lesions, rapidly accumulating CA. On PET/CT with ^{18}F-choline axial (**b**, **c**) and sagittal projection (**e**, **f**), the lesions are characterized by increased RP accumulation

16 Colorectal Cancer (CRC)

Colorectal cancer (CRC) is a general term determining the concepts of *colon cancer* and *rectal cancer*. It combines malignant epithelial tumors of the cecum, colon, rectum, and anal canal; varies by their form, location, and histological structure; and constitutes 15% of all primary tumors diagnosed.

According to the World Health Organization, more than 900,000 new cases of colorectal cancer (CRC) are diagnosed in the world each year. The highest incidence is observed in the USA, Canada, Western Europe, and Russia. An increase in the incidence by 14.7% in men and 18.0% in women was noted from 3 to 1997 in Russia (Martyniuk 2000). Subsequent studies showed that this trend continues from 2003 to 2008, and the incidence increased by 11.6% in men and 13.4% women (Davydov and Axel 2010). According to forecasts, in Russia in years to come, CRC will be leading among tumors of the gastrointestinal tract, as is currently the case in most developed countries.

Mortality from colorectal cancer remains high. The largest mortality from CRC is reported in the Czech Republic, Hungary (34.3 per 100,000 people), and New Zealand (26.4), while the lowest (15.2) is in the USA (Khanevich et al. 2008). In Russia, CRC occupies the third place in terms of mortality from all malignant tumors. In Western Europe, due to active screening programs, about 80% of patients have tumors that can be surgically removed (Vogel et al. 2000). The five-year survival in colorectal cancer is about 60% in developed countries and less than 40% in resource-limited countries.

A major factor in the development of colorectal cancer is advanced age: the likelihood of CRC substantially increases after the age of 55 years and becomes the highest after 70–75 years of age (Boyle and Leon 2002; Faivre et al. 2002; Papapolychroniadis 2004), although patients in 7% of cases are younger than 50 years old. According to various sources, the hereditary factor plays a role in 6–30% of cases: familial adenomatous polyposis or hereditary nonpolyposis colorectal cancer (Lynch syndrome). Among other factors associated with an increased risk of colorectal cancer, there are chronic inflammatory diseases of the colon—ulcerative colitis and Crohn's disease with colon involvement. However, according to Burt et al. (1990), in 75%, CRC occurs without any known predisposing factors.

Colorectal cancer most often metastasizes to the lungs (10–20%) and liver (20–30%), less often to the spine, uterus, adrenal glands, pancreas, and brain (Patanaphan and Salaazar 1993; Tan et al. 2009). According to Graf et al. (1988), CRC metastases comprise 1.8–4.8% of all metastatic brain lesions. According to other authors, the incidence of secondary brain involvement reaches 10% in patients with colorectal cancer (Temple et al. 1982). The median interval from CRC diagnosis to detection of metastases in the brain is 22–33 months. In our sample, patients with colorectal cancer metastases in the brain made up 5.4% of all metastatic lesions of this type of cancer.

The probability of brain metastases (including micrometastases) cannot be ruled out in patients with localized forms of gastrointestinal cancer. Thus, according to Vogel et al. (2000), tumor cells circulating in the blood were found in 40%, while micrometastases in the bone marrow were detected in 39% of patients with stage I–II colon cancer. This substantiates the advisability of adjuvant drug therapy after a curative surgery for colorectal cancer in order to improve long-term results of the treatment.

A native (without contrast enhancement) CT study of colorectal cancer metastases visualizes rounded lesions with isodense or slightly decreased density. It is often difficult to establish a clear boundary between the tumor edge and a perifocal edema. In small tumor lesions, it can be identified by a possible presence of indirect signs—edema of the brain substance, accompanying the tumor. The accumulation of the contrast agent by the metastasis helps clearly visualize its

M. Dolgushin et al., *Brain Metastases*, DOI 10.1007/978-3-319-57760-9_16

external borders and allows to differentiate it from the brain tissue edema; CRC metastases accumulate radiopaque contrast agents well.

Despite pronounced CA accumulation by the solid part of colorectal cancer metastases, CBV values in such cases appeared to be significantly lower and quantitatively similar to CBV of those for metastases of breast cancer and uterine and lung cancer (CBV = 8.14 ± 3.71 (ml/100 g)). Average CBF values in colorectal cancer metastases (as well as in renal cancer metastases) are low and quantitatively similar, CBF = 72.13 ± 35.35 (ml/100 g/min), but with a large dispersion of individual values. MTT values obtained (7.72 ± 3.26 s) were not specific for CRC as compared to MTT values in metastatic tumors with another morphogenesis.

As noted, the use of CT perfusion imaging in follow-up studies after radiosurgery performed for colorectal cancer metastases in the brain may be useful not only in terms of assessing the effectiveness of the treatment but also, in some of the cases, allowing to determine the presence of continued growth of the metastatic lesion, not detectable with MRI.

MRI in colorectal cancer is the preferred alternative to CT. The contrast agent accumulation in MRI in colorectal cancer metastases is pronounced, with fairly clear, sometimes bumpy contours; however, the lesion borders are always well determined. An MR picture on T1-weighted MRI + Gd of colorectal cancer metastases in the brain somewhat resembles that in metastases of uterine cancer.

Particularly noteworthy are metastases of colorectal adenocarcinoma, which were characterized by a hypointense signal on T2-weighted MRI in the majority (83%) of cases in our clinical material. Some of them showed signs of moderate central necrosis, characterized by a higher signal on T2-weighted MRI. Perifocal edema in the area of colorectal cancer metastases is quite expressed, which indicates active growth of the tumor. As indicated above, such MR tissue characteristics with an iso-hypointense signal on T2-weighted MRI were obtained in cases of pigmented melanoma metastases in the brain, which was due to the paramagnetic properties of melanin, but no evidence of increased signal on T1-weighted MRI was observed in colorectal cancer metastases. In metastases from other primary tumors, this pattern was not encountered, and, in case of an unknown primary tumor site, it allowed to suspect the source of metastases. It is assumed that changes in MR characteristics of colorectal adenocarcinoma metastases were associated with mucin content, having paramagnetic properties. However, this hypothesis requires further investigation.

The use of SWI (SWAN) to verify vascular changes in the structure of colorectal cancer metastases in the brain is not informative (as in melanomas), unlike metastases of other histogenesis and primary brain tumors. A characteristic diffuse decrease in MR signal on SWI (SWAN) for CRC metastases in the brain does not allow to use the method as an expert one to evaluate the hemorrhagic component of these tumors. The signal on SWI (SWAN) MRI from CRC metastases, according to our data, was homogeneously reduced in 85% of cases, which distinguishes these metastases from other secondary tumor lesions of the brain.

In the diagnosis of colorectal cancer metastases in the brain, MR spectroscopy identified common findings for metastases of different histogenesis: in the central part of metastases (typically, this is an area of tumor tissue degradation), before the treatment, there is an increase in the peaks of lactate and lipids in all cases; in 10% of cases, there is a moderate choline peak. No MRI spectroscopy findings specific for colorectal cancer metastases in the brains were obtained.

On DWI images, solid components of CRC metastases had an iso-hypointense, homogeneous MR signal; ADC is lower on the border of the metastasis and perifocal edema than in primary brain tumors ($p < 0.15$).

The complexity of the diagnosis in case of detecting the areas with increased RP accumulation (^{18}F-FDG) in the projection of the intestines is that a PET picture is not specific for tumor lesions, but displays local inflammatory changes, diverticula, erosions, ulcers, and symptoms of diabetes. Therefore, a prerequisite is colonoscopy to obtain a biopsy and a histological examination of the latter. A study of tumor markers (CEA or CA) is also mandatory. When colorectal cancer metastases are large enough, they are well differentiated on the background of intact brain substance.

16.1 Clinical Cases

See Figs. 16.1, 16.2, 16.3, 16.4, 16.5, 16.6, 16.7, 16.8, 16.9, 16.10, 16.11, 16.12, 16.13, 16.14, 16.15, 16.16, 16.17, and 16.18.

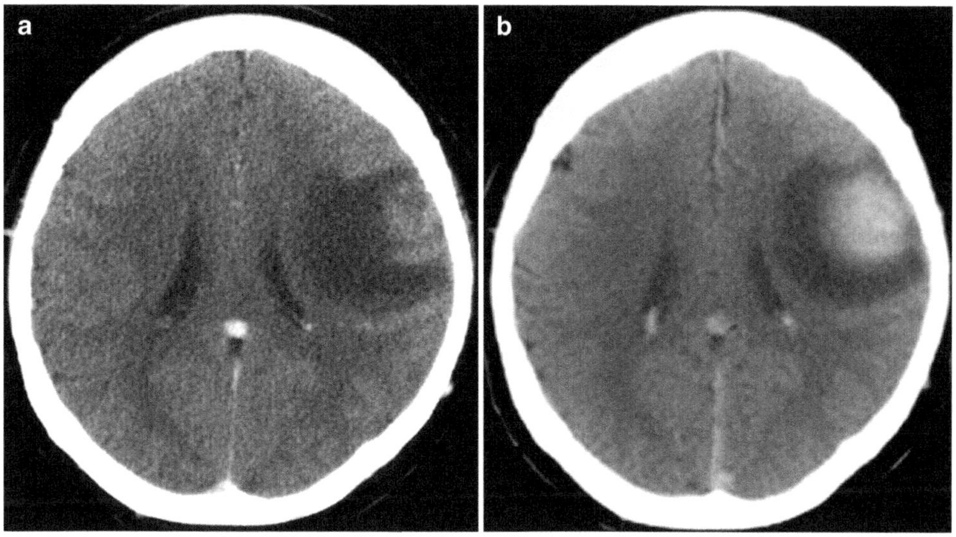

Fig. 16.1 Colorectal cancer metastases in the brain. On a CT scan in the axial projection, there is a large, isodense tumor lesion (**a**) intensely and homogeneously accumulating the contrast agent on the background of the expressed perifocal edema (**b**), convexitally, in the left frontal region

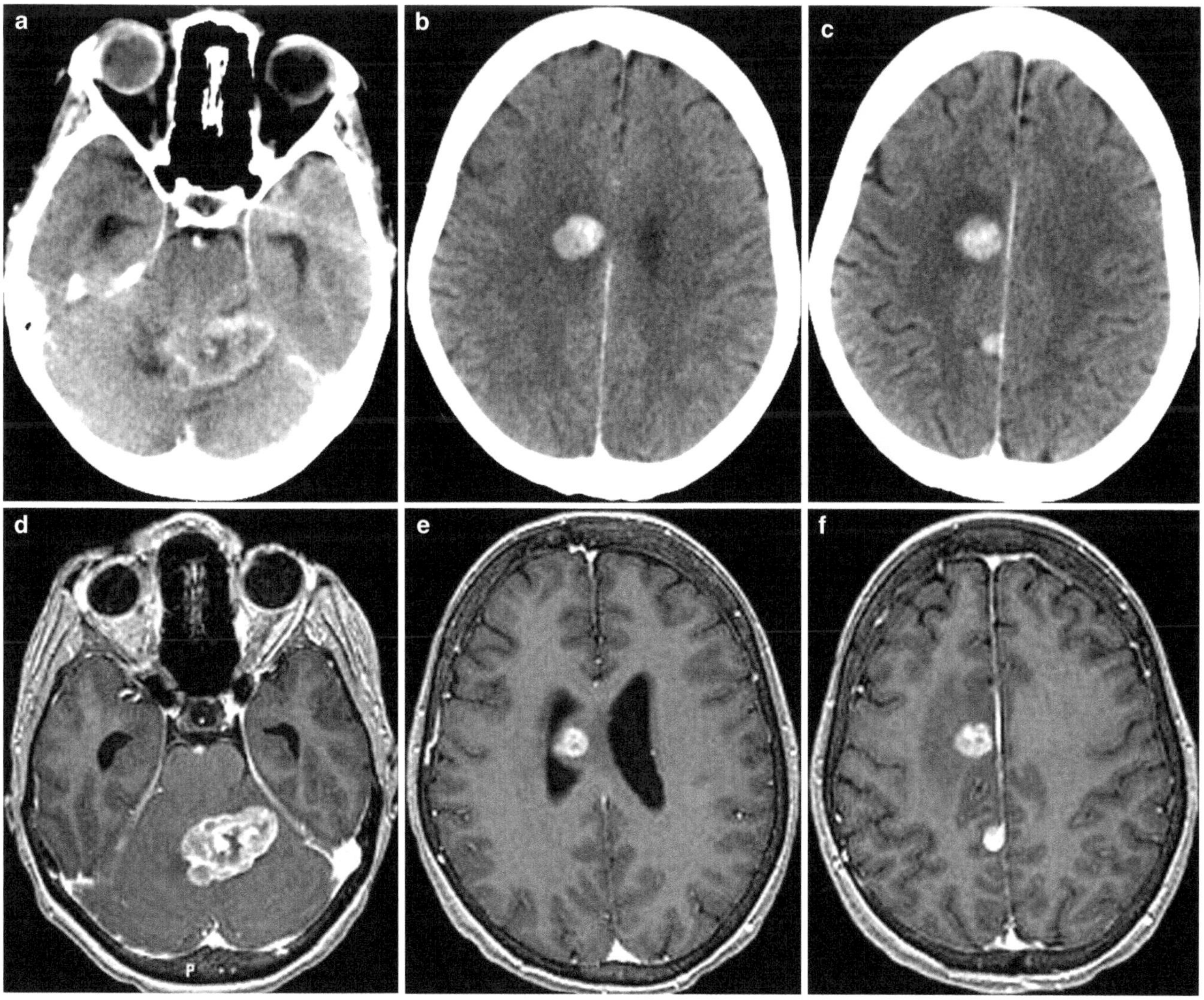

Fig. 16.2 Multiple metastases of colorectal cancer in the brain. A three-level study. On CT and MRI on T1-weighted fat sat MRI after intravenous CA administration, there are multiple space-occupying lesions with signs of a moderate perifocal edema, rapidly and unevenly accumulating the contrast agent in the left hemisphere of the cerebellum (**a**, **d**), as well as in the deep sections of the right frontal region (**b**, **e**) and parasagittal sections of the right frontoparietal region (**c**, **f**)

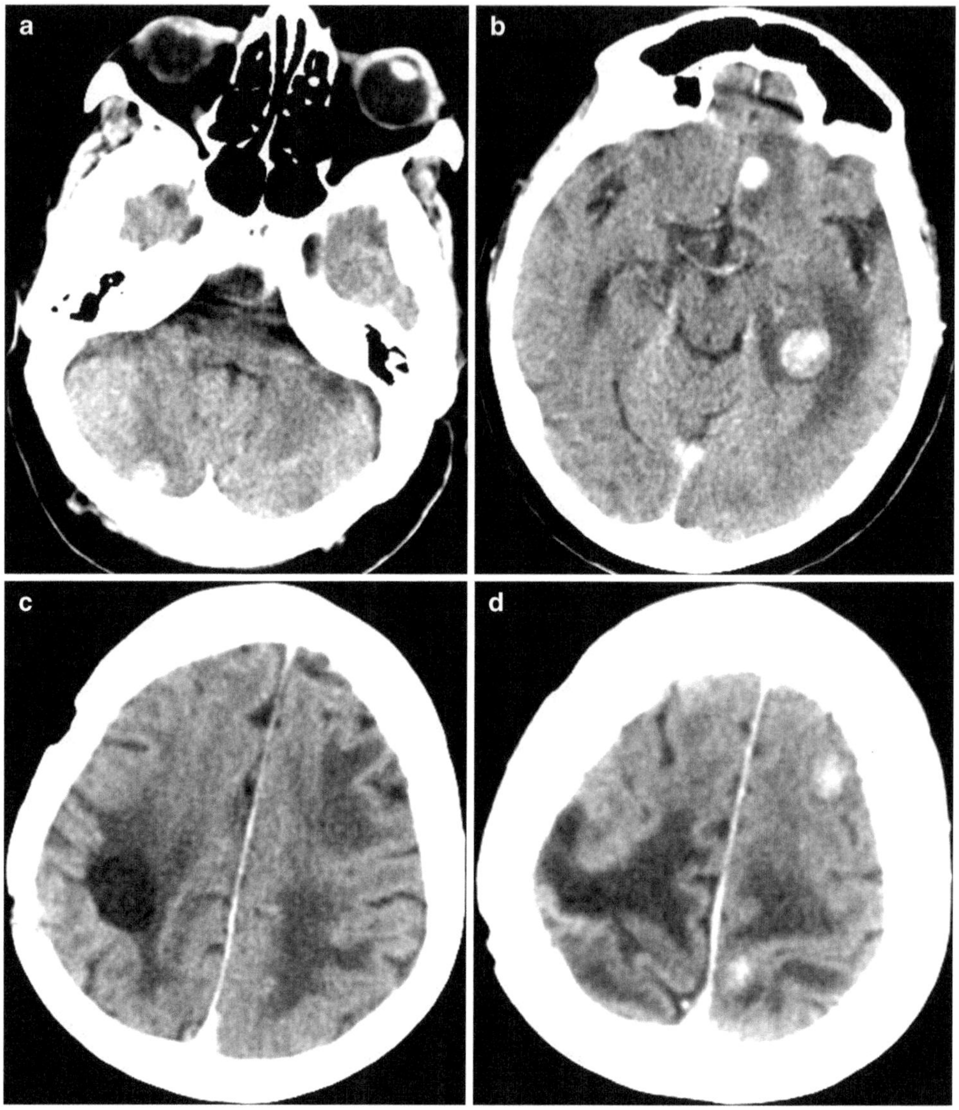

Fig. 16.3 Multiple metastases of colorectal cancer in the brain. A four-level study. Condition after surgical removal of the metastasis in the right frontoparietal region. On a CT scan after intravenous CA administration, there are multiple space-occupying lesions with an expressed area of perifocal edema, rapidly and unevenly accumulating CA in the convexital sections of the right hemisphere of the cerebellum (**a**) and in the deep sections of the left temporal region and basal and convexital sections of the left frontal region (**b**, **d**). In the right parietal region, a postoperative fluid-containing cyst with perifocal edema and no signs of tumor recurrence (**c**) is observed

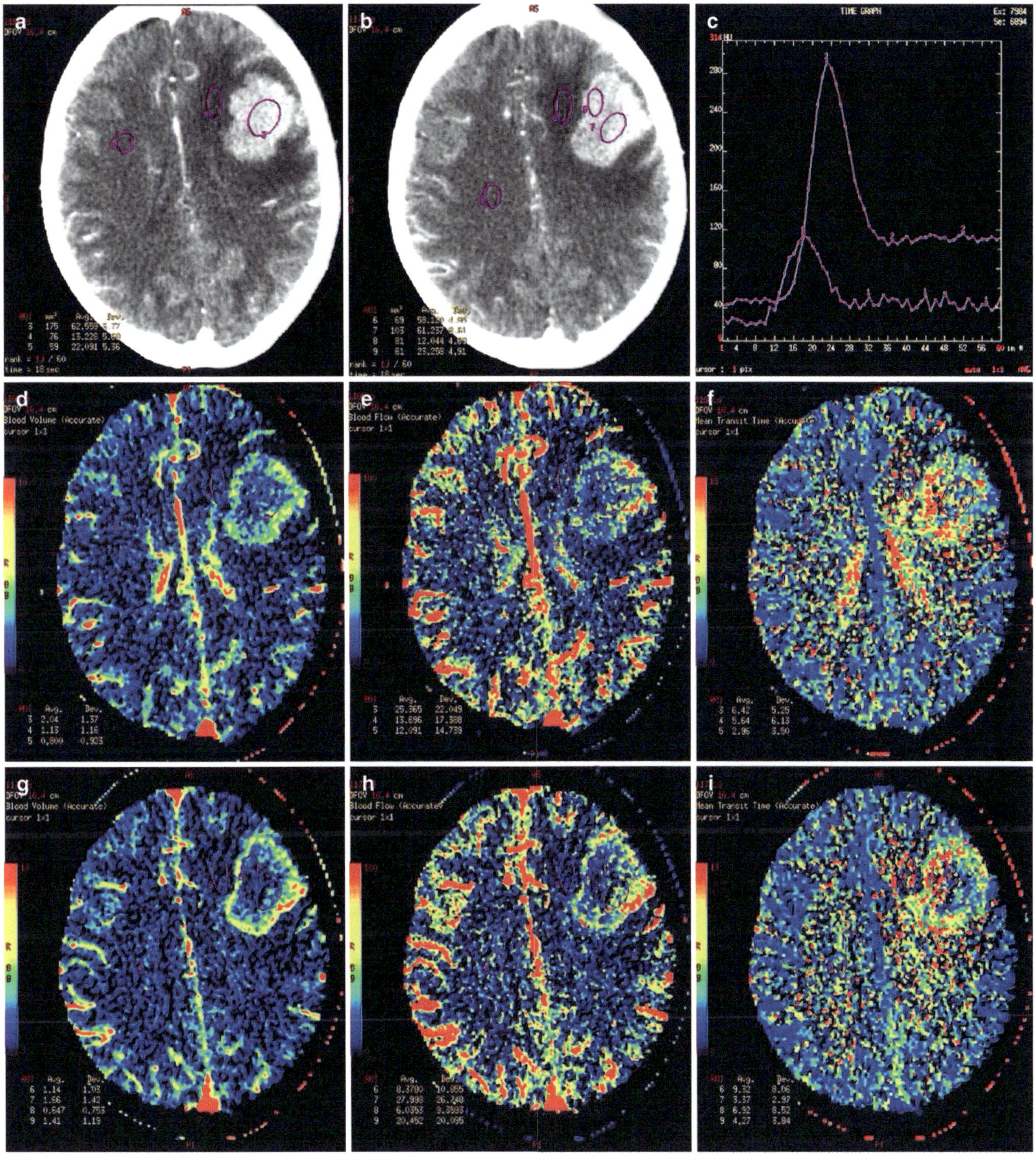

Fig. 16.4 Colorectal cancer metastases in the brain. On CT images with contrast enhancement (**a**, **b**), there is a space-occupying lesion that intensely and uniformly accumulates CA, with a pronounced perifocal edema (low-density area) in the left frontal region; ROIs are highlighted. The graph of correlation between arterial and venous peaks of contrast agent transit for calculation of perfusion values (**c**). On two-level CT perfusion maps, the lesion is characterized by high levels of CBV (**d**, **g**), CBF (**e**, **h**), and MTT (**f**, **i**); of note are higher perfusion parameters along the periphery of the metastasis, with homogeneous contrast enhancement of the entire metastasis on routine CT scans

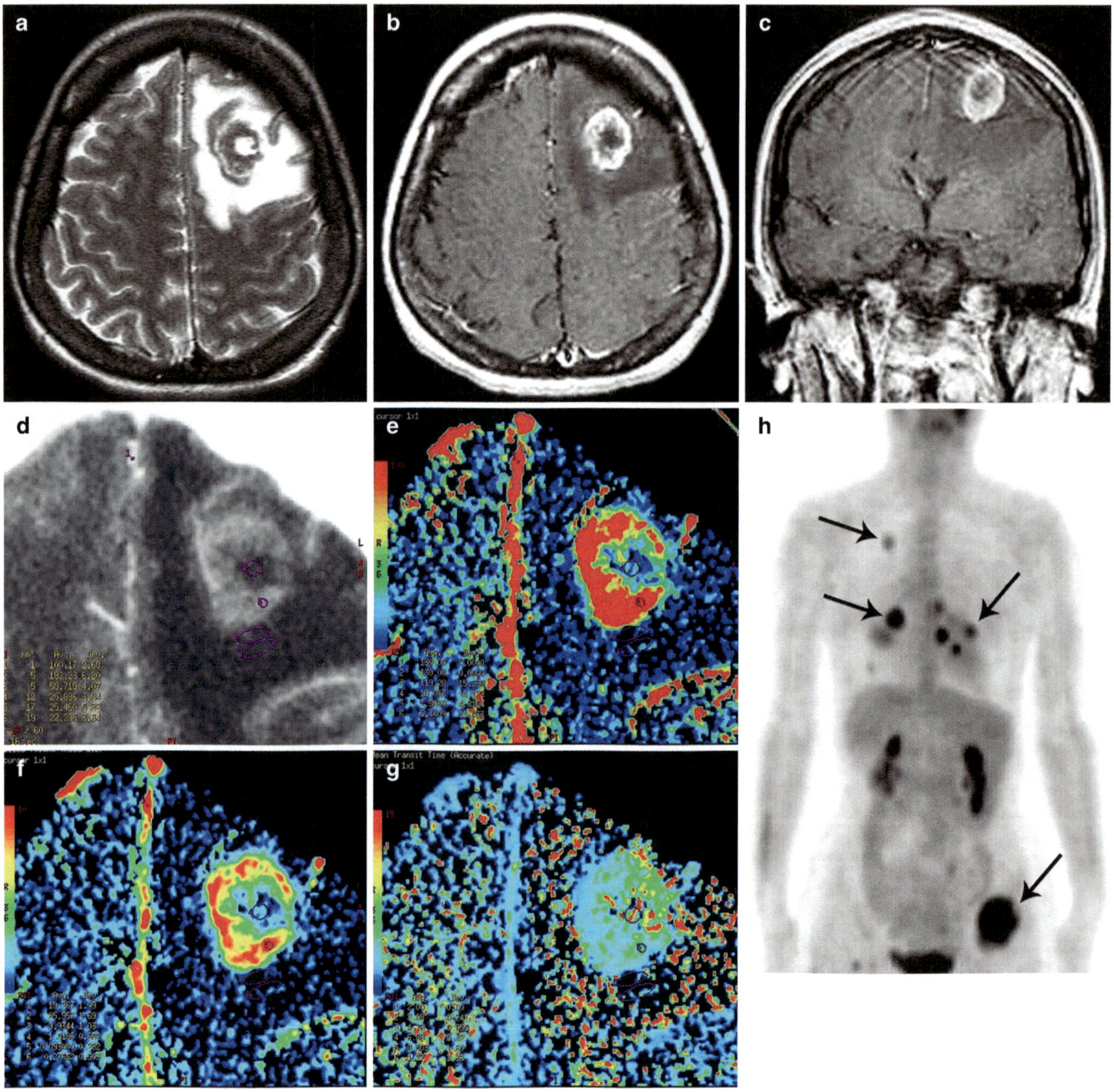

Fig. 16.5 Colorectal cancer metastases in the brain. In the left frontal region, there is a rounded lesion with an isointense signal on T2-weighted MRI (**a**) with a pronounced perifocal edema. After the contrast agent administration, its intense accumulation is noted in the solid structure of the tumor (**b**, **c**), and the area of central necrosis is well visualized. On contrast-enhanced CT, the tumor also accumulates CA (**d**). On CT perfusion maps, the lesion is characterized by high levels of CBV (**e**), CBF (**f**), and moderately increased MTT values (**g**). On the PET MIP image (**h**), there are multiple foci with increased accumulation of ^{18}F-FDG in the lungs and lymph nodes in the mediastinum and ilium (metastases) (the *arrows*)

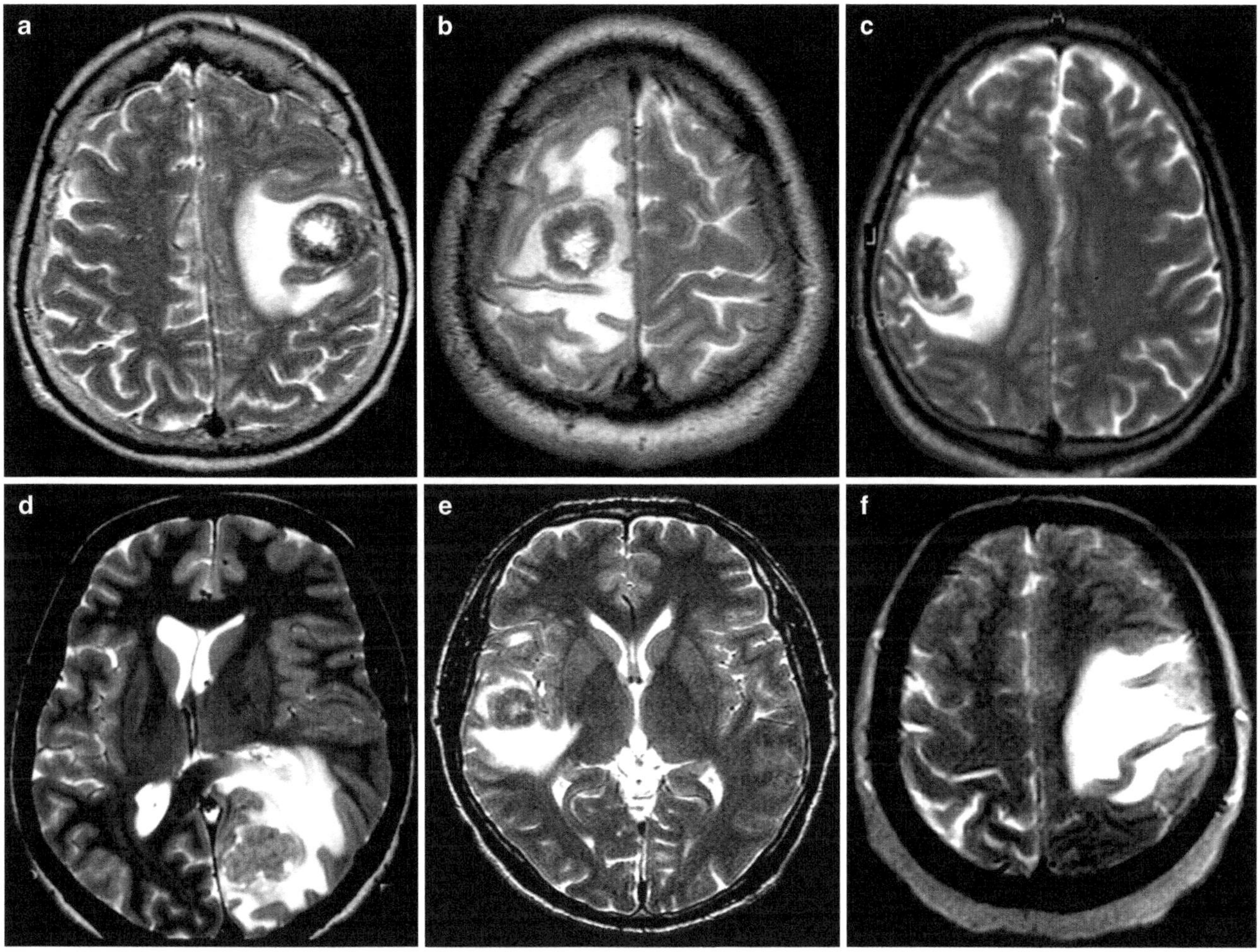

Fig. 16.6 Colorectal cancer metastases in the brain. The images are presented from studies carried out in several colon cancer patients with metastases in the brain. All focal cerebral lesions are characterized by a hypointense signal on T2-weighted MRI and a pronounced perifocal edema (**a**–**f**). According to our findings, in 85% of cases, colorectal cancer metastases are characterized by a decreased signal on T2-weighted MRI

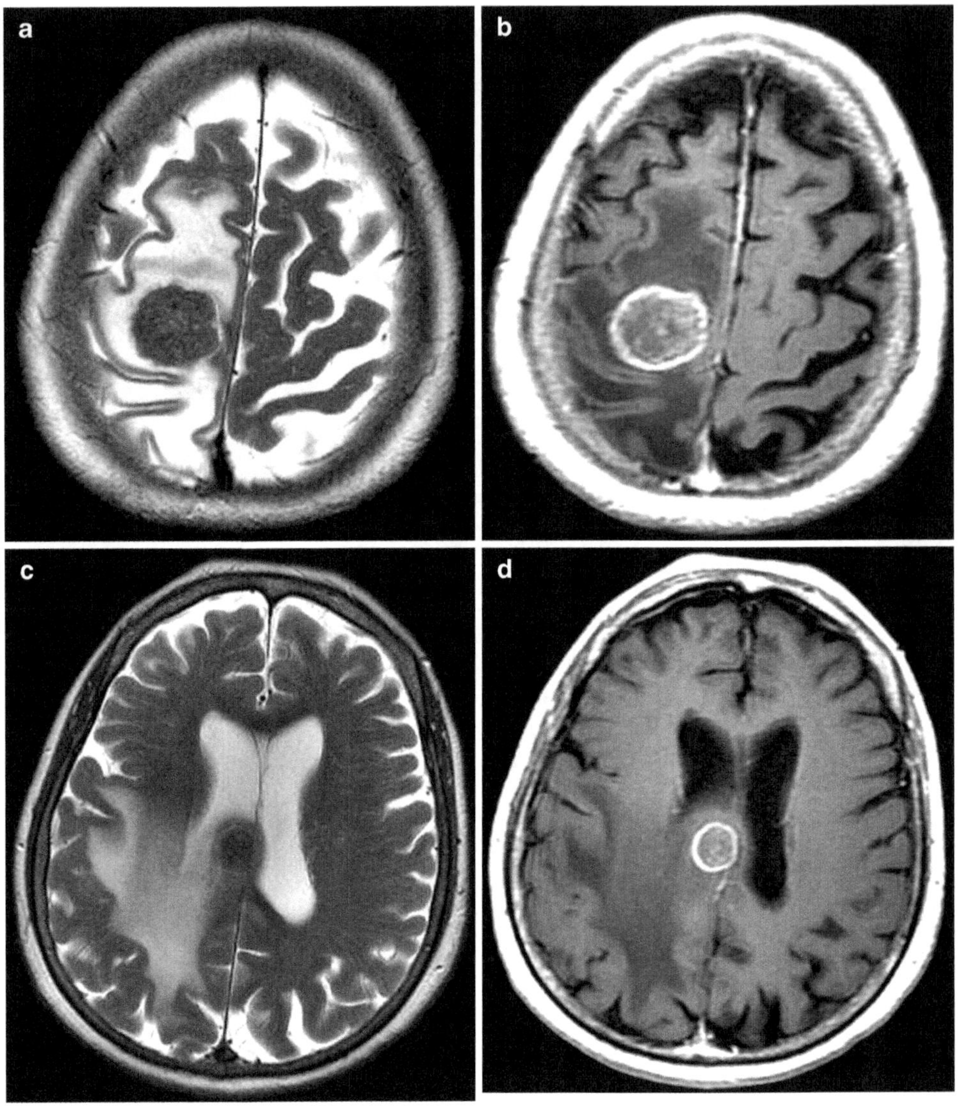

Fig. 16.7 Multiple colorectal cancer metastases in the brain. A two-level study. In the right frontoparietal region and in the region of the corpus callosum on T2-weighted MRI (**a**, **c**), there are two space-occupying hypointense lesions with signs of a pronounced perifocal edema and compression of the posterior horn of the lateral ventricle. After intravenous administration of the contrast agent on T1-weighted MRI (**b**, **d**), there is its intense and uneven (mostly along the periphery) accumulation in these lesions

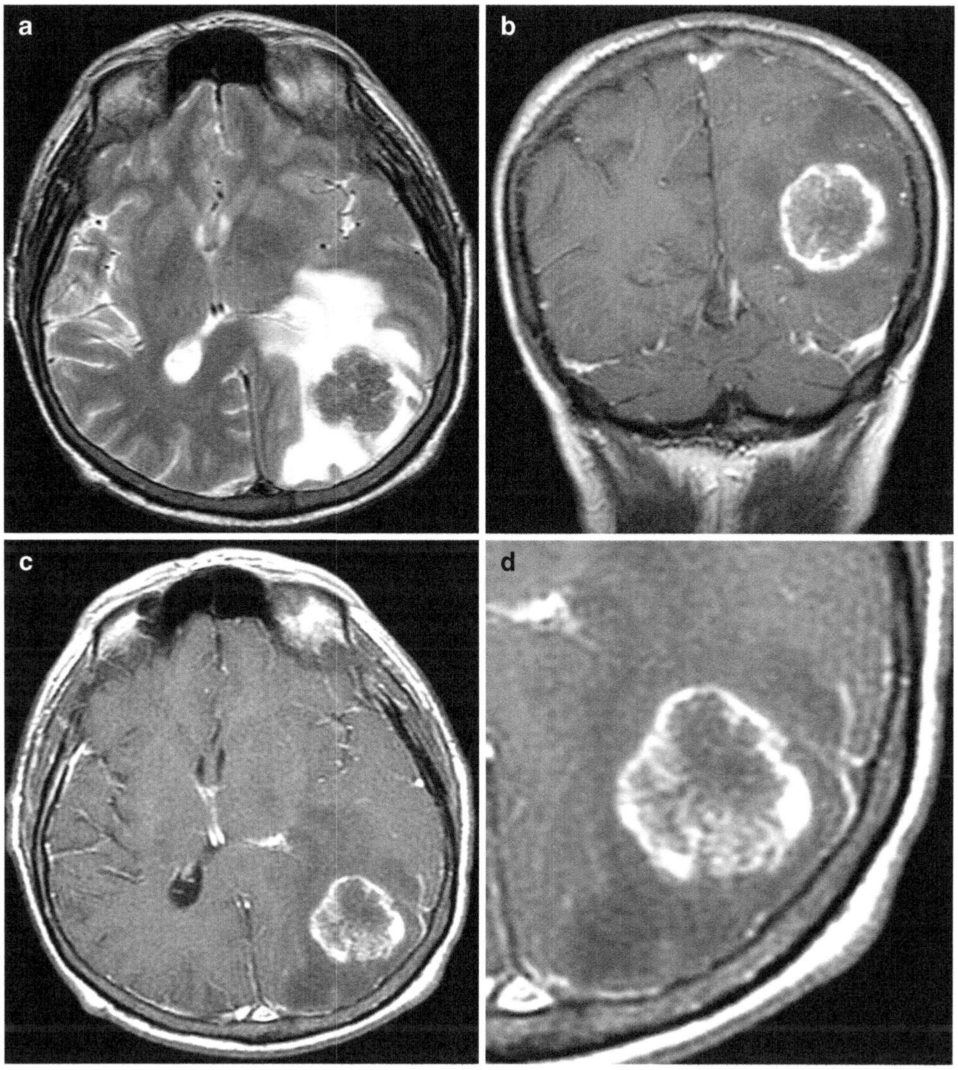

Fig. 16.8 Colorectal cancer metastases in the brain. In the left parietal lobe, there is a large homogenous space-occupying lesion with a moderately low signal on T2-weighted MRI (**a**) with a pronounced area of perifocal edema and a mass effect in the form of compression of the posterior horn of the left lateral ventricle and displacement of the midline structures. Following intravenous CA administration on T1-weighted MR images in the coronary (**b**) and axial (**c**, **d**) projections, there is its intense and uneven accumulation, more pronounced in the peripheral regions of the tumor

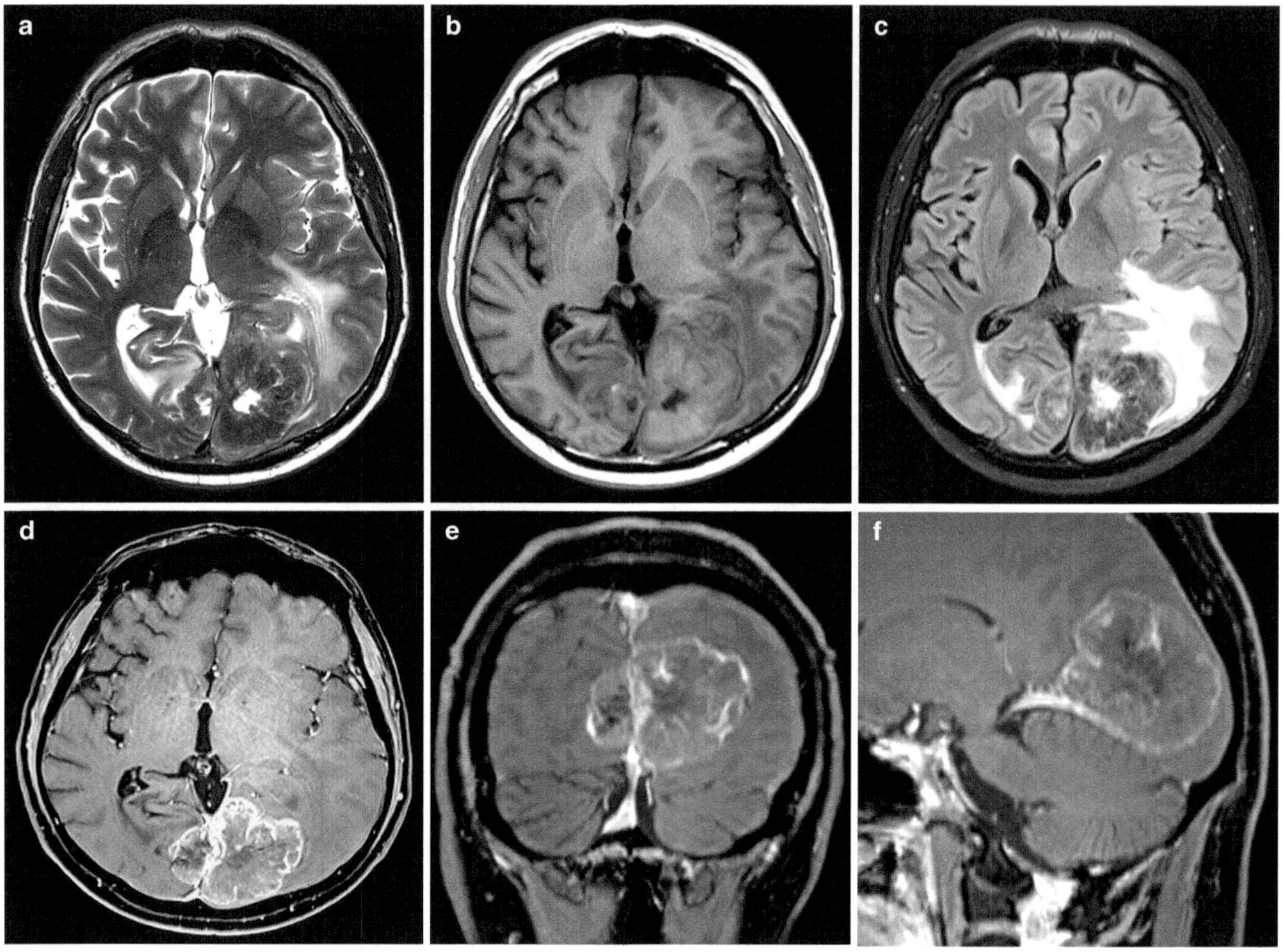

Fig. 16.9 A colorectal cancer metastases in the brain. In the occipital region with the spread to the falx, there are two large, confluent, heterogeneous lesions with an iso-hypointense signal on T2-weighted and T2-FLAIR MRI (**a**, **c**) and an isointense signal on T1-weighted MRI (**b**). Following intravenous CA administration on T1-weighted fat sat MRI (**d**–**f**), its intense and inhomogeneous accumulation (mostly along the periphery) is observed in the tumor. In the sagittal projection, infiltrative tumor growth into the cerebellar tentorium is well visualized

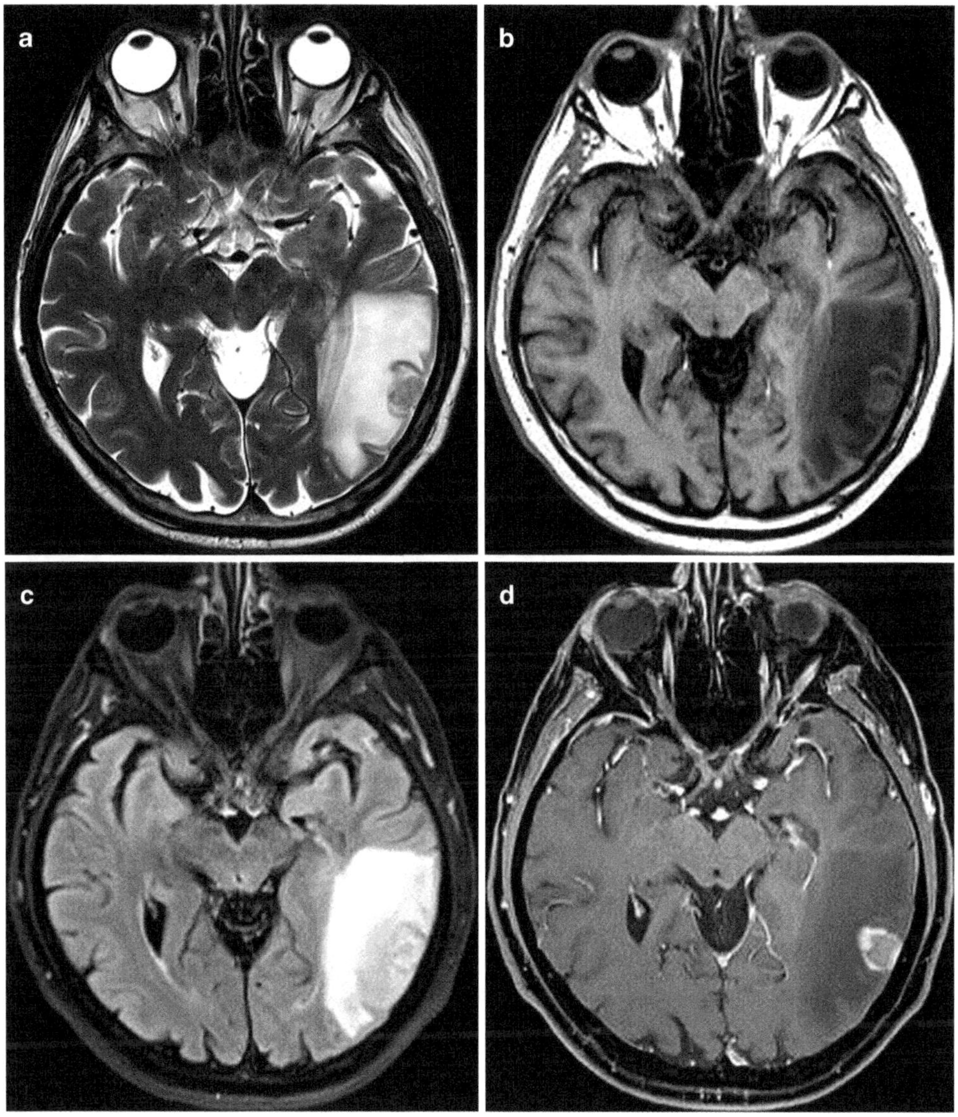

Fig. 16.10 Colorectal cancer metastases in the brain. In convexital sections of the left posterior temporal region, there is a space-occupying lesion, closely adjacent to the dura mater. On T2-weighted (**a**) and T2-FLAIR MRI (**c**), the metastasis has an increased signal and is accompanied by a pronounced perifocal edema. On T1-weighted MRI (**b**), the lesion is characterized by an isointense signal. After intravenous CA administration on T1-weighted fat sat MRI (**d**), the tumor intensely and inhomogeneously accumulates CA (mostly on the periphery)

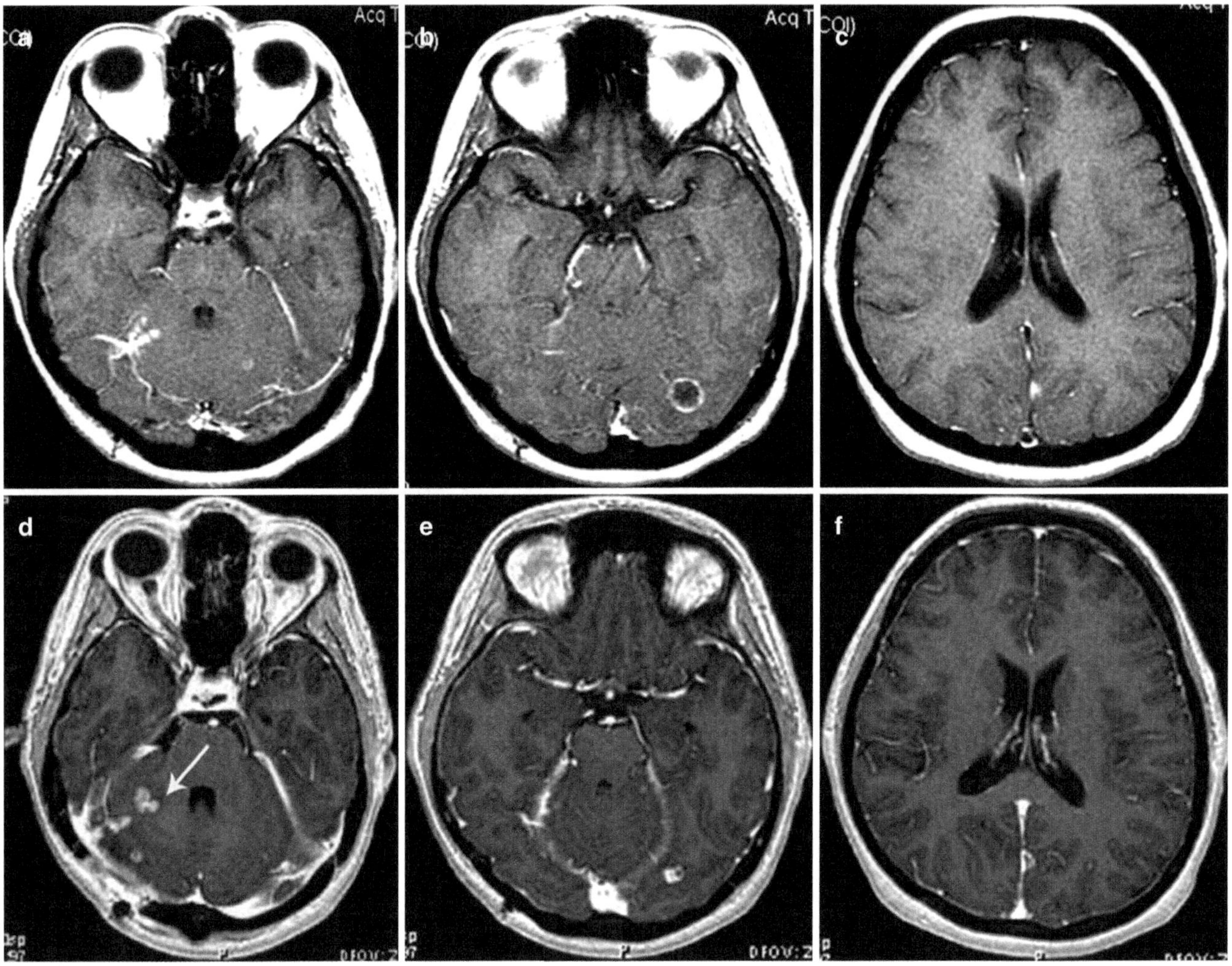

Fig. 16.11 Multiple colorectal cancer metastases in the brain. A follow-up study before and after radiosurgery. Axial sections at three levels. In the brain matter, there are multiple small foci with no obvious signs of perifocal edema in the left hemisphere of the cerebellum (**a**), in the left occipital region (**b**), and in parasagittal sections of the left occipital region (**c**). These lesions intensely and homogeneously accumulate CA after its intravenous administration on T1-weighted MRI (mostly on the periphery). On T1-weighted MRI with contrast enhancement 1 month after the radiosurgery, a decrease in the size of lesions is noted in the left hemisphere of the cerebellum and in the left occipital region (**d**, **e**). The metastasis in parasagittal sections of the left occipital region is slightly increased (**f**). The emergence of "new" metastases is also noted in the right hemisphere of the cerebellum (**d**) (*arrow*)

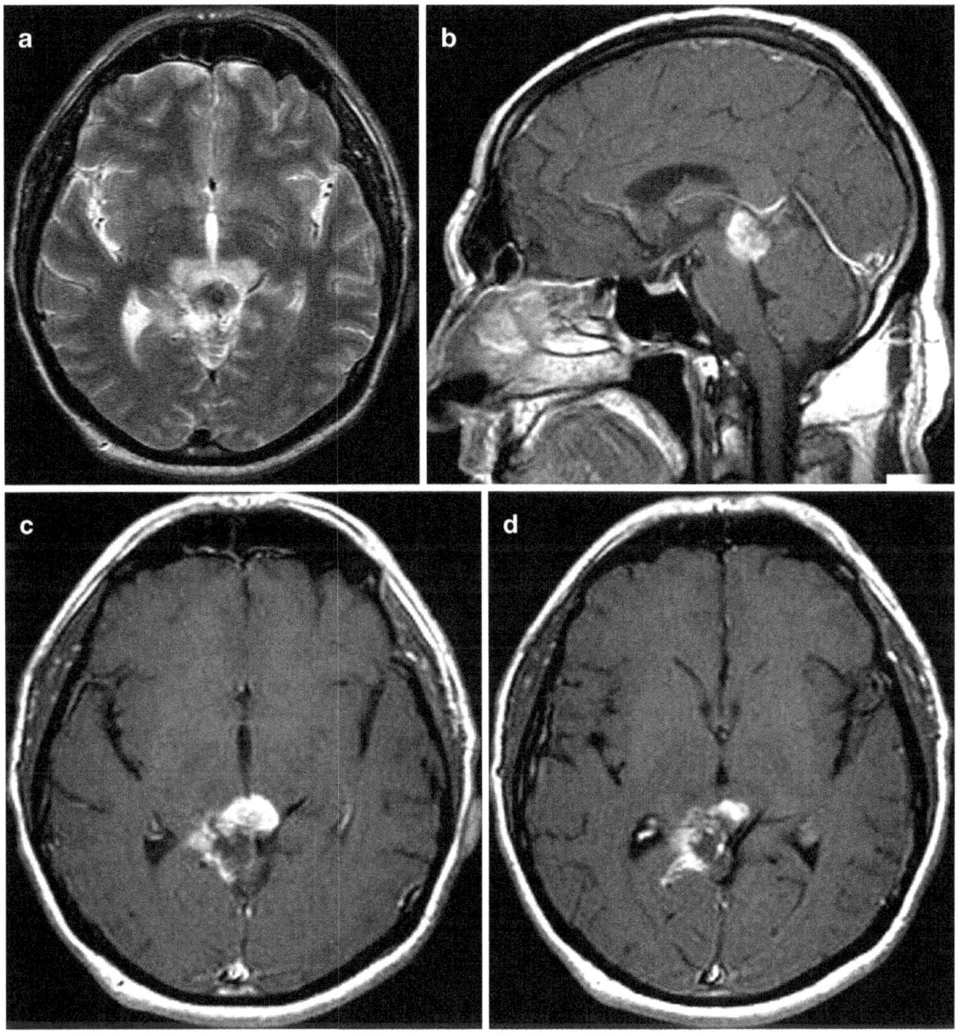

Fig. 16.12 Colorectal cancer metastases in the brain. In the pineal region on T2-weighted MRI (**a**), there is a space-occupying iso-hypointense lesion with signs of a moderate perifocal edema. Following intravenous CA administration on T1-weighted MRI in the sagittal (**b**) and axial (**c**, **d**) projections, its intense and inhomogeneous accumulation in the lesion is noted, with the spread of the tumor to the quadrigeminal plate

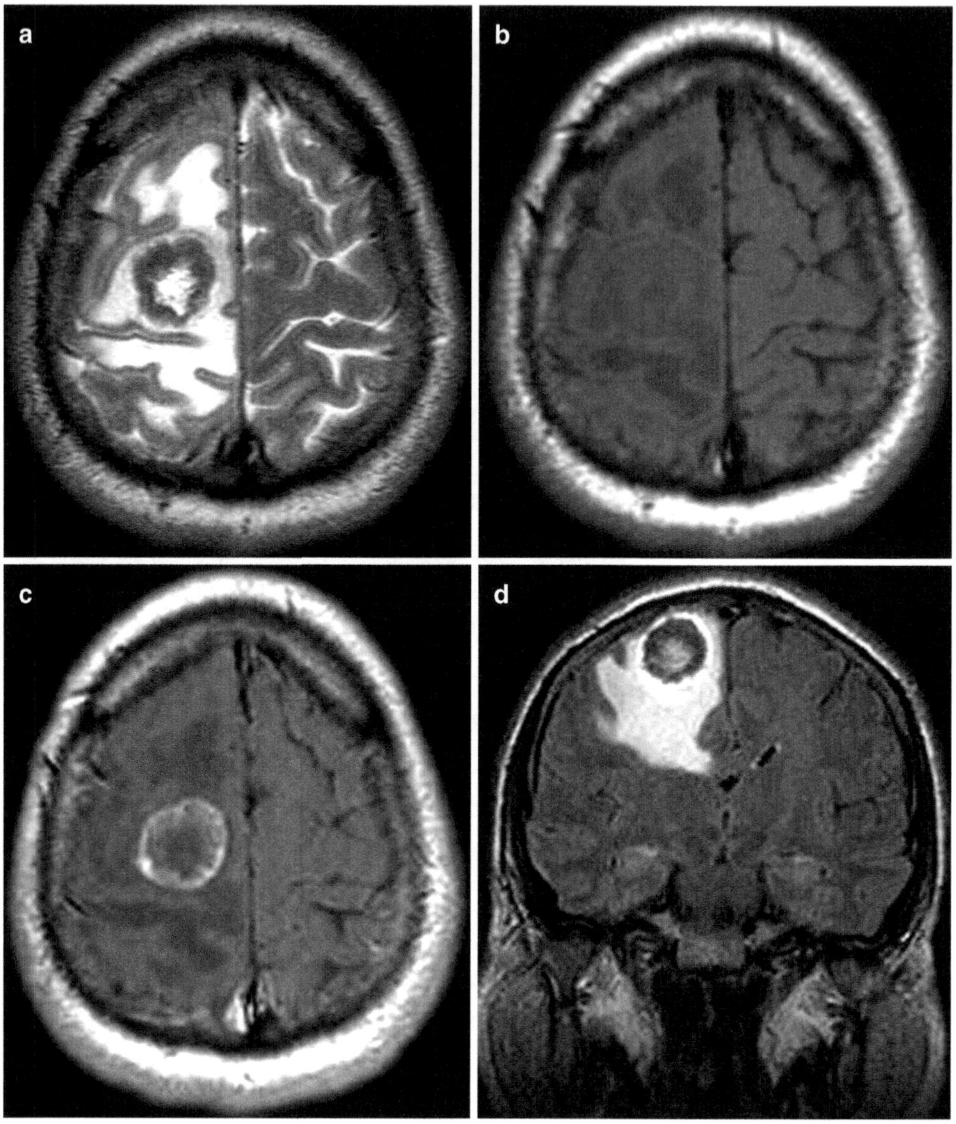

Fig. 16.13 Colorectal cancer metastases in the brain. In the right frontoparietal region, there is a space-occupying, heterogeneous lesion with signs of central necrosis (a hyperintense area on T2-weighted (**a**) and T2-FLAIR (**d**) MRI) with an expressed area of perifocal edema and intense CA accumulation on the periphery of the tumor (**c**)—ring enhancement. On T1-weighted MRI (**b**), the signal from the lesion is isointense, due to which the lesion is not differentiated on the background of edema

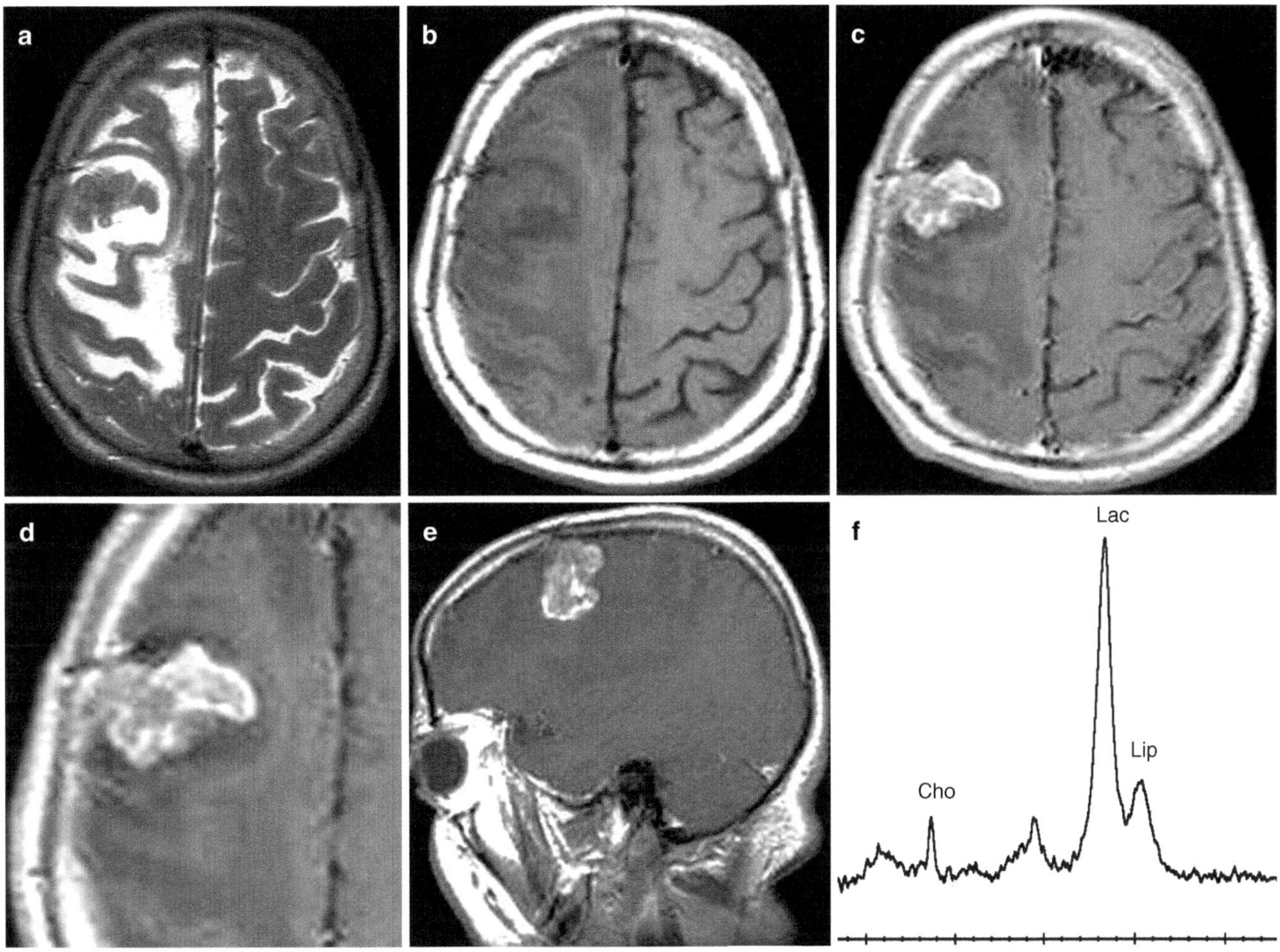

Fig. 16.14 Colorectal cancer metastases in the brain. In the right frontal lobe, there is a space-occupying lesion with an irregular shape and isointense signal on T2- and T1-weighted MRI (**a**, **b**), with a pronounced perifocal edema. After intravenous CA administration, on T1-weighted MRI in the axial (**c**, **d**) and sagittal (**e**) projections, its intense accumulation in the tumor is noted. On MR spectrum (**f**), there is an increase in the Lip-Lac complex and a moderate increase in the Cho peak

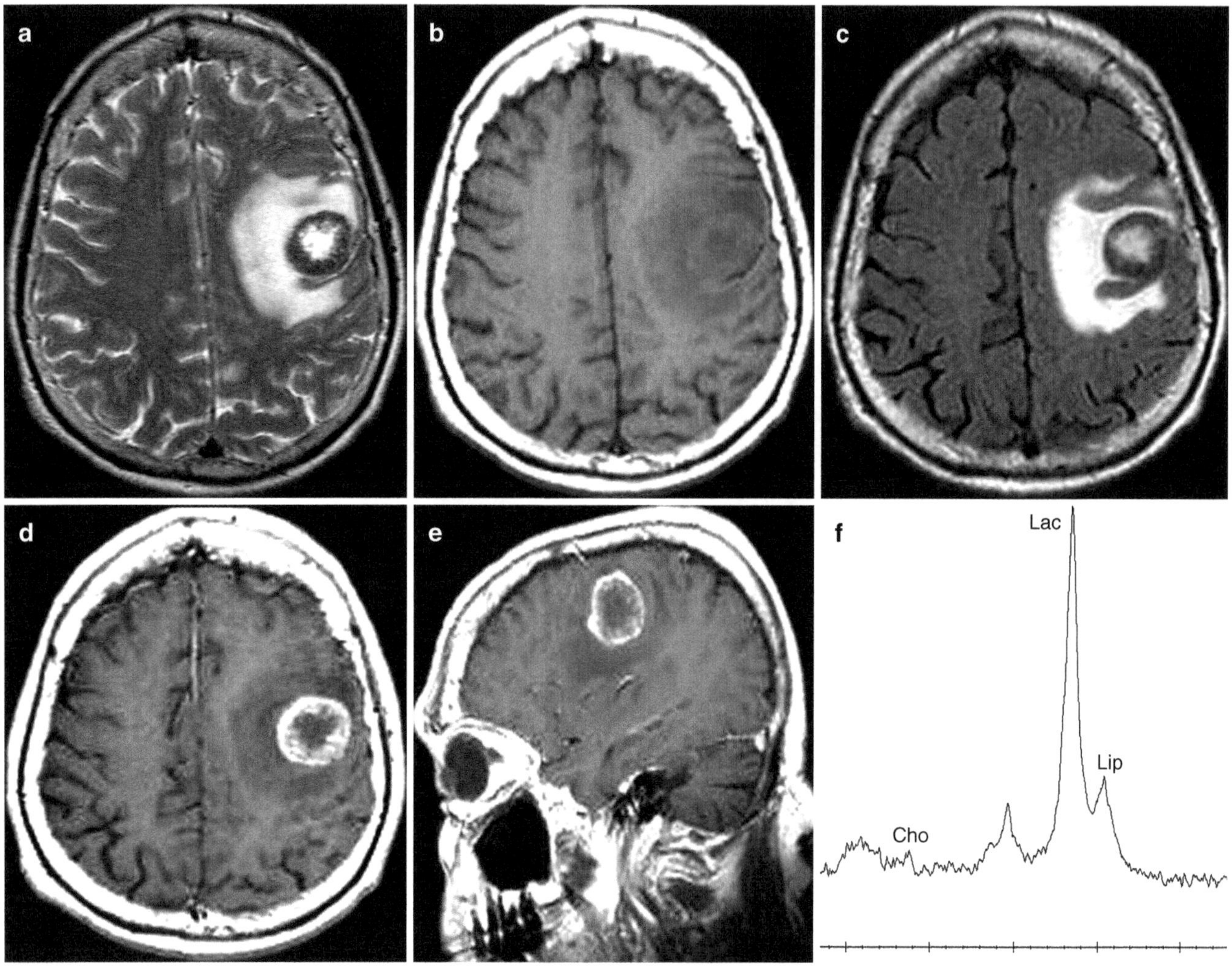

Fig. 16.15 Colorectal cancer metastases in the brain. In the left post-frontal region, there is an iso-hypointense lesion on T2-weighted MRI (**a**) with signs of central necrosis and an area of a pronounced perifocal edema. On T1-weighted MRI (**b**), the signal from the solid part of the lesion is isointense, while on T2-FLAIR MRI (**c**), it is significantly reduced. Following intravenous CA administration on T1-weighted MRI in axial T1 (**d**) and sagittal (**e**) projections, its intense and inhomogeneous accumulation (mostly along the periphery) is observed in the tumor. On the spectrum (**f**), a marked peak of the Lip-Lac complex is noted; other peaks, including Cho peak, are leveled

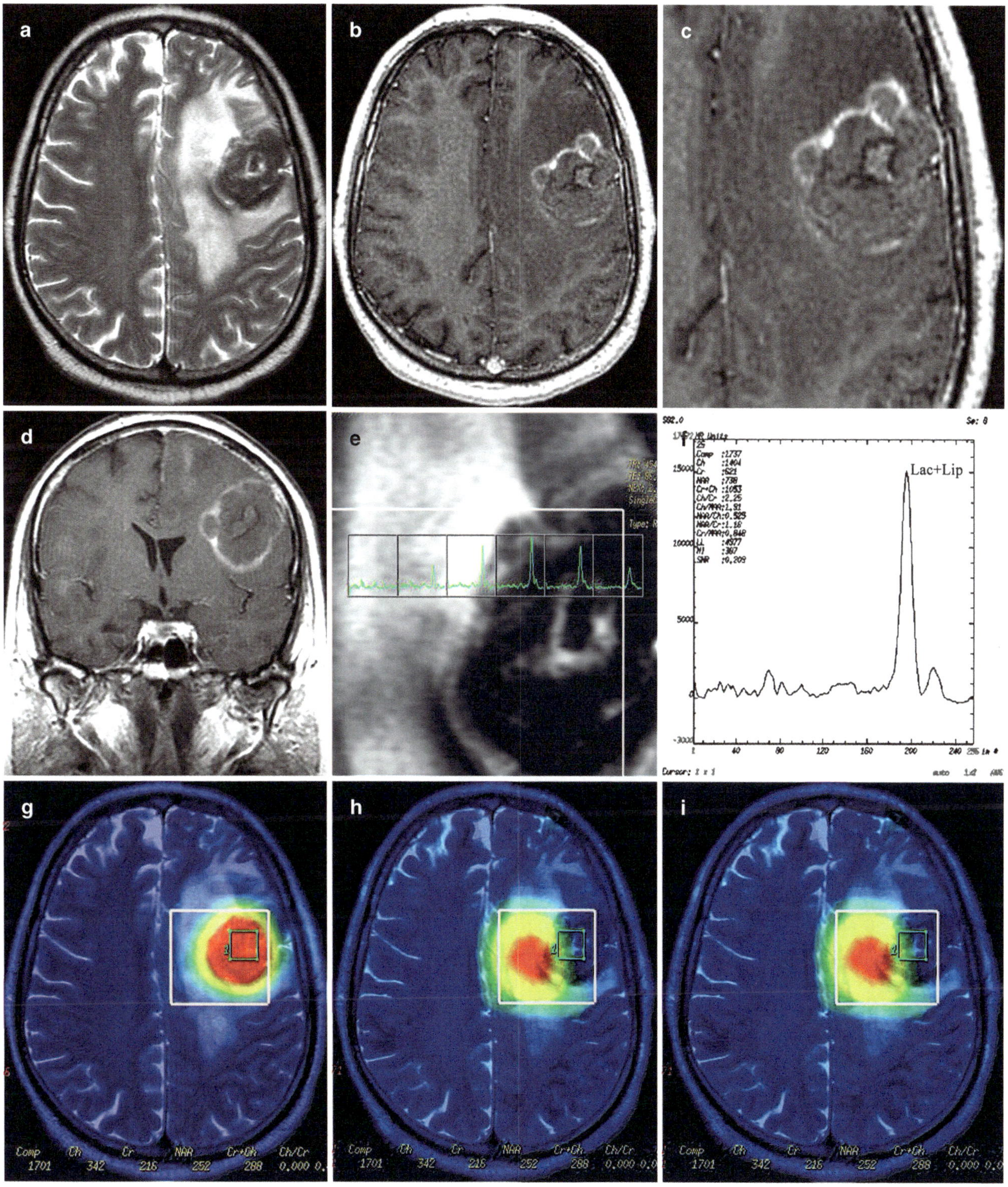

Fig. 16.16 Colorectal cancer metastases in the brain. Condition after radiosurgical treatment. In the left frontal region, there is a large space-occupying lesion, hypointense on T2-weighted MRI (**a**), with signs of central necrosis and a pronounced perifocal edema. After intravenous CA administration on T1-weighted MRI in the axial (**b**, **c**) and coronal (**d**) projections, there is its weak, inhomogeneous accumulation, more pronounced on the periphery of the lesion. On multi-voxel MR spectroscopy (**e**, **f**), the Lip-Lac complex prevails in the central parts of the metastasis. On the color maps of metabolite distribution (Lip-Lac, Cho, NAA), the boundary between Cho and NAA is clearly visualized (**g**–**i**)

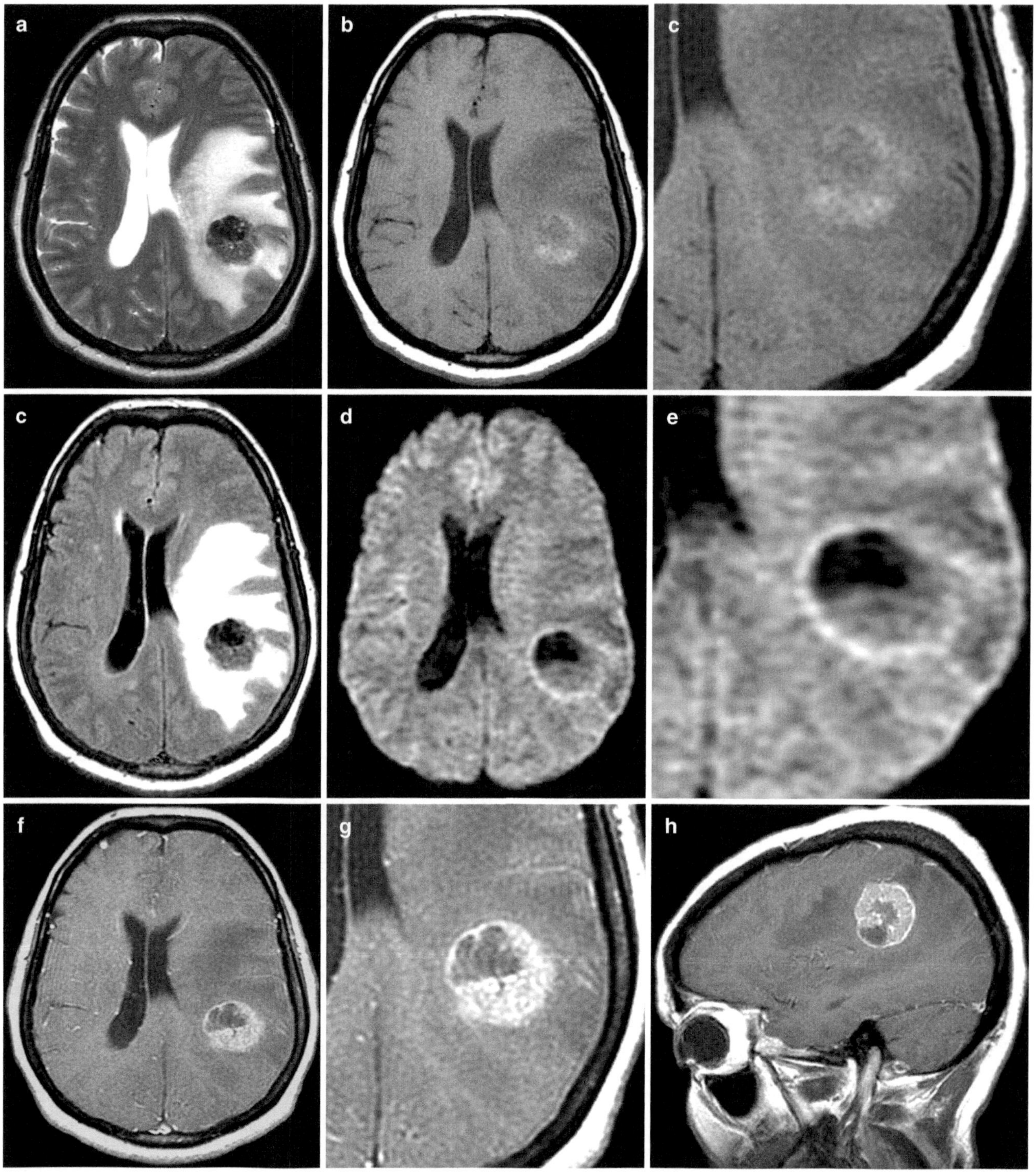

Fig. 16.17 Colorectal cancer metastases in the brain. In the left frontoparietal region, there is a large space-occupying lesion, heterogeneously hypointense on T2-weighted (**a**) and T2-FLAIR (**c**) MRI with a pronounced perifocal edema (a hyperintense zone) and mass effect, in the form of compression of the left lateral ventricle. On T1-weighted MRI (**b**, **c**), there are small hyperintense inclusions in the structure of the metastasis. On DWI MRI (**d**, **e**), on the anterior pole of the lesion, a hypointense site is clearly differentiated. After intravenous CA administration, on T1-weighted MRI in the axial (**f**, **g**) and sagittal (**h**) projections, its intense accumulation is noted along the contour of the lesion; a necrosis area is well differentiated along the anterior contour of the metastasis

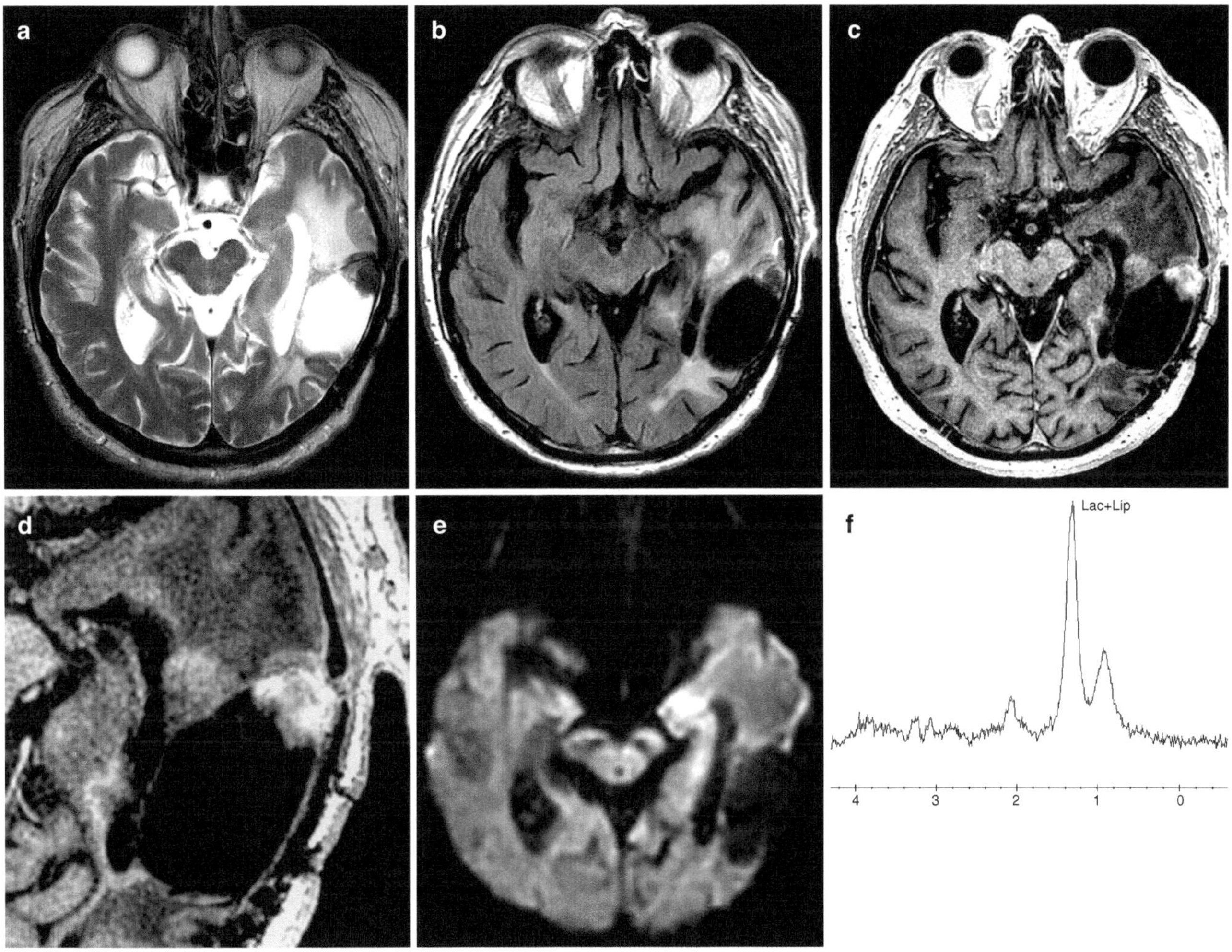

Fig. 16.18 Metastasis of colon cancer. Recurrence after surgical removal. In the left temporal lobe, anteriorly to the postoperative cavity, there is a space-occupying lesion characterized by a hypointense signal on T2-weighted (**a**), T2-FLAIR (**b**), and DWI (**e**) MRI. A quite severe edema of the brain substance persists in the left temporal region. After intravenous CA administration, on T1-weighted MRI (**c**, **d**), there is its intense accumulation in the tumor. On MR spectroscopy (**f**), there is a spectrum typical for the metastatic tumor—a high Lip-Lac complex

17 Stomach Cancer (SC)

In men, stomach cancer is detected two times more often than in women. According to IARC, the maximum incidence of stomach cancer was observed in men in Japan (Kutuki et al. 1996; Fan et al. 2004). In Russia, SC is second only to lung cancer, 48.8 thousand new cases of gastric cancer are reported annually, and 45,000 patients die from this disease each year. According to Davydov and Axel (2014), mortality from gastric cancer is one of the highest in Russia, ranking second among men (12.0%) after lung cancer and in women (10.0%) after breast cancer. Patients with SC have lower survival rates as compared to lung cancer, breast cancer, and kidney cancer (Go et al. 2011). In Western Europe and the USA, the 5-year survival rate ranges within 25%. In Japan, known for success in the treatment of gastric cancer, the figure is 66% among patients with primary gastric cancer and 68.2% among patients who underwent radical surgery (Verlato et al. 2012).

Most stomach carcinomas are adenocarcinomas and signet ring cell carcinomas. In 75% of newly diagnosed patients, the disease is identified in stages III–IV; the frequency of detection of early forms of gastric cancer does not exceed 10–20%. One of the potentially important markers that reflect the activity of metastases of stomach cancer is nm23 protein (nonmetastatic cell protein) (Ji et al. 2002; Lee et al. 2003).

The final destination of regional metastatic gastric cancer, regardless of the tumor site, is a para-aortic lymph collector. Even with a small depth of tumor invasion into the stomach wall, for example, to the level of its muscle membrane or submucosal layer, the frequency of lymphogenic metastases may increase from 15 to 40% (Lewis et al. 2008).

Stomach cancer metastasizes to the brain even more often than colorectal cancer. Kim (1999) noted the development of metastatic brain lesions in only 13 (0.2%) of 8080 patients with gastric carcinoma. In turn, York (1999) reported a 0.7% frequency of SC metastases to the brain in 23 of 3320 patients. Gastric cancer patients with brain metastases amount to not more than 1% of all cases of brain metastases, both according to autopsy findings and clinical manifestations (Zimm et al. 1981; Graf et al. 1988). Metastases in the brain develop 1–23 months after the diagnosis of gastric cancer, with the overall survival of patients of about 9 weeks. In our study, the proportion of stomach cancer metastases in the brain was 0.4% of all metastatic lesions.

There are no specific radiological signs that would allow to differentiate gastric cancer metastases in the brain from secondary tumors from other primary sites.

17.1 Clinical Cases

See Figs. 17.1, 17.2, 17.3, 17.4, 17.5, 17.6, 17.7, 17.8, 17.9, 17.10, and 17.11.

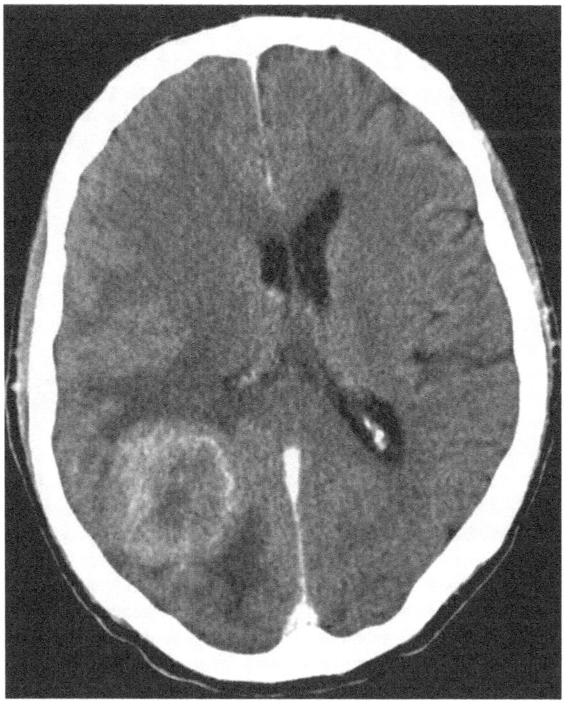

Fig. 17.1 A stomach cancer metastasis in the brain. On axial CT after intravenous CA administration, in the right parietal-occipital region, there is a large heterogeneous space-occupying lesion with an intense and uneven contrast media accumulation mainly on the periphery, with signs of a pronounced perifocal edema in the form of low-density areas (ring enhancement). The lateral ventricles are deformed

M. Dolgushin et al., *Brain Metastases*, DOI 10.1007/978-3-319-57760-9_17

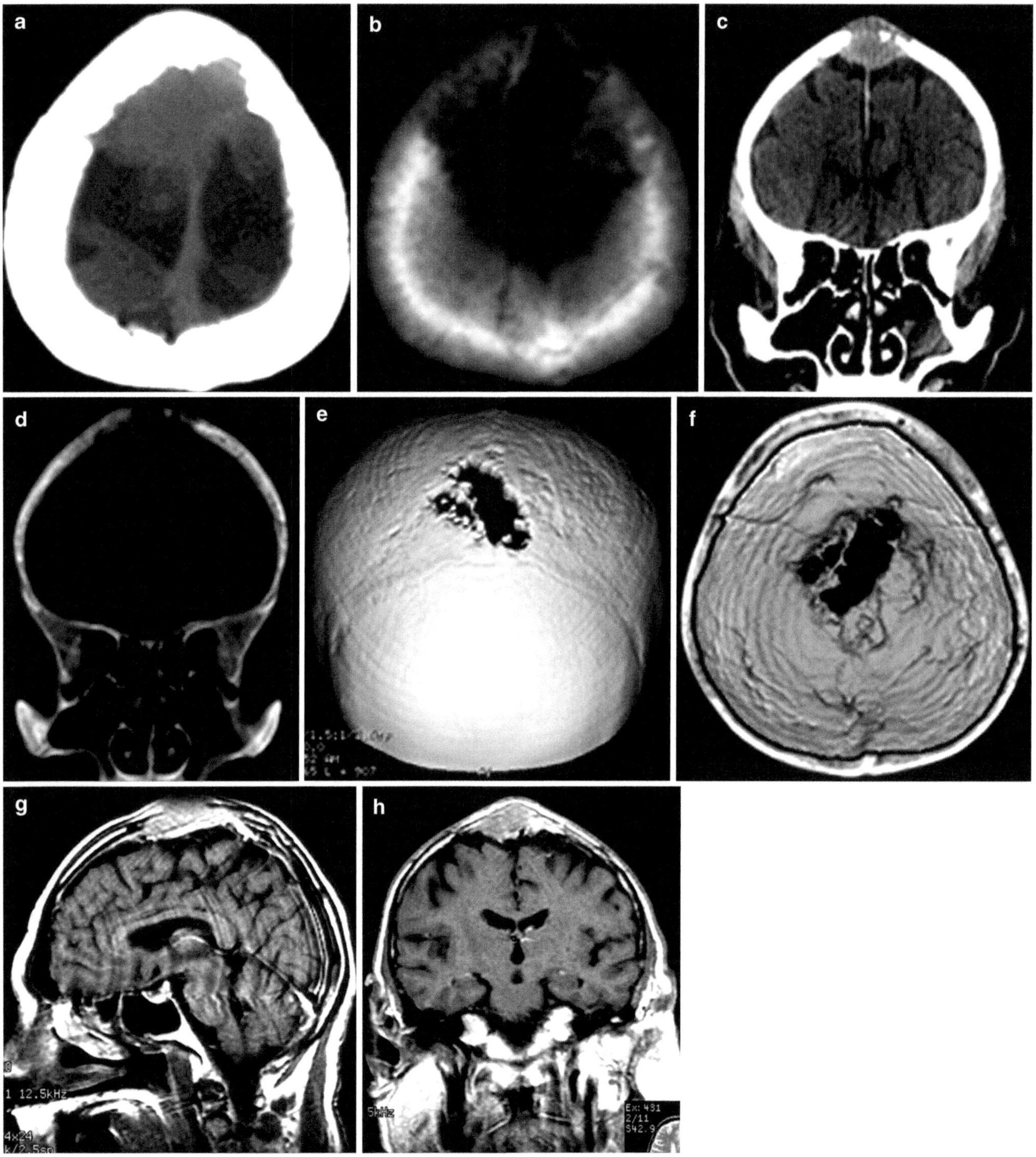

Fig. 17.2 A stomach cancer metastasis in the brain. A space-occupying lesion with an irregular shape, unclear contours, and intra- and extracranial spread, with the involvement of the dura mater and the superior sagittal sinus, is identified in the posterior part of the squama of the frontal bone. On CT in the axial (**a**, **b**) and coronary (**c**, **d**) projections, as well as on the 3D reconstruction (**e**, **f**), a portion of osteodestruction is determined. After intravenous CA administration on CT (**c**) and T1-weighted MRI in the sagittal (**g**) and coronary projections (**h**), there is intense accumulation of the contrast agent in the soft tissue of the metastasis. The metastasis grows into the superior sagittal sinus

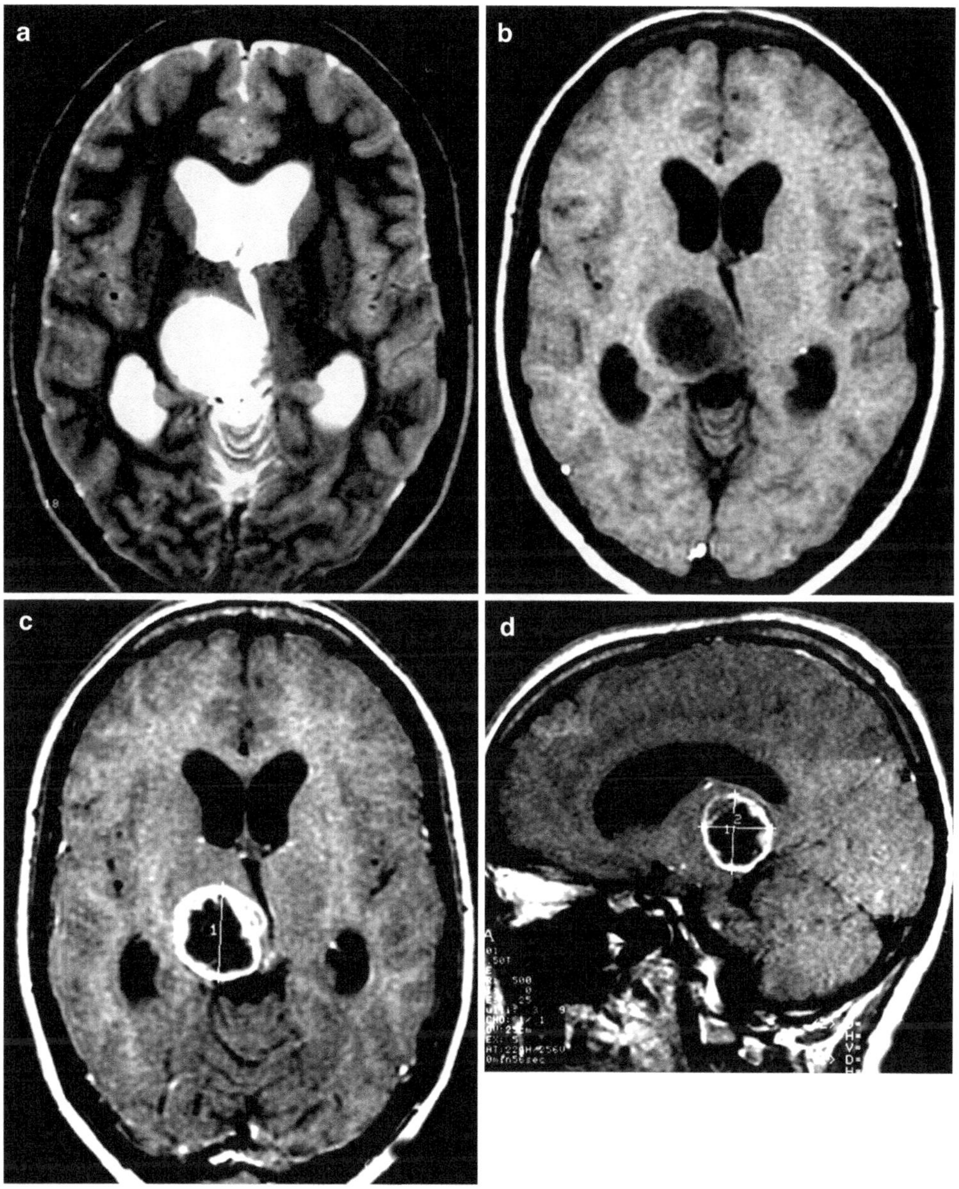

Fig. 17.3 A stomach cancer metastasis in the brain. In the projection of the right thalamus, there is a rounded space-occupying lesion with signs of central necrosis. On T2-weighted MRI, the lesion has a high signal (**a**); there is no perifocal edema. On T1-weighted MRI (**b**), the solid part of the metastasis has a moderately low signal, while its cystic part has a hypointense signal. After CA administration (**c**, **d**), the solid part of the tumor is intensely contrast enhanced

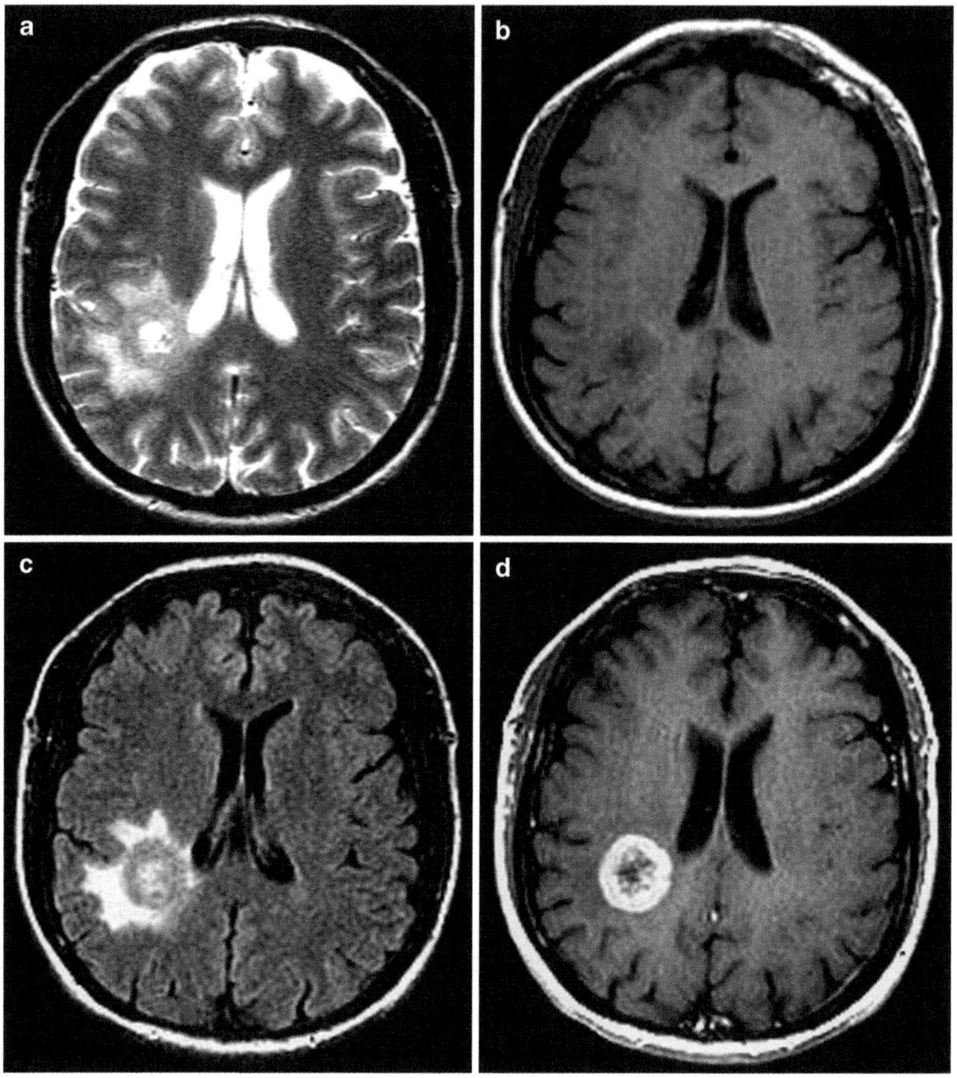

Fig. 17.4 A stomach cancer metastasis in the brain. A rounded, space-occupying lesion is detected in the deep parts of the right frontoparietal region. On T2-weighted (**a**) and T2-FLAIR (**c**) MRI, there is a hyperintense area with perifocal edema—a picture of ring enhancement. On T1-weighted (**b**) MRI, the signal from the solid part of the tumor is reduced. Following intravenous CA administration on T1-weighted MRI (**d**), its intense and inhomogeneous accumulation (mostly along the periphery) is observed in the metastasis tissue

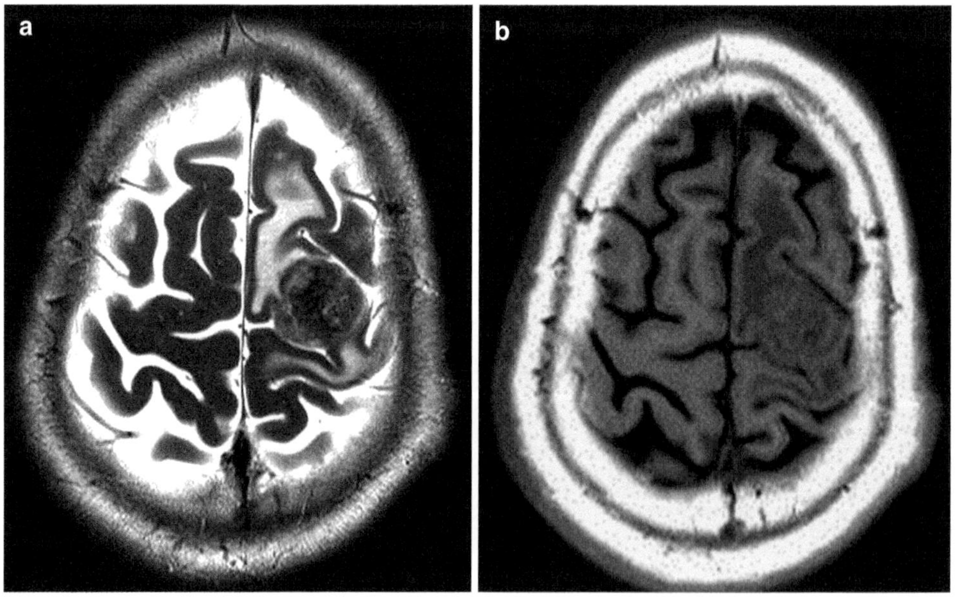

Fig. 17.5 A stomach cancer metastasis in the brain. In the left frontal region on T2-weighted MRI (**a**), there is a hypointense space-occupying lesion with a hyperintense area with an expressed perifocal edema on T2-weighted (**a**) and T2-FLAIR MRI (**c**). Before CA administration on T1-weighted MRI (**b**), the lesion has an isointense MR signal and is poorly differentiated. After intravenous CA administration on T1-weighted fat sat MRI (**d**), its intense and inhomogeneous accumulation is observed in the tumor

Fig. 17.5 (continued)

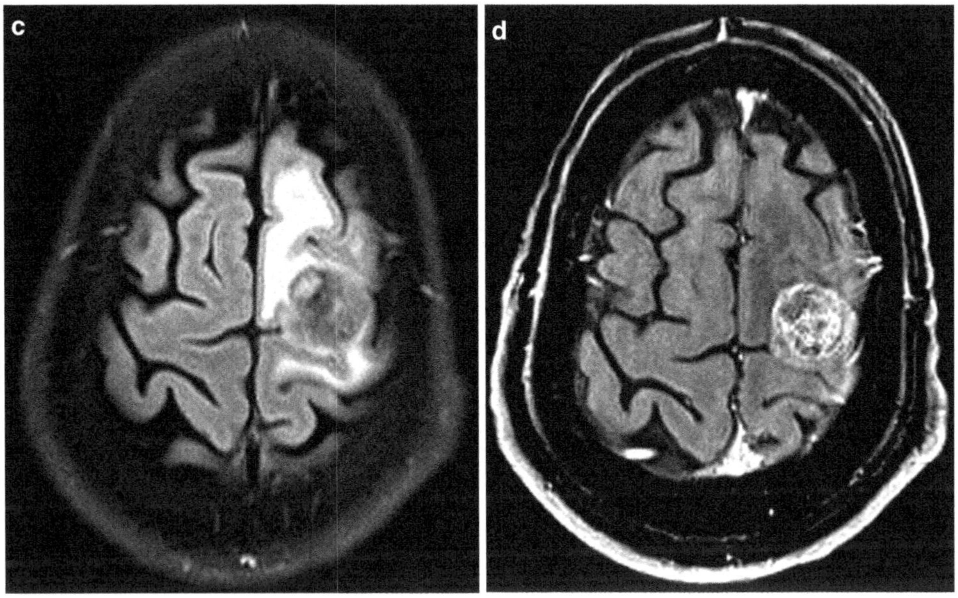

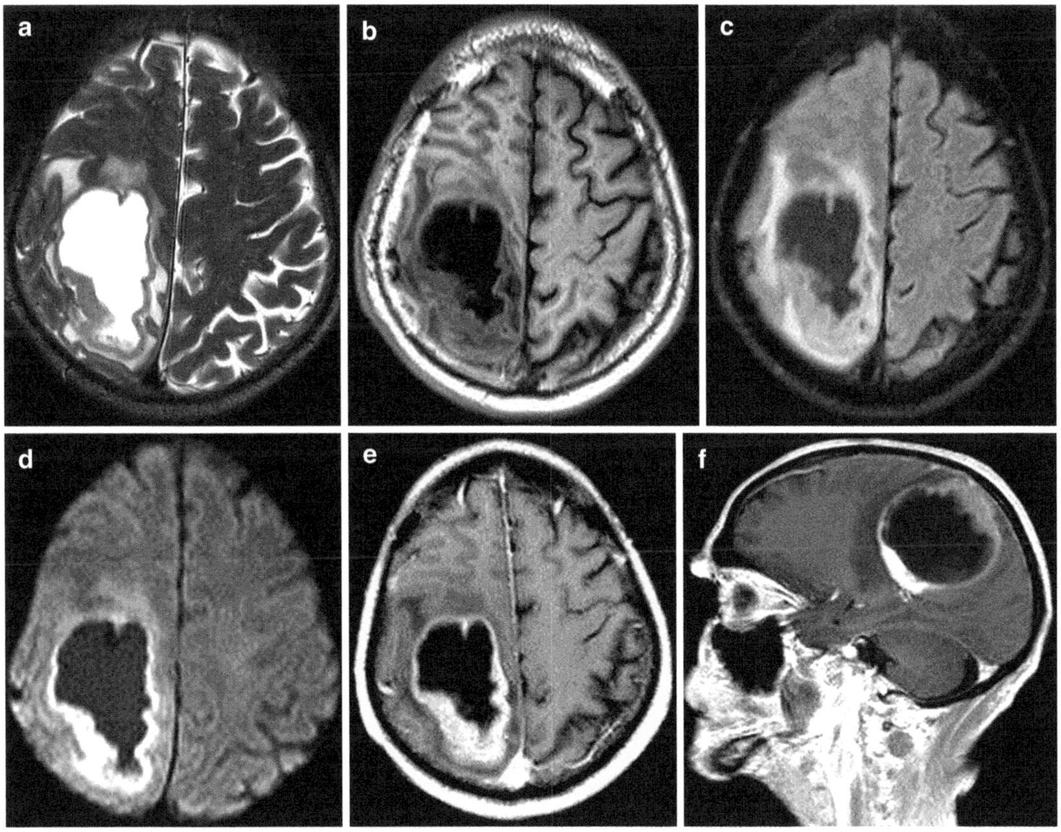

Fig. 17.6 A stomach cancer metastasis in the brain. In the right frontoparietal region, there is a large solid-cystic nodule with signs of a mild perifocal edema on T2-weighted and T2-FLAIR MRI (**a**, **c**). The solid part of the lesion, the most pronounced on the anterior and posterior pole of the metastasis, is characterized by a hypointense signal on T1-weighted MRI (**b**), a moderately hyperintense signal on T2-weighted and T2-FLAIR MRI (**a**, **b**), and a hyperintense signal on DWI MRI (**d**). Following intravenous CA administration on T1-weighted MRI in the axial (**e**) and sagittal (**f**) projections, its intense accumulation is observed in the solid component of the tumor

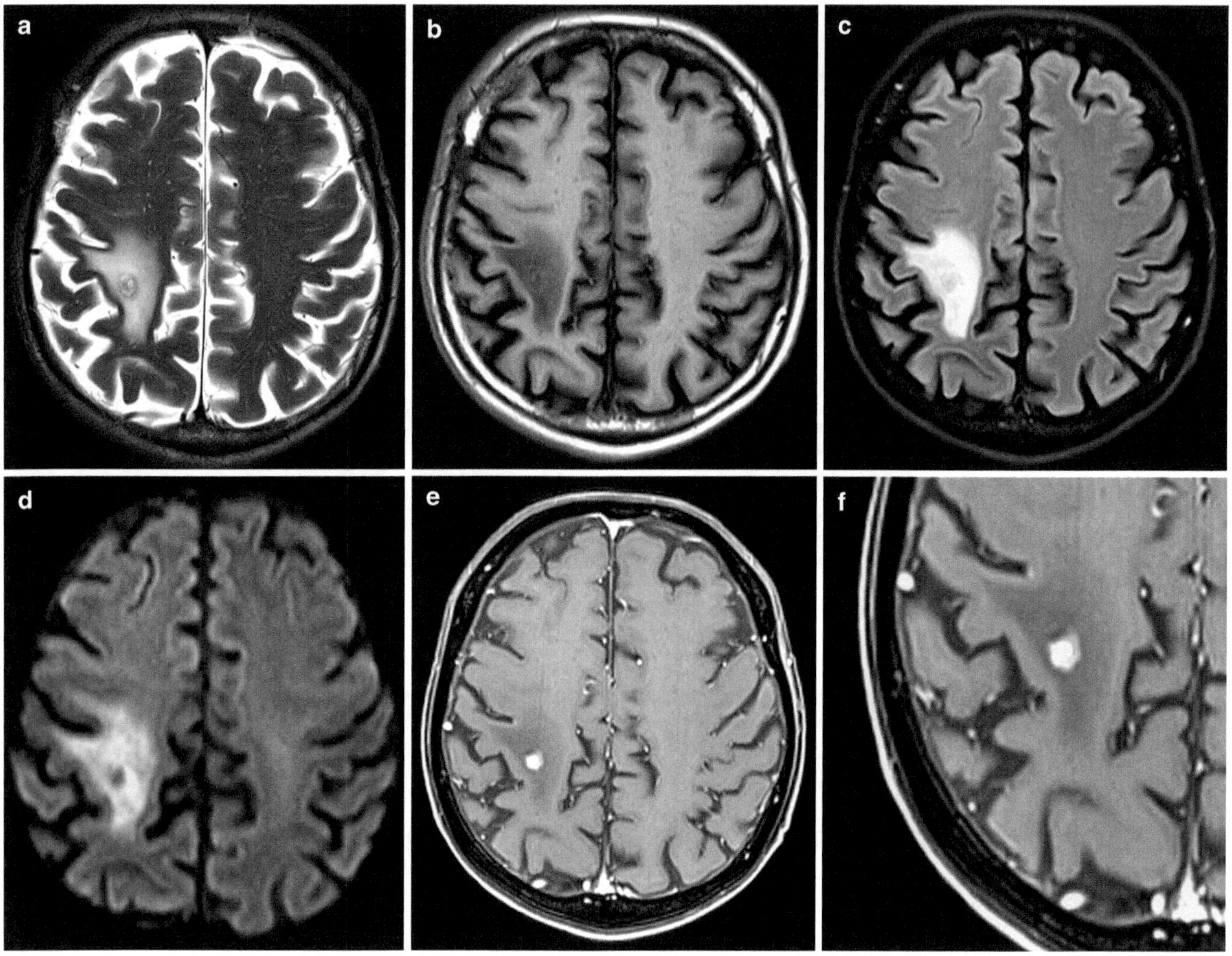

Fig. 17.7 A stomach cancer metastasis in the brain. In the deep parts of the right parietal region, there is an individual small focal lesion with an expressed area of perifocal edema on T2-weighted and T2-FLAIR MRI (**a**, **c**). The tumor lesion is characterized by a hypointense signal on T1-weighted (**b**) and DWI MRI (**d**). Following intravenous CA administration on T1-weighted fat sat MRI (**e**, **f**), its intense and relatively uniform accumulation in the tumor is observed

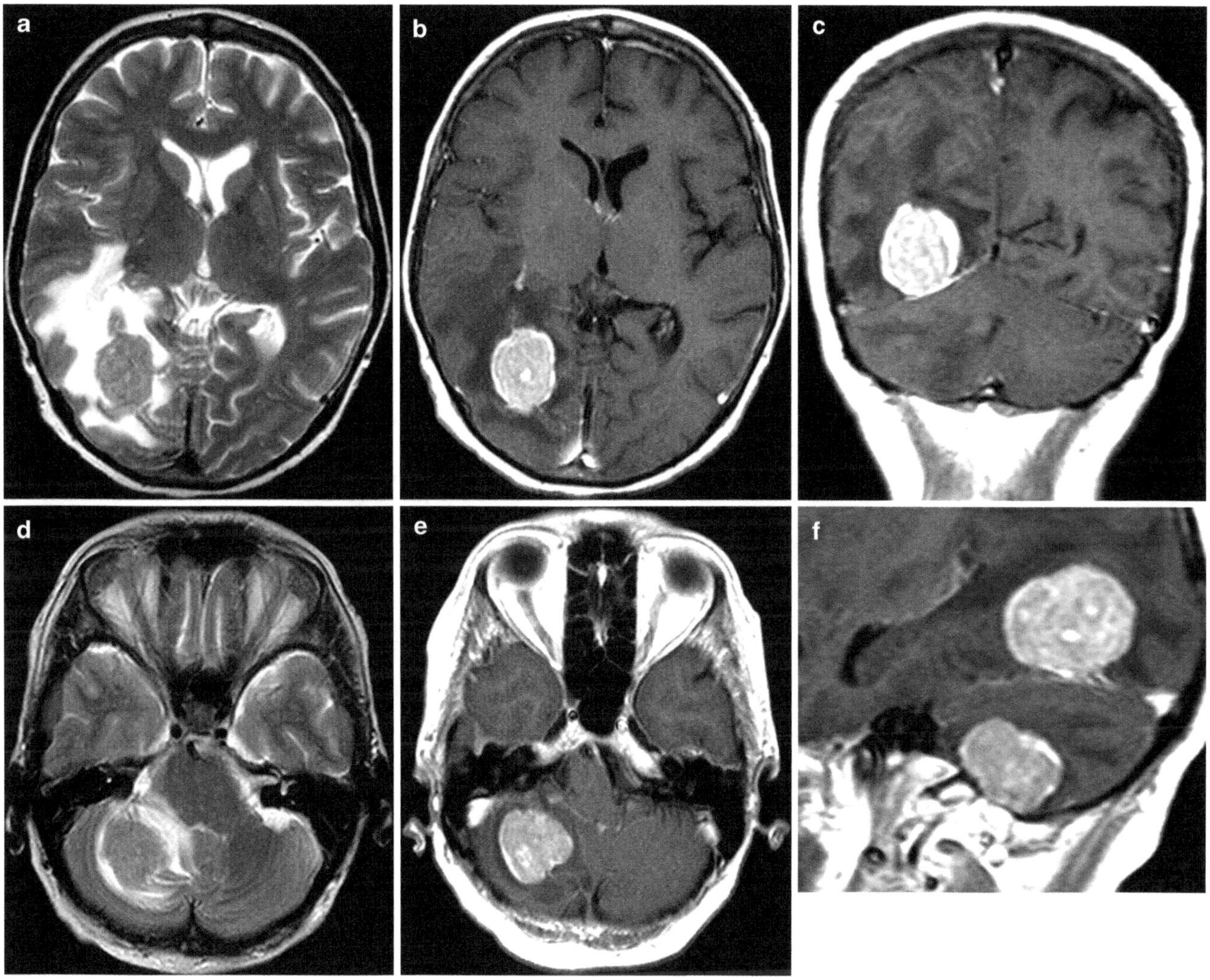

Fig. 17.8 Multiple stomach cancer metastases in the brain. A two level study. In the right hemisphere of the cerebellum and in the right occipital region, there are two large space-occupying lesions with a slightly increased signal on T2-weighted MRI (**a, d**) with signs of a pronounced perifocal edema. After intravenous CA administration, on T1-weighted MRI in the axial (**b**, **e**), coronary (**c**), and sagittal (**f**) projections, there is its intense and relatively homogeneous accumulation in the tumor lesions, with the "upper" metastasis having signs of infiltration of the cerebellar tentorium and formation of a "tail." There is no area of central necrosis

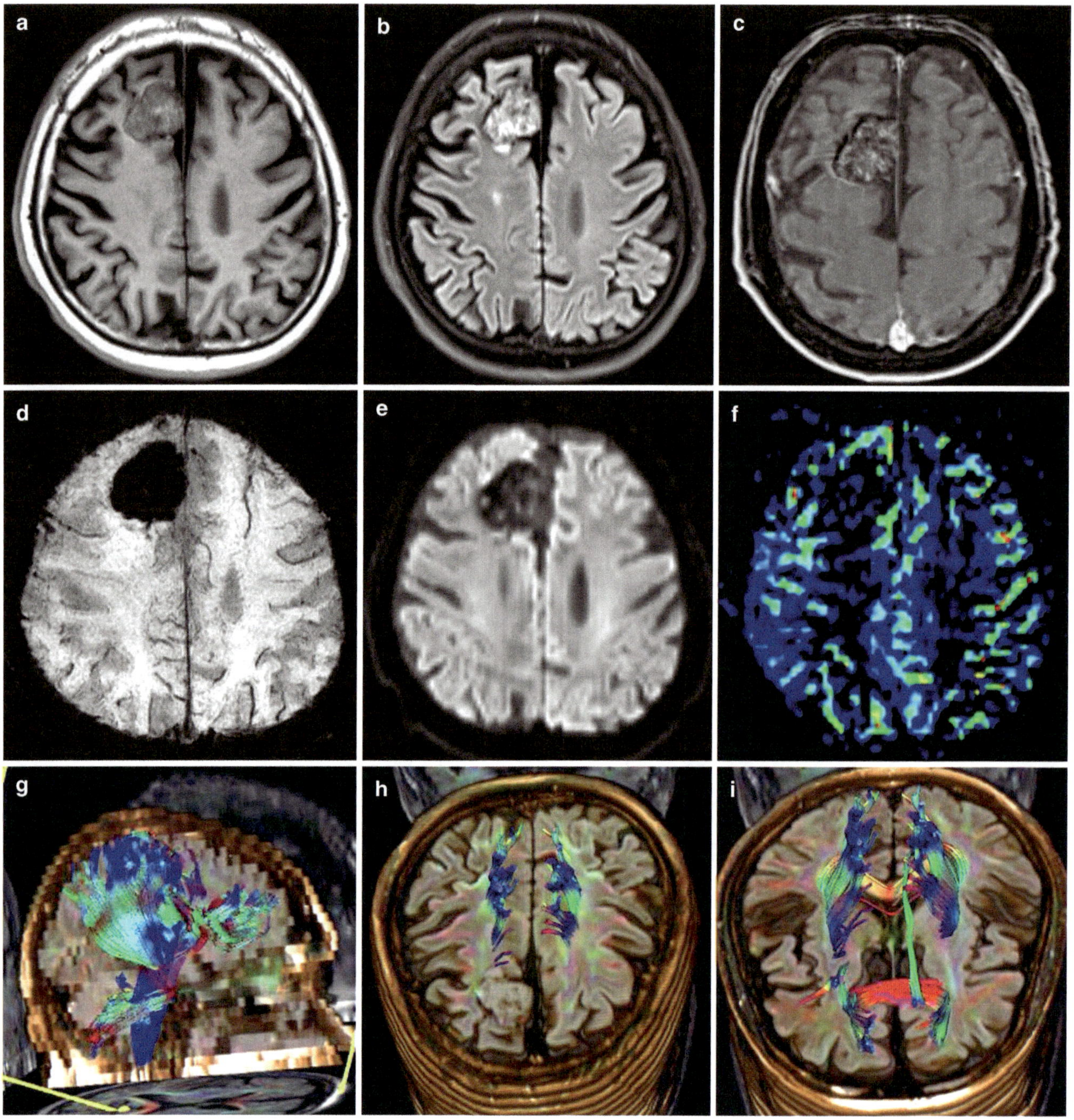

Fig. 17.9 A metastasis of gastric cancer. Condition after radiosurgical treatment. In the right frontal lobe, there is a large space-occupying lesion, tightly adjacent to the falx, with no apparent signs of perifocal edema. The lesion is characterized by a hypointense signal (with the presence of small hyperintense fragments) on T1-weighted MRI (**a**) and a moderately high signal on T2-FLAIR MRI (**b**). Following intravenous CA administration on T1-weighted fat sat MRI (**c**), its insignificant fragmentary accumulation in the tumor is observed. On SWI (**d**) and DWI MRI (**e**), the signal from the lesion is sharply reduced. On ASL MRI, in the structure of the lesion, the decreased perfusion is decreased (**f**). On MR tractography (**g**, **h**, **i**), the deformation of the conductive pathways is determined along the periphery of the tumor; the conductive pathways downward from the tumor are intact

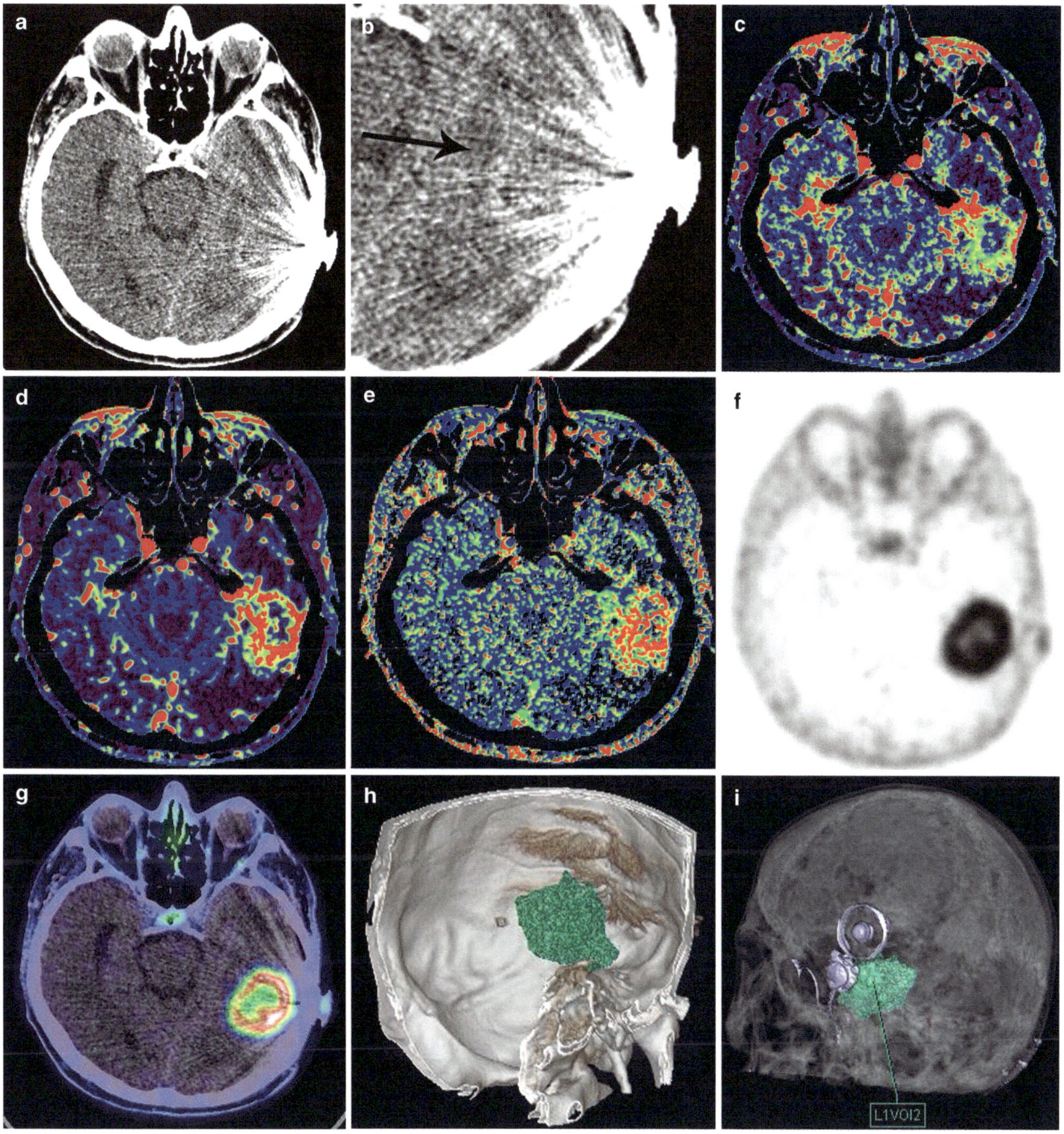

Fig. 17.10 A stomach cancer metastasis in the brain. On CT (**a**), on the background of artifacts from the hearing aids, only posterior portions of the tumor are weakly visualized in the left temporal region (**b**)—the *arrow*. On CT perfusion maps, the lesion is characterized by high levels of CBV (**c**), CBF (**d**), and MTT (**e**). On PET/CT with intravenous administration of ^{18}F-choline, there is high RP accumulation (**f**). In superimposed PET/CT images (**g**), the artifact from the metal construction is smoothed, while on 3D reconstructions (**h**, **i**), the relation of metastasis to the bone structures of the skull and the hearing aid is well visualized

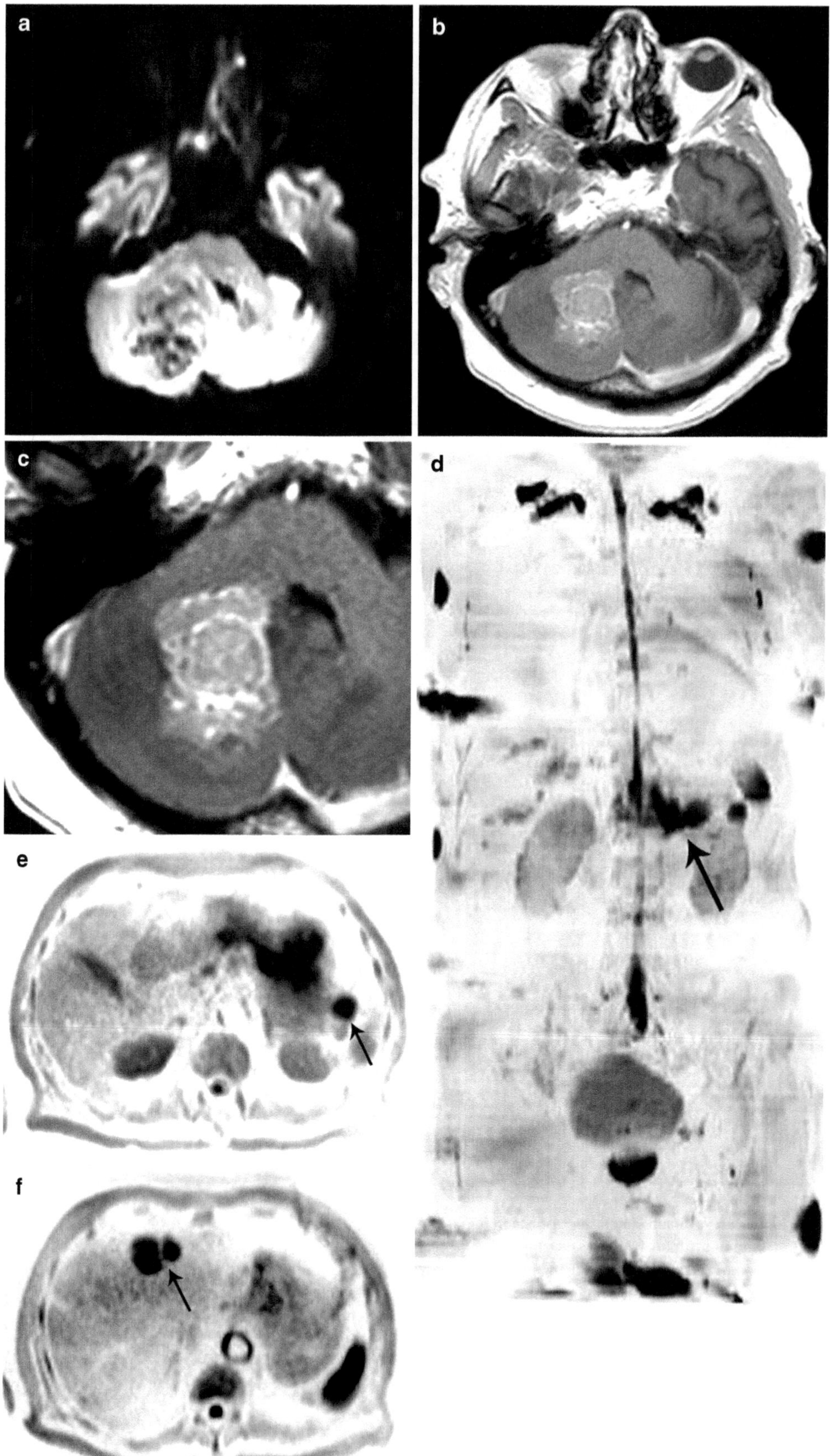

Fig. 17.11 A stomach cancer metastasis in the brain. In the right hemisphere of the cerebellum, there is a large space-occupying lesion with an iso-hypointense signal on DWI MRI (**a**); after CA administration, its intense accumulation in the metastasis (**b**, **c**) is noted. Of note is the presence of two sites of tumor growth anteriorly and posteriorly from the main rounded tumor lesion. In the whole-body MR-DWI study (**d**–**f**), there is an increased signal area in the projection of the cardia, in precardiac lymph nodes, and in the liver parenchyma, consistent with a tumor in the stomach with metastases in the regional lymph nodes and liver (the *arrows*)

18 Esophageal Cancer (EC)

Esophageal cancer (EC) is a malignancy that is also relatively rare in the European part of Russia; however, in recent years, according to Lagergren and Lagergren (2002), its incidence is increasing. The annual incidence of EC in Russia is more than 7000 people. The disease develops predominantly in men (over two times more often than in women). Most esophageal cancer patients belong to the age group over 60 years. Its histological types include squamous cell EC, accounting for 90% of cases, and adenocarcinoma; small cell carcinoma, carcinosarcoma, etc. are very rarely diagnosed. The prognosis for two main histological types of EC is unfavorable—the 5-year survival rate is 10–15% (Sundelof et al. 2002).

EC metastasizes to the brain, according to Weinberg et al. (2003) and Song et al. (2014), who studied large groups of patients with EC ($n = 1588$ and $n = 1612$, respectively), in 1.7% and 1.6% of cases. Thus, Song et al. noted that squamous cell EC metastasizes to the brain more frequently than adenocarcinoma. In most cases, brain metastases develop in patients with large primary esophageal tumors and metastatic involvement of distant lymph nodes. Intracranial EC metastases account for less than 1% of all malignant tumor metastases in the brain. We observed esophageal cancer metastases in the brain in four patients (less than 1%).

18.1 Clinical Cases

See Figs. 18.1 and 18.2.

M. Dolgushin et al., *Brain Metastases*, DOI 10.1007/978-3-319-57760-9_18

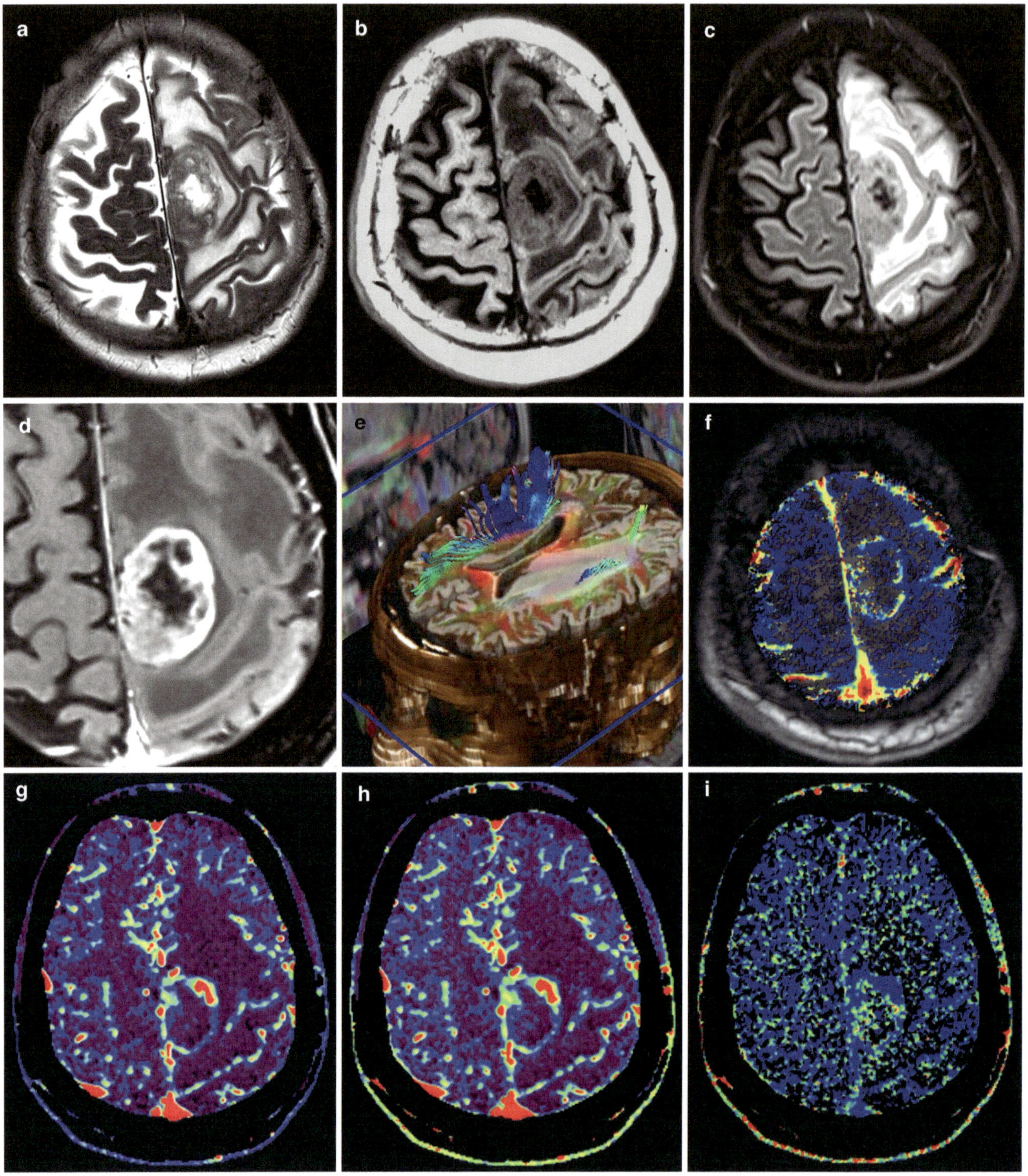

Fig. 18.1 An esophageal cancer metastasis in the brain. In convexital portions of the left postfrontal area, there is a large space-occupying heterogeneous lesion, partially adjacent to the falx, with signs of central necrosis. On T2-weighted and T2-FLAIR MRI (**a**, **c**), the signal from the lesions is heterogeneous; the hyperintense area with an expressed perifocal edema is well visualized. The solid part of the lesion is characterized by a moderately low signal on T1-weighted MRI (**b**) and an isointense signal on T2-FLAIR MRI (**c**). Following intravenous CA administration, on T1-weighted fat sat MRI (**d**), its intense and inhomogeneous accumulation is observed in the solid part of the metastasis. On MR tractography (**e**), there is deformation of the conductive paths in this region. On Ktrans maps (**f**), its higher values are observed along the periphery of the lesion. On CT perfusion maps of CBV (**g**) and CBF (**h**), along the anterior pole of the metastasis, an increased perfusion area is observed, and MTT (**i**) values are reduced. On CT without contrast enhancement, the lesion is not clearly visualized on the background of the expressed perifocal edema (**j**). On PET/CT with ^{18}F-tyrosine (**k**, **l**), there is its intense accumulation in the solid component of the tumor and no accumulation in the central area of necrosis

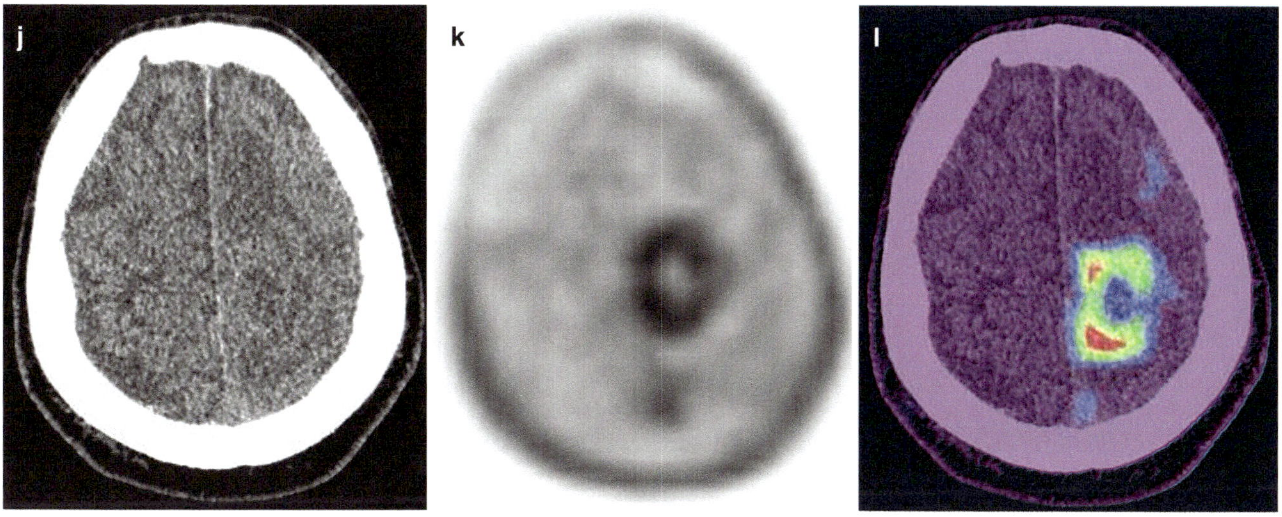

Fig. 18.1 (continued)

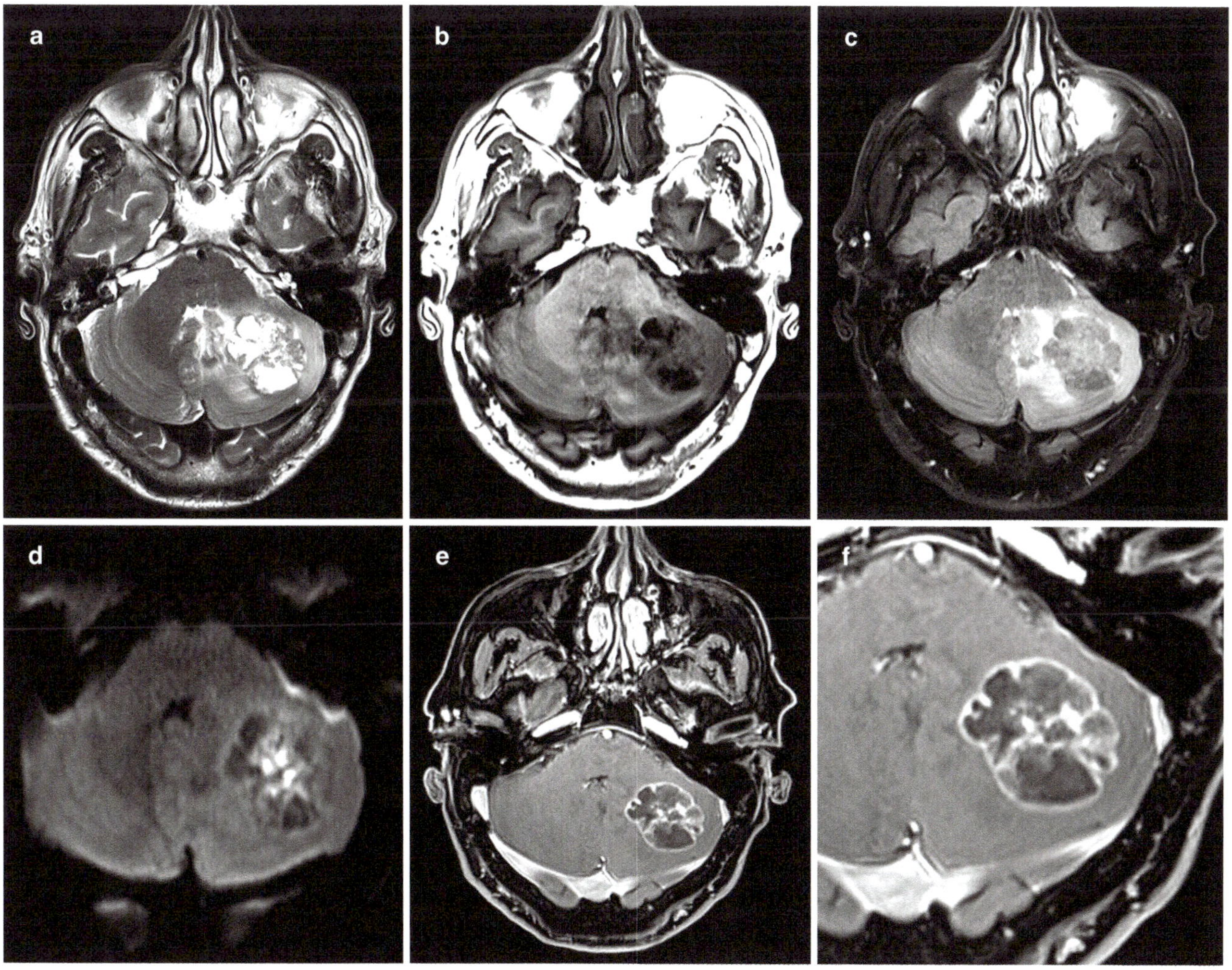

Fig. 18.2 A metastasis of esophageal cancer. In the left hemisphere of the cerebellum, there is a heterogeneous lesion with an iso-hyperintense signal on T2-weighted (**a**), T2-FLAIR (**c**), and DWI (**d**) MRI and an iso-hypointense signal on T1-weighted MRI (**b**), with a hyperintense area of perifocal edema on T2-weighted (**a**) and T2-FLAIR (**c**) MRI. Following intravenous CA administration on T1-weighted fat sat MRI (**e**, **f**), there is its intense accumulation in the solid part of the tumor, with multiple trabeculae being differentiated in the metastasis structure. There is an area with reduced perfusion in the structure of the lesion on ASL (**g**). On SWI MRI (**h**, **i**), in the metastasis structure, there are multiple pinpoint areas with a low signal

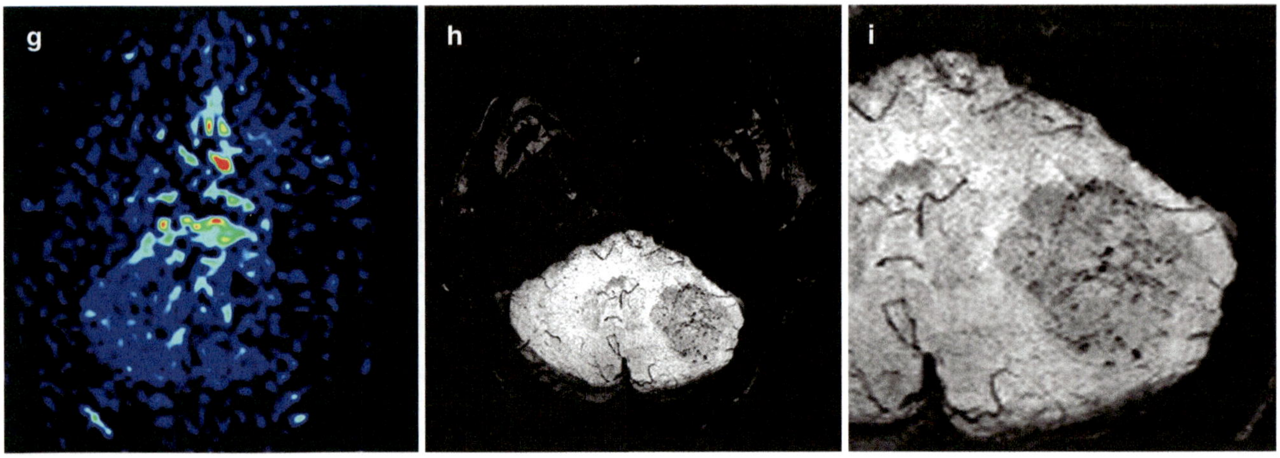

Fig. 18.2 (continued)

19 Pancreatic Cancer (PC)

Pancreatic cancer (PC) is a highly aggressive disease, accounting for up to 3% of malignant tumors. In Russia, more than 14,000 cases of pancreatic cancer are diagnosed each year. According to Lemke et al. (2013), the 5-year survival rate is only 5%. More than 90% of pancreatic cancer is represented by cancer that develops from the pancreatic ductal epithelium (mainly adenocarcinoma) and 10.5% by cancer arising from islet cells. The prognosis for these patients is extremely unfavorable. Pancreatic carcinomas are primarily characterized by the lymphogenous spread to the regional lymph nodes and lymph collectors around the celiac trunk and aorta (Pneumaticos et al. 2009). Hematogenous metastases of pancreatic cancer affect the liver (80% of cases), peritoneum (50%) (Schneider et al. 2005), lungs (17%) (Sancho-Chust 2009), less frequently muscles (Wafflart et al. 1996), kidneys (Martino et al. 2004), skin (Otegbayo et al. 2005), heart (Robinson et al. 1982), pleura (Turiaf et al. 1969), stomach (Takamori et al. 2005), and prostate (Merseburger et al. 2005).

The spread of tumor cells to colonize distant organs is a major factor in deaths of cancer patients (Steeg et al. 2016).

Pancreatic cancer rarely metastasizes to the brain (El Kamar et al. 2004; Lemke et al. 2013; Matsumoto and Yoshida 2015). According to the literature, a total of 18 cases were described of pancreatic cancer with brain metastases since 1978 (Table 19.1). Park et al. (2003) identified metastases to the brain in only four patients (0.3%) in the group of 1229 patients with pancreatic cancer; the median survival in this group was 2.9 months (Table 19.1). In our clinical sample, pancreatic cancer metastases developed in six cases (less than 1%).

Multiple brain metastases in prostate cancer may be localized both supra- and subtentorially. Most of them have a cystic nature and manifest with annular accumulation of the contrast medium. The presence of cystic metastases of pancreatic cancer was observed in the majority of case series from various authors. In our material, the metastatic prostate cancer in the brain manifested in the form of a single node, with clearly separated, intensely contrast-enhanced capsule and small areas of CA accumulation in the central parts. Such an X-ray picture can be typical for intracerebral tumors; in addition, the presence of a clearly differentiated capsule in these cases does not exclude an inflammatory origin of abnormalities (e.g., abscess). Using additional methods, including CT perfusion, helps establish the correct diagnosis; however, identification of tumors is often achieved only by a biopsy.

M. Dolgushin et al., *Brain Metastases*, DOI 10.1007/978-3-319-57760-9_19

Table 19.1 Localization of pancreatic cancer metastases in the brain structures

	Author (No.)	Year	Number of patients	Sex/age	Site of metastases in the brain
1	Ferreira Montero V. et.al.	1983	1	M/62	No data available
2	Shangaĭ V.A.	1984	1	M/57	No data available
3	Kuratsu jun-ichi et.al.	1990	2	M/56	Thalamus
				M/58	vermis cerebelli
4	Ohira et al.	1991	1	M/25	bilateral temporal
5	Tsuji et al.	1996	1	F/62	Multiple
6	Ferreira Filho et al.	2001	1	M/49	Carcinomatous meningitis
7	Yamada K. et.al.	2002	1	M/62	Multiple
8	Park K.S. et al.	2003	4	M/48	Multiple
				M/51	L. frontal lobe
				M/52	L. parietal lobe
				M/62	L. frontal, L. basal ganglia
9	El Kamar FG	2004	1	M/56	hemispheres and pons
10	Caricato M. et.al.	2006	1	M/67	Cerebellum
11	Kimura et al.	2008	1	M/50	Multiple
12	Naugler C. et.al.	2008	1	F/66	Pinus
13	Zaanan et al.	2009	1	M/57	Multiple
14	Matsumura T. et.al.	2009	1	M/64	No data available
15	Marepaily et al.	2009	1	F/36	Cerebellum
16	Shah SU et al.	2011	5	F/75	L. choroid
				F/43	R. choroid
				M/54	R. choroid
				F/73	L. choroid
				F/79	R. choroid
17	Lemke et al.	2011	2	F/48	Cerebellum
				M/66	R. parietal lobe
18	Chiang et al.	2012	1	M/54	L. frontal lobe
19	Rajappa et al.	2013	1	M/71	R. occipital lobe
20	Rao et al.	2013	1	M/57	Multiple
21	Matsumoto H. et al.	2015	1	M/68	R. temporoparietal region
22	Kumar A. et al.	2015	8	?/49-70	L. parieto-occipital region
					R. parietal lobe
					Multiple, CN XII
					Multiple
					Clivus, pituitary stalk, CNVI
					Cerebellar vermis, fourth ventricle
					Choroid
					Multiple
23	Dolgushin	2015	1	F/66	Brainstem

1. Ferreira MV, Eiras AJ, Gómez PR, Montori LM, Valero PM. Cerebral metastasis, idiopathic pneumoperitoneum and obstructive jaundice as clinical manifestations of carcinoma of the pancreas. Rev Esp Oncol. 1983;30(3):399–409.
2. Shangaĭ VA, Gavrik I. Metastasis of pancreatic cancer to the brain. Vrach Delo. 1984;11:77.
3. Kuratsu J, Murakami M, Uemura S, Ushio Y. Brain and skull metastases of hepatic or pancreatic cancer—Report of six cases. Neurol Med Chir (Tokyo). 1990;30:476–82.
4. Ohira Y, Kaga K, KodamaA. A case of bilateral sudden hearing loss and vertigo caused by bilateral temporal bone metastasis from pancreatic carcinoma – Comparison of clinical findings and temporal bone pathological findings. Nihon Jibiinkoka Gakkai Kaiho. 1991;94:9–15.
5. Tsuji Y, Ohigashi H, Ishikawa O, Yasuda T, Nakano H, Nakamori S, et al. A case of non-resectable pancreatic cancer surviving more than 4 years by intra-arterial infusion chemotherapy with angiotensin-II. Gan To Kagaku Ryoho. 1996;23:1617–20.
6. Ferreira Filho AF, Cardoso F, Di Leo A, Awada A, da Silva VD, Tovar RB, Schwartsmann G. Carcinomatous meningitis as a clinical manifestation of pancreatic carcinoma. Ann Oncol. 2001;12:1757–59.
7. Yamada K, Miura M, Miyayama H, Sakashita N, Kochi M, Ushio Y. Brain metastases from asymptomatic adenocarcinoma of the pancreas: an autopsy case report. Surg Neurol. 2002;58(5):332–36.
8. Park KS, Kim M, Park SH, Lee KW. Nervous system involvement by pancreatic cancer. J Neurooncol. 2003;63:313–16.

9. El Kamar FG, Jindal K, Grossbard ML, Mizrachi HH, Kozuch PS. Pancreatic carcinoma with brain metastases: case report and literature review. Dig Liver Dis. 2004;36(5):355–60.
10. Caricato M, Borzomati D, Ausania F, Garberini A, Rabitti C, Tonini G, Coppola R. Cerebellar metastasis from pancreatic adenocarcinoma. A case report. Pancreatology. 2006;6:306–8.
11. Kimura H, Furukawa Y, Kuwada Y, Hananoki M, Matsumoto N, Yamamoto M, et al. A patient with pancreatic cancer associated with brain and skin metastases. Suizou. 2008;23:74–82.
12. Naugler C, Xu Z. Pancreatic adenocarcinoma metastatic to the pineal gland. J Clin Neurosci. 2008;15(11):1284–86.
13. Zaanan A, Lequoy M, Landi B, Lievre A, Franco D, Taïeb J. Brain metastases from pancreatic adenocarcinoma. BMJ Case Rep. 2009;2009.
14. Matsumura T, Ohzato H, Yamamoto T, Ota K, Mabuchi E, Miwa H, et al. A case of postoperative brain metastasis originated from pancreatic cancer which was successfully treated by resection and postoperative irradiation. Gan To Kagaku Ryoho. 2009;36:2433–5.
15. Marepaily R, Micheals D, Sloan A, Hatfield J, Adsay V, Joyrich R, et al. Octreotide uptake in intracranial metastasis of pancreatic ductal adenocarcinoma origin in a patient with a prolonged clinical course. Dig Dis Sci. 2009;54:188–90.
16. Shah SU, Shields CL, Bianciotto CG, Shields JA. Pancreatic cancer metastasis to choroid. Ophthalmology. 2011;118(7):1483.
17. Lemke J, Barth TF, Juchems M, Kapapa T, Henne-Bruns D, Kornmann M. Long-term survival following resection of brain metastases from pancreatic cancer. Anticancer Res. 2011;31:4599–603.
18. Chiang KC, Yu CC, Chen JR, Huang YT, Huang CC, Yeh CN, Tsai CS, Chen LW, Chen HC, Hsu JT, et al. Oncocytic-type intraductal papillary mucinous neoplasm (IPMN)-derived invasive oncocytic pancreatic carcinoma with brain metastasis—A case report. World J Surg Oncol. 2012;10:138.
19. Rajappa P, Margetis K, Wernicke G, Ginter P, Cope W, Sherr DL, et al. Stereotactic radiosurgery plays a critical role in enhancing long-term survival in a patient with pancreatic cancer metastatic to the brain. Anticancer Res. 2013;33:3899–903.
20. Rao R, Sadashiv SK, Goday S, Monga D. An extremely rare case of pancreatic cancer presenting with leptomeningeal carcinomatosis and synchronous intraparenchymal brain metastasis. Gastrointest Cancer. Res. 2013;6:90–2.
21. Matsumoto H, Yoshida Y. Brain metastasis from pancreatic cancer: A case report and literature review. Asian J Neurosurg. 2015;10:35–9.
22. Kumar A, Dagar M, Herman J, Iacobuzio-Donahue C, Laheru D. CNS involvement in pancreatic adenocarcinoma: a report of eight cases from the Johns Hopkins Hospital and review of literature. J Gastrointest Cancer. 2015;46(1):5–8.
23. Rotin DL, Dolgushin MB, Pronin IN, et al. Brain metastasis of ductal pancreatic adenocarcinoma. Oncosurgery. 2011;3:78–81.

19.1 Clinical Cases

See Figs. 19.1 and 19.2.

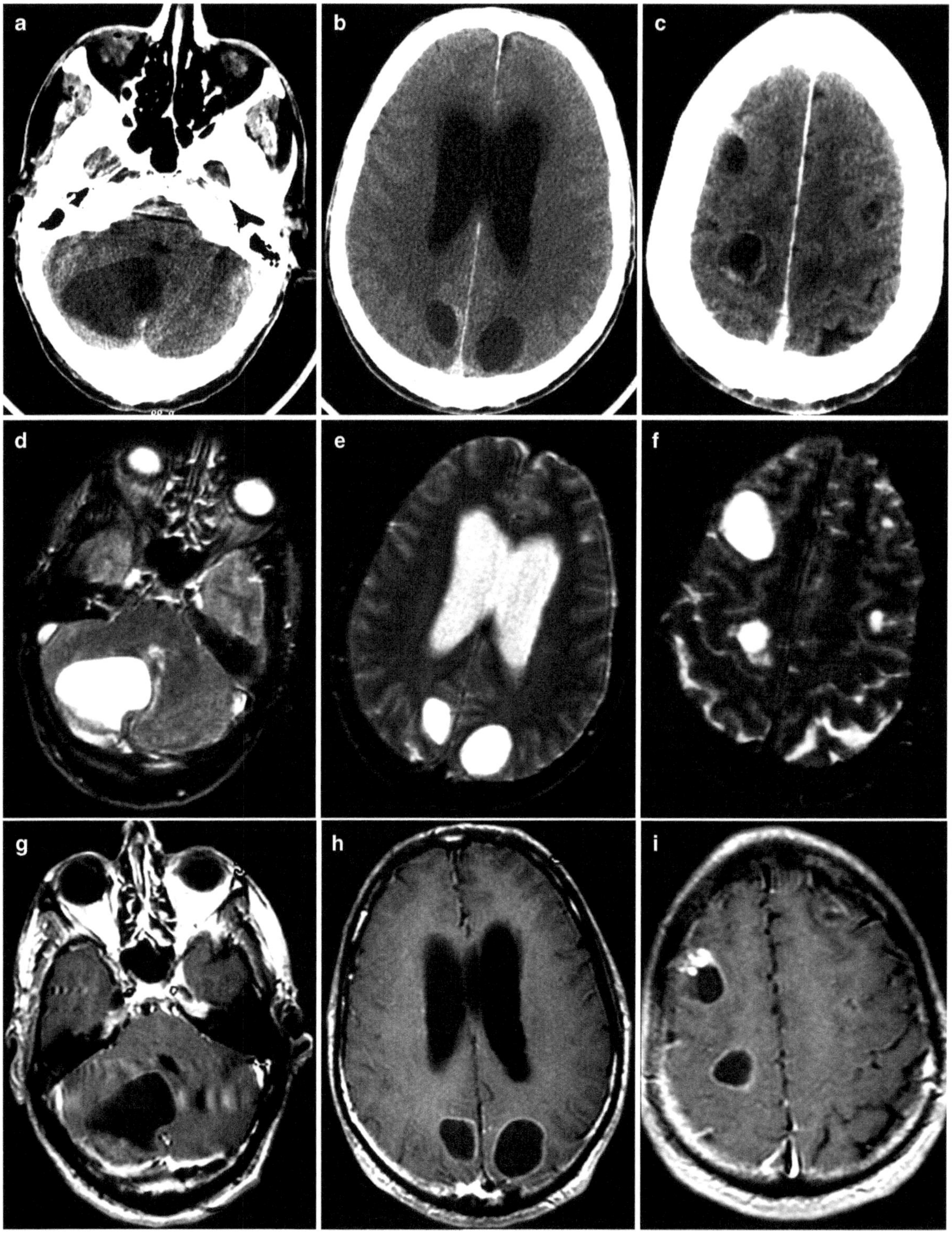

Fig. 19.1 Multiple pancreatic cancer metastases in the brain. A three-level study. On CT (**a–c**) and T2-weighted MRI (**d–f**), in the brain matter, there are multiple rounded cysts with clear contours, with a very weakly expressed or non-expressed hyperintense area of perifocal edema; after CA administration, on T1-weighted MRI (**g–i**), its intensive accumulation is noted along the contour of metastases

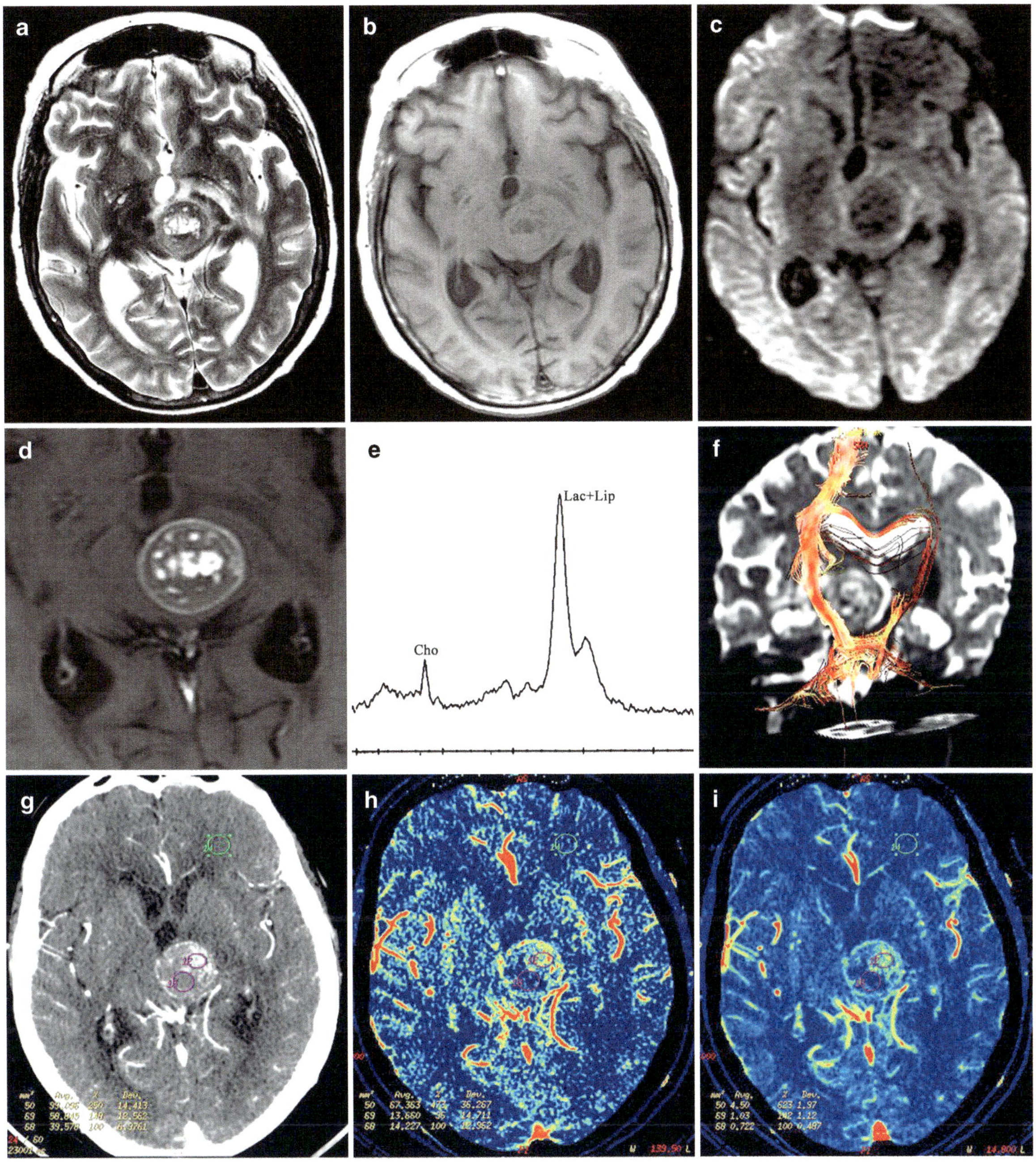

Fig. 19.2 A pancreatic cancer metastasis in the brain. In the projection of the left cerebral peduncle with transition to the thalamus, there is a rounded space-occupying lesion with clear margins, a heterogeneously increased signal on T2-weighted MRI (**a**), an isointense signal on T1-weighted MRI (**b**), and a hypointense signal on DWI MRI (**c**). After CA administration (**d**), its intense lumpy accumulation is noted in the central parts of the metastasis, as well as accumulation in the form of a thin rim. On the spectrum (**e**), there is a pronounced prevalence of the Lip-Lac complex peak and a small Cho peak. On tractography (**f**), the lateral dislocation of conductive pathways is well differentiated. On contrast-enhanced CT (**g**), the metastasis intensely accumulates the contrast agent. On CT perfusion, there is a marked increase in CBV (**h**) and CBF values (**i**), mostly along the anterior pole of the metastasis

20 Prostate Cancer (PrC)

Prostate cancer (PrC) is the most common solid tumor in men and the second by mortality rate in male population (Jeman et al. 2007). According to Jemal et al. (2011), the estimated number of PrC cases in 2016 in the USA will reach nearly 181,000 people, which makes up 21% of all cancers in men, and 126,000 will presumably die from this disease (8%). In Russia, almost 27,000 males develop PrC annually. According to Davydov and Axel (2014a, b), in the structure of morbidity of malignant neoplasms, PrC amounts to 12.1% and is the leader by an increase in its incidence rate in the male population (35.8%).

Although the incidence and survival rates vary widely in different EU countries, mortality rates do not differ significantly. PrC mortality tends to decrease, both in the USA and in the EU. The survival rate has increased, probably due to more active implementation of early diagnostic procedures and screening programs. Thus, the 10-year and 15-year survival rate has already reached 93% and 77%, respectively. Studies showed that men diagnosed with PrC in the early stages had a minimal risk of death from cancer during 20 years after the diagnosis. PrC in elderly men is a greater problem in the developed countries, where the percentage of relatively older men is higher. Thus, according to Steliarova-Foucher and Parkin (2011), PrC accounts to about 15% of cancers in men in developed countries, whereas it is only 4% in developing countries. It should be noted that the incidence of PrC varies considerably depending on the region. For example, according to the data published by the Swedish National Board of Health and Welfare, Stockholm, in this country, characterized by a high life expectancy and a relatively low mortality from diseases associated with smoking, PrC accounted for 37% of all new cancer cases in 2004.

PrC most often metastasizes to the bones, liver, lungs, and lymph nodes and rarely to the brain. According to different authors, bone tissue metastases in PrC amount from 54 to 85%. Thus, according to Ganova et al. (2014), who studied PrC metastases in young and middle-aged men, more than 80% of the lesions are located in the bones of the pelvis and the lumbar spine. The authors noted that 73% of patients were aged 54–59 years.

PrC metastases to the bones are mostly multiple, often of an osteoblastic type, though there are also lytic lesions. Note that bone involvement occurs in 95% of PrC patients with brain metastases. Concomitant involvement of the bones and lungs accounts for 31% of cases, while of the bones, lungs, and liver accounts for 19%.

Metastases to the brain in the presence of concomitant visceral metastases indicate an active process in the internal organs. The combination of metastatic brain lesions with other organ involvement is typical of PrC. Prostate cancer metastasizes to the brain 28 months after the initial diagnosis.

Prostate cancer metastasizes to the brain in 0.6–6% (Catane et al. 1976; Castaldo et al. 1983; Khanson and Imyanitov 2001; Tremont-Lukats et al. 2003; Hatzoglou et al. 2014). According to Catane et al. (1976), based on the analysis of diagnostic findings in a series of autopsies with MTSs to the brain (n = 1202), PrC metastases were found only in 0.8% of cases. According to Lynes et al. (1986), at autopsies of 856 cases, PrC metastases to the brain were identified in 1.3% (n = 11). When analyzing a large clinical sample (n = 6107) in patients with secondary metastatic brain lesions, Sutton et al. (1996) identified PrC metastases in 0.9%, with 0.6% of them being diagnosed in vivo. In our material, PrC metastases to the brain amounted to no more than 1% (9 patients).

Prostate cancer metastasizes to CNS via both hematogenous and mixed lymphohematogenous routes. By the lesion location in the brain structures, Kalkun (1963) noted their most frequent location in the brain substance (78%), less frequently in the dura (18%) and pia (4%) mater. According to Lynes et al. (1986), in a group of patients with prostate adenocarcinoma (n = 55), metastases were observed in the meninges in 67%, in the hemispheres in 25%, and in the

M. Dolgushin et al., *Brain Metastases*, DOI 10.1007/978-3-319-57760-9_20

cerebellum in 8%. Prostate cancer often metastasizes to the orbital bones, the greater wing of the sphenoid bone, significantly increasing the size of the orbit and causing a secondary sclerotic bone response.

A neuroimaging picture of metastatic brain lesions in PrC does not differ from that in cerebral metastases from other organs: in most cases, a decreased density dominates on CT, a decreased MR signal is observed in native (T1-weighted) images, and an increased signal is predominant in T2-weighted images. An increase in the density and an increase in the intensity of MR signal characteristics are often associated with the presence of hemorrhages in metastatic lesions and protein-containing and calcified inclusions. Lesions often accumulate the contrast agent with a pronounced ring enhancement and an increased CT density (a high intensity of MR signal), which is explained by the presence of necrosis in the central part of the lesion and its rich vascularization on the periphery.

As noted above, PrC is one of the cancers that often (like breast cancer) metastasizes to the cranial bones. In case metastases are located in the bone structures of the skull base, their visualization can be difficult. The use of additional methods in such studies may facilitate their identification and, in general, a correct diagnosis. In their study, Nemeth et al. (2007) noted the low sensitivity of DWI method in the evaluation of metastatic involvement of the skull bones in PrC, in contrast to secondary tumors of another origin.

20.1 Clinical Cases

See Figs. 20.1, 20.2, 20.3, and 20.4.

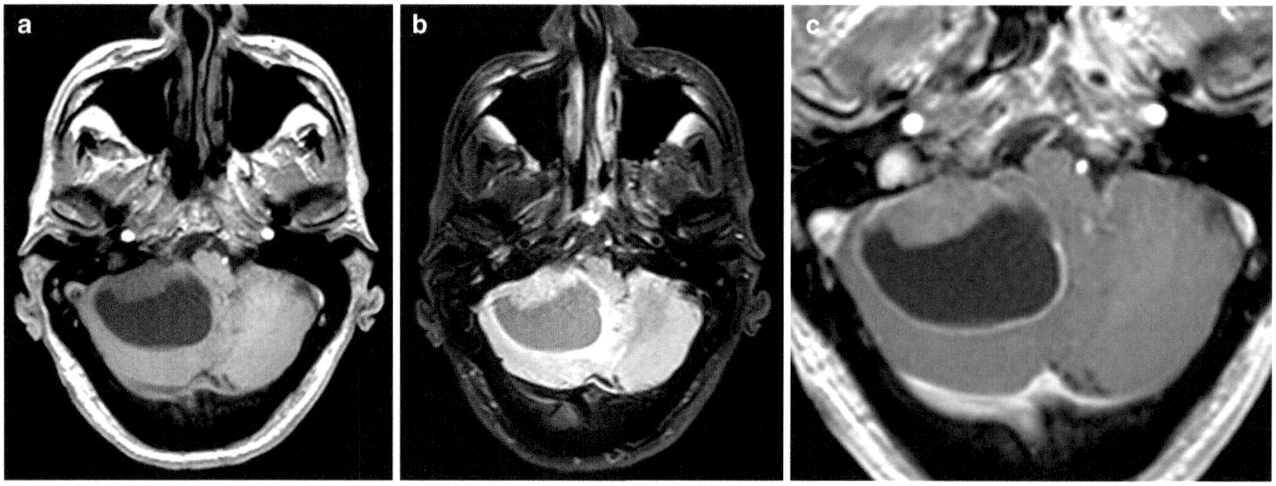

Fig. 20.1 A prostate cancer metastasis in the brain. In the right cerebellar hemisphere, there is a large, space-occupying, solid-cystic lesion with a decreased signal on T1-weighted MRI (**a**), showing signs of a mild perifocal edema (**b**), accumulating the contrast agent on the periphery as a thin rim and a thickening along the front contour (**c**). In the whole-body DWI MRI study (**d**–**g**), there are high-signal areas in the prostate gland, in nodules lateral to the right kidney, in the hilum of the right lung, and around the left kidney (the *arrows*), consistent with the changes identified on T2-weighted TIRM MRI (**h**–**j**): prostate tumors with metastatic involvement of the retroperitoneal lymph nodes and the hilum of the right lung

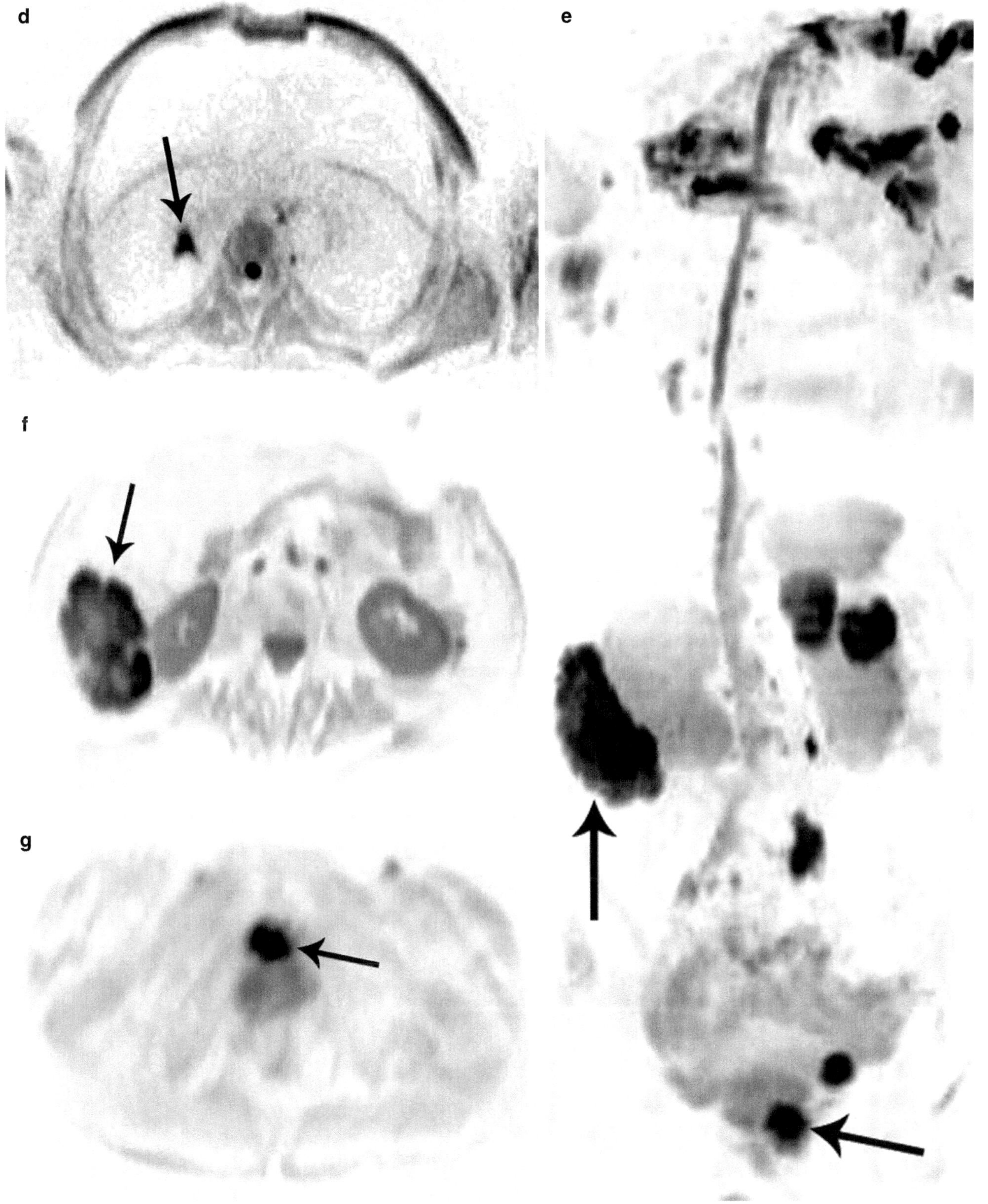

Fig. 20.1 (continued)

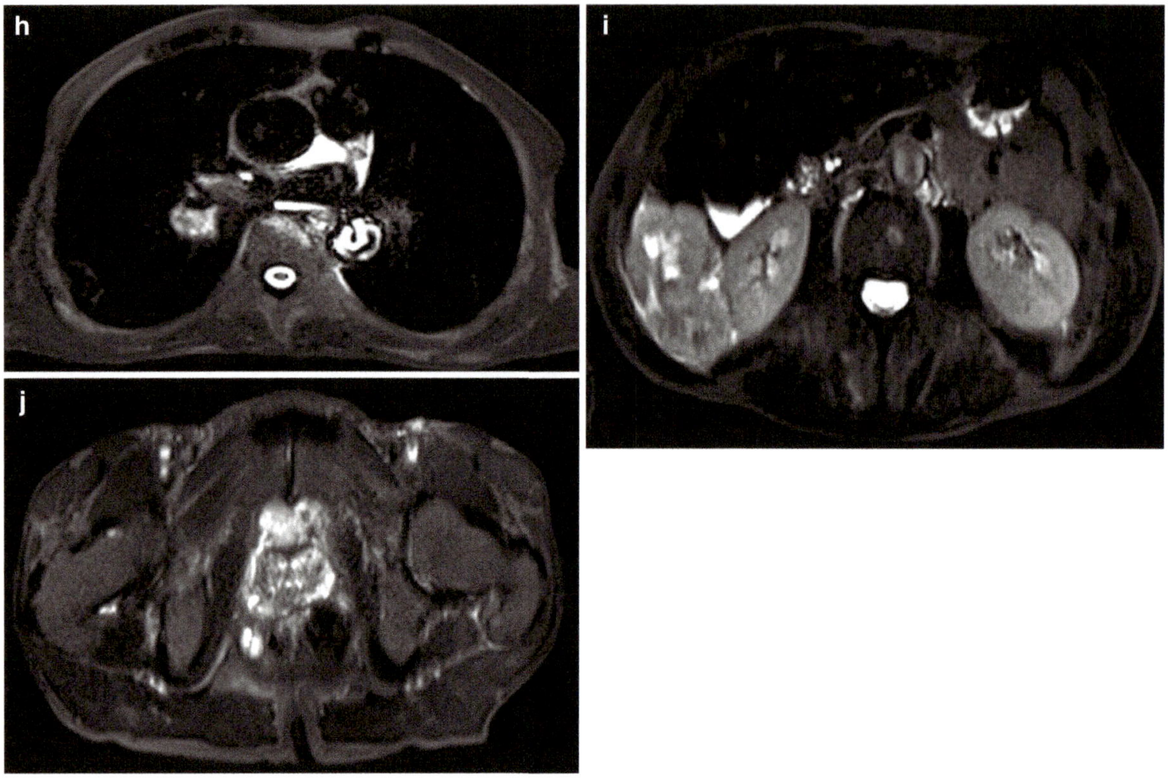

Fig. 20.1 (continued)

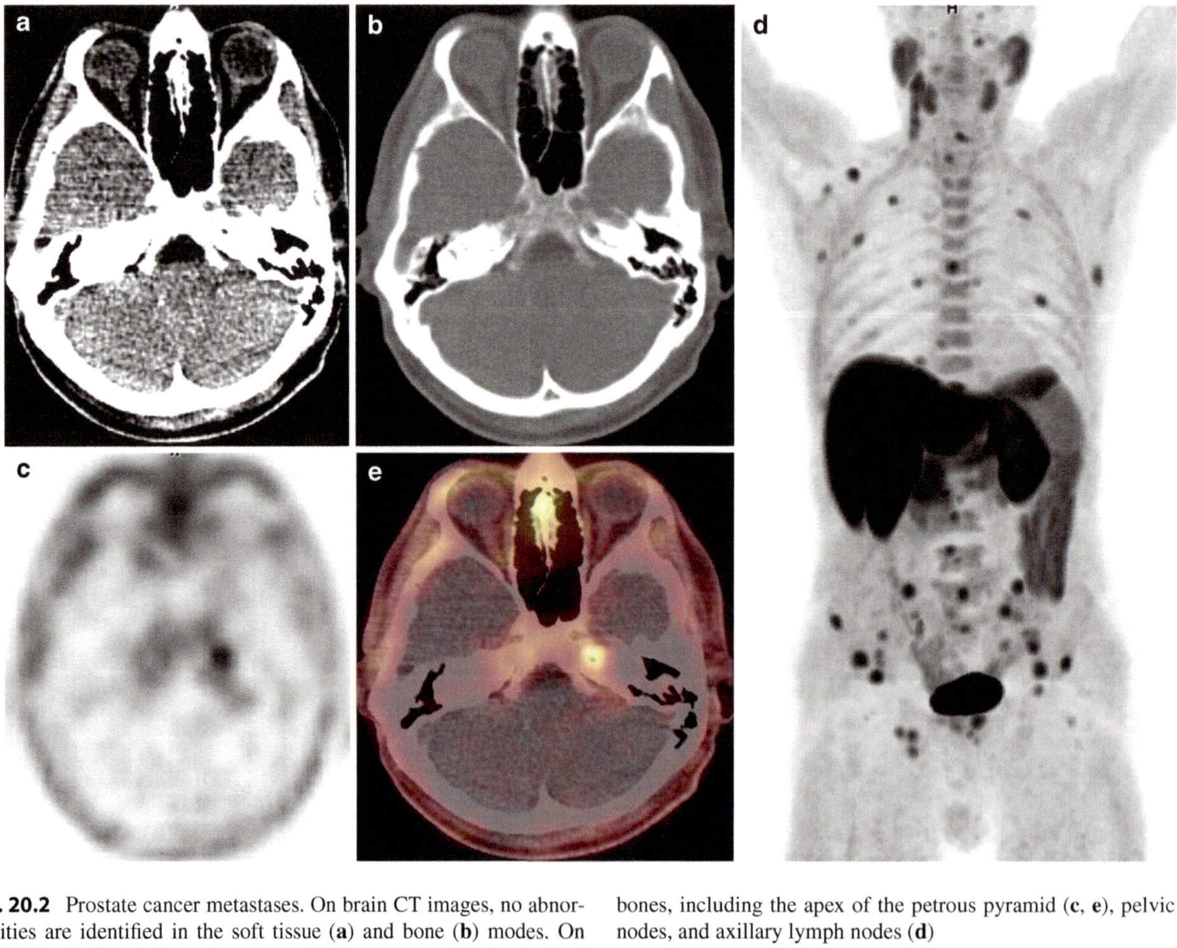

Fig. 20.2 Prostate cancer metastases. On brain CT images, no abnormalities are identified in the soft tissue (**a**) and bone (**b**) modes. On PET/CT with ^{18}F-choline, there are multiple metastases in the skeletal bones, including the apex of the petrous pyramid (**c**, **e**), pelvic lymph nodes, and axillary lymph nodes (**d**)

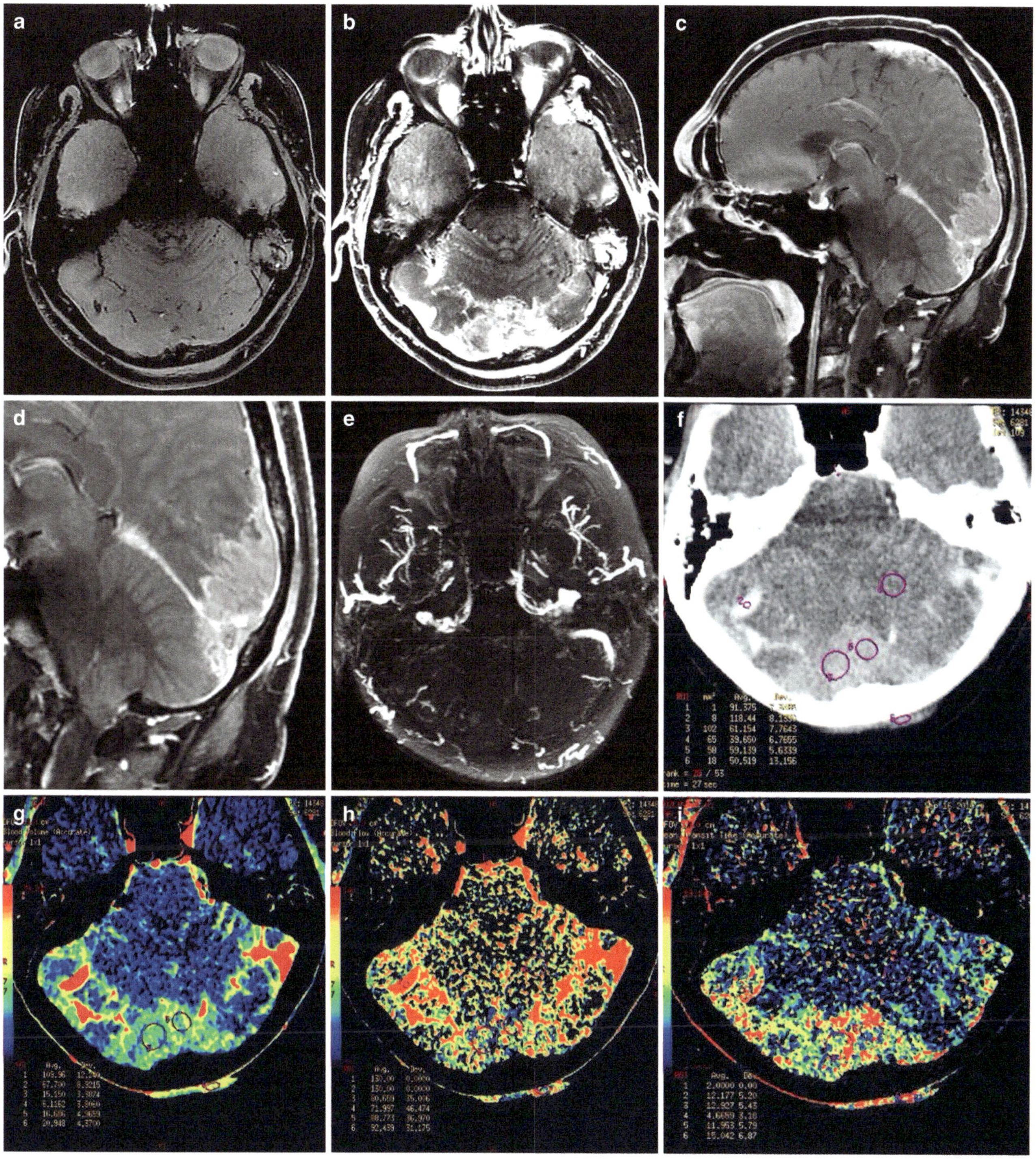

Fig. 20.3 Multiple prostate cancer metastases in the brain. Along the meninges, in the occipital regions, there is a space-occupying lesion, isointense on T1 fatsat (**a**), intensely accumulating the contrast agent on T1-weighted fat sat images (**b**, **c**, **d**). Noteworthy is the infiltrative tumor spread along the dura and pia mater. On MR venography (**e**), the lumina of transverse sinuses are not visualized. Intense accumulation of the contrast agent is also observed in the tumor (**f**) on CT. On CT perfusion, an increase in perfusion parameters (CBF, CBV, MTT) is observed in the affected area (**g**–**i**)

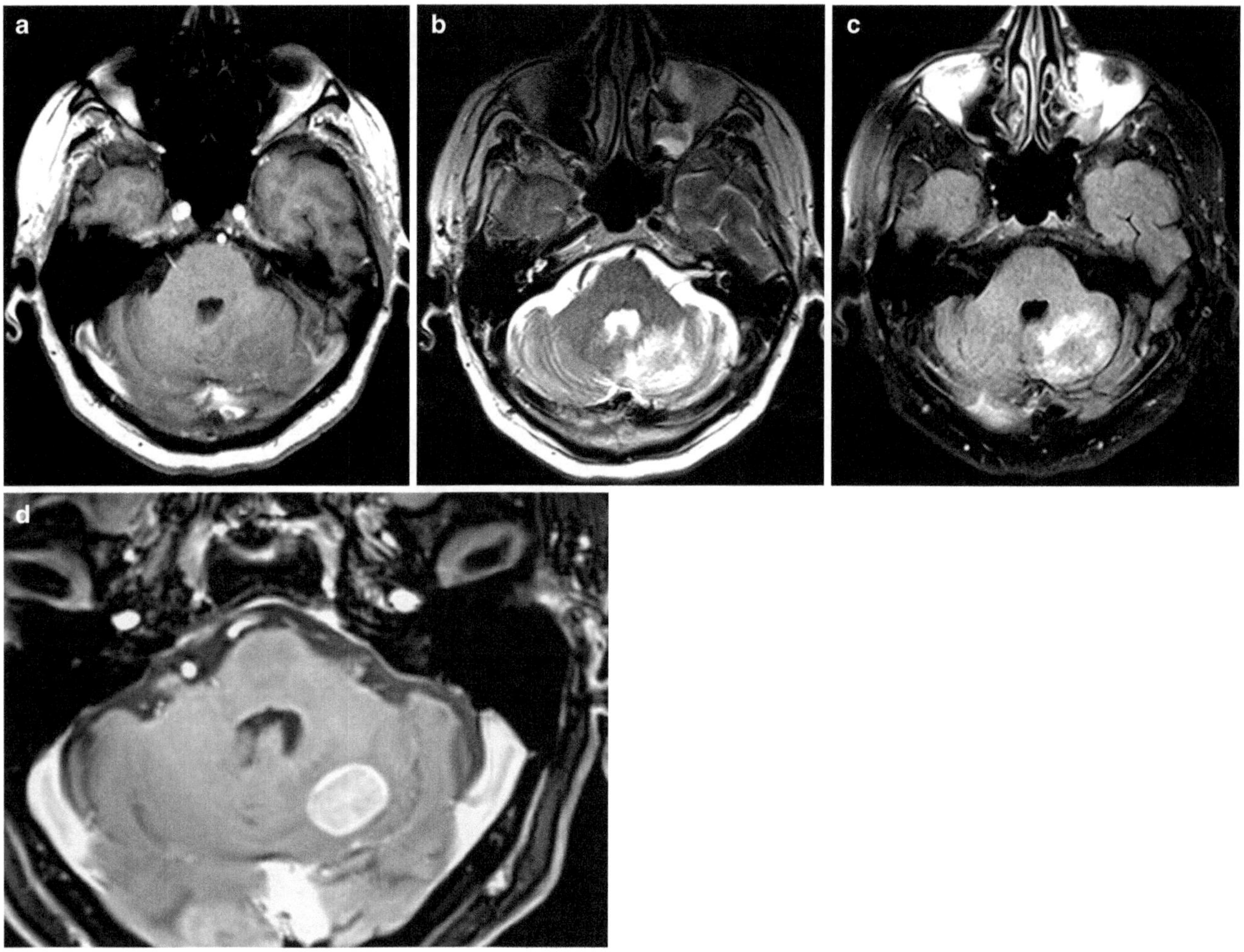

Fig. 20.4 A prostate cancer metastasis in the brain. In the left cerebellar hemisphere, there is a solid, space-occupying lesion with a moderately decreased signal on T1-weighted (**a**) MRI, showing a slight perifocal edema on T2 and T2-FLAIR images (**b**, **c**), that homogeneously intensely accumulates the contrast agent (**d**)

21 Testicular Cancer

Testicular cancer does not exceed 2% by the frequency of metastases in the brain (Guenot 1994). The clinical picture of metastatic lesions in PrC and testicular cancer is not different from the clinical picture of metastases of cancers from other sites in the brain. We observed two cases of brain involvement in this cancer (less than 1%).

CT studies conducted in patients with cerebral metastases of testicular cancer did not identify any specific radiological characteristics and pathognomonic symptoms as compared to those in metastatic brain lesions of other primary tumors. In a series of similar cases, the authors noted that solitary metastases were found at the site of the primary tumor in the pelvic area (86%)—prostate and urinary bladder—in the half of cases. The metastatic lesions identified have the density identical to or lower than that of the brain; however, in case of an isodense structure, the presence of a metastatic lesion can be confirmed by the edema area surrounding the tumor. The contrast agent accumulation has a ring-shaped character with the adjacent tissue component—"ring + tissue."

MRI for suspected metastases in the brain should be performed according to the standard protocol to obtain the images in the axial (T1-weighted, T2-weighted, T2-FLAIR) and sagittal (T1-weighted) planes and contrast-enhanced T1-weighted sequences in three perpendicular planes or SPGR (VIBE).

The tissue MRI characteristics of cerebral metastases of testicular cancer are not specific and do not differ from the majority of metastatic tumors with different histogenesis.

21.1 Clinical Cases

See Figs. 21.1 and 21.2.

M. Dolgushin et al., *Brain Metastases*, DOI 10.1007/978-3-319-57760-9_21

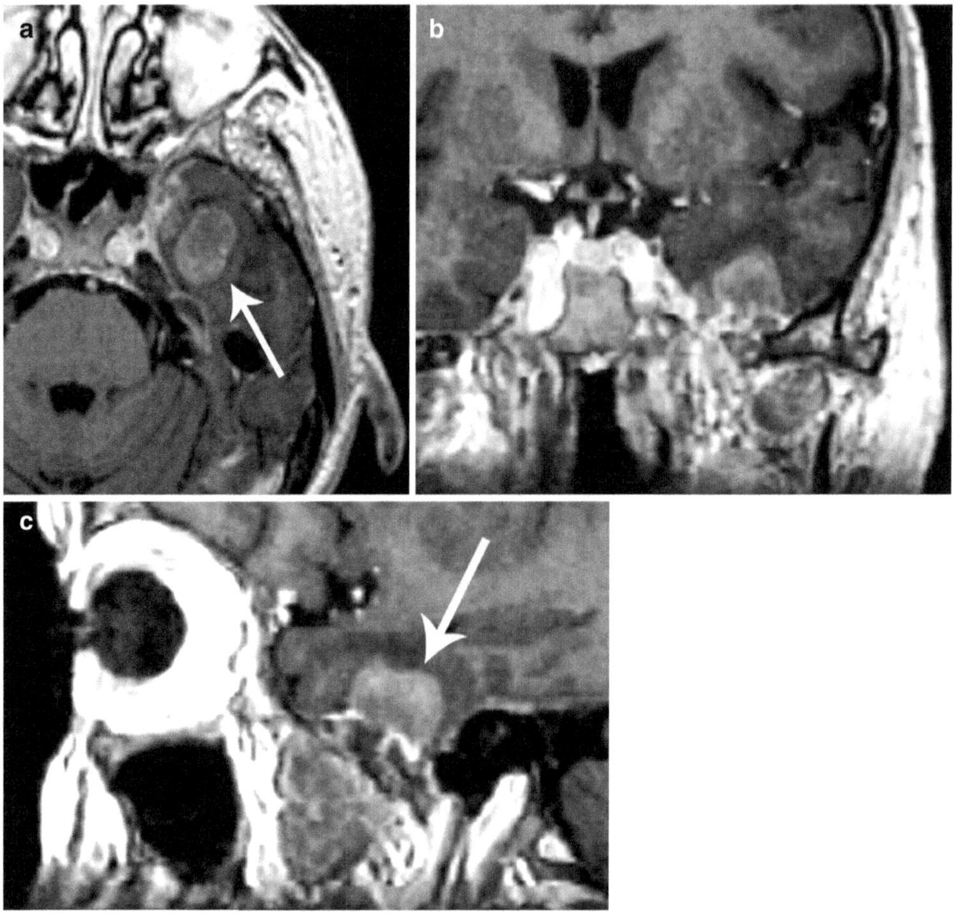

Fig. 21.1 A metastasis of testicular cancer in the brain. On T1-weighted MRI after intravenous CA administration in the axial (**a**), frontal (**b**), and sagittal (**c**) projections, in the left basal portions of the left temporal area, a small tumor is identified that is widely attached to the membranes of the middle cranial fossa (the *arrows*). Contrast enhancement of dural “tails” on either side of the tumor is visualized

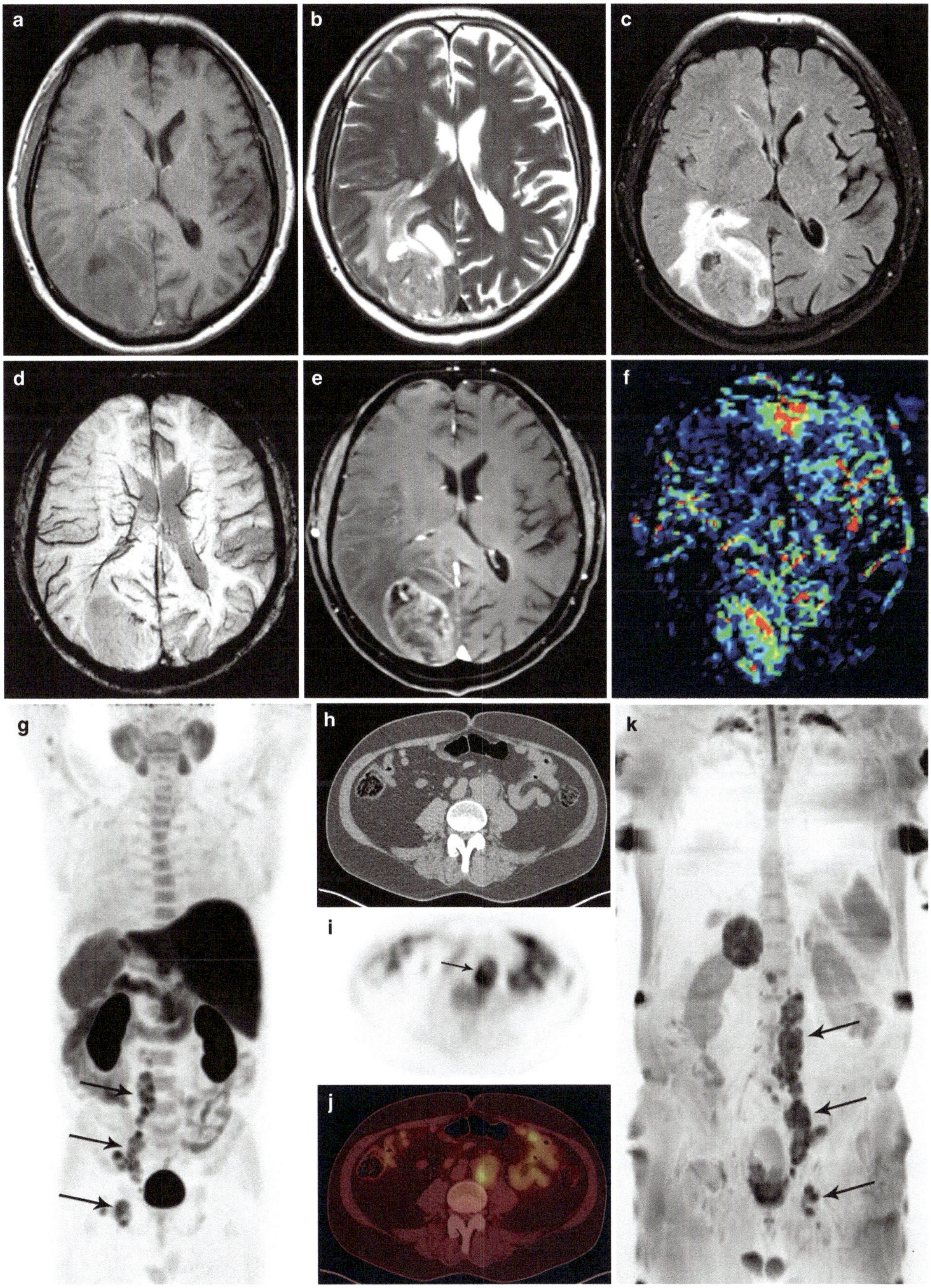

Fig. 21.2 Testicular cancer metastases. In the right occipital region, there is a space-occupying lesion with a moderately decreased signal on T1-weighted MRI (**a**) and an increased signal on T2-weighted MRI (**b**) with signs of an expressed perifocal edema on T2-FLIAR (**c**). On SWI (SWAN) MRI (**d**), no hypointense inclusions were identified in the tumor structure. After CA administration, its intense accumulation in the metastasis is observed (**e**). On ASL maps (**f**), the lesion is characterized by an increased blood flow. On PET/CT with 18F-choline (**g**–**j**) and whole-body DWI MRI (**k**), areas of abnormal RP accumulation and increased signal areas are observed in the enlarged iliac and para-aortic lymph nodes on the left (the *arrows*)

22 Uterine Cancer (UC)

Malignant tumors of the female genital organs occupy a special place in the clinical oncology, since they are the most common malignancies in women. Of the 12.7 million of new cases with various forms of cancer reported each year in the world, almost 1 million account for gynecologic tumors. In Russia, in 2010, the number of newly diagnosed female genital tumors was 47 700 thousand, which was 17% of all malignant tumors (Jemal et al. 2011).

Cervical cancer is one of the most common malignancies, ranking seventh among all malignant cancers and fifth in the structure of cancer incidence in women in the Russian Federation, after breast cancer and gastrointestinal cancer. In 2012 more than 15.3 thousand cervical cancer patients and 7.37 thousand deaths were reported in Russia. According to Davydov and Axel (2014), during the period from 2007 to 2012, an increase in the absolute number of cases of cervical cancer was 11.2%, defining the fourth place by the increase rate among malignant tumors. In the structure of malignant neoplasms in the female population of Russia, the proportion of cervical cancer decreased from 7.0% in 1989 to 5.3% in 2012.

In developed countries, standardized incidence rates (9.0 per 100,000) are two times lower than in developing countries (17.8 per 100,000), accounting for 78% of cases of cervical cancer, while its proportion is 15% of all malignancies in women (4.4% in developed countries). Disturbing is an increase in the incidence of cervical cancer in Russia from 12.5 per 100,000 of female population in 2007 to 13.9 per 100,000 in 2012. The maximum age-standardized incidence rates of cervical cancer were reported in the age group of 50–64 years old—31–32 per 100,000. Cervical cancer is the leading cause of death among all malignant tumors in women aged 15–40 years old, reaching 19.5%. In the age category of 40–54 years, cervical cancer moves to second place, accounting for 9.7%.

In developed countries, the incidence of uterine cancer (UC) (12.9–100,000 of female population) was 2.2 times higher than in developing countries (5.9 per 100,000). In the structure of cancer incidence among the female population in the Russian Federation (2012), UC ranked second (7.5%) after breast cancer (20.7%). During the period from 2007 to 2012, an increase in the absolute number of cases was 8.7%. The incidence of UC increased in all age groups, starting from 25 years, and reached the maximum values (91.9—100,000) for the age group of 60–64 years (Axel 2012).

The average age of patients with gynecologic cancer in Russia decreased by 6 years—from 58 years in 1989 to 52 in 2010. An important factor is insufficient mass implementation of screening programs in Russia as compared with Western European countries, allowing to diagnose precancerous conditions and early forms of cancer.

Survival rates vary: good predictions are noted in the USA, 72%; in European countries, 60%; and in developing countries, 48%. The lowest survival rate was registered in Eastern Europe.

According to literature, cerebral metastases of cervical cancer, uterine cancer, and ovarian cancer are, on average, 0.5–1.2%, 0.6%, and 0.49–2.2%, respectively (Aalders et al. 1984; Ikeda and Yamada 1998; Chura et al. 2007; Ogava 2008; Setoodeh et al. 2012; Sierra et al. 2015). Spinal metastases of cervical and ovarian cancer are detected in 6% and 0.1–0.12% of cases, respectively (Matsuyama et al. 1989; Tiwari 2007).

The time interval from the detection of primary cancer to the detection of metastatic brain lesions of cervical cancer can reach up to 8 years. According to Kim et al. (2015), who analyzed a group of patients with cerebral metastases of malignant gynecologic tumors ($n = 61$) from 2002 to 2012, the average interval for cervical, uterine, and ovarian cancer was found to be 33.1 months, 27.8 months, and 21.6 months, respectively. The survival rates for patients with brain metastases of cervical, uterine, and ovarian cancer were 8.8 months, 23.3 months, and 14.1 months, respectively.

Although cerebral metastases are rare, according to Martinez-Manas et al. (1998), well-differentiated endometrial carcinoma with signs of vascular invasion can metastasize to the brain even before clinical manifestations of the primary tumor occur. According to Piura and Piura (2015),

M. Dolgushin et al., *Brain Metastases*, DOI 10.1007/978-3-319-57760-9_22

cerebral metastasis of endometrial carcinoma is so rare that authors found only 115 cases in the analysis of 35 studies.

In our cases, UC metastases in the brain were detected in 7% of cases, which greatly exceeds the data from literature.

On CT and MRI, cerebral metastases of UC manifest both as single and multiple tumors. Lesions are often solid, but we often diagnosed metastases with a solid-cystic structure. Almost always an expressed area with a perifocal edema is visualized. Accumulation of the contrast agent by the solid part of the metastasis significantly increases its density on the periphery; therefore, a "target" type of accumulation is often observed.

Although the vast majority of cases of cerebral metastases have a characteristic perifocal edema, we also diagnosed large lesions without any perifocal edema in our studies. These lesions had a dense solid structure with irregular contours.

The solid part of UC metastases has almost similar low values of cerebral blood volume, CBV and CBF, such as metastatic breast cancer. UC metastases have the lowest MTT values = 5.36 ± 0.74 (s), which indicates a rapid blood flow through their parenchyma in comparison with other cerebral metastases.

22.1 Clinical Cases

See Figs. 22.1, 22.2, 22.3, 22.4, 22.5, 22.6, 22.7, 22.8, 22.9, 22.10, and 22.11.

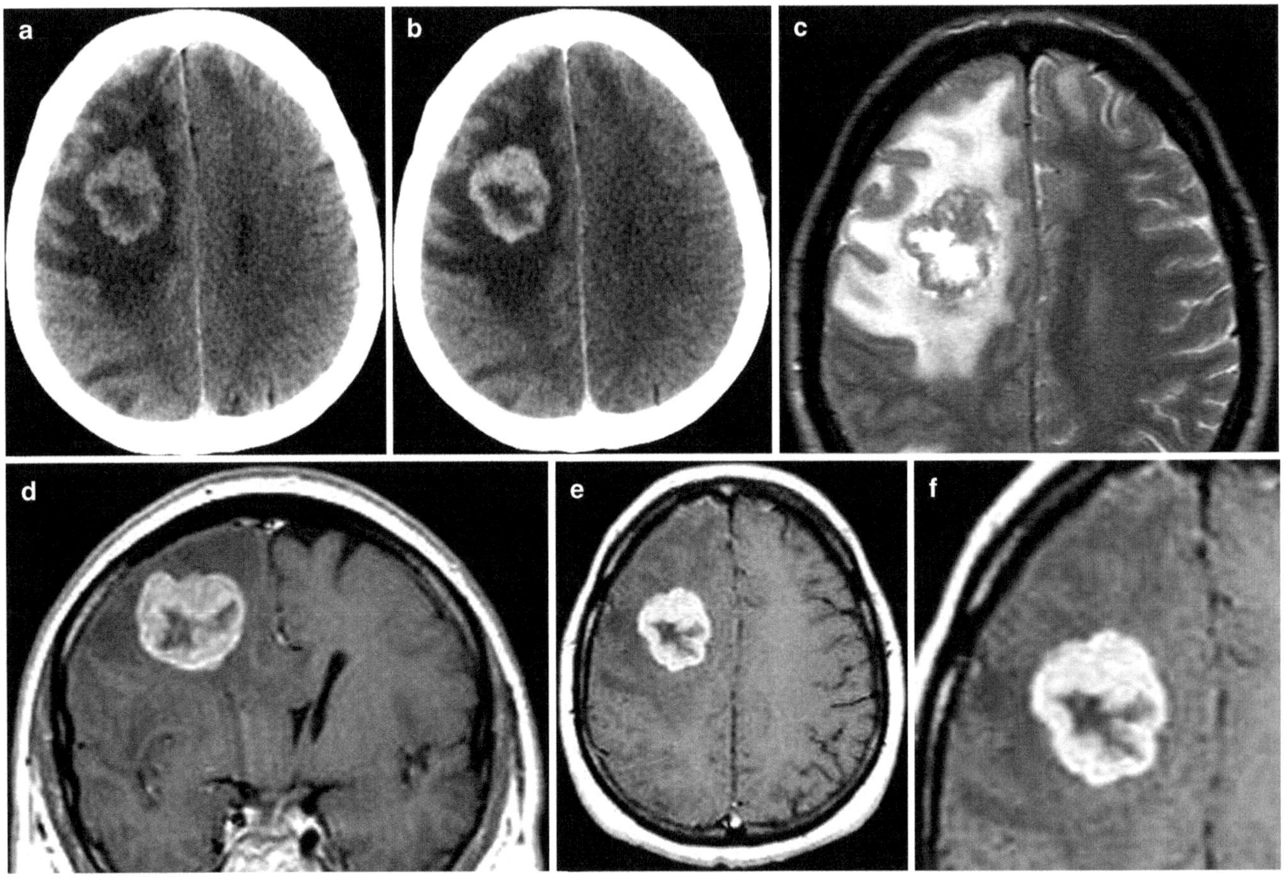

Fig. 22.1 A uterine cancer metastasis. On CT, in the right frontal lobe, there are space-occupying lesion with a moderately high density, an area of necrosis in the central parts, and a perifocal edema (**a**). The metastasis intensely accumulates the radiopaque agent (**b**). On T2-weighted MRI, the solid part of the tumor has an iso-hypointense signal (**c**), while the central necrosis has an increased signal. There is intense accumulation of the contrast agent in the solid structure of the tumor (**d–f**)

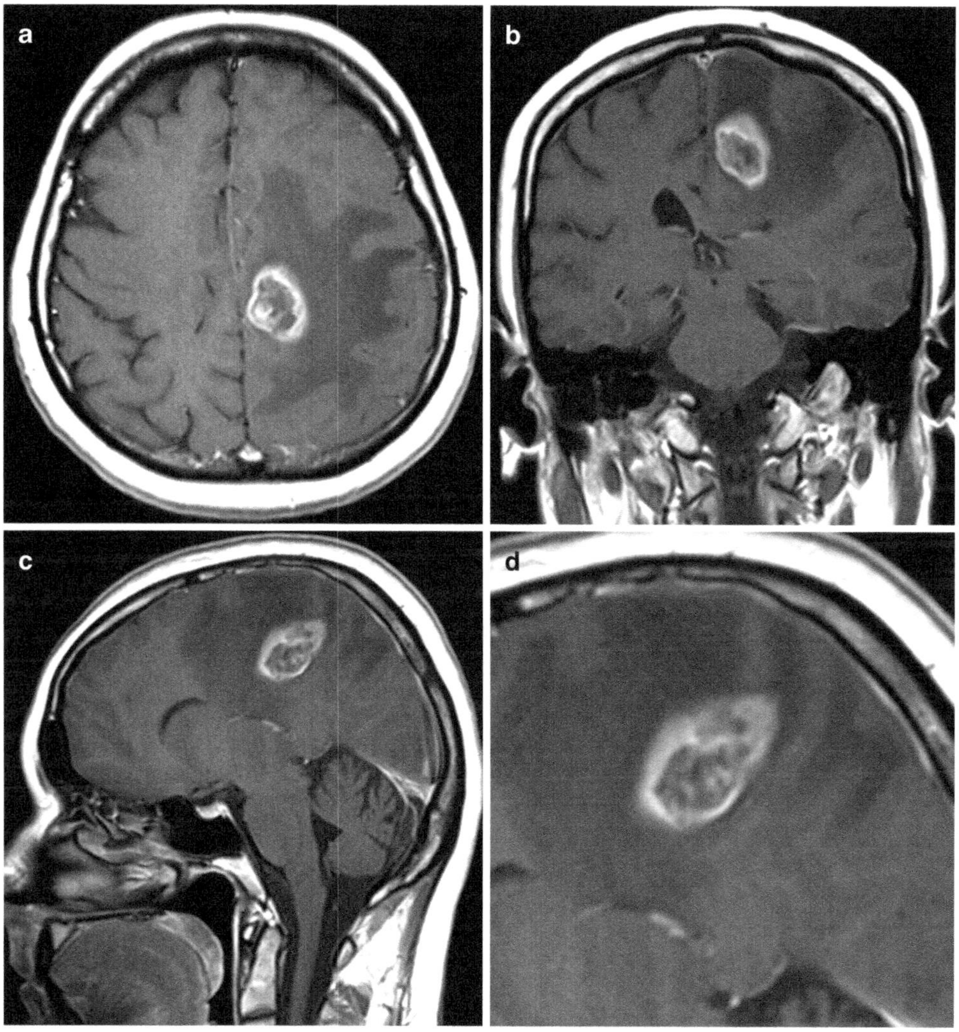

Fig. 22.2 A uterine cancer metastasis in the brain. On T1-weighted MRI with contrast enhancement in axial (**a**), coronal (**b**), and sagittal (**c**, **d**) projections, in the deep parts of the left frontoparietal region, an oblong lesion is detected with a pronounced perifocal edema, unevenly accumulating CA. The left lateral ventricle is drastically compressed

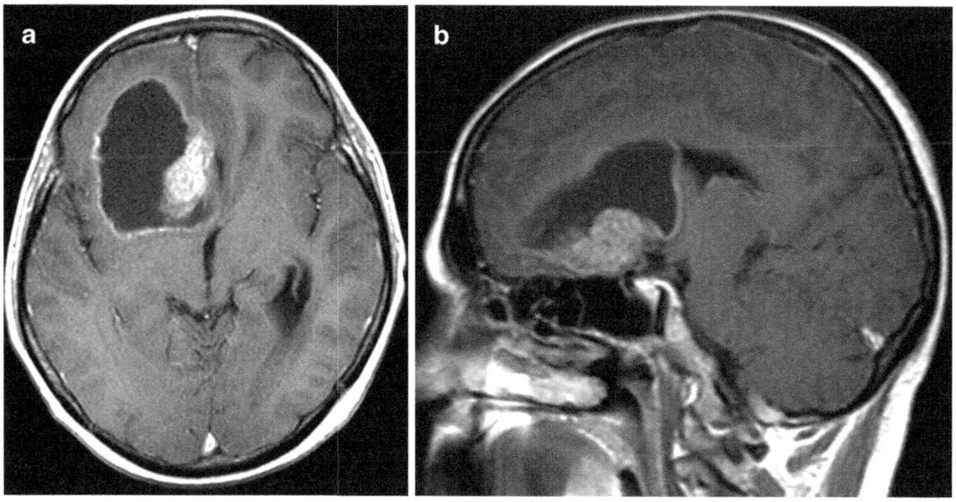

Fig. 22.3 A uterine cancer metastasis. On T1-weighted MRI with contrast enhancement in axial (**a**), sagittal (**b**), and coronal (**c**, **d**) projections, in the right frontal region, there is a space-occupying solid-cystic lesion accumulating the contrast agent along the contour of the cystic component with the formation of a node in the most expressed solid part of the tumor (lower medial tumor segments). The lateral and third ventricles are deformed

Fig. 22.3 (continued)

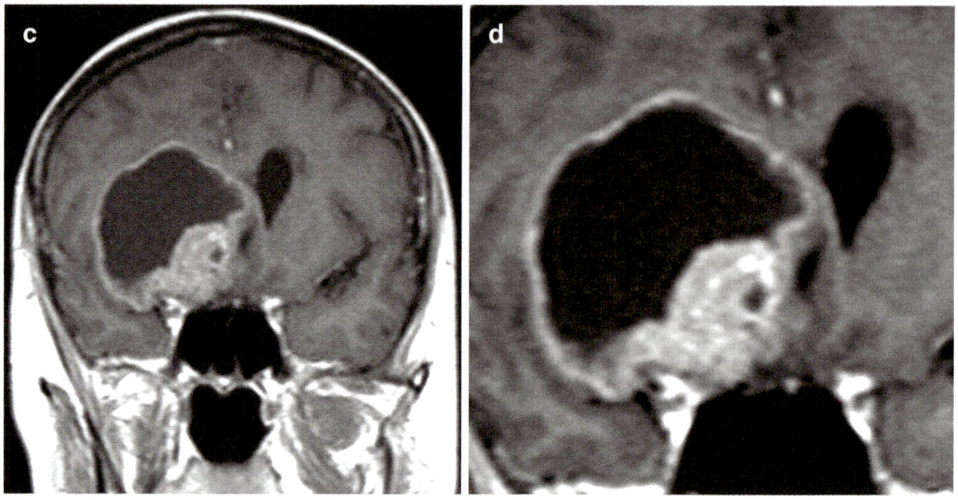

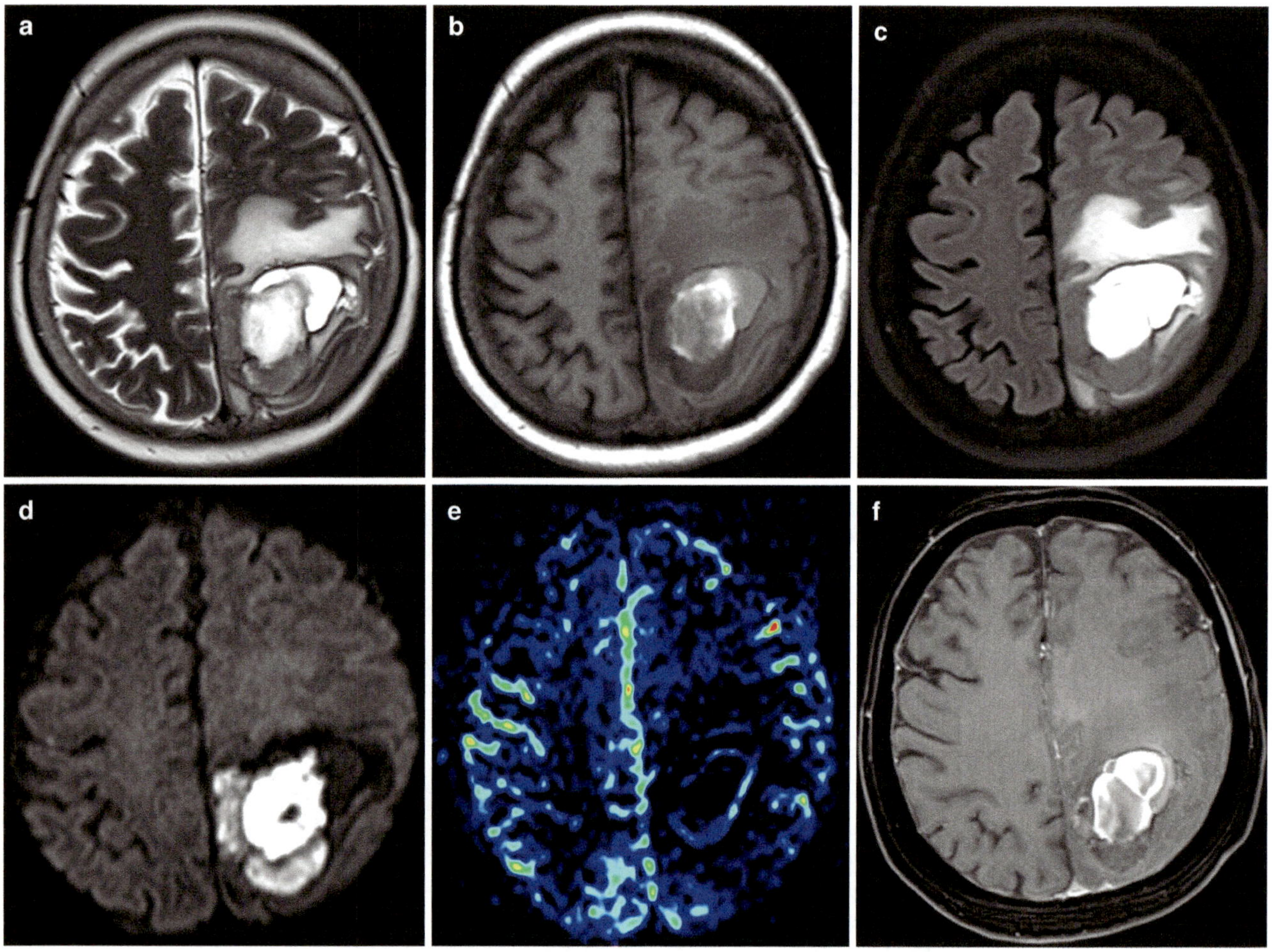

Fig. 22.4 A uterine cancer metastasis in the brain. In the left parietal lobe, there is a space-occupying lesion, heterogeneous on T2-weighted (**a**), T1-weighted (**b**), and DWI (**d**), with signs of a hemorrhage—a bright signal on T1-weighted images (**b**) and a pronounced perifocal edema (**a**, **c**). On non-contrast-enhanced MR perfusion, there is a slight increase in CBF along the lesion contour (**e**). Following intravenous CA administration, its inhomogeneous accumulation along the contour of the metastasis is observed (**f**)

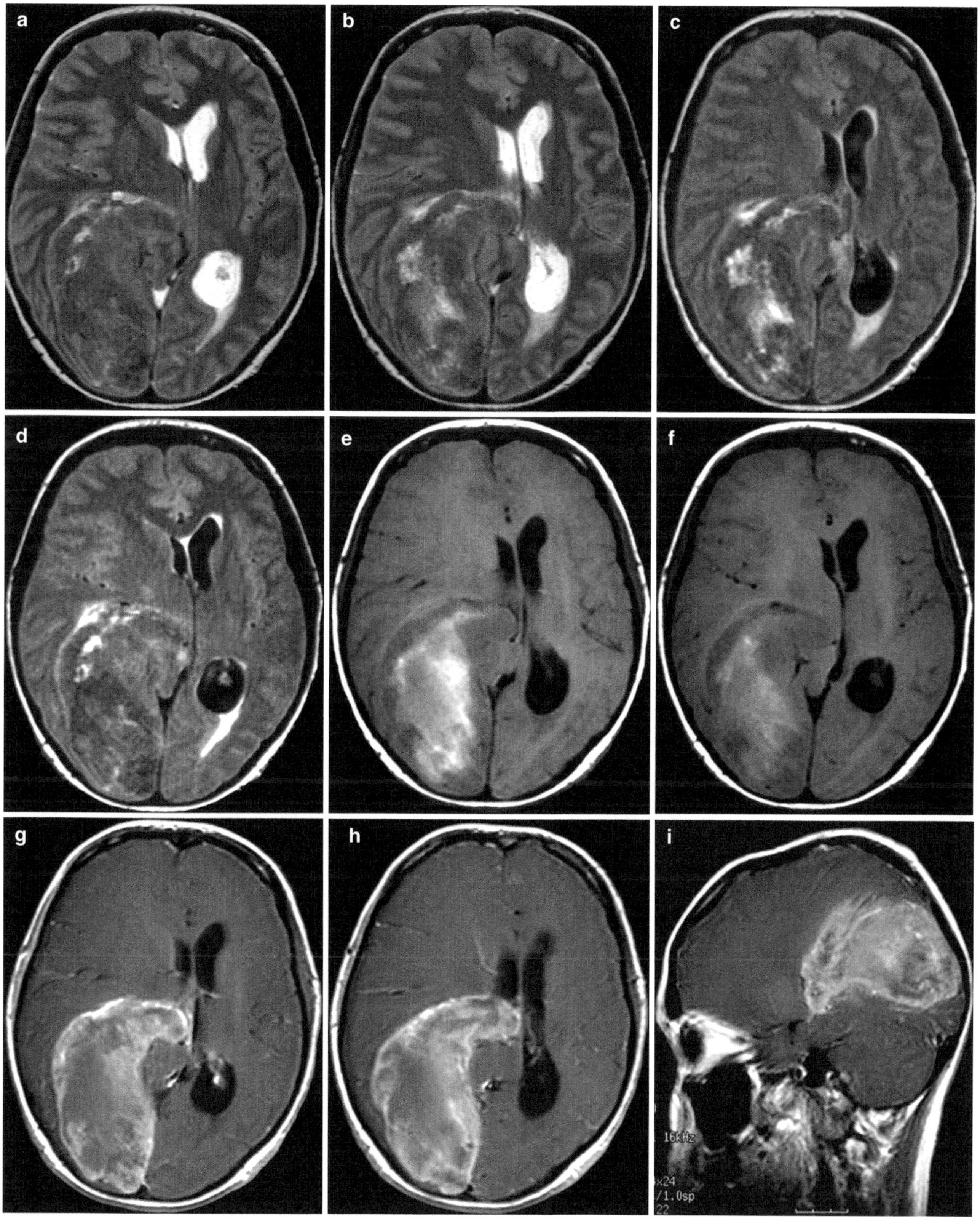

Fig. 22.5 A uterine cancer metastasis in the brain. A two-level study. On MRI in the right parietal-occipital region, there is a huge tumor with hemorrhagic and necrotic components; an iso-hyperintense signal on T2-weighted (**a**, **b**) MRI, and T2-FLAIR MRI (**c**, **d**); and an irregularly increased signal on T1-weighted MRI (**e**, **f**). After CA accumulation, on T1-weighted MRI (**g**, **h**) in the axial projection (**i**, **j**), in the sagittal projection, and (**k**, **l**) in the frontal projection, its intense accumulation in the structure of metastasis, with almost no perifocal edema

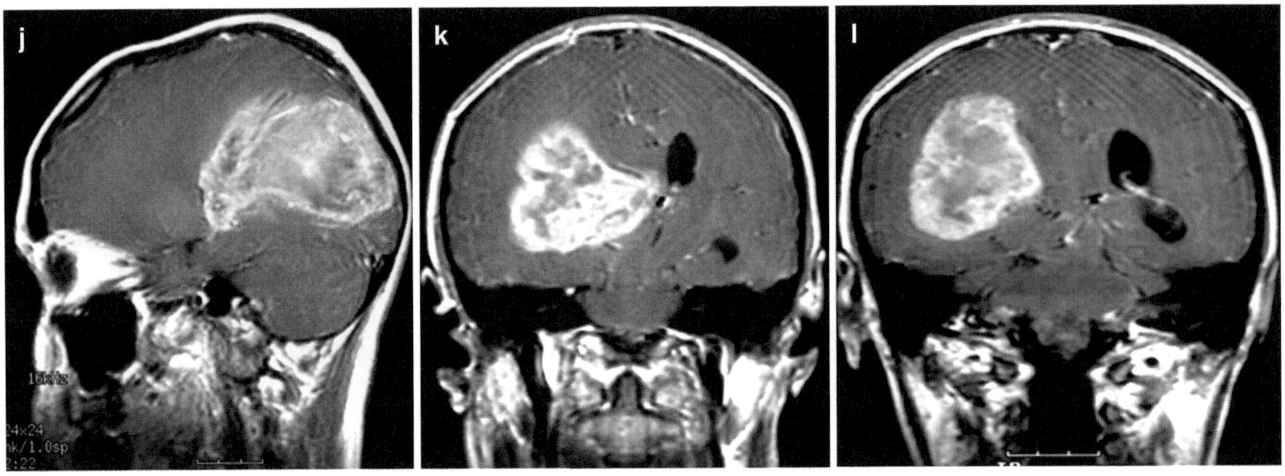

Fig. 22.5 (continued)

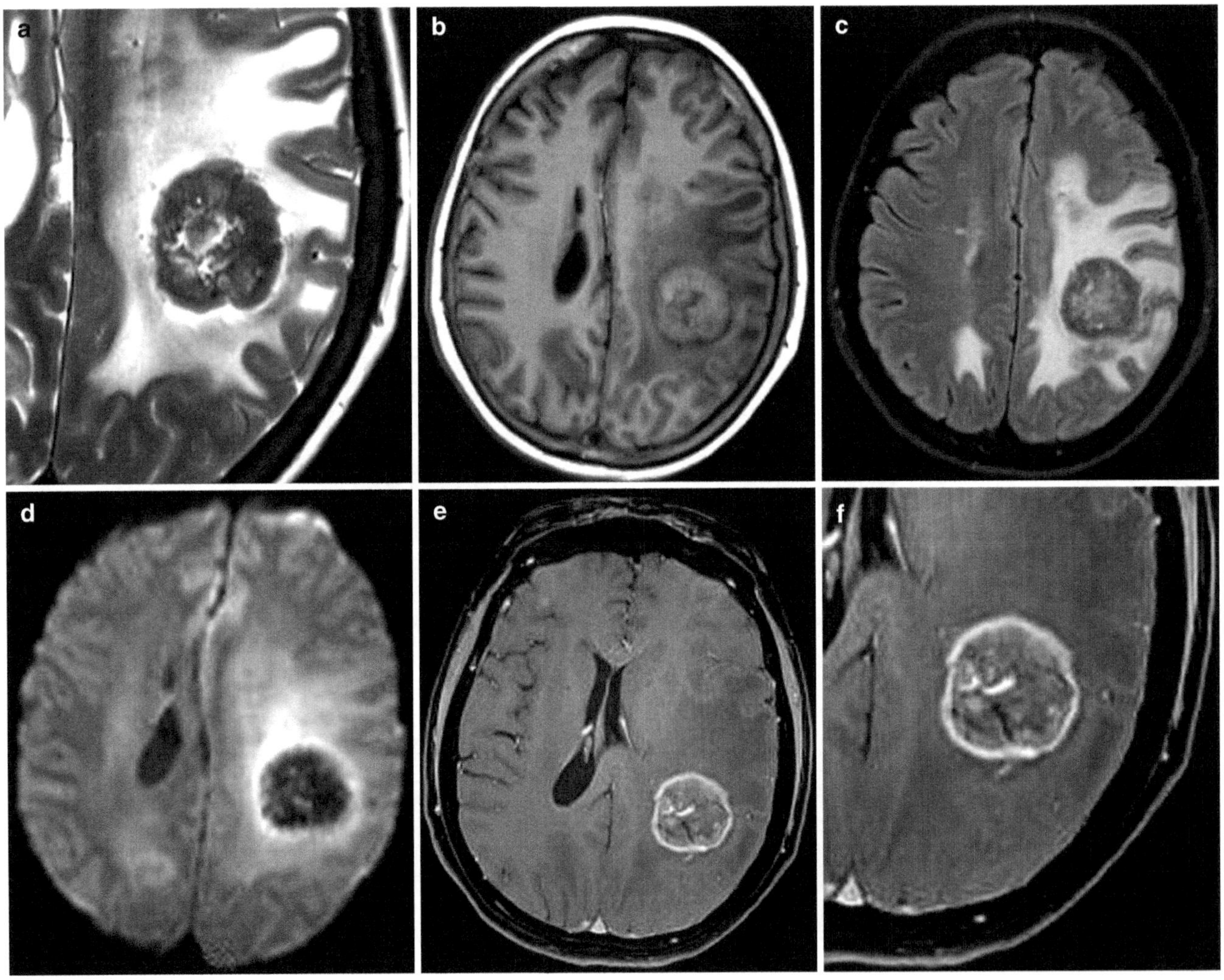

Fig. 22.6 Multiple uterine cancer metastases in the brain. In the left frontoparietal region, there is a large lesion with a hypo-isointense MR signal on T2-weighted MRI (**a**), an isointense signal on T1-weighted MRI (**b**), an iso-hypointense signal on T2-FLAIR (**c**), and a hypointense signal on DWI MRI (**d**). Perifocal edema is significant. After intravenous CA administration, the lesion accumulates CA throughout the entire area but more intensely in the form of a thin rim on the periphery (**e**, **f**)

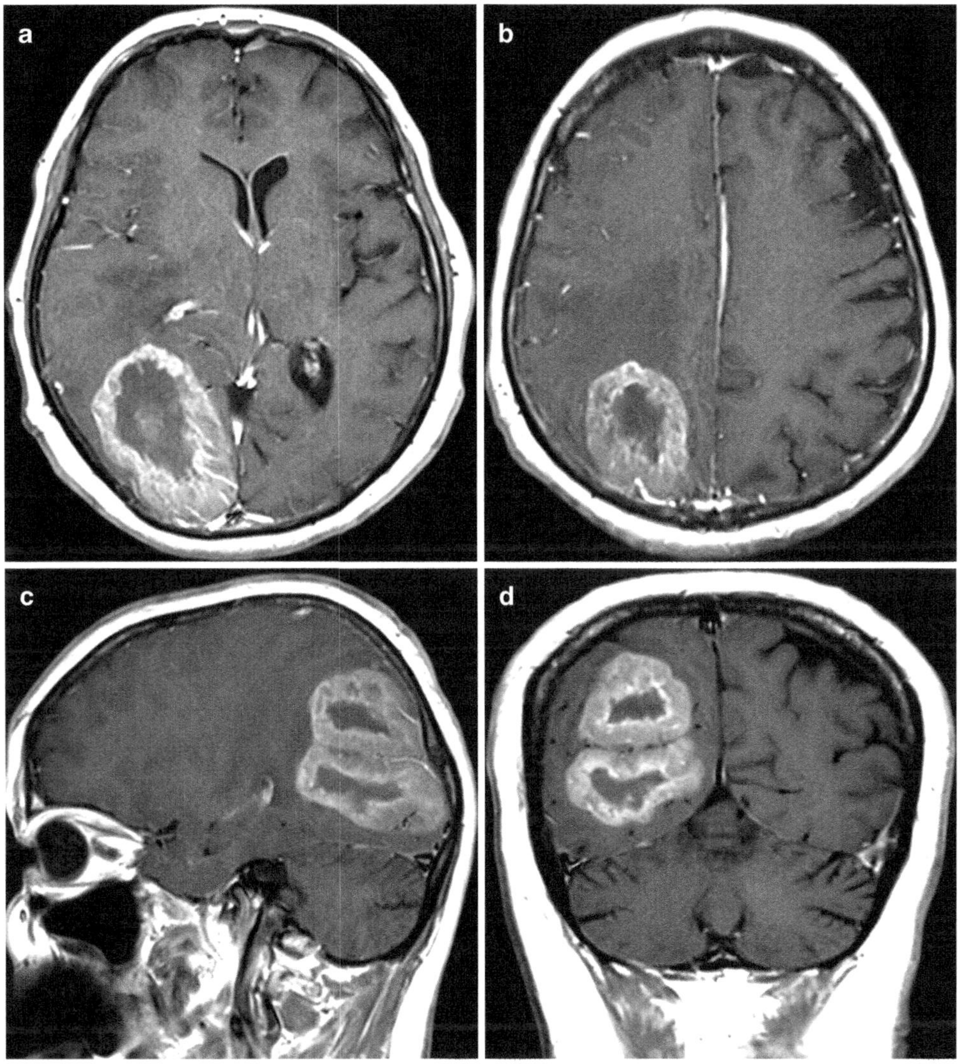

Fig. 22.7 Multiple uterine cancer metastases in the brain. On T1-weighted MRI, in the axial (**a**, **b**), sagittal (**c**), and frontal (**d**) projections after intravenous CA administration, there is a multinodular lesion in the right parietal-occipital region, with signs of intense accumulation of the contrast agent in the form of thick rolls. The central parts of tumor are represented by necrosis. The corpus callosum and the median brain structures are deformed

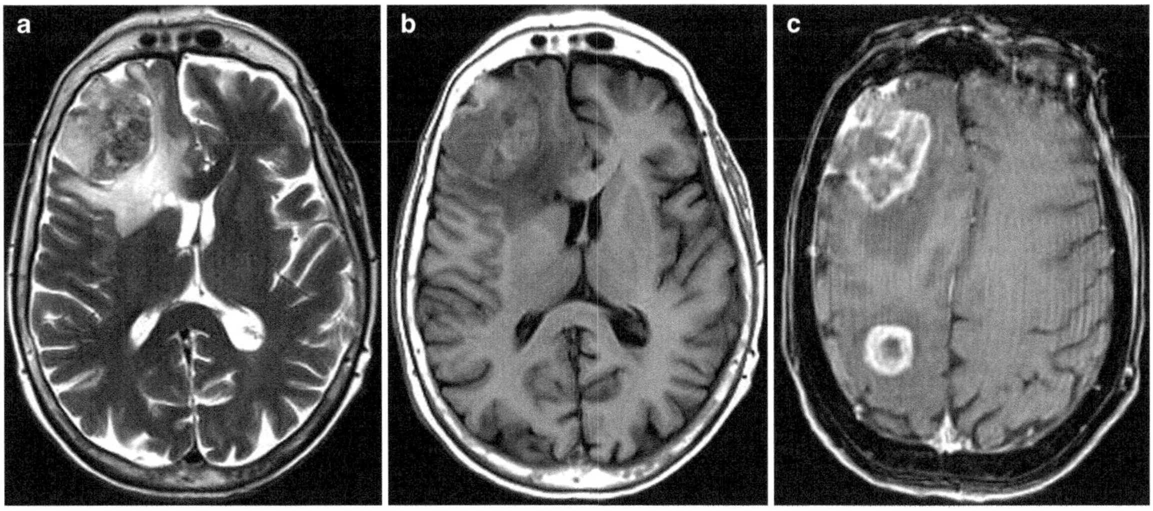

Fig. 22.8 Multiple uterine cancer metastases in the brain. A two-level study. On T2-weighted MRI (**a**, **d**), in the right frontal and frontoparietal regions, there are large tumor lesions with a low decreased signal with signs of a moderate perifocal edema. On T1-weighted MRI (**b**, **e**), the signal from the lesions is moderately reduced. Following intravenous CA administration (**c**), both lesions rapidly accumulate the contrast agent. On DWI MRI (b = 1000), the signal from the lesion is reduced (**f**)

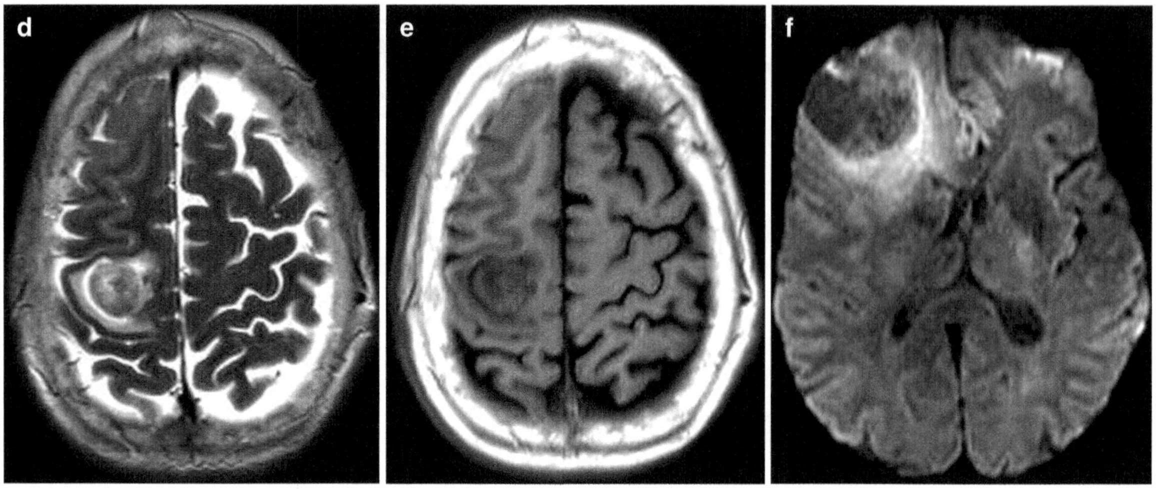

Fig. 22.8 (continued)

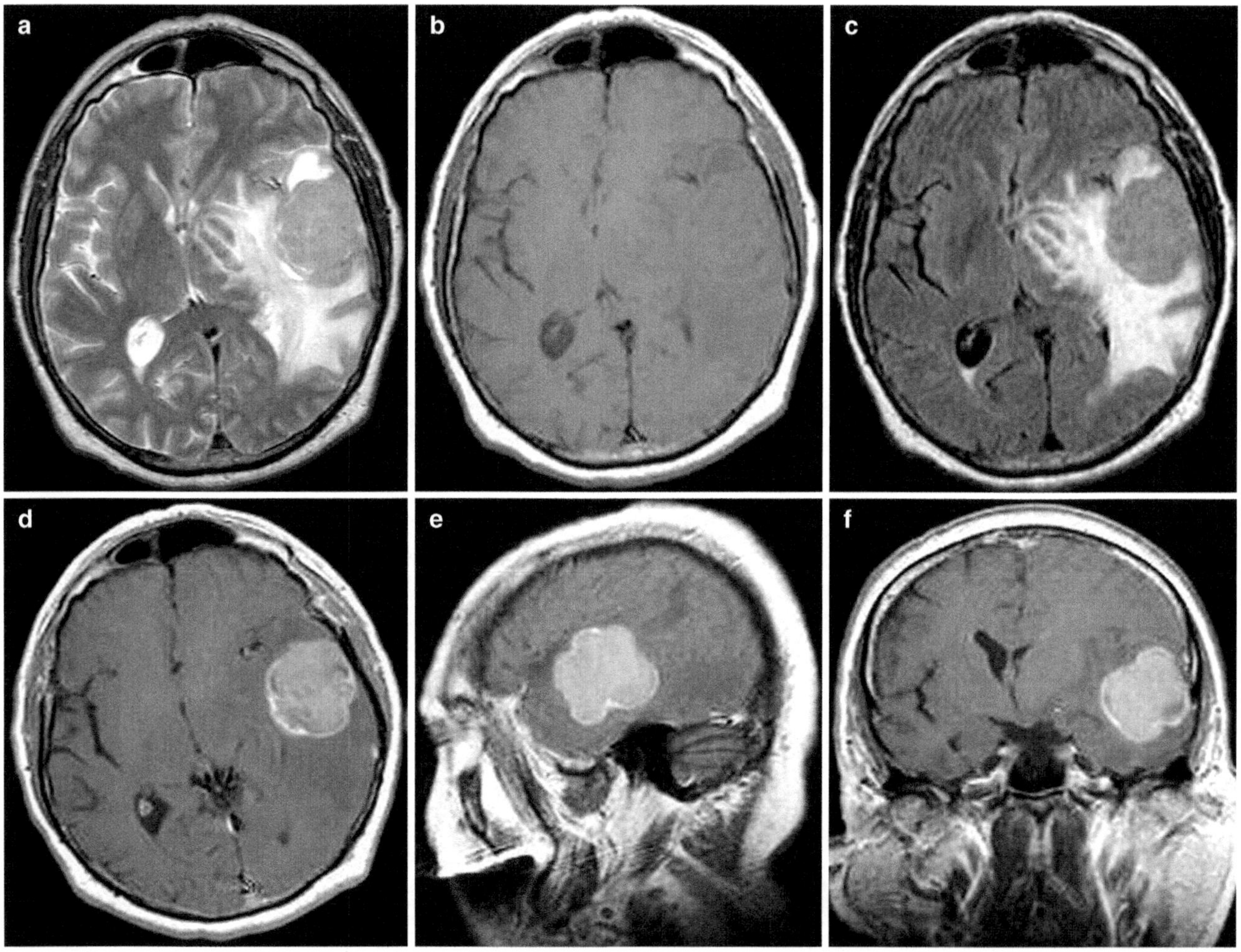

Fig. 22.9 A uterine cancer metastasis in the brain. In the left temporal region, there is an iso-hyperintense signal on T2-weighted and T2-FLAIR MRI (**a**, **c**) with a pronounced area of perifocal edema. On T1-weighted MRI (**b**), the signal from the lesion is isointense. After CA administration in the axial (**d**), sagittal (**e**), and frontal (**f**, **g**) projections, its intense, homogeneous accumulation is noted, somewhat more pronounced on the periphery and less intense and uniform in the central parts of the tumor. Despite the tumor being closely adjacent to the meninges, no evidence of the "tail" symptom was found. On MR spectroscopy (**h**, **i**), there is a marked peak of Lip-Lac complex and a well-defined Cho peak

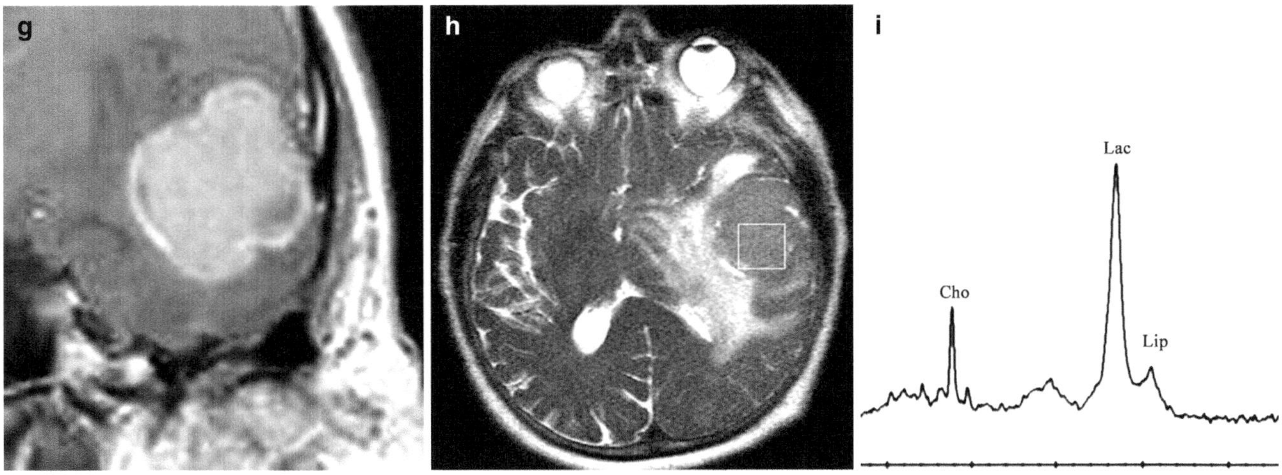

Fig. 22.9 (continued)

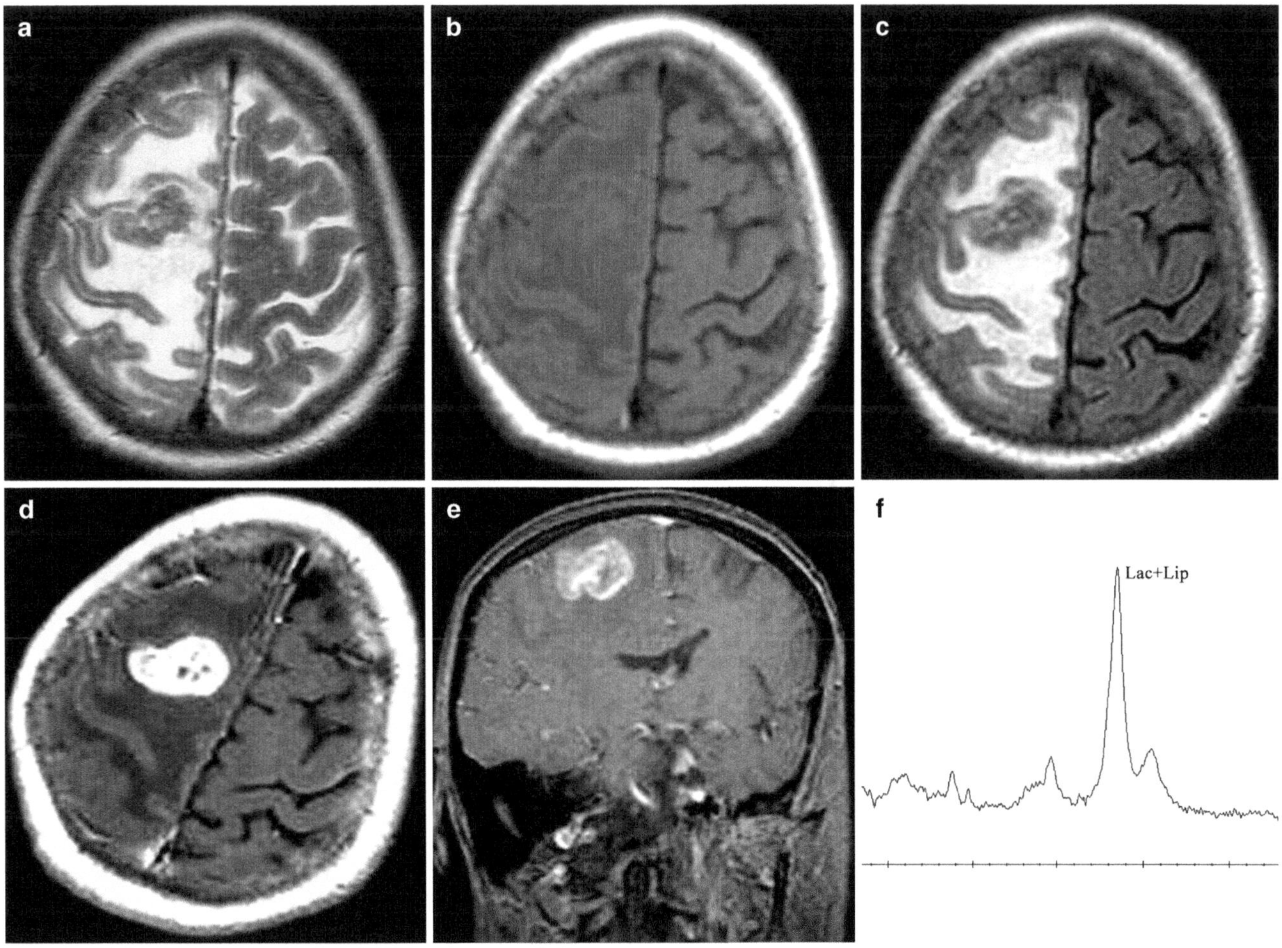

Fig. 22.10 A uterine cancer metastasis in the brain. In the right frontal region, there is a solid lesion, hypo-isointense on T2-weighted MRI (**a**) and isointense on T1-weighted MRI (**b**) and T2-FLAIR MRI (**c**), with a pronounced perifocal edema. Following intravenous CA administration, the metastasis intensely accumulates it (**d**, **e**). On MR spectroscopy, there is a pronounced prevalence of the Lip-Lac complex (**f**)

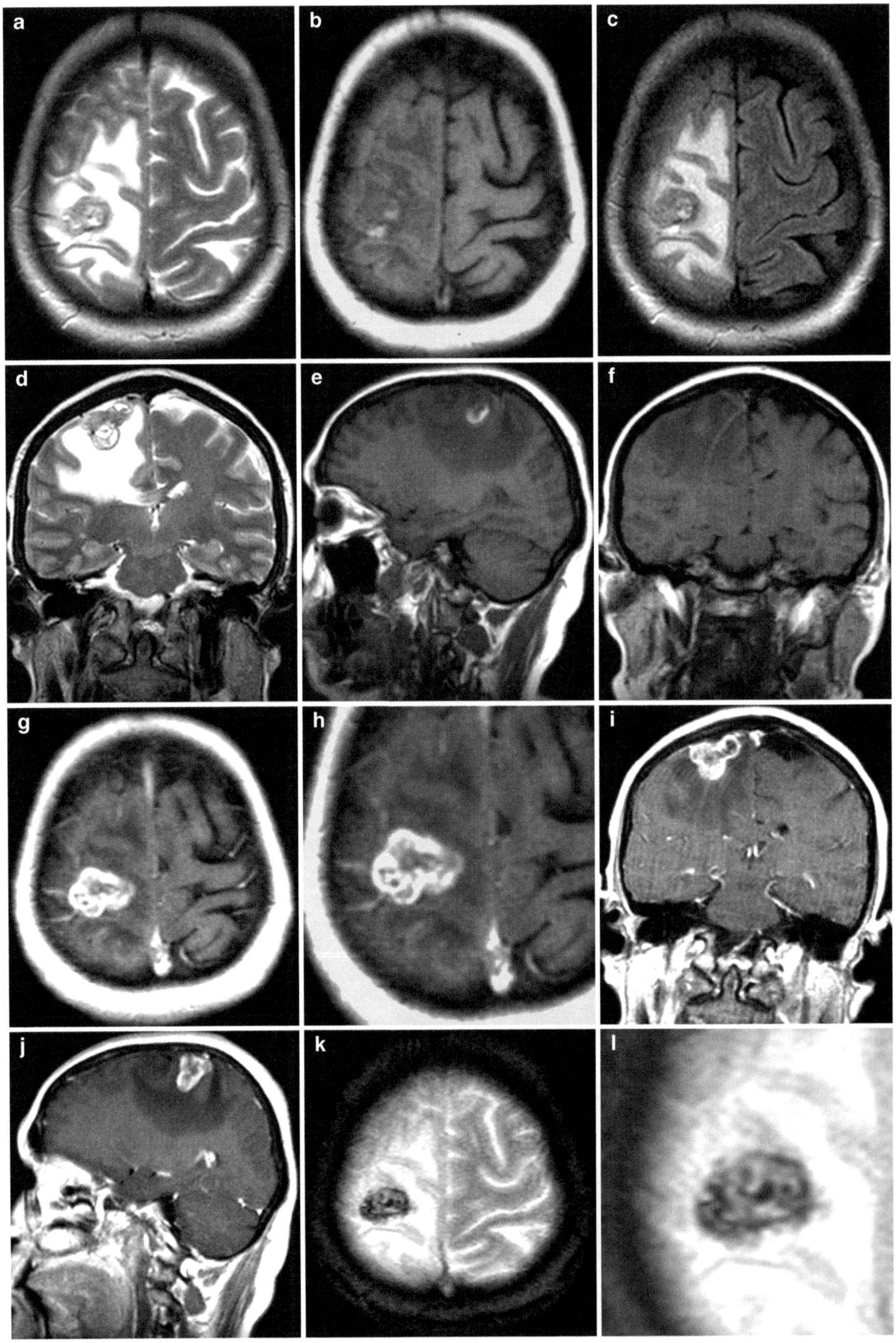

Fig. 22.11 A uterine cancer metastasis in the brain. In convexital parts of the right postfrontal area, there is a tumor lesion with a heterogeneously increased signal on T2-weighted (**a**) and T2-FLAIR MRI (**c**), with areas of hemorrhages—hyperintense inclusions—on T1-weighted MRI (**b**, **e**, **f**) and a pronounced perifocal edema (**c**). After intravenous CA administration, its intense accumulation is noted in the tumor (**g**–**j**); the tumor fragment involving the meninges is well visualized. On T2 GRE MRI, the signal from the lesion is nonuniformly reduced (**k**, **l**)

22.2 Post-radiation Changes

See Fig. 22.12.

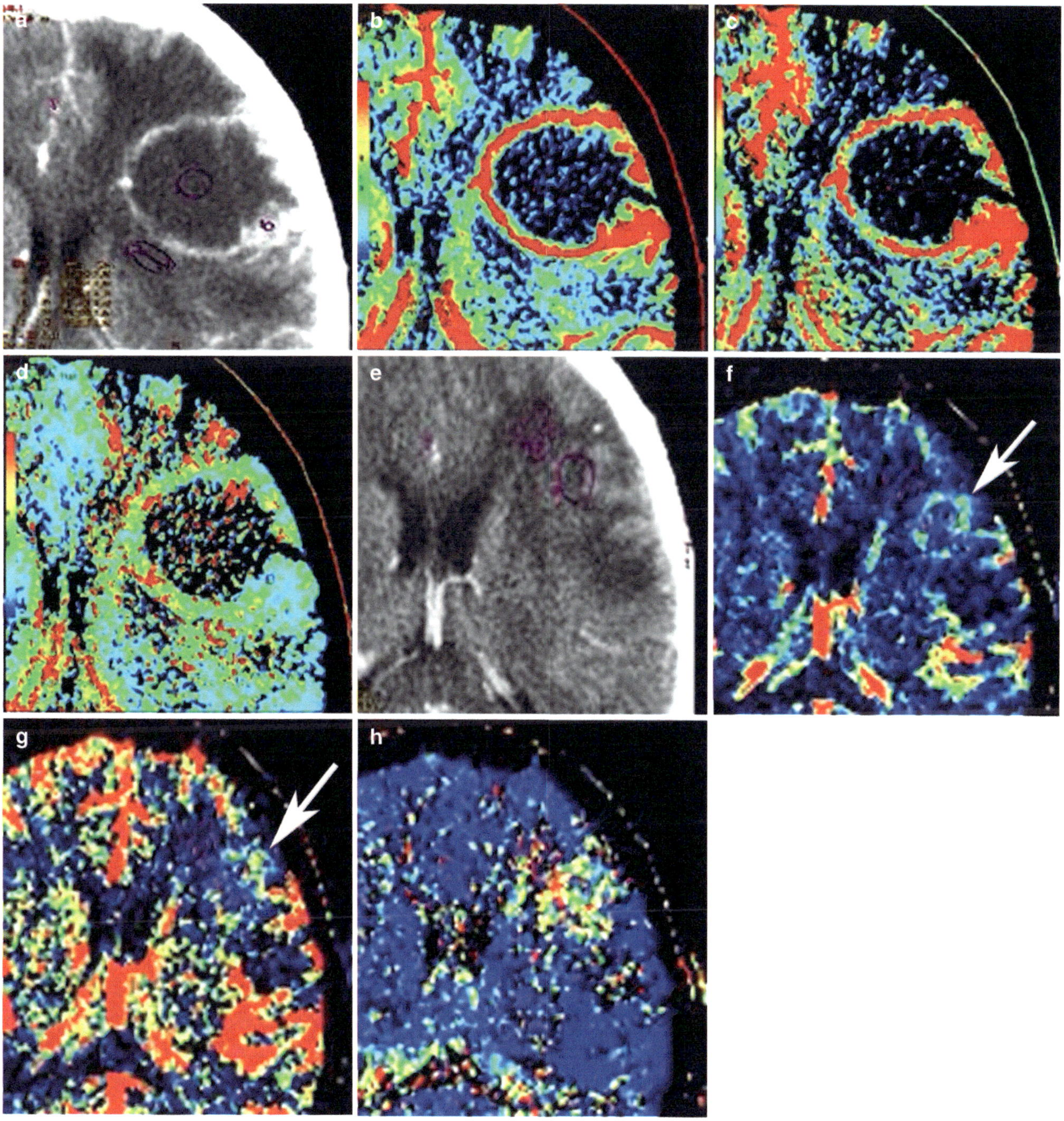

Fig. 22.12 A uterine cancer metastasis in the brain. A follow-up study before and after radiosurgery. The patient had a pacemaker; therefore, MRI could not be performed. In the left frontal lobe, there is a space-occupying solid-cystic lesion accumulating the contrast agent in the CT study (**a**) and having increased CBV (**b**), CBF (**c**), and MTT (**d**) values on CT perfusion maps. In the control study, there is a significant reduction in the tumor size (**e**); however, a portion remains with moderately elevated CT perfusion values along the anterior pole (**f**, **g**)—a residual tumor—and increasing of the MTT values (**h**)

23 Ovarian Cancer

According to Hardy and Harvey (1989), the analysis of a small group of ovarian carcinoma cases detected metastases in the brain in 11.6% of cases. Bruzzone et al. (1993) identified metastatic brain lesions only in 2.2% of cases among 413 patients with ovarian carcinoma treated with platinum-based therapy from 1981 to 1989. Mayer et al. (1978) found brain metastases in 0.9% of 567 autopsies of patients who died from ovarian cancer. In another large study by Pectasides et al. (2006), during 22 years in the analysis group ($n = 1450$ patients with ovarian cancer), only 17 (1.17%) developed brain metastases.

In our material, the proportion of ovarian cancer metastases in the brain was 1.8%, and there was a tendency to its increase in recent years.

Most ovarian cancer metastases in the brain manifest as single lesions. Lesions have a solid-cystic structure with a predominance of the cystic component. Almost always an area with a perifocal edema is visualized. The accumulation of the contrast agent by the solid part of the metastasis is expressed; the solid component of metastases is well visualized on MRI. When lesions are multiple, metastases may have different forms and can be detected by the presence of necrosis. Hemorrhages in the structure of ovarian cancer metastases are rare.

On SWI (SWAN) MRI, ovarian cancer metastases have a small number of hypointense inclusions. On the spectrum, there is a Lip-Lac complex typical of all metastases. On ASL images, the blood flow activity is directly proportional to the volume of the solid tumor, while the tumor is not visualized when its cystic component is prevalent.

The solid part of ovarian cancer metastases showed the lowest CBV values (5.34 ± 1.45 ml/100 g). Metastatic ovarian cancer is also characterized by the lowest CBF (49.51 ± 19.6 ml/100 g/min) values and mean MTT values (10.58 ± 6.27 s). Based on CT perfusion findings that identified perfusion indices specific to this type of metastases, the primary source of metastases can be assumed.

Despite the complexity of the diagnosis related to the close location of the pelvic organs and the presence of concomitant non-oncological diseases (tubo-ovarian abscesses, cysts, endometriosis), PET allows quite accurately the identification of the initial site of the primary tumor and its spread.

Grigsby et al. (2001), based on the data of the comparative analysis of the results from a survey in women with cervical and ovarian carcinoma (101 cases) by CT and PET, found that even single-organ PET was three times more effective than CT in detecting metastatic lesions of the pelvic lymph nodes (67 and 20%, respectively). Also, PET additionally identified metastatic involvement of supraclavicular lymph nodes in 8% of patients in this series.

The use of PET with ^{18}F-FDG for the primary diagnosis of metastatic brain lesions in ovarian cancer is impractical, both due to the predominantly cystic structure of such metastases and due to relatively low RP accumulation by the solid part of the tumor that merges with the image of the intact brain substance, since it physiologically accumulates the radiopharmaceutical.

23.1 Clinical Cases

See Figs. 23.1, 23.2, 23.3, 23.4, 23.5, 23.6, 23.7, 23.8, and 23.9.

M. Dolgushin et al., *Brain Metastases*, DOI 10.1007/978-3-319-57760-9_23

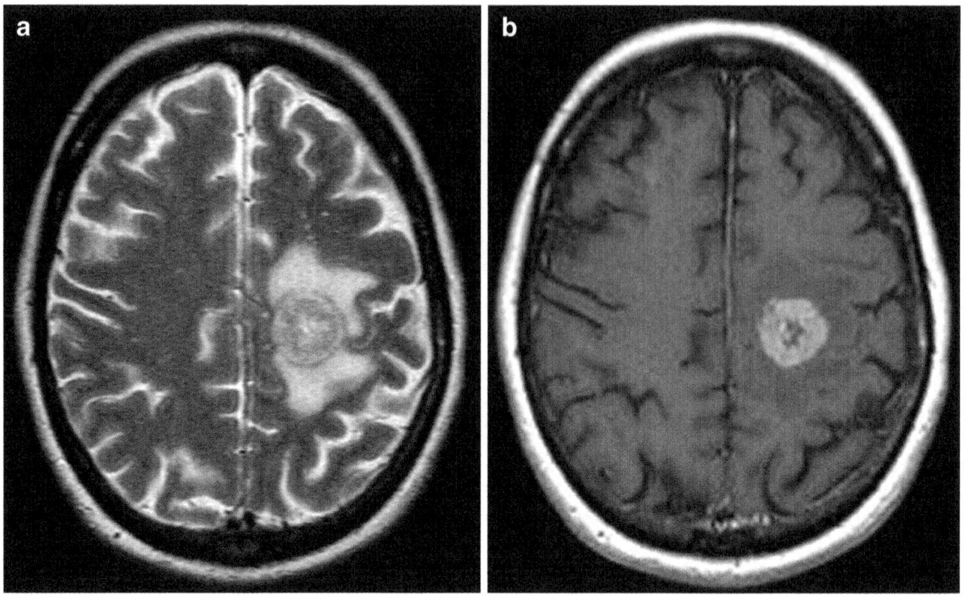

Fig. 23.1 An ovarian cancer metastasis in the brain. On MRI in the left frontal region, there is a rounded tumor lesion with an increased signal and signs of a perifocal edema on T2 images (**a**), intensely accumulating the contrast agent (**b**)—ring enhancement

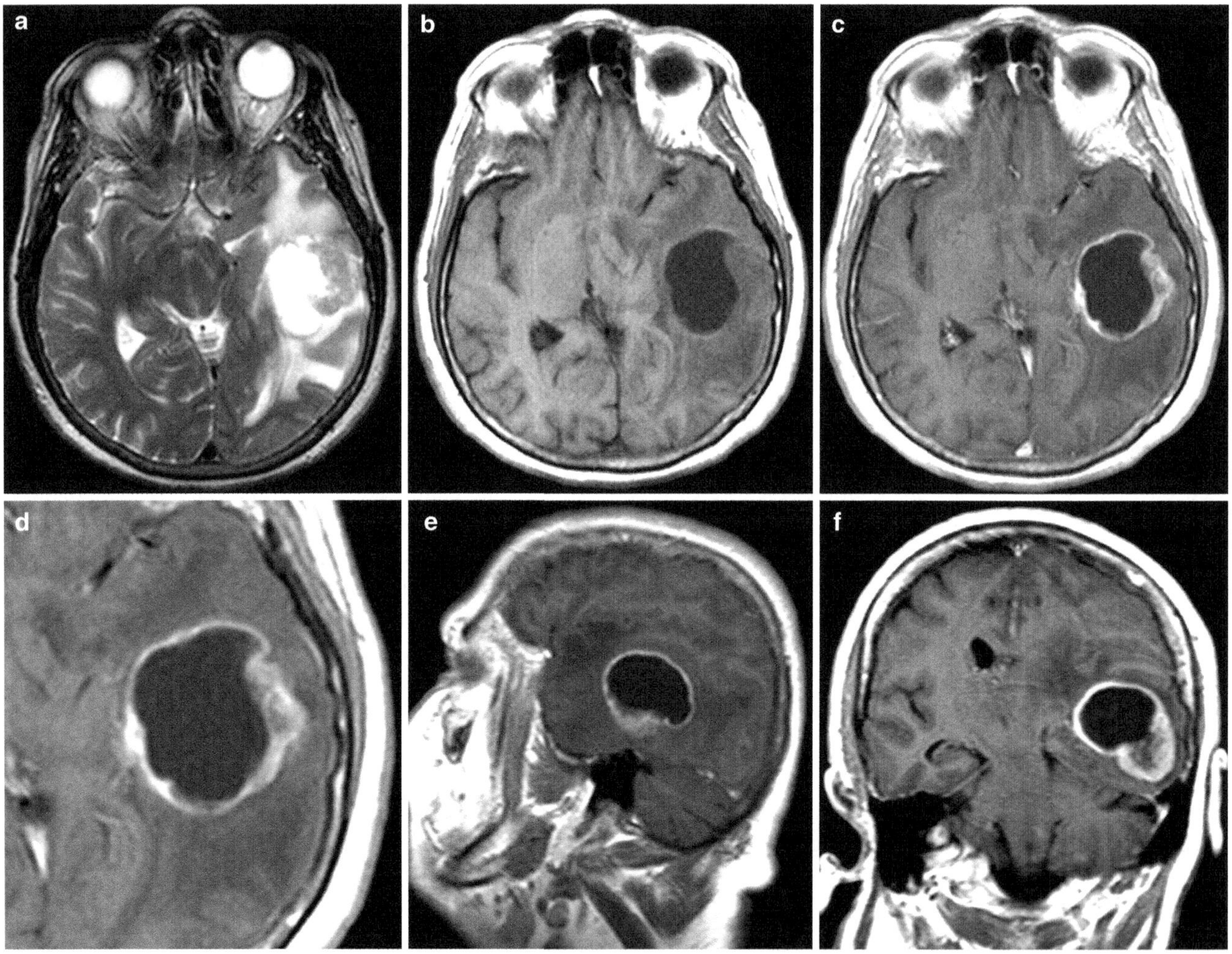

Fig. 23.2 An ovarian cancer metastasis in the brain. In the left temporal region, there is a solid-cystic lesion with a heterogeneously high signal on T2-weighted MRI (**a**) with an area of a pronounced perifocal edema and an isointense signal in the solid portion on T1-weighted MRI (**b**). The solid part of the tumor rapidly accumulates the contrast agent (**c**–**f**)

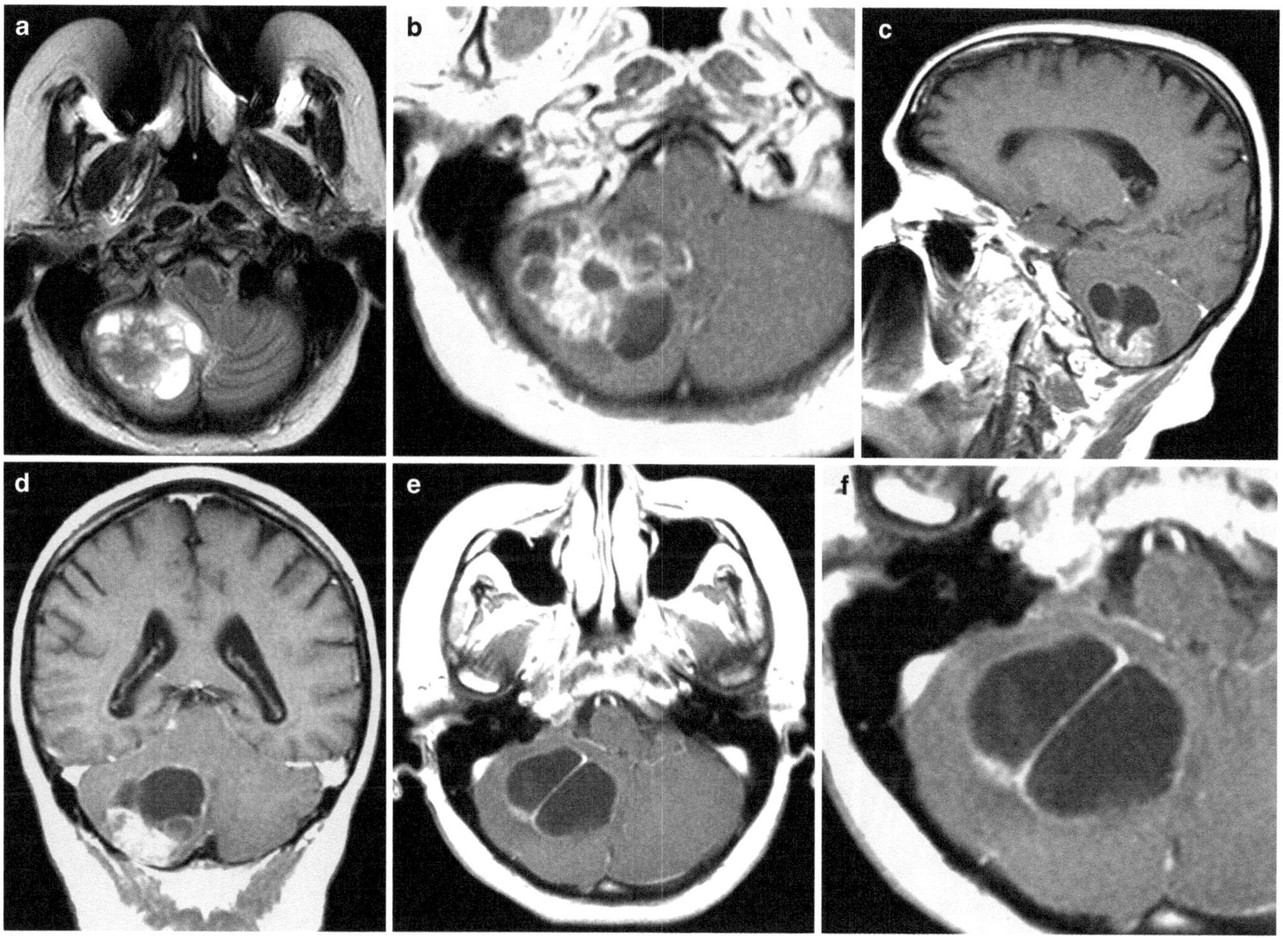

Fig. 23.3 An ovarian cancer metastasis in the brain. A two-level study. In the right hemisphere of the cerebellum, there is a solid-cystic lesion with a heterogeneously increased signal on T2-weighted MRI (**a**), intensely inhomogeneously accumulating the contrast agent in the solid parts of the tumor (**b–d**) and in the form of a thin rim—along the contour of cystic inclusions in the upper portions of the metastasis (**e**, **f**), with well-differentiated intratumoral trabeculae

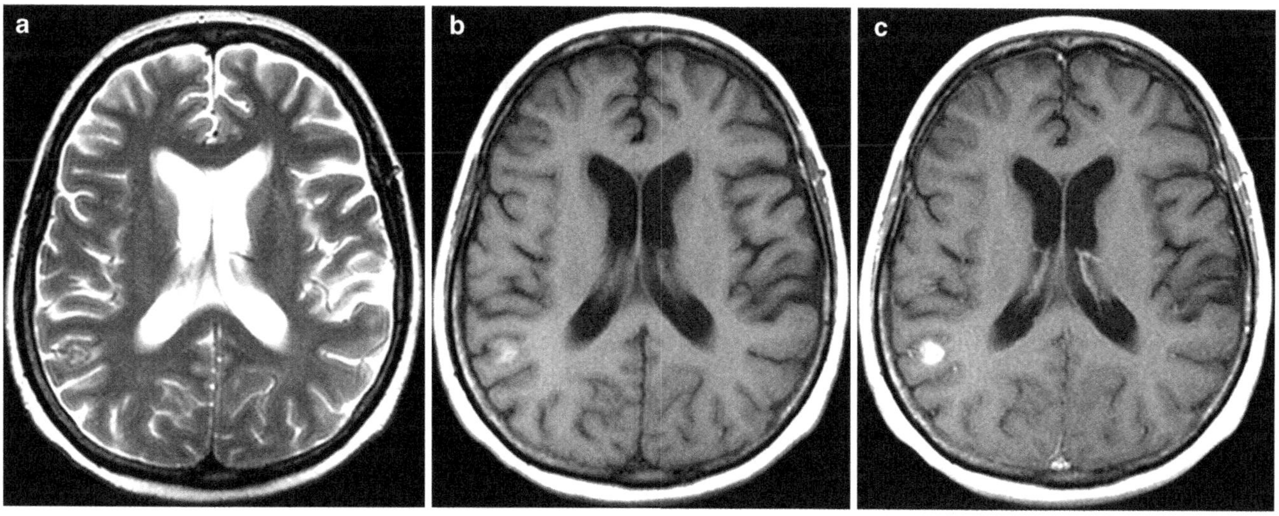

Fig. 23.4 An ovarian cancer metastasis in the brain. In the right parietal region, there is a small lesion with an iso-hyperintense signal on T2-weighted MRI (**a**) with no signs of a perifocal edema and with hemorrhagic inclusions, as evidenced by an increased signal on T1-weighted MRI (**b**); the lesion intensely accumulates the contrast agent (**c–f**). Upward from the lesion, there is a small portion of vascular origin that also intensely accumulates the contrast agent (**f**)—venous angioma (the *arrow*)

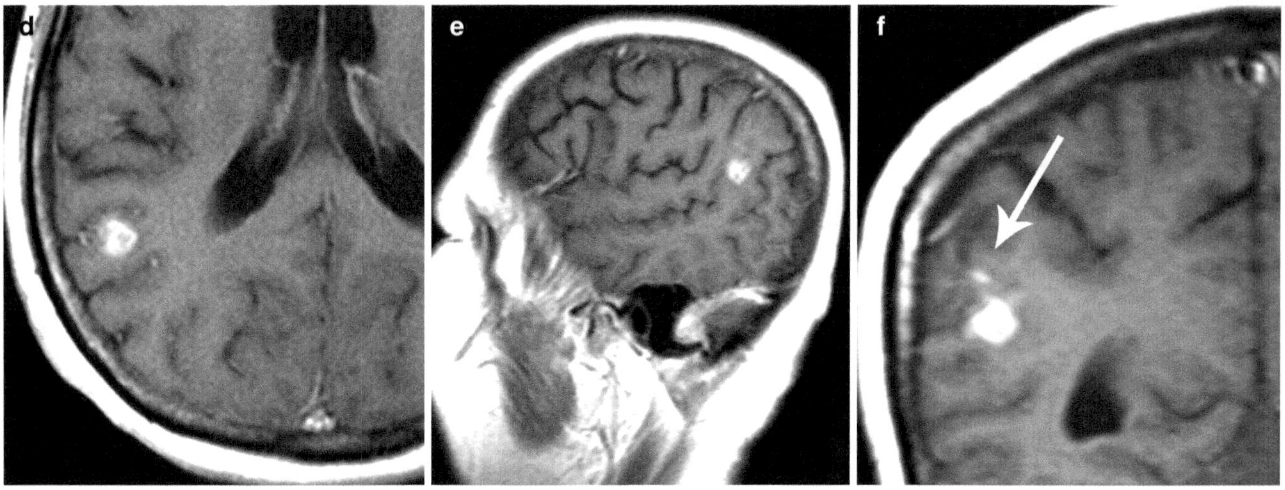

Fig. 23.4 (continued)

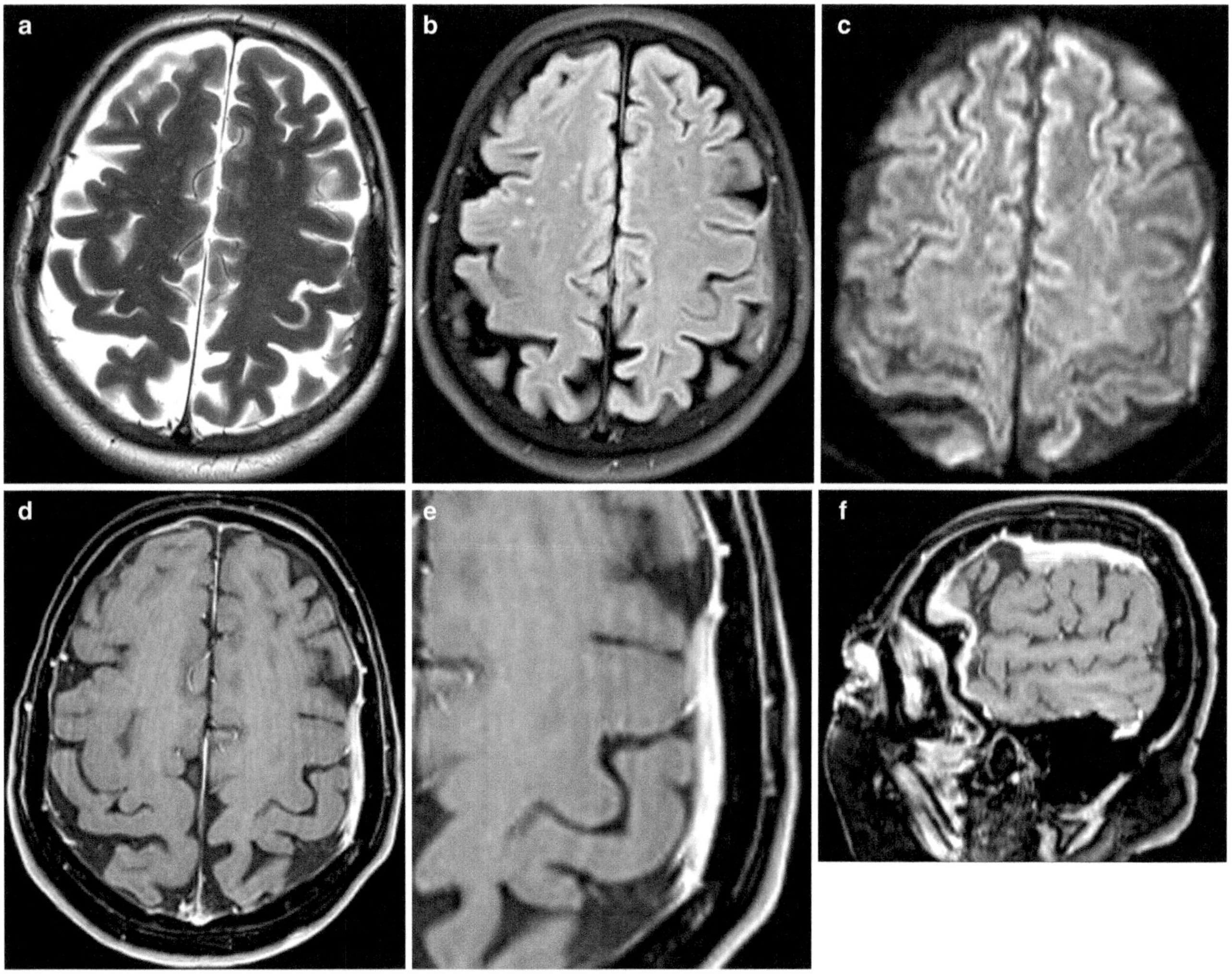

Fig. 23.5 Ovarian cancer metastases in the brain. Along the meninges in the left frontoparietal region, there is a space-occupying lesion with an iso-hypointense signal on T2-weighted (**a**) and T2-FLAIR MRI (**b**). On DWI MRI, the signal from the tumor is heterogeneously increased (**c**). The lesion intensely accumulates the contrast agent (**d**, **e**); the tumor spread into the region of the middle cranial fossa is visualized on sagittal constructs (**f**)

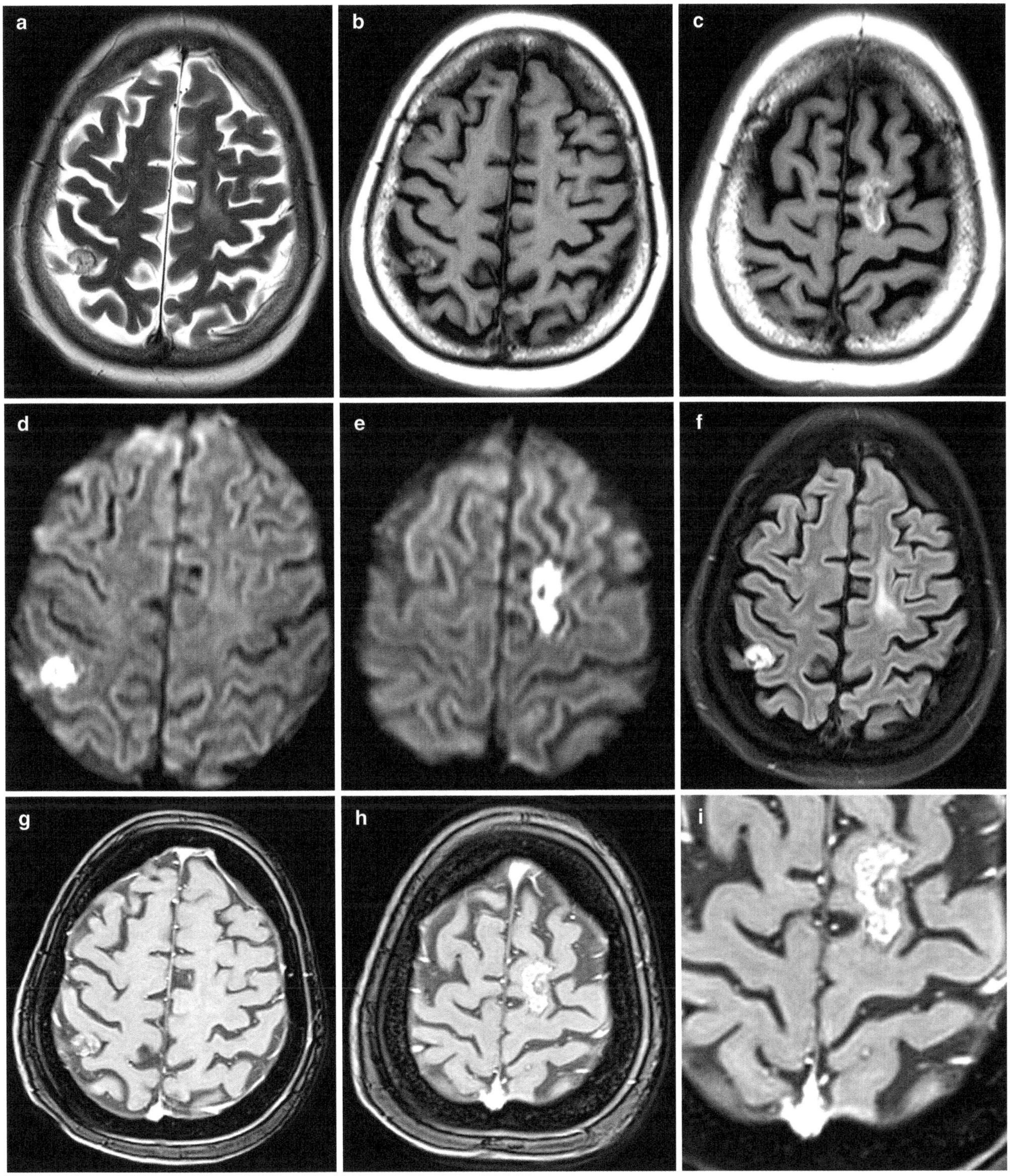

Fig. 23.6 Multiple ovarian cancer metastases. Condition after radiosurgery. A two-level study. MRI revealed abnormal lesions in the convexital parts of the right parietal region and a lesion in the left frontoparietal region similar by its signal intensity—a decreased signal on T2-weighted MRI (**a**), a heterogeneously increased signal on T1-weighted MRI (**b**, **c**), and a drastically increased signal on DWI (**d**, **e**) and T2-FLAIR MRI (**f**). Hemorrhagic changes have a high signal on T1-weighted MRI. Following intravenous administration, CA lesions weakly and fragmentarily accumulate the contrast agent (**g**–**i**)

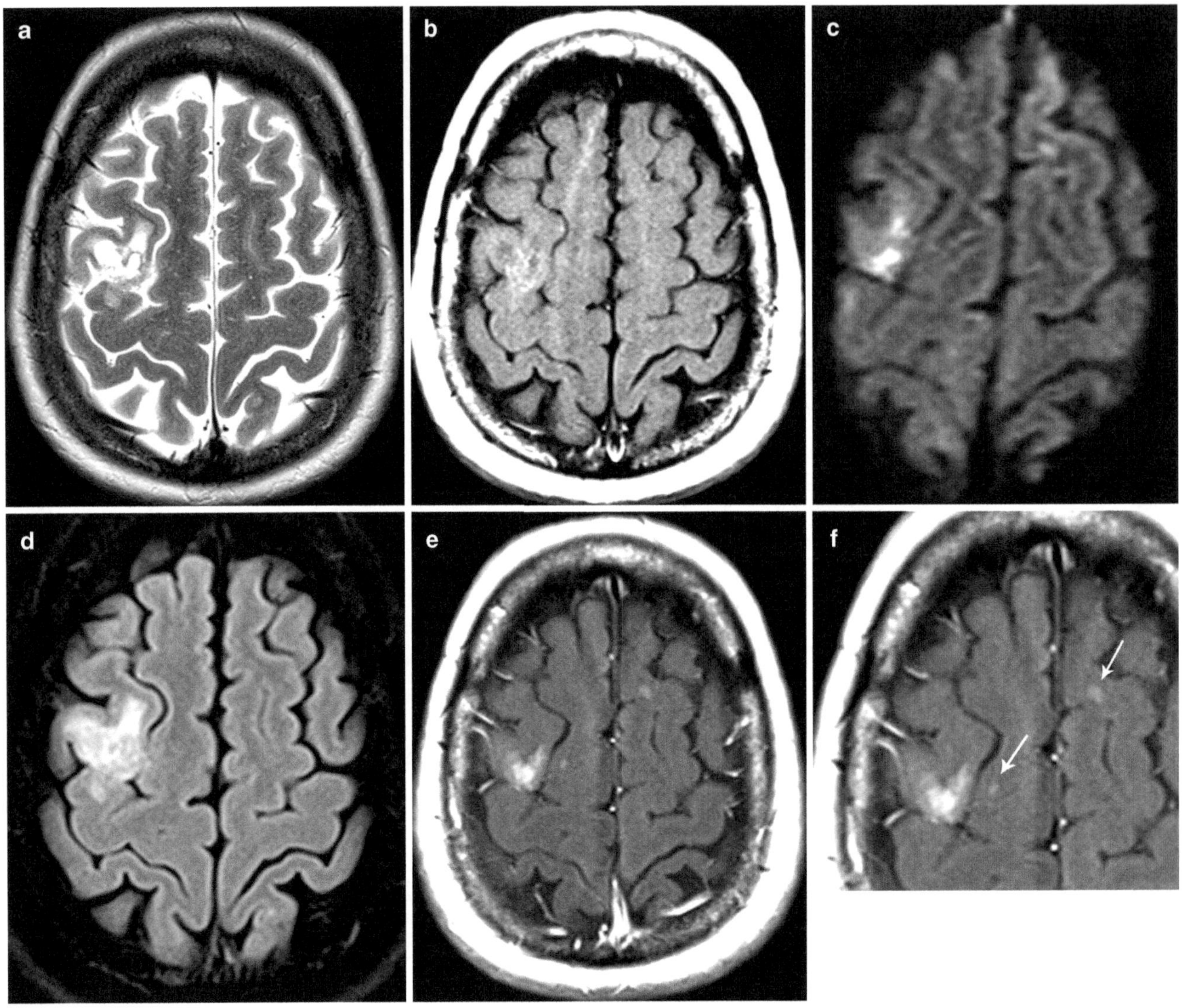

Fig. 23.7 Multiple ovarian cancer metastases in the brain. In the convexital portions of the right postfrontal region, there is a lesion with an increased signal on T2-weighted (**a**), T1-weighted (**b**), and DWI MRI (**c**), with an area of a moderate perifocal edema on T2-FLAIR images (**d**). Following intravenous CA administration, the lesion intensely accumulates the contrast agent; there are also contrast agent accumulation areas medially to the lesion and in the contralateral lobe (**e**, **f**) (the *arrows*)

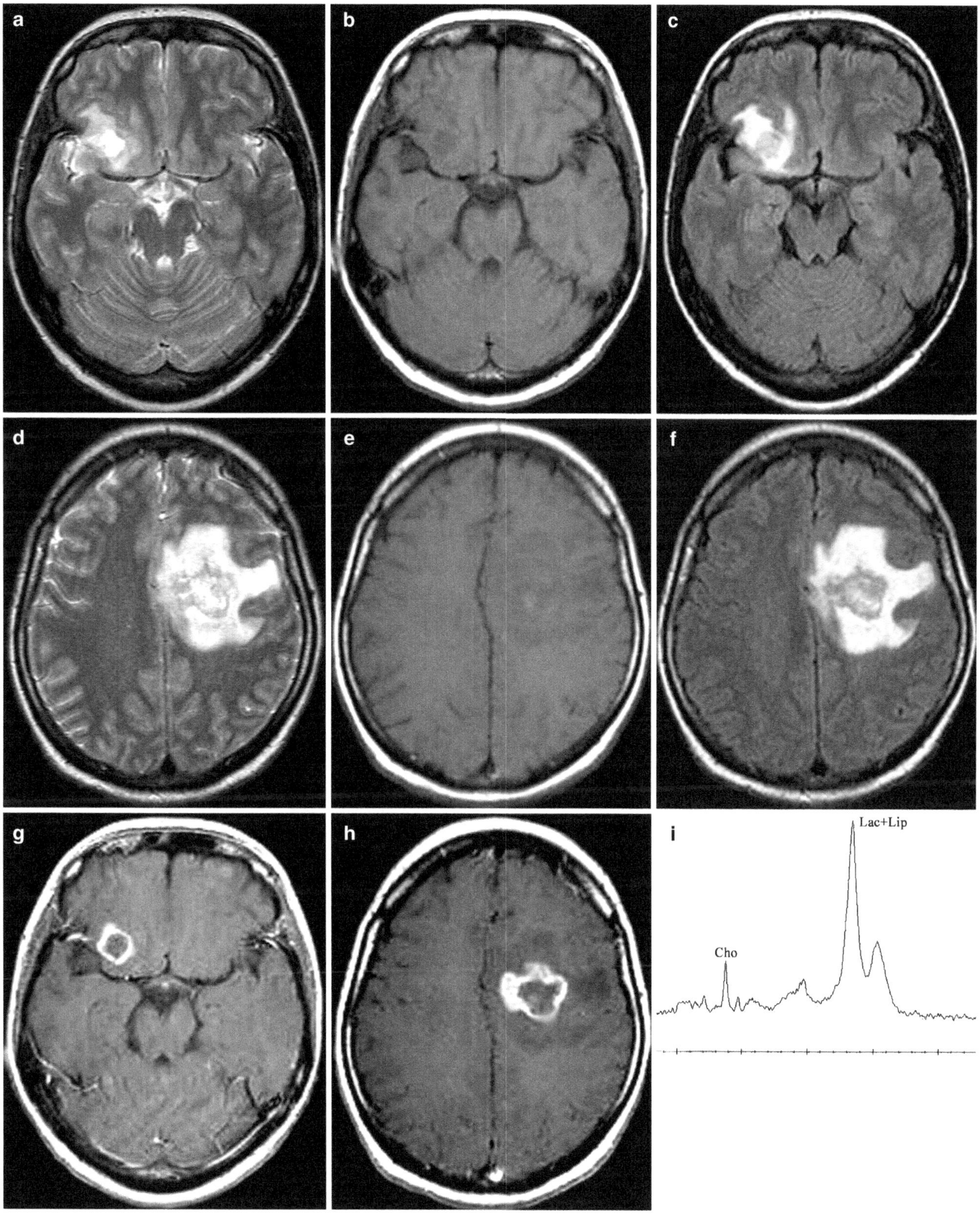

Fig. 23.8 Multiple ovarian cancer metastases in the brain. A two-level study. In the basal portions of the right frontal region, there is a lesion with a heterogeneous structure on T2-weighted MRI (**a**) and a hypo-isointense signal on T1-weighted MRI (**b**) with an area of a moderate perifocal edema (**c**). A similar lesion is located in the left frontal region (**d–f**). Following intravenous CA administration, all lesions actively accumulate the contrast agent on the periphery, with irregular contours (**g, h**). Both are characterized by central necrotic changes. On MR spectroscopy (**i**), there is an increase in the Lip-Lac complex and a moderate increase in the Cho peak

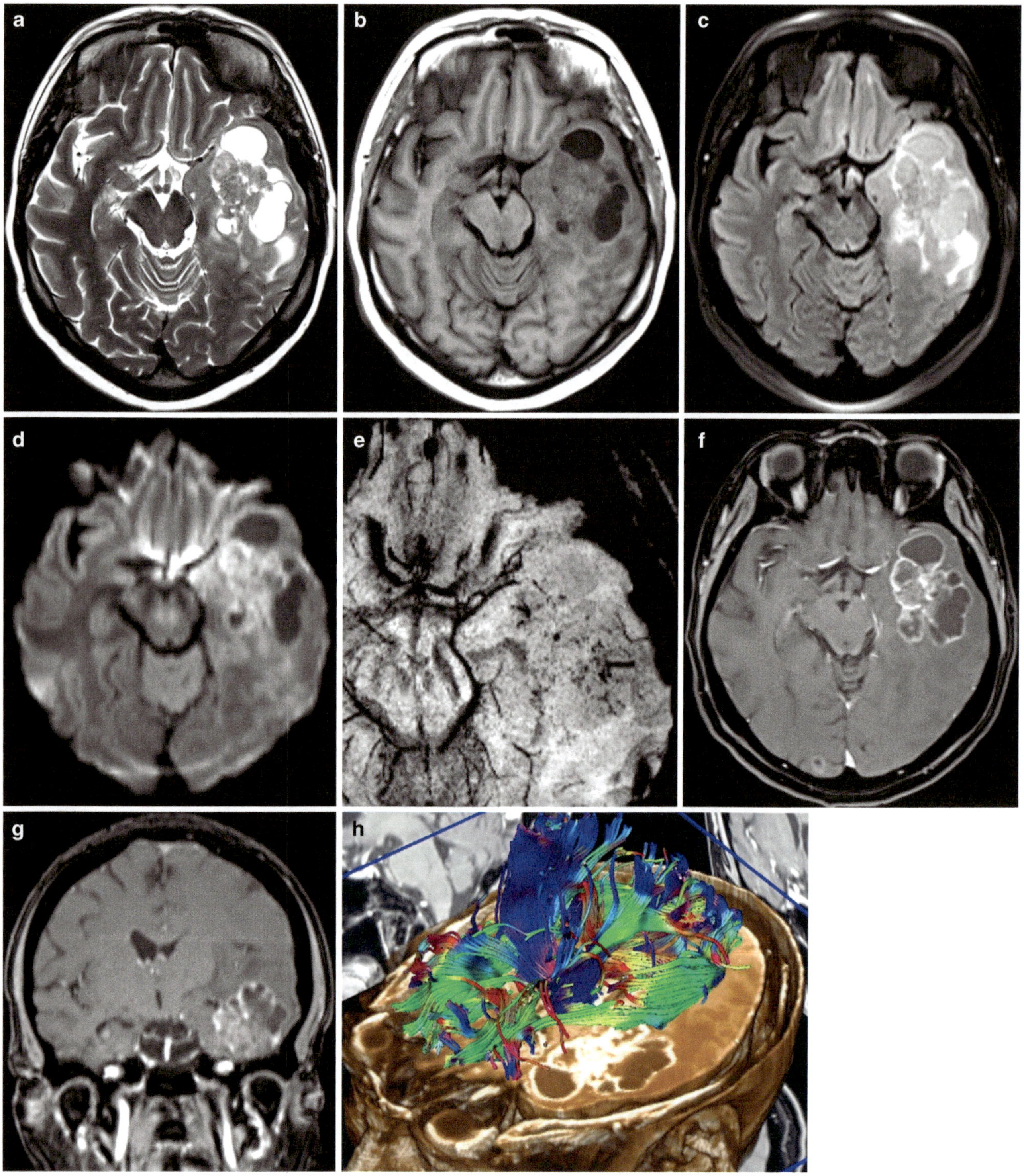

Fig. 23.9 An ovarian cancer metastasis in the brain. In the left temporal region, there is a solid-cystic lesion with a heterogeneously increased signal on T2-weighted MRI (**a**) and an iso-hypointense signal on T1-weighted MRI (**b**) with a moderate perifocal edema area (**c**). On DWI MRI (**d**), the signal from the lesion is heterogeneous due to the plurality of cystic inclusions. On SWI MRI (**e**), individual pinpoint inclusions with a low signal are determined in the metastasis structure. Following intravenous CA administration, the lesion intensely and inhomogeneously accumulates it (**f**, **g**); cystic components of the tumor are well visualized on the background of solid elements. On MR tractography, a deformation of adjacent conductive pathways (**h**) is observed

24 Thyroid Cancer

Thyroid cancer (TC) is the most common tumor of the endocrine system and amounts to 1–3% in the overall structure of cancers. The incidence of thyroid cancer has been steadily increasing within the past two decades, especially in industrialized countries. In Europe, the average rates are 1.2–3 per 100000 population. In Russia, more than 10000 patients are diagnosed with thyroid cancer every year. According to Davydov and Axel (2012), an increase in the incidence of thyroid cancer amounted to 6.2% in 2007–2012. The increased incidence of thyroid cancer is prevalent in the female population. Women make up 86% of all thyroid malignancies identified (Paches 2000a, b).

Factors contributing to the development of thyroid cancer include hyperplastic processes and disorders of endocrine regulation, radiation exposure and occupational hazards, stay in the areas of radiation accidents, and thyroid injuries.

Papillary carcinoma is a common tumor of the thyroid gland. It accounts for about 70% of all malignant tumors of the thyroid gland and usually develops in the third and fourth decade of life. Papillary carcinoma is characterized by lymphogenous metastasizing, while hematogenous metastasizing occurs relatively infrequently, with the typical location of metastases being lungs. Follicular thyroid cancer amounts to 15–20% and occurs in older age. The incidence of lymphogenous metastasizing of follicular carcinoma is 2–10%; hematogenous metastases occur in 20% of cases, typically in bones. Both forms of cancer are characterized by rather slow growth and a favorable prognosis. The 5- and 10-year survival rate in papillary and follicular thyroid carcinomas is 95.3% and 94.2% and 90.1% and 85.7%, respectively. According to Pacini et al. (2008), despite the increase in its incidence, mortality from thyroid cancer, in general, and from papillary thyroid carcinoma, in particular, remained stable both in 1973 and 2002 and amounted to 0.5 deaths per 100000 patients.

The proportion of other malignant thyroid tumors (medullary carcinoma, undifferentiated/anaplastic cancer) does not exceed 8–15%, while that of squamous cell carcinoma is 3.1%. Squamous thyroid cancer is characterized by early and extensive metastasizing, a severe clinical course and a poor prognosis. Non-differentiated thyroid cancer is also characterized by a severe clinical course with a median survival of 5–6 months (Paches and Propp 1995; Valdina 2006).

The incidence of metastatic brain lesions with thyroid cancer, according to different authors, is 0.1–5% (Parker et al. 1986; Jyothirmayi et al. 1995; Altimari-Romero et al. 1997; Salvati et al. 2001; Mazzaferri et al. 2006; Al-Dhahri et al. 2009). On the other hand, Pemberton (1939) found metastases in 4–9% in the analysis of a series of 774 patients with thyroid cancer. In a retrospective database study for the period from 1976 to 2011, Tsuda et al. (2013) found metastases of papillary carcinoma in the brain only in five cases. The time from the detection of the primary tumor to the detection of metastases of thyroid cancer in the brain is 2.8 years for papillary cancer and 1.2 years for anaplastic cancer (Salvati et al. 1995).

In our sample, metastases of thyroid cancer were identified in 0.8% of cases.

Thyroid cancer metastases in the brain are presented as a supra- and subtentorial lesions. In our cases, we also noted metastatic involvement of the skull with intracranial spread. No significant invasion of adjacent meninges was

M. Dolgushin et al., *Brain Metastases*, DOI 10.1007/978-3-319-57760-9_24

noted, while the destruction of bone structures infiltrated by the tumor was total. The contrast agent accumulation in the TC metastasis stroma in the brain is homogeneous, in several cases microhemorrhagic inclusions were observed in the form of increased signal portions on T1-weighted MRI.

MRI provides for a study according to the standard protocols—T2-weighted, T1-weighted, T2-FLAIR, and T1-weighted + Gd MRI. Additional methods—3D SPGR, SWI (SWAN), spectroscopy, and ASL—did not show any significant differential diagnostic signs.

24.1 Clinical Cases

See Figs. 24.1, 24.2, 24.3, 24.4, and 24.5.

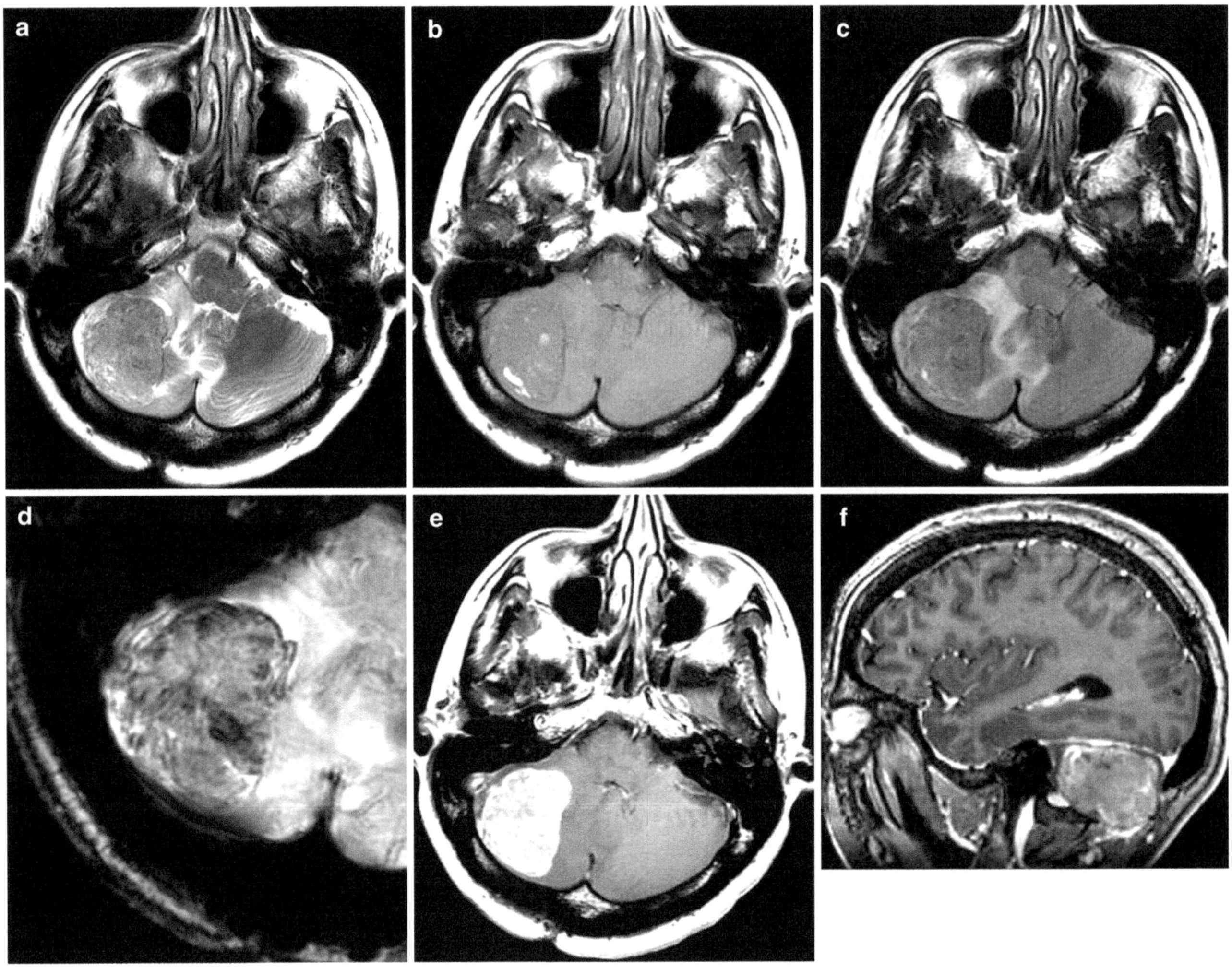

Fig. 24.1 A thyroid cancer metastasis in the brain. In the right cerebellar hemisphere, there is large solid lesion with an increased signal on T2-weighted MRI (**a**), with areas of hemorrhagic changes—an increased signal on T1-weighted MRI (**b**) and a moderately pronounced perifocal edema (**c**). On SWI MRI, individual blurred inclusions with a decreased signal are identified in the tumor (**d**). After CA administration, its intense homogeneous accumulation is observed in the lesion (**e**, **f**); the fourth ventricle is compressed

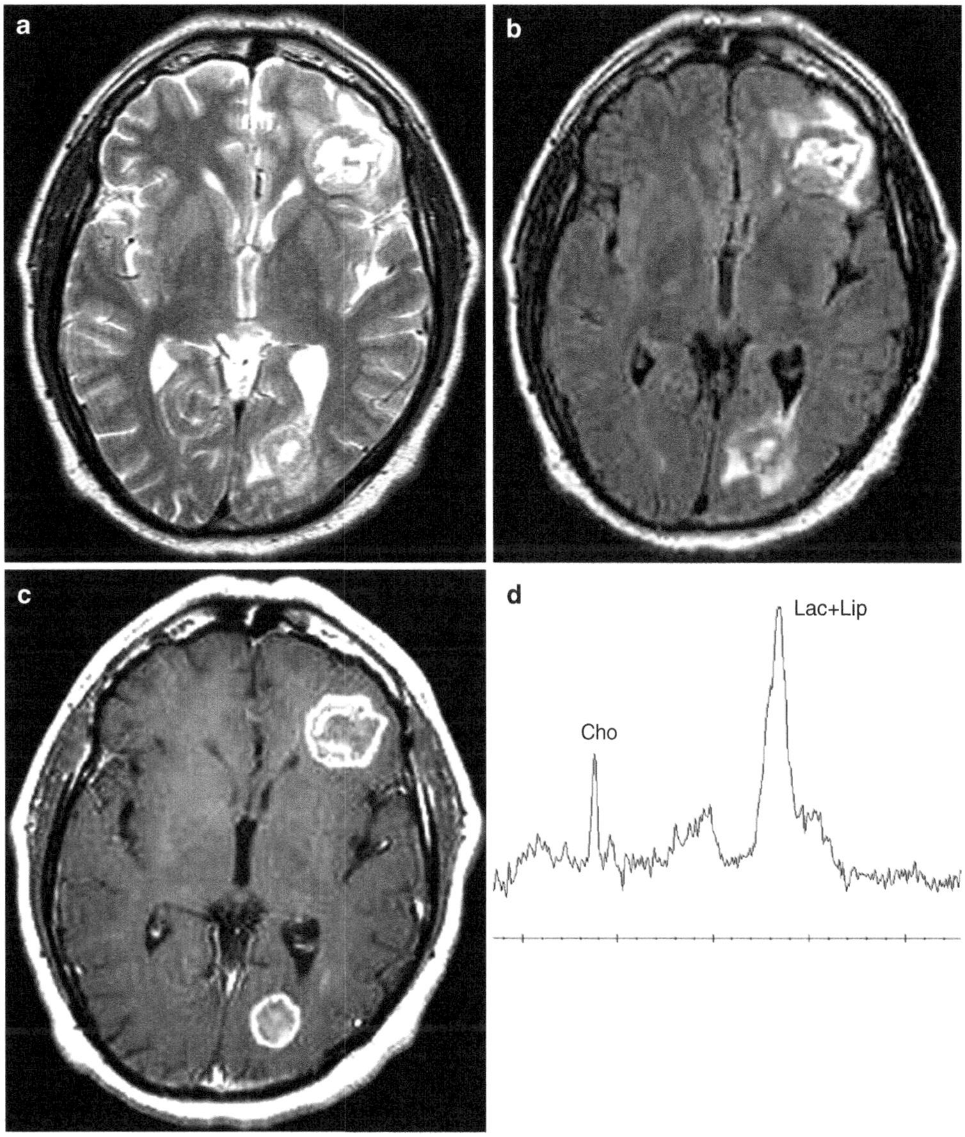

Fig. 24.2 Multiple thyroid cancer metastases. In the left frontal and occipital areas, there are lesions with a heterogeneous structure on T2-weighted and T2-FLAIR MRI (**a**, **b**) with a moderate perifocal edema. After CA administration, its intense inhomogeneous accumulation is observed predominantly on the periphery of metastases (**c**). MR spectroscopy shows an increase in the peak of the Lip-Lac complex as well as a fairly high Cho peak (**d**)

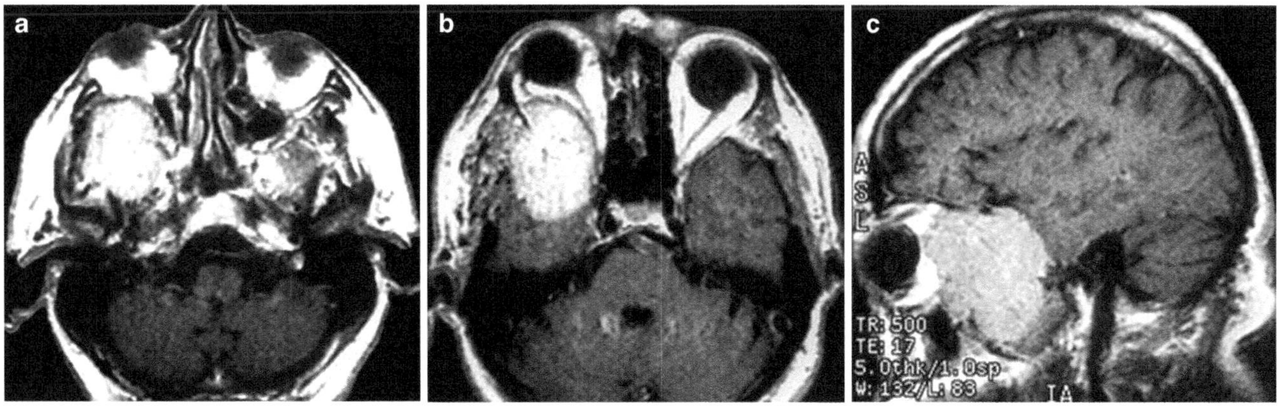

Fig. 24.3 A metastasis of thyroid cancer. On T1-weighted MRI with contrast enhancement in the axial (**a**, **b**) projection at two levels and sagittal (**c**) projection, there is a tumor lesion located in the lateral parts of the right orbit with the spread into the infratemporal fossa. A vast area of destruction of the orbital walls is observed. The optic nerve is displaced medially; exophthalmos is present

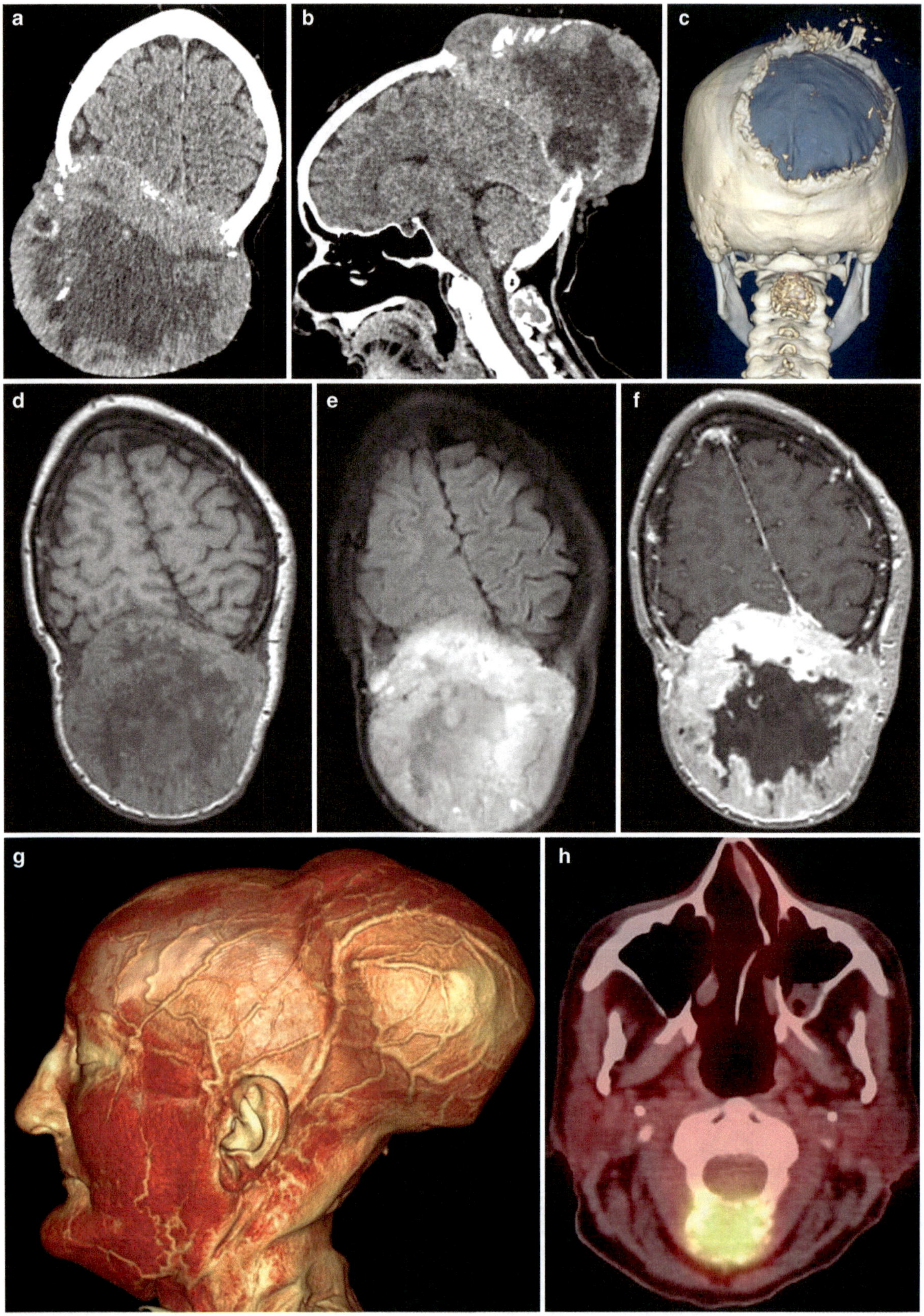

Fig. 24.4 A metastasis of thyroid cancer (before treatment). On CT in the parietal-occipital areas (mostly on the right), there is a large lesion with extra-intracranial spread; marked destruction of the cranial bones is noted with the dislocation of bone fragments (**a**–**c**). The lesion is characterized by an iso-hypointense signal on T1-weighted MRI (**d**) and an increased signal on T2-FLAIR MRI (**e**). After CA administration, its intense accumulation is noted in the solid part of the metastasis (**f**); central parts of the tumor are presented by necrosis. On 3D-CT reconstructions (**g**), dilated surface veins and arteries of soft tissues of the head are well visualized. On a PET/CT study, there are areas with abnormal RP accumulation in the area of the spinous process and C2 vertebral arch (**h**, **j**) and in the lateral lesions in the sacrum on the right (**i**, **j**)

Fig. 24.4 (continued)

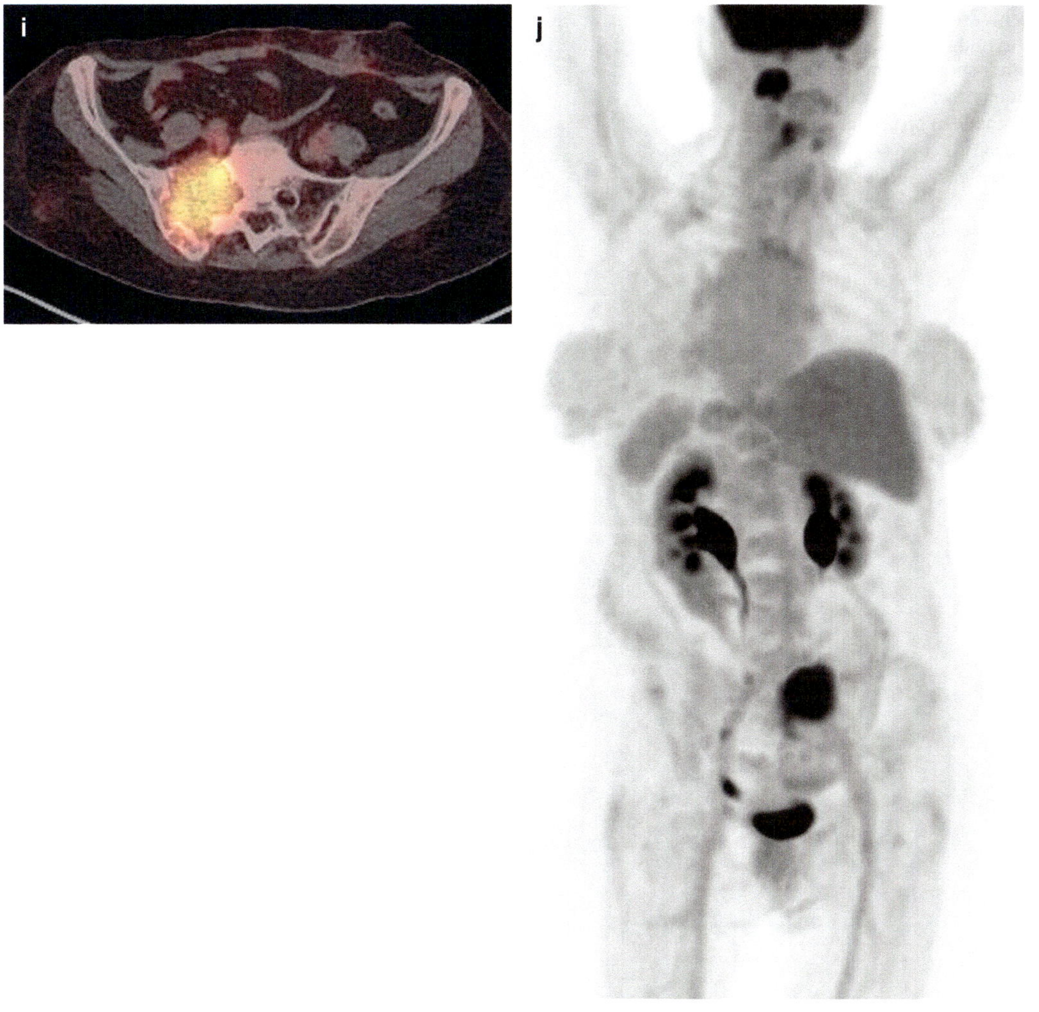

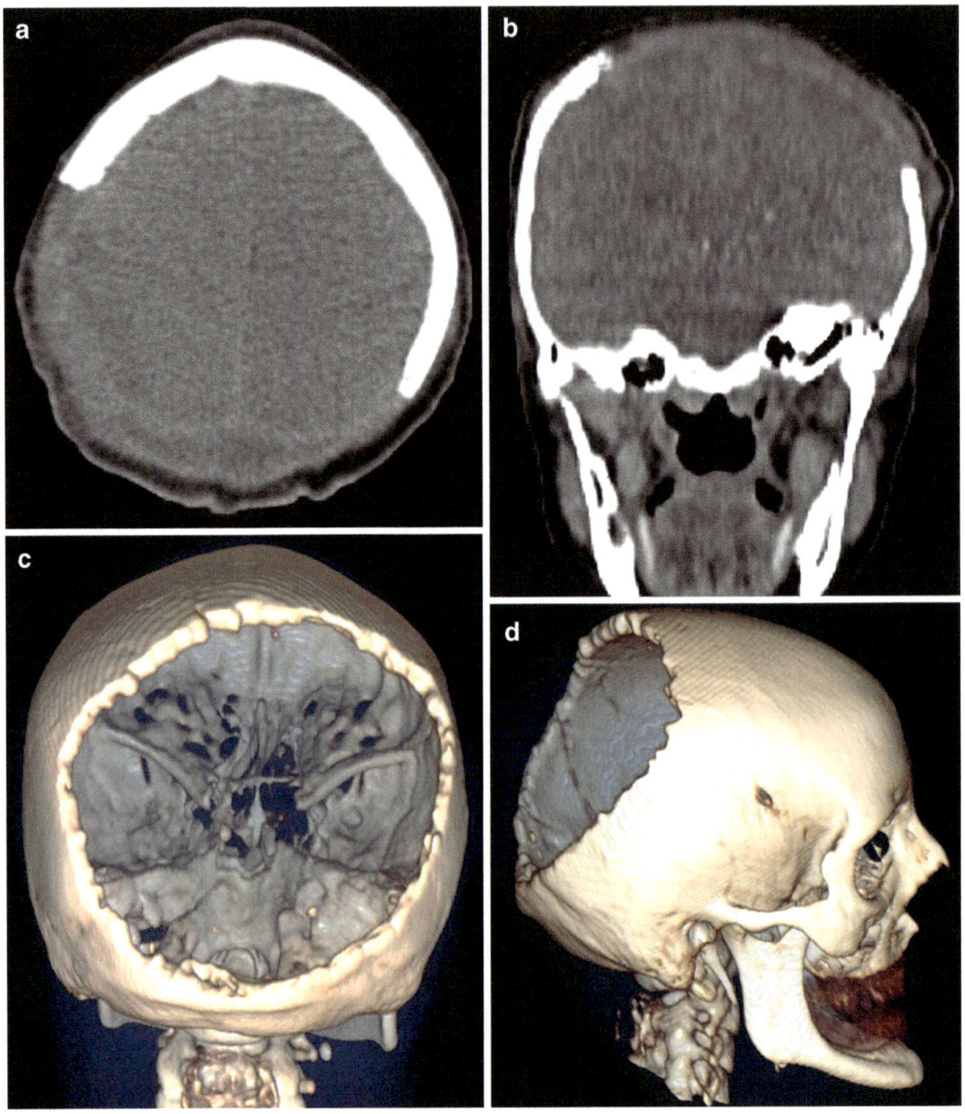

Fig. 24.5 A metastasis of thyroid cancer. Condition after surgical removal of the tumor. On CT in axial (**a**) and frontal (**b**) projections and 3D reconstruction (**c**, **d**), there is an extensive bone defect in the area of the removed metastasis

25 Rare Forms of Cancer with Metastases in the Brain

In most cases, metastatic tumors classified as "rare forms of cancer" also did not show any specific diagnostic characteristics that would differentiate them from other metastases, but we find we have to present this small group of cases.

25.1 Cancer of the Parotid Salivary Gland

The most common tumor of the salivary glands is a pleomorphic adenoma—a benign mixed tumor consisting of both epithelial and mesenchymal tissues—and accounts for about 70% of all tumors of the salivary glands (Gnepp et al. 2001; Som et al. 2003). Most of these tumors are located laterally to the area of the facial nerve. Mostly, these are well-separated painless tumors; they occur in middle-aged patients. Malignant forms of ductal carcinoma are the most common malignant variant of salivary gland tumors. In 25% of cases, if untreated, they can metastasize with involvement of meninges (Thackray and Lucas 1983; Peel and Gnepp 1985; Som et al. 1988; Olsen and Lewis 2001). Malignant neoplasms are accompanied by severe pain and are identified in the elderly; infiltrative spread to the salivary gland tissue is possible. The 5-year survival is only about 50% (Som and Brandwein 2003), with the cause of death being metastases, including to the brain. The brain involvement is combined with involvement of the lymph nodes in the neck. Since the spread of the tumor occurs mainly by a hematogenous route, distant metastases are found in 44% of cases (Olsen and Lewis 2001). They usually affect the lungs, pleura, kidneys, and choroid. We observed three cases of intracranial metastases of the parotid gland tumor.

Metastases of the parotid gland cancer in the brain are often cystic, with the solid component rapidly accumulating the contrast agent. No reliable differential diagnostic characteristics have been identified using additional methods. No hemorrhages were observed (Figs. 25.1 and 25.2).

25.2 Neuroendocrine Tumors (NETs)

Neuroendocrine tumors (NETs) heterogeneously group of epithelial tumors developing from APUD system cells, characterized by a positive immunohistochemical reaction to specific markers (chromogranin A, synaptophysin) and the ability to produce a variety of peptide hormones and biogenic amines. Standardized incidence rates for NETs in different countries vary within 0.71–1.36 per 100000 patient-year (Gulec et al. 2002). The most common site of NETs is the gastrointestinal tract (73.7%) and the bronchopulmonary system (25.1%). Within the gastrointestinal tract, most tumors are located in the small intestine (28.7%), the appendix (18.9%), and the rectum (12.6%). The overall 5-year survival of patients with NETs, regardless of their site, is 67.2–82% (Bektas et al. 2002).

NET metastases in the brain, including those of intracranial nature (pituitary tumors), are extremely rare (our clinical material includes two cases, one of which is presented below).

In most cases, NETs have no clinical symptoms to complications or to the development of carcinoid syndrome. Therefore, in most cases, a primary tumor and metastases are difficult to diagnose. The degree of differentiation of APUD cells and their functional activity and synthesis of hormones affect the rate and characteristics of tumor growth and its ability to metastasize. The principal method of treatment for NETs of the abdominal cavity and retroperitoneal space is surgery. Most authors have quite a unanimous opinion on the treatment strategy: a local excision can be performed for tumors smaller than 2.0 cm; radical operations are performed for larger tumors (subtotal resection of the stomach, small intestine resection, and hemicolectomy (Neumann et al. 2002; Soga 2003)). For conservative treatment, hormonal and chemotherapeutic drugs are used (6-methylprednisolone, ACTH, Endoxan, 5-fluorouracil). The effect of their use is low and short term.

M. Dolgushin et al., *Brain Metastases*, DOI 10.1007/978-3-319-57760-9_25

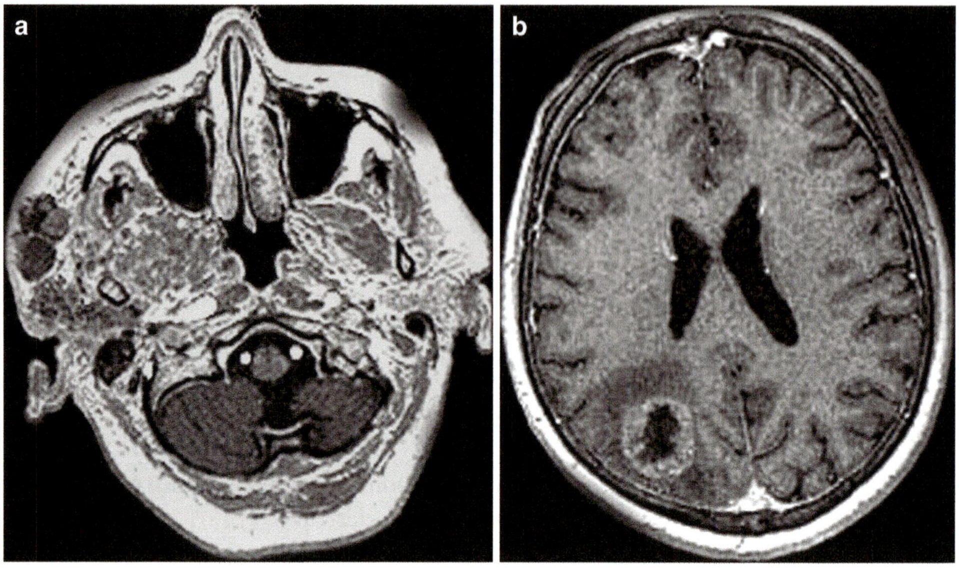

Fig. 25.1 Metastases of parotid gland cancer. A two-level study. On T1-weighted MRI with contrast enhancement, multiple tumor lesions are identified in the soft tissues of the right malar area (**a**). In the right parietal lobe region, there is a solitary rounded lesion that intensely accumulates the contrast agent of in the form of ring enhancement (**b**)

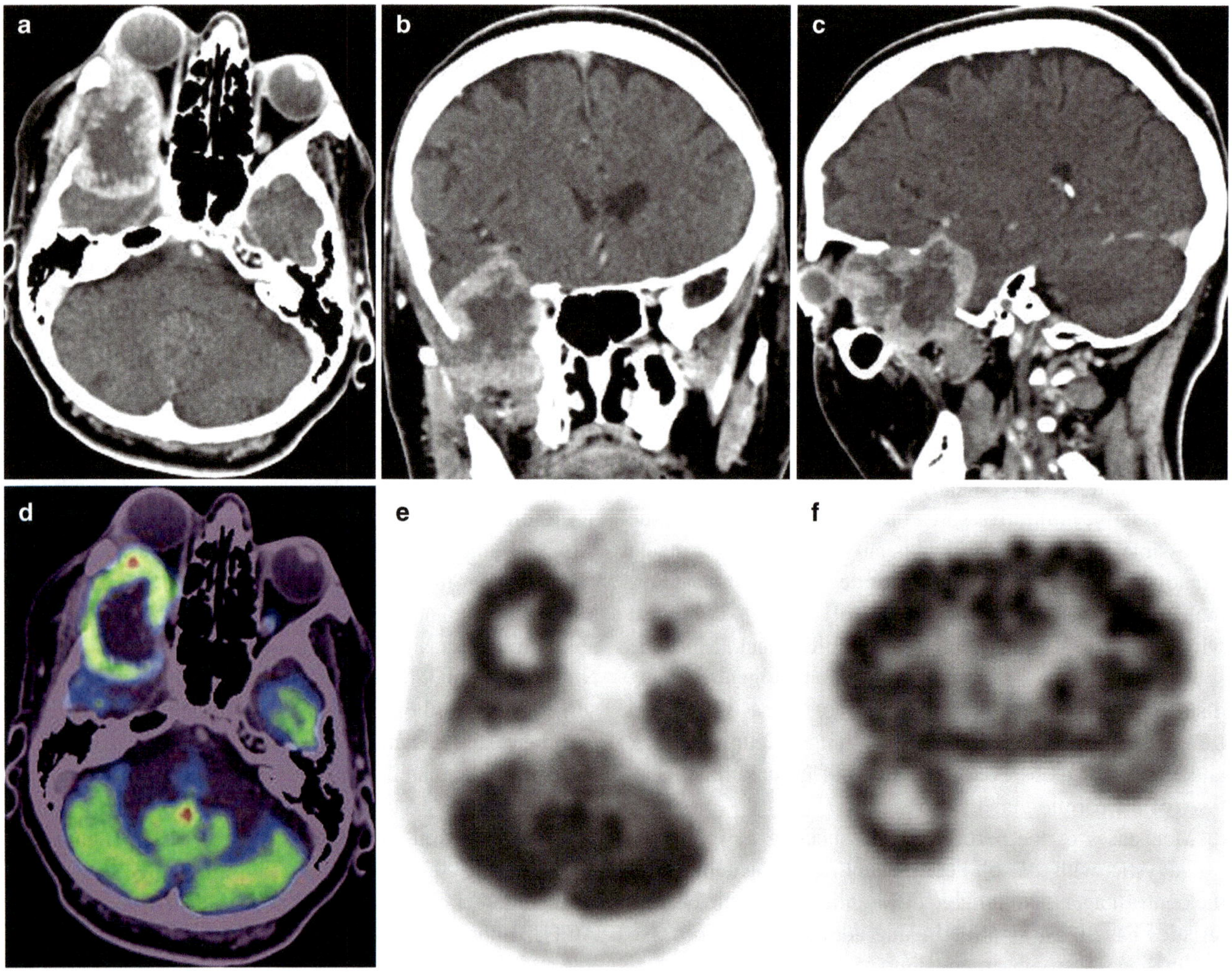

Fig. 25.2 A metastasis of parotid gland cancer in the brain. In the basal right temporal region, there is a lesion destroying the adjacent bone structures and extending to the region of the right orbit, infratemporal fossa, as well as intracranially, deforming the temporal lobe and shifting it upward (**a–c**). On a PET/CT study with ^{18}F-FDG, there is an increase in SUV along the contour of the tumor (**d–f**)

Today, there are various methods for NET diagnosis: CT, MRI and ultrasound methods; lately, radioisotope methods are widely used—SPECT/CT with ^{111}In-octreotide and PET/CT with ^{68}Ga-DOTA (TOC, TATE, NOC). These drugs allow to evaluate the tumor receptor activity; therefore, they are highly specific in the diagnosis of NETs (Fig. 25.3).

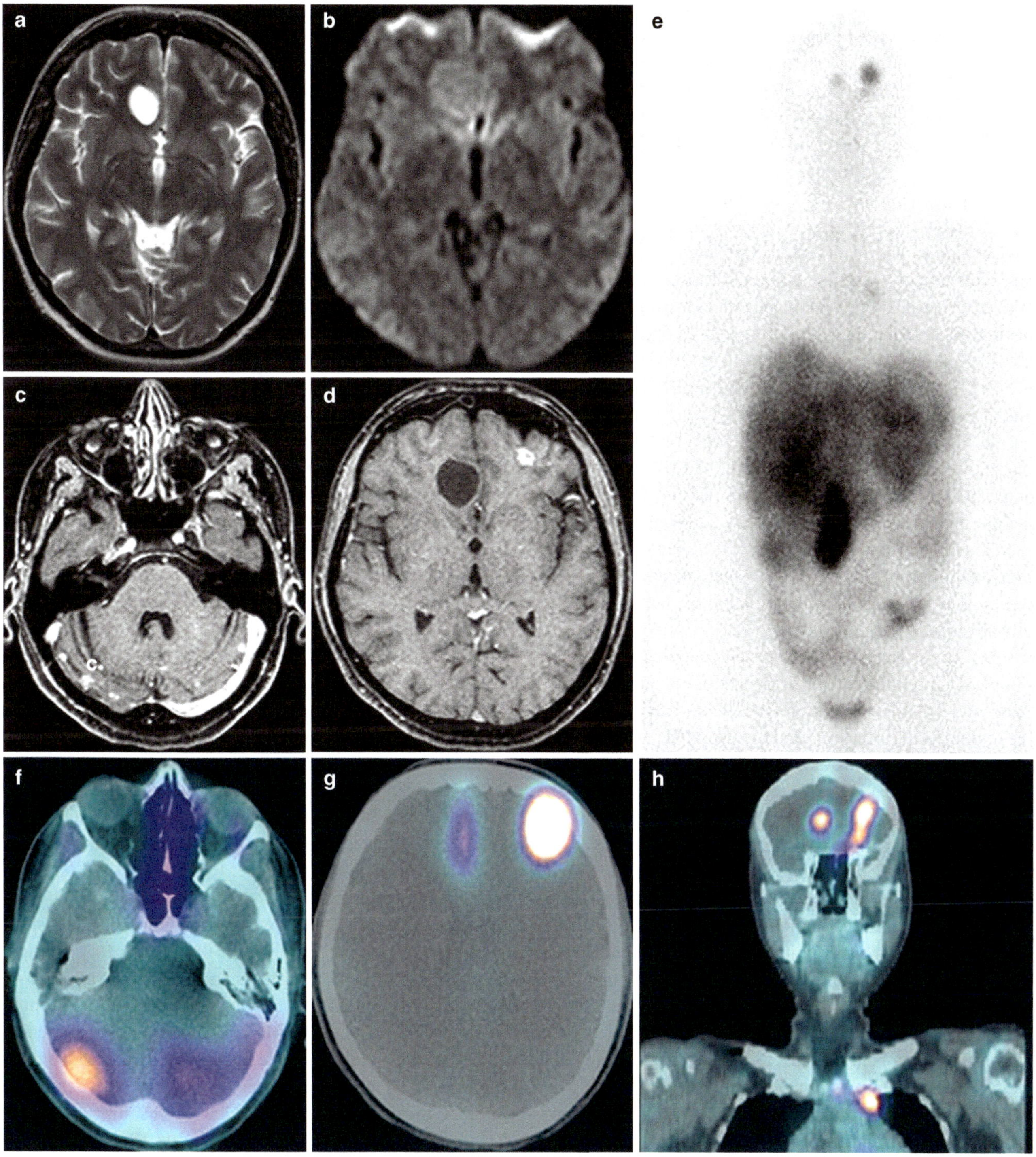

Fig. 25.3 Multiple neuroendocrine tumor metastases in the brain. Sub- and supratentorially, there are multiple lesions with various sizes. In the right frontal region, there is the largest cystic lesion with an increased signal on T2-weighted MRI (**a**), a moderately high signal on DWI MRI (**b**), that weakly accumulates the contrast agent along its contour (**d**). Small metastases in the left frontal region and in the hemispheres of the cerebellum have a mainly solid structure and intensely accumulate the contrast agent (**c**, **d**). There is no perifocal edema. A radionuclide study with ^{111}In-octreotide on whole-body scans in the frontal projection (**e**) shows lesions with increased RP accumulation in the frontal areas of the brain, the hilum of the left lung, and the liver. On SPECT images in the axial (**f**, **g**) and frontal (**h**) projections, the cystic lesion in the right frontal region is characterized by a smaller area of increased RP accumulation than the small solid lesion in the left frontal region. Multiple pinpoint metastases in the cerebellum exhibit diffuse accumulation. A tumor site in the upper mediastinum is additionally identified (**h**) (the image is courtesy of Professor Shiryaev, S.V.)

25.3 Sarcoma (Fibrosarcoma)

Sarcoma (fibrosarcoma) is a malignant tumor of soft tissues that is formed from the immature fibrous connective tissue. It is often located in the muscles of extremities (hip, shoulder) or torso. Brain sarcomas are quite rare, occur with a frequency of up to 2%, and are usually located in the craniofacial area. There are infantile fibrosarcoma (in children under 10 years of age) and adult fibrosarcoma (common in children older than 10 years of age and in adults, more often at the age of 40–55 years old) (Toro et al. 2006).

Brain sarcoma has all the properties of a malignant tumor—aggressive rapid growth and the ability to grow into normal tissues and metastasize. Sarcomas are characterized by predominantly hematogenous metastasizing in 90% (Friedrichs et al. 2006), with not less than two third of patients having affected the lungs, less frequently bones, brain, pancreas, liver, and kidneys (Ottaiano et al. 2005). Warren and Meyer (1938) and then a number of other authors (Taylor and Nathanson 1942; Willis 1952; Pack and Ariel 1958) suggested the possibility of lymphatic metastasizing of sarcomas; however, it accounts for no more than 10% (Behranwala et al. 2004; Yanagawa et al. 2014). In our material, sarcomas are presented by two cases of intracranial metastases.

CT and MRI manifestations of craniofacial sarcoma are indistinguishable from those other malignancies growing in this area. By the time of primary diagnosis, the tumor is usually advanced.

On CT, this is a soft tissue space-occupying lesion, causing the destruction of bone structures in the anterior cranial fossa and craniofacial region. Presence of petrifications in the tumor stroma is uncharacteristic. An MRI pattern depends on the predominant histological structure. On T1-weighted images, this is usually an isodense lesion as compared to the brain; on T2-weighted images, the MR signal is variable from hypo- to slightly hyperintense.

Osteogenic sarcoma causes bone destruction with an aggressive periosteal reaction and formation of bony growths, often observed in the lower jaw. On CT, this lesion has an increased density with a periosteal reaction and a solid component accumulating the contrast agent. On T1-weighted MRI, in case of high mineralization, this is a heterogeneous lesion with a low-intensity MR signal; if the soft tissue component prevails, the signal has medium intensity. If the tumor has a soft tissue structure, on T2-weighted MRI, a high MR signal prevails; if intense mineralization is observed, the MR signal is low (Yamaguchi et al. 2004) (Figs. 25.4, 25.5, and 25.6).

25.4 Laryngeal Cancer

In the general structure of morbidity of malignant tumors, laryngeal cancer (LC) occupies the ninth place and accounts for 1.8–2.2% (Paches 2000a, b). In 2000, the number of newly diagnosed LC cases was 7.7 per 100000 of Russian population, while 65% of them were of working age (Chissov et al. 2000). The disease predominantly develops in men (96%) aged 50–70 years old (Kozhanov et al. 2008; Daykhes et al. 2009).

In recent years, there is a trend to steady growth in the incidence of this disease in women. According to Davydov and Axel (2014a, b), the standardized increase in the incidence of LC in the female population of the Russian Federation for the period from 2007 to 2012 was 14.3%, determining the second place (in terms of an increase rate) in the structure of malignant tumors in women. In the male population, in contrast, a downward trend in this parameter was observed (−4.1%).

In the world population, the leading place in the LC incidence belongs to Thailand and Poland. A high incidence was noted in the countries of Western Europe—Italy, Spain, and France. A more favorable situation was observed in the Scandinavian countries and Japan, where the incidence is two persons per 100000.

The leading etiological factor of LC development is the combination of smoking and alcohol abuse. According to many authors, up to 98% of patients have many years of history of smoking (Brennan et al. 1995). A certain role plays chronic inflammatory processes in the larynx.

Malignant neoplasms of the larynx usually develop from the surface epithelium and, in general, are presented by squamous cell carcinoma (95%). Sarcomas, adenocarcinomas, and other neuroendocrine cancers develop in the larynx extremely rare. It should be noted that laryngeal cancer occupies the first place among malignant tumors of the upper respiratory tract by its incidence.

Regional metastases in LC are found in 35–60% of cases (Vokes et al. 1993; Ushakov and Ivanov 2003). The risk of distant metastasizing increases in the presence of multiple regional metastases. Metastases to distant organs occur in 1–9% of cases, mainly by a lymphogenous route and more often in younger patients. Most often the lungs are affected and less frequently the mediastinum, pleura, and liver. Metastases of laryngeal cancer in the brain are extremely rare: the incidence of distant LC metastases, including cerebral metastases, does not exceed 1% (de Bree et al. 2001; Ghosh and Prabhash 2011) (Figs. 25.7 and 25.8).

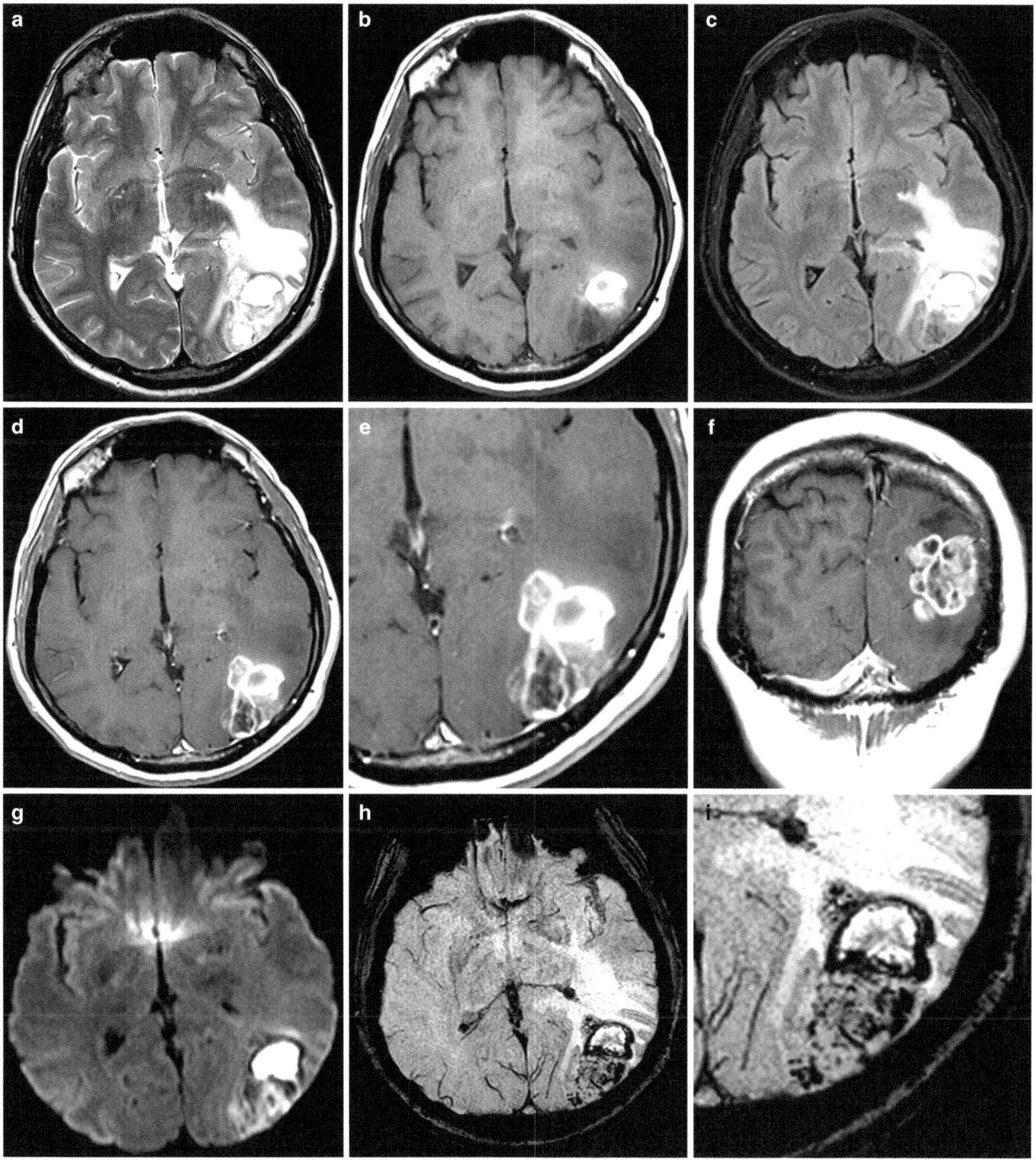

Fig. 25.4 A sarcoma metastasis in the brain. On MRI, in the left parietal-occipital region, there is a multinodular lesion with a solid-cystic structure, with a high signal on T2-weighted MRI (**a**), with hemorrhagic changes, as evidenced by hyperintense inclusions on T1-weighted MRI (**b**) and hypointense inclusions on SWI MRI (**h**, **i**), surrounded by a severe edema (**c**). There is intense, inhomogeneous accumulation of the contrast agent by the solid areas and along the contour of the tumor cystic components (**d**–**f**). On DWI, there is an inhomogeneous increase in the signal from the tumor (**g**) due to the hemorrhagic component

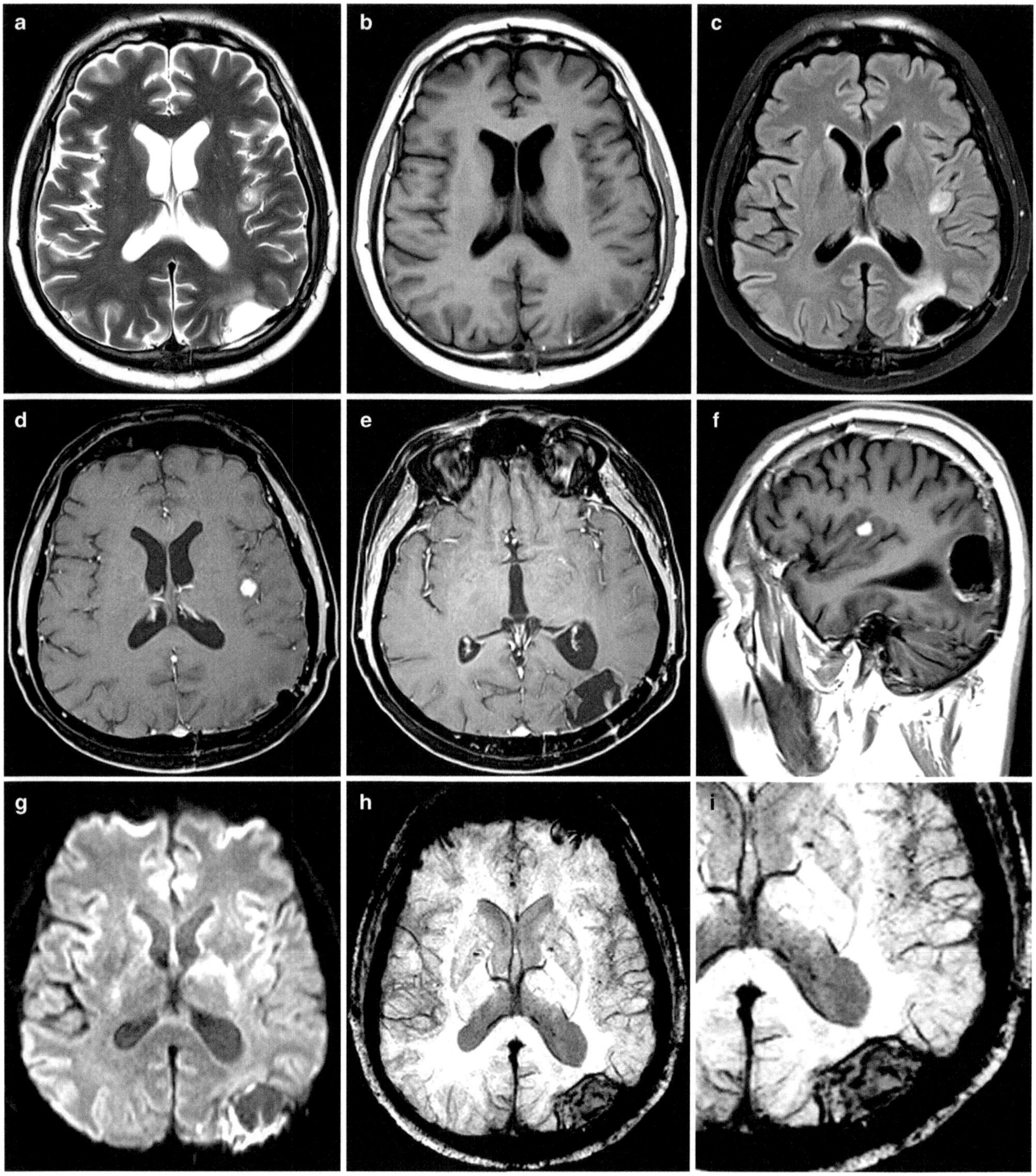

Fig. 25.5 A sarcoma metastasis in the brain. Condition after surgical removal, recurrence, and disease progression. On the background of postoperative changes in the left occipital region, there is a postoperative cavity (**a**, **b**, **c**) along the inferior contour, where a small linear portion of abnormal accumulation of the contrast agent is observed (**e**, **f**). In the left temporal region, there is a lesion with a high MR signal on T2-weighted (**a**) and T2-FLAIR MRI (**c**), uniformly intensely accumulating the contrast agent (**d**, **f**). On DWI MRI, there is an increase in the signal from the abovementioned areas (**g**). On SWI MRI, the lesion in the left temporal region is not visualized; there is an extensive area of an inhomogeneously decreased signal (**h**, **i**) in the left occipital region

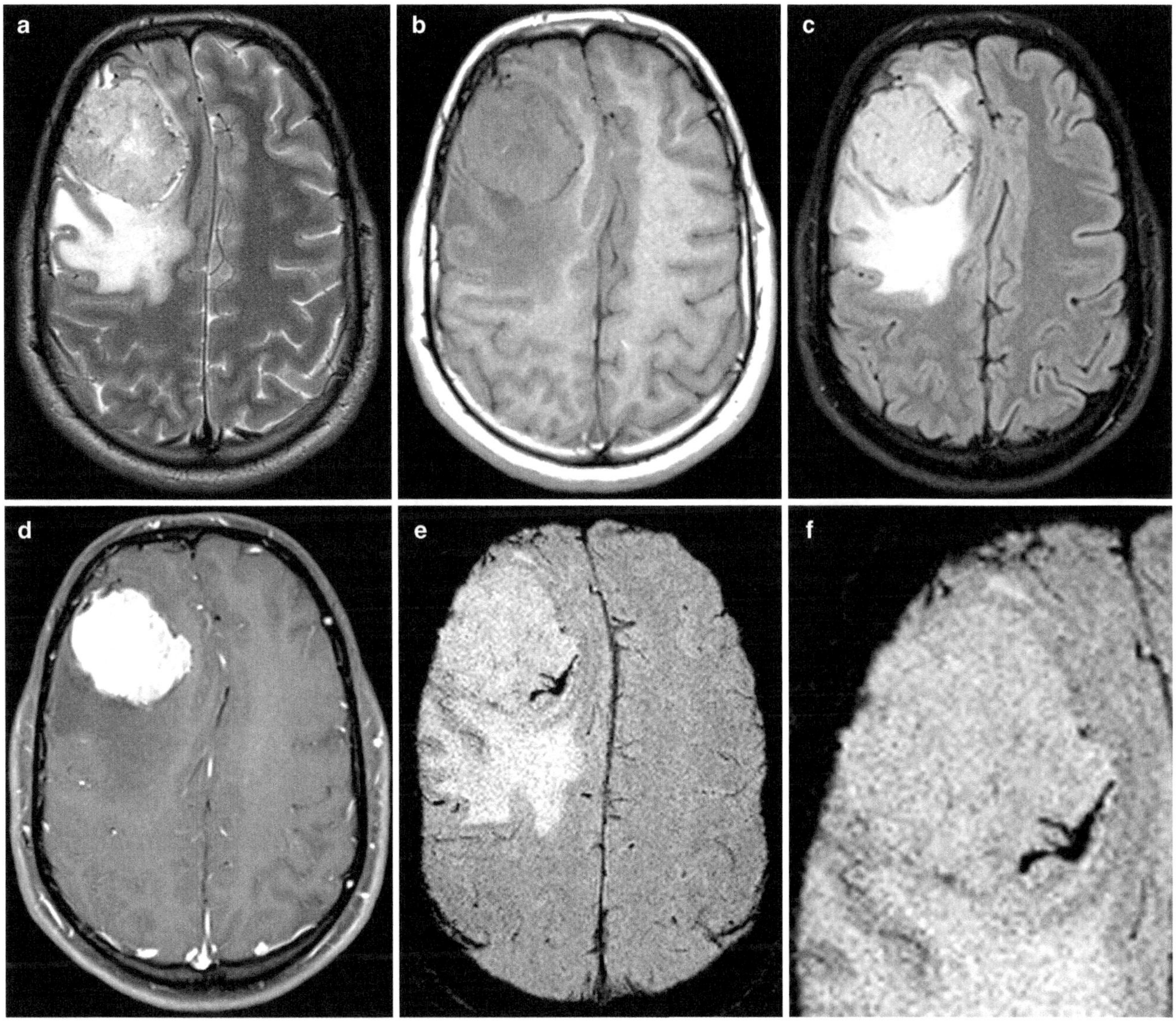

Fig. 25.6 A sarcoma metastasis in the brain. In the right frontal region, there is a large space-occupying lesion with an increased signal on T2-weighted and T2-FLAIR MRI (**a**, **c**), surrounded by a region with a perifocal edema. Noteworthy is the presence of a CSF cleft along the periphery of the metastasis. On T1-weighted MRI, the signal from the lesion is homogeneous, weakly hypointense (**b**). Following intravenous CA administration, the lesion intensely and uniformly accumulates it (**d**). On SWI MRI, the signal from the main mass of the lesion is homogeneous and increased, except for the medial contour, where a hypointense portion is observed, representing venous vessels (**e**, **f**)

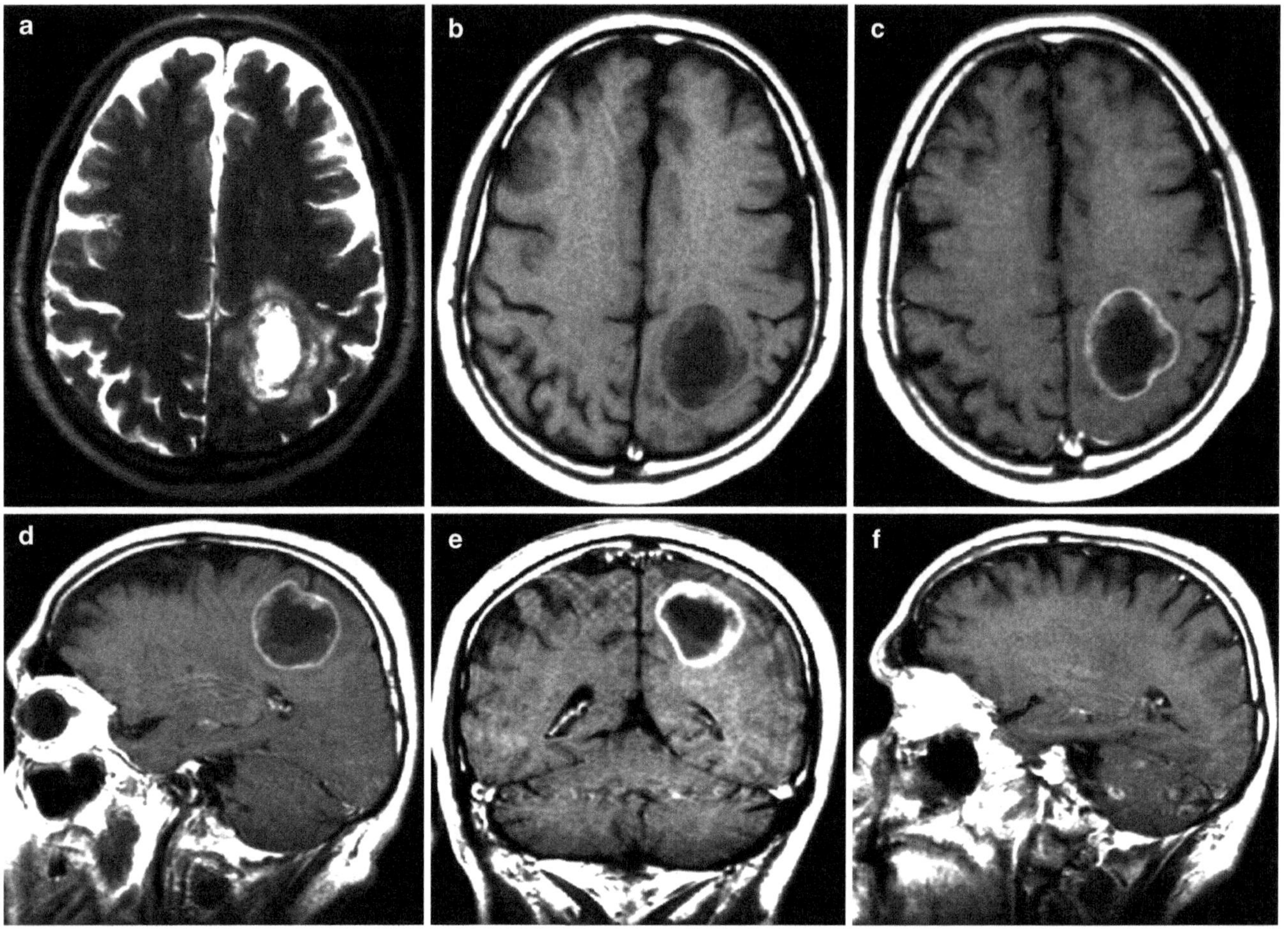

Fig. 25.7 Multiple laryngeal cancer metastases in the brain. In the left parietal region, there is a solid-cystic nodule with a heterogeneously increased signal on T2-weighted MRI (**a**) with a small hyperintense area of perifocal edema. The lesion is iso-hypointense on T1-weighted MRI (**b**). After intravenous CA administration on T1-weighted MRI in the axial (**b**), sagittal (**d**), and coronal (**e**) projections, there is intense accumulation of the contrast agent on the periphery (in the solid component) of the tumor. Multiple small lesions are identified in the cerebellum, in the sagittal projection (**f**)

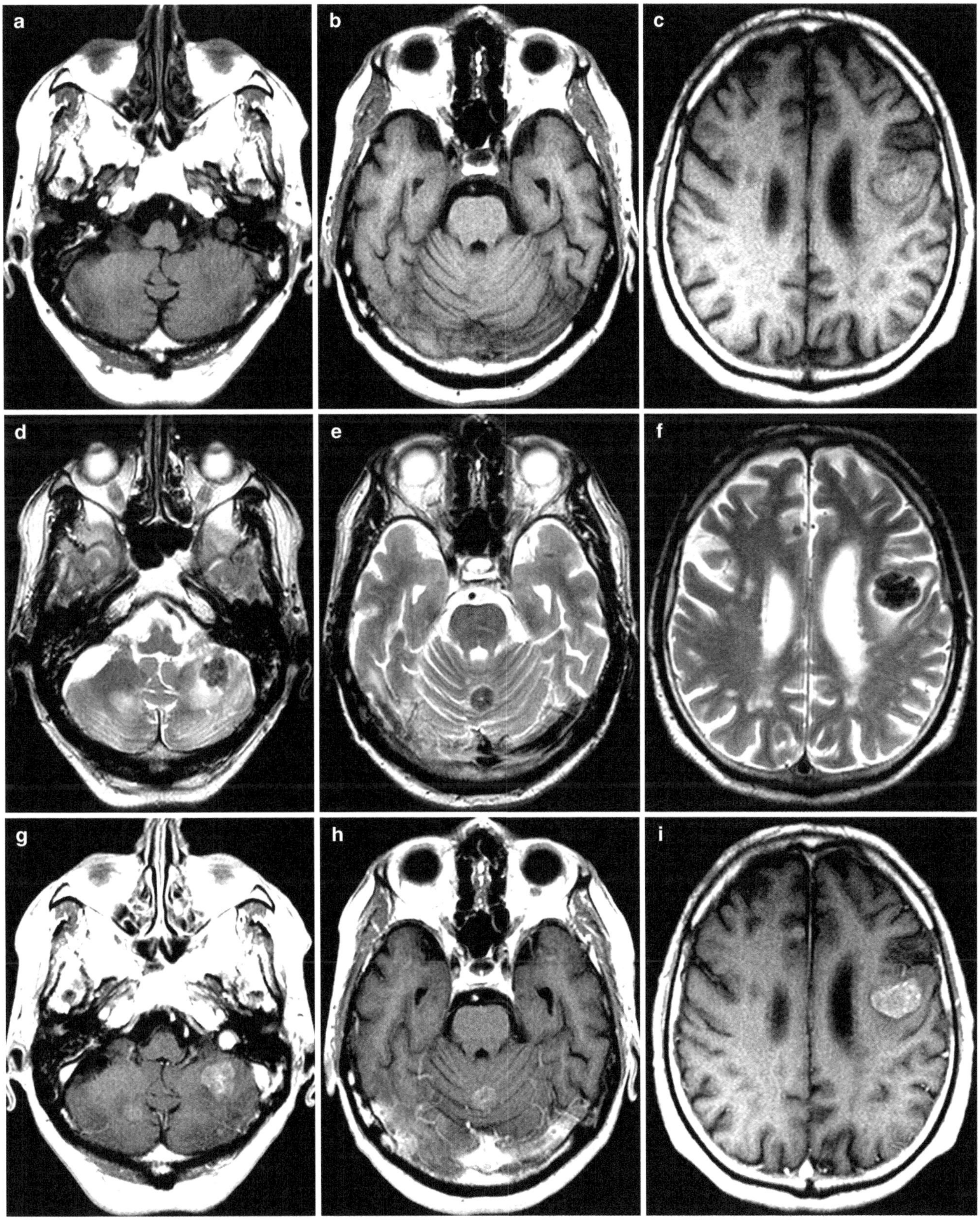

Fig. 25.8 Multiple laryngeal cancer metastases in the brain. A three-level study. On T1-weighted MRI, multiple space-occupying lesions with an isointense signal are identified in the brain matter (**a**–**c**). Noteworthy is a markedly decreased signal on T2-weighted MRI (**d**–**f**) with a mild area of perifocal edema, which is also observed in colorectal cancer metastases. After IV administration of the contrast agent on T1-weighted MRI (**g**–**i**), there is its weak and inhomogeneous accumulation in these lesions

Metastases in the Brain from an Unknown Primary Origin

26

There is still quite a large group of patients, in whom secondary brain involvement is the only manifestation of cancer. In this case, metastasis of unknown primary origin (cancer of unknown primary origin, CUP) is suggested, which does not mean that it actually does not exist. The importance of solving the issue of specifying the diagnosis of metastases of unknown primary origin cannot be overestimated. In a large frequency of cases, where the clinical picture of metastatic involvement of the brain is the only manifestation of a malignant tumor of unknown primary origin, often inaccessibility of metastatic lesions for a biopsy to obtain the tissue samples for morphological identification of the tumor does not allow to provide adequate medical care for such patients. The development of modern technologies gives us more and more new diagnostic possibilities in this regard; however, so far, this does not give any grounds for reasonable optimism. The incidence of CUPs does not decrease; often the primary source is detected only in an autopsy. This group of patients proves again that many aspects related to the mechanisms of emergence and development of human cancers have not yet been identified.

Statistical data on the incidence of tumors of unknown primary origin in patients with proven metastases in the brain is quite variable, with the latter being, according to various estimates, 10–40% and 10–15% (Campos et al. 2009, Zimm et al. 1981, Gramada et al. 2011). Indeed, it affects the life expectancy of these patients, although the prognosis is similar both for patients with known and unknown primary origin (Rudà et al. 2001).

The picture of multifocal brain involvement suggests the metastatic origin of neoplasms.

In case of a solitary lesion, the differential diagnosis with glioblastoma is carried out before a biopsy or a surgical removal of the tumor, because of the similarity of their X-ray pictures. Very important is correct taking of medical history, since glioblastoma transformed from glial tumors grade 2–grade 3 may have a long duration with mild transient symptoms (impaired speech, dizziness, numbness in the fingers, loss of consciousness, inadequate behavior), which is often observed by the patient's relatives. Metastases grow more aggressively; the clinical picture develops rapidly.

On the other hand, in case of multifocal lesions, there is a risk of misdiagnosis, since up to 20% (Campos et al. 2009) of glioblastoma cases manifest by multifocal lesions and multicentrically in 2.4%, with involvement of the contralateral hemisphere of the brain (Shakur et al. 2013). Multifocal brain lesions are also diagnosed in lymphoma, demyelinating diseases, parasitic infestation, etc.

In most cases with no primary lesion detected, metastases in the brain occur in highly differentiated adenocarcinoma (50–70% of all CUPs), poorly differentiated cancers (20–25%), squamous cell carcinoma (about 10–5%), and neuroendocrine tumors (about 1%) (Mayor 2010; Seyedin and Geffen 2014).

The use of PET in the majority of cases (83%) allows to identify the primary source of metastatic brain lesions, which justifies its use at the first stage of diagnosis. The resolution capability of PET is 5–6 mm, which certainly limits its possibilities; therefore, in no case, it eliminates the use of other methods of radiation diagnosis. A subsequent biopsy of abnormal extracranial lesions identified by PET or other methods of diagnosis is also mandatory.

26.1 Clinical Cases

In this case, glioblastoma can be assumed due to the presence of one large lesion in the right frontal region (Figs. 26.1 and 26.2).

These are presumably metastases of melanoma.

M. Dolgushin et al., *Brain Metastases*, DOI 10.1007/978-3-319-57760-9_26

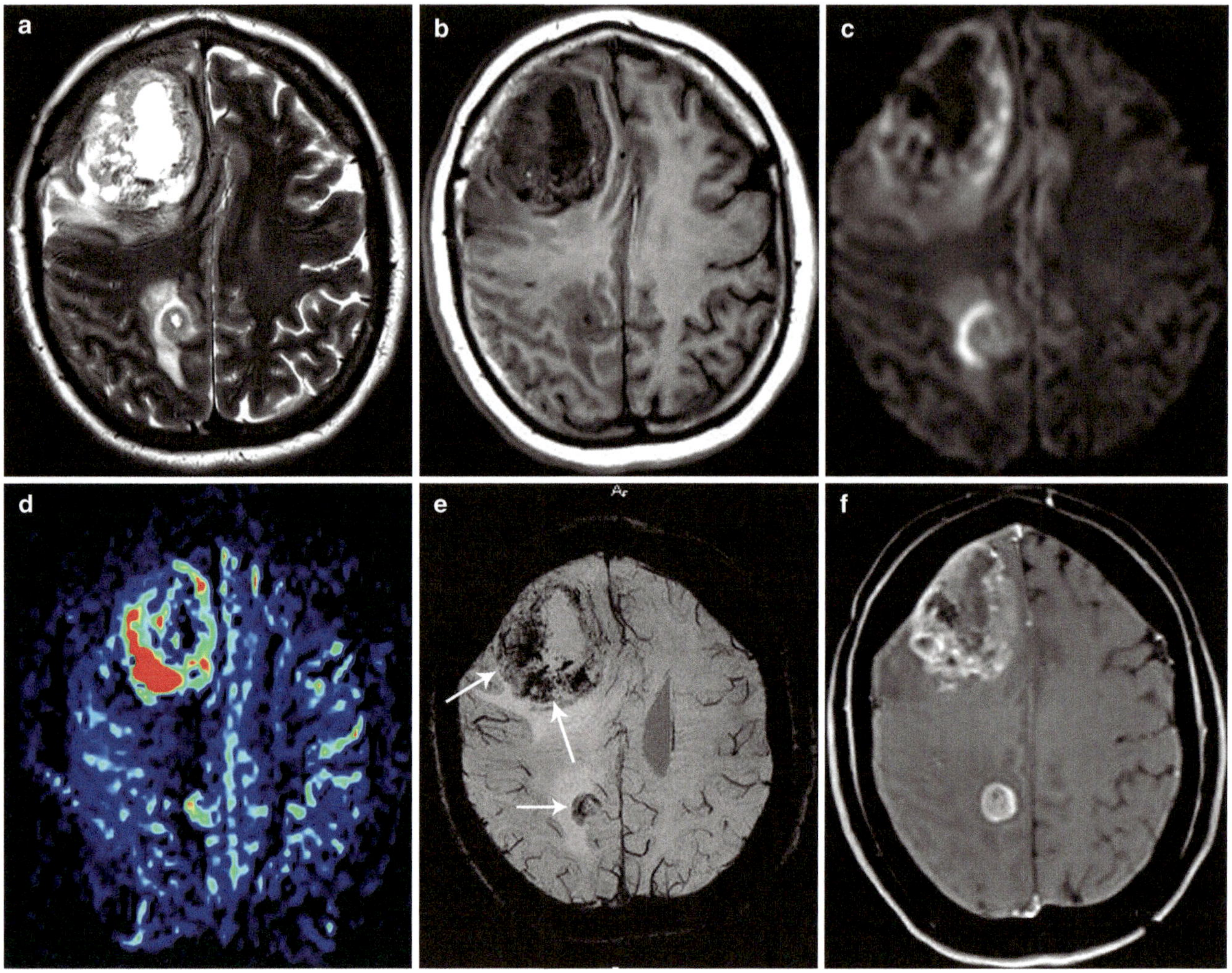

Fig. 26.1 Metastases of unknown primary origin. On MRI in the right frontal and parietal areas, there are space-occupying lesions with various sizes. The largest tumor is located in the right frontal regions, with signs of a weak perifocal edema (**a**), central necrosis, and a hypointense signal on T1-weighted MRI (**b**). The solid portion of the tumor has a heterogeneous signal on DWI MRI (**c**) and an increased blood flow on ASL MRI (**d**). There are quite a large number of hypointense inclusions in the structure of lesions (*arrows*) on SWI MRI (**e**). After intravenous administration of the contrast medium (**f**), its intense accumulation in tumors is noted. These are presumably uterine cancer metastases

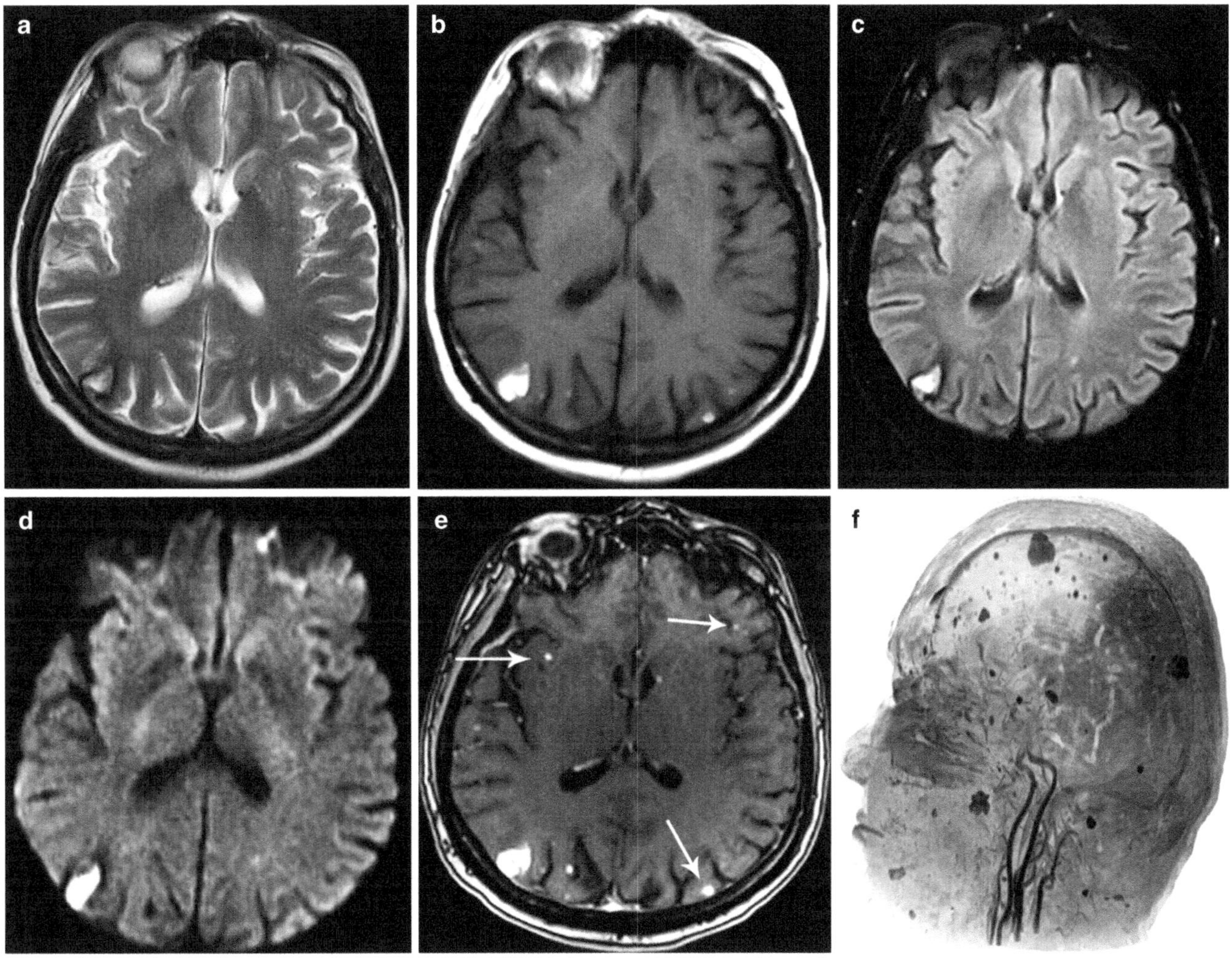

Fig. 26.2 Metastases of unknown primary origin. On MRI of the brain substance, there are multiple space-occupying lesions with various sizes. The largest tumor with signs of a hemorrhage, as evidenced by a decreased signal on T2-weighted MRI (**a**) and an increased signal on T1-weighted MRI (**b**), T2-FLAIR MRI (**c**), and DWI MRI (**d**), is located in the right parietal region. There are no signs of perifocal edema. Small pinpoint multiple lesions are also characterized by an increased signal on T1-weighted MRI (**b**, the *arrows*). After intravenous administration of the contrast medium, its intense accumulation in tumors is noted (**e**). In the inversion 3D image reconstruction of T1vibe images, multiple lesions are well visualized (**f**)

Part IV

Differential Diagnosis of Metastases of Extracranial Malignant Tumors in the Brain and Other Lesions

27 Introduction to Differential Diagnosis of Metastases in the Brain and Other Lesions

Currently, the issue of interpretation of neuroradiological findings in the differential diagnosis of metastatic brain lesions, particularly in solitary (single) lesions, causes great difficulties. With the development of imaging methods, from direct angiography to magnetic resonance imaging and positron emission tomography, the perplexity of differential diagnosis between primary and secondary brain tumors is still in the spotlight. Most metastatic lesions do not have any specific neuroimaging characteristics when using standard diagnostic approaches. They can be solid and cystic, contain in their structure areas of necrotic decay or hemorrhages, and, in case of multiple metastatic lesions, may be characterized by all of the above at the same time. There are a number of neoplastic and nonneoplastic lesions in the brain that have similar clinical and radiological manifestations. In this section, we will review some abnormal conditions and lesions of the brain, which, from the point of view of a radiologist, cause the greatest difficulty in the differential diagnosis with metastatic brain lesions from primary extracranial malignant tumors.

Perifocal edema of the brain substance not always has a clear dependence on the size of a metastatic tumor lesion, which does not allow to differentiate metastases with certainty, for example, from primary brain tumors, especially in case of a single lesion (Fig. 27.1). Moreover, as shown in the previous section, metastases of various malignant tumors in the brain, even from a single source, may have different tissue characteristics, including different character of contrast medium accumulation, different type of contrast enhancement picture. The factor of multiplicity of brain lesions, even if the patient has a known history of cancer, is either not a pathognomonic characteristic reflecting metastatic involvement (Fig. 27.2).

New high-tech CT and MRI methods, developed and implemented into clinical practice, allowing to improve the specificity and assess the structural component of abnormal lesions and surrounding brain tissue, have already found their application in routine practice. They have become the methods of choice for some nosological forms. An in-depth, detailed study of an abnormal processes in the brain based on these methods provides additional possibilities in the differential diagnosis. Determination of differential diagnostic criteria and algorithms in metastatic brain damage based on the use of both standard and additional methods plays a key role in making a diagnosis in modern clinical practice.

In this chapter, we aimed to describe the diversity of various manifestations of tumors in the brain, which can mimic its metastatic involvement.

M. Dolgushin et al., *Brain Metastases*, DOI 10.1007/978-3-319-57760-9_27

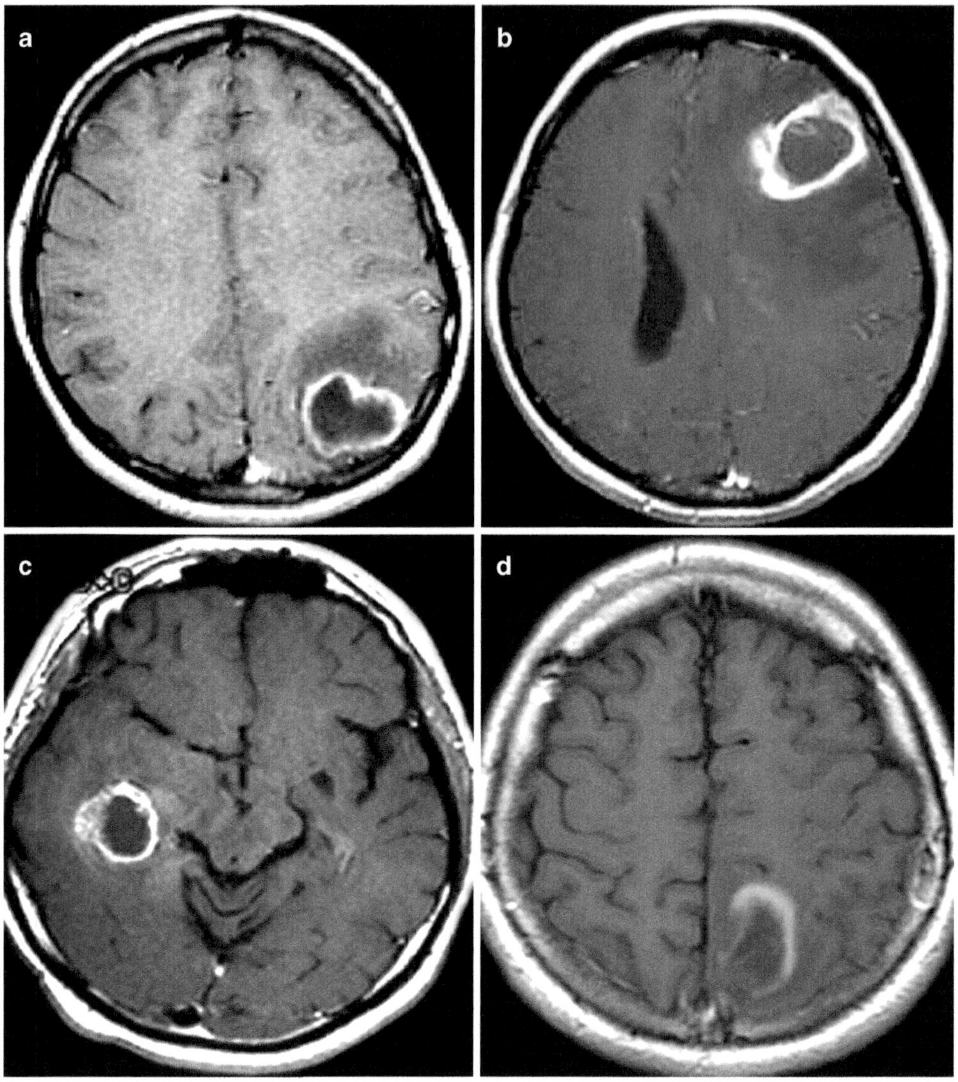

Fig. 27.1 Verified solitary lesions in the brain: abscess (**a**), glioblastoma (**b**), oligodendroglioma (**c**), and multiple sclerosis (**d**). At the stage of specifying diagnosis, differential diagnosis between these lesions is difficult: all solitary lesions are characterized by intense accumulation of the contrast agent on the periphery, central necrosis, and perifocal edema—ring enhancement

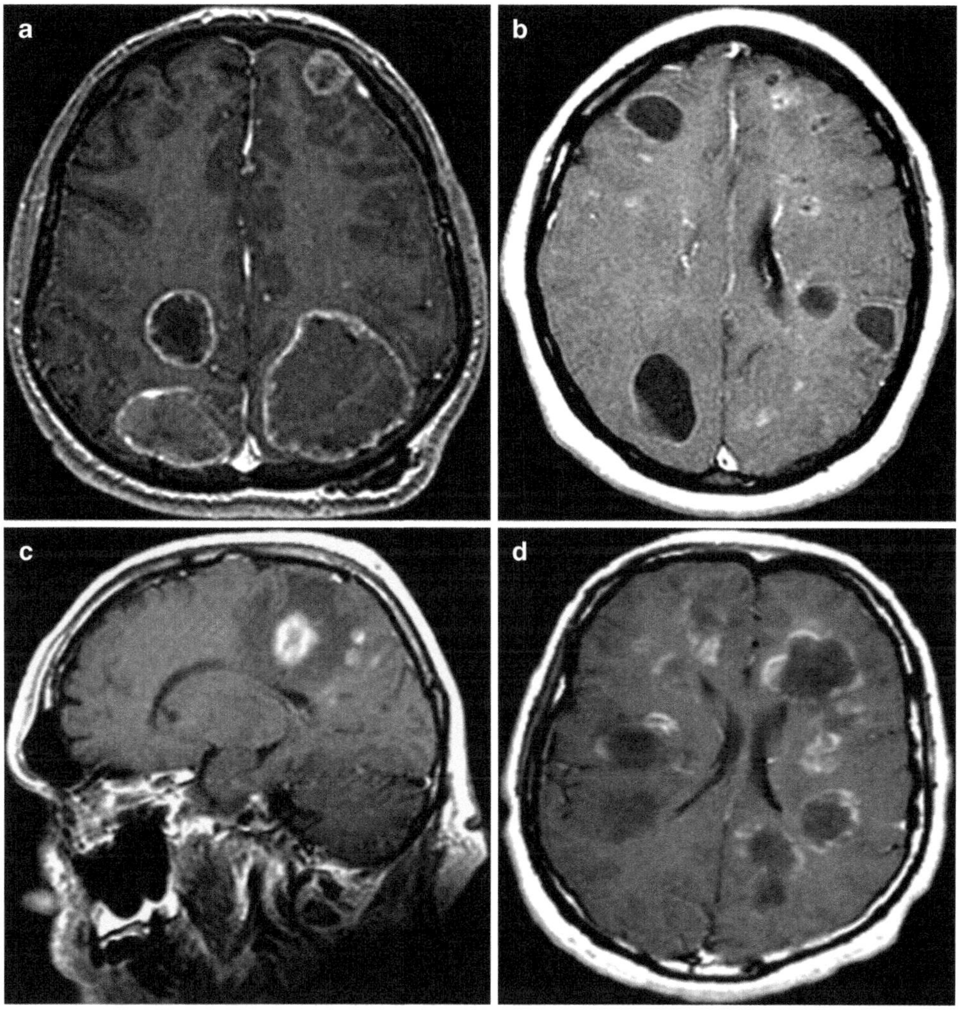

Fig. 27.2 Multiple brain lesions. Verified cases of lung cancer metastases (**a**), cysticercosis (**b**), fungal infections (**c**), and acute disseminated encephalomyelitis (**d**). Identification of these lesions at the stages of specifying diagnosis is difficult: multiple lesions in each case have various sizes and structures, but all are characterized by intense accumulation of the contrast agent

Gliomas

28

Various glial tumors, due to their predominant involvement of brain structures, are the main reason of difficulties in the differential diagnosis with intracranial metastases. According to Russell and Rubinstein (1989), gliomas account for 40–45% of all intracranial tumors, forming a heterogeneous group of brain tumors, which consists of both relatively benign forms and tumors with a severe degree of malignancy.

In the truncated version of WHO classification (2016), brain tumors are divided into:

Diffuse astrocytic and oligodendroglial tumors (diffuse astrocytoma (low grade), anaplastic (malignant) astrocytoma, glioblastoma (variant—gliosarcoma), oligodendroglioma, anaplastic oligodendroglioma, oligoastrocytoma)
Other astrocytic tumors: pilocytic astrocytoma (variant—pilomyxoid astrocytoma), pleomorphic xanthoastrocytoma, and subependymal giant cell astrocytoma
Ependymal tumors (ependymoma, anaplastic ependymoma, myxopapillary ependymoma, subependymoma)
Tumors of the choroid plexus
Neuronal and mixed neuronal-glial tumors
Tumors of the pineal region
Embryonic tumors
Meningiomas
Mesenchymal tumors
Melanotic tumors
Lymphomas
Histiocytosis
Germinomas
Tumors of the sellar region

Glial tumors, diverse by their histological structure, have different CT and MRI manifestations. Many of them have tissue characteristics similar to those of metastases.

Astrocytic tumors (ASTs) are divided into two large categories: these are prognostically unfavorable, *diffusely growing (or diffuse) tumors* accounting for up to 75% of all astrocytic tumors and *localized tumors* with a more favorable prognosis. The first category includes tumors with an increasing degree of anaplasia (from astrocytoma with a low degree of malignancy to glioblastoma), characterized by the absence of clear macro- and microscopic boundaries with the surrounding brain substance. Glioblastoma often mimics solitary metastatic lesions. The second category consists of pilocytic astrocytomas, pleomorphic xanthoastrocytomas, and subependymal giant cell astrocytomas that have macro- and microscopic isolation from the brain substance but develop much rarer and at a younger age. The peak incidence of supratentorial astrocytomas is between the ages of 20 and 50 years, which is generally 10 years younger than that for glioblastomas. These tumors can develop in any part of the brain, with relatively smaller involvement of the occipital lobes. When the tumor is located in the deep parts, there may be a bilateral invasion. The abnormal process affects both white and gray matter.

Low-grade astrocytomas (LGASC) are a group of diffuse tumors that constitute about 10–15% of all gliomas. LGASC affects mainly young adults (20–40 years of age). The life expectancy of patients with astrocytomas ranges from 2.5–15 years.

LGASCs by their radiological characteristics do overtly not qualify for the differential diagnosis with metastases, despite the fact that native CT and MRI scans can show characteristics similar to those in metastases in some cases. On CT, LGASCs are visualized as hypodense lesions without clear boundaries with the surrounding brain substance. There are also isodense forms of tumors, which in some cases may result in a delayed diagnosis, if they are investigated only using CT. Intravenous administration of a contrast medium in most cases does not change their CT density or exhibits individual portions of increased density on the background of a hypodense area.

It is believed that perifocal edema is not typical for this type of tumors. At the same time, CT or MRI does not allow to differentiate between the tumor and perifocal edema due to their similar densities and signal characteristics. The use of additional intravenous contrast enhancement facilitates iden-

M. Dolgushin et al., *Brain Metastases*, DOI 10.1007/978-3-319-57760-9_28

tification of the tumor structure on the background of edema. It is well known that benign, diffusely growing hemispheric ASCs, for the most part, do not accumulate the contrast agent.

We must not forget that approximately 10–12% of cases may be characterized by *cystic or atypical* diffuse ASC forms (Fig. 28.1), with focal and even intense contrast enhancement, which may have signs similar to those in metastases (Fig. 28.2).

It should be noted that infiltrative growth of ASCs results in the tumor spread beyond the signal change area visible on T2-weighted and T2-FLAIR images. On DWI MRI (with b = 1000), low-grade ASCs have the signal strength equal to or slightly lower than that of the normal white matter. The average ADC values for LGASCs, based on the results of our studies, are 1.52 ± 0.4 mm^2/s. MR tractography provides additional information on the structure of the nerve fibers of the white matter in the area of ASC growth. The tumor causes destructive changes in the conductive tracts of the brain; however, in some cases, they can be traced in the tumor tissue. On perfusion MRI or CT studies, ASCs are characterized by similar parameters of local cerebral blood supply (CBV) and local cerebral blood flow (CBF) in comparison with the surrounding brain substance. The specificity of spectroscopic characteristics of LGASCs is low; however, a decrease in the NAA/Cr and Cho/Cr peak ratio is detected on MR spectrograms (Fig. 28.3). The absence of a lactate peak and low Cho peak values are indicative of the benign nature of the brain lesion with equal other CT and MRI manifestations of the tumor in relation to the assessment of the degree of malignancy.

Gradual transformation of benign ASC into an anaplastic form, well known in the clinical practice, can be demonstrated by follow-up CT or MRI studies. Moreover, the presence or appearance in the LGASC structure of an area of the contrast

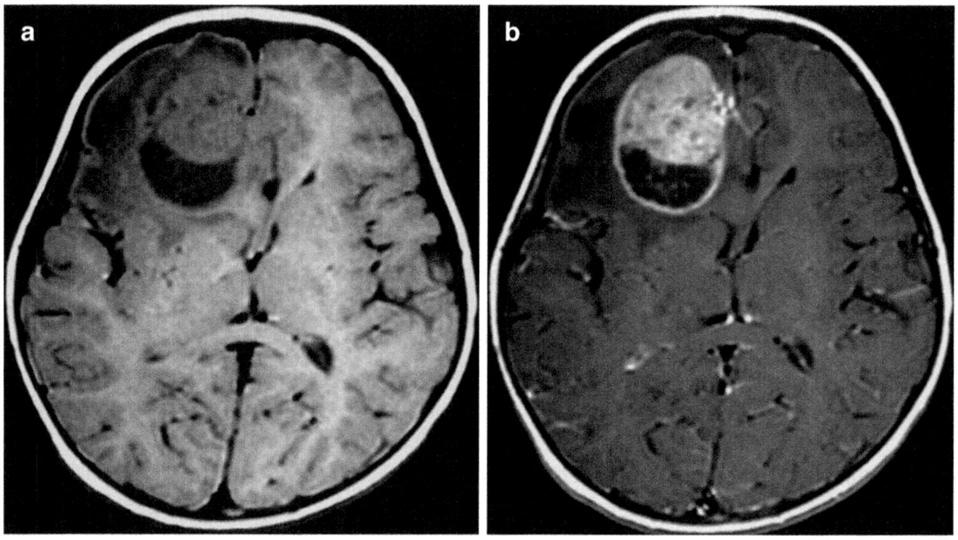

Fig. 28.1 Fibrillar astrocytoma. In the right frontal area on T1-weighted MRI (**a**), there is a solid-cystic space-occupying lesion that has characteristics close to those of the gray matter in the solid part and a reduced signal from the cystic component located in the posterior pole. The structure of the tumor and its borders are well differentiated after contrast enhancement (**b**)

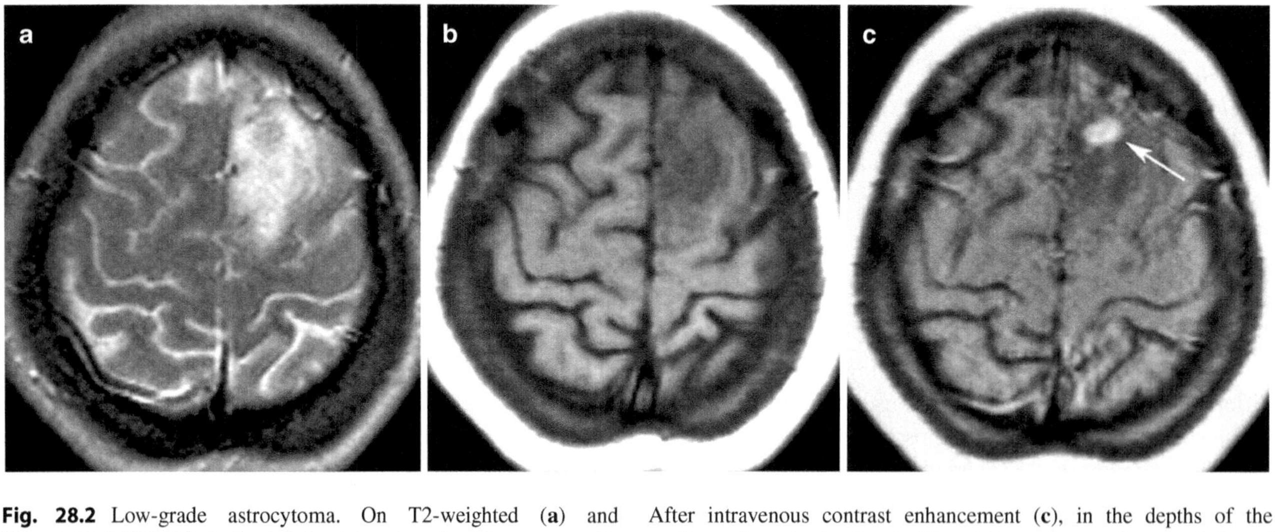

Fig. 28.2 Low-grade astrocytoma. On T2-weighted (**a**) and T1-weighted MRI (**b**), in the left frontal region, there is an area with diffuse abnormal changes in the signal. Adjacent sulci are compressed. After intravenous contrast enhancement (**c**), in the depths of the portion, a focus is visualized with an intense abnormal accumulation of the contrast agent (the *arrow*)

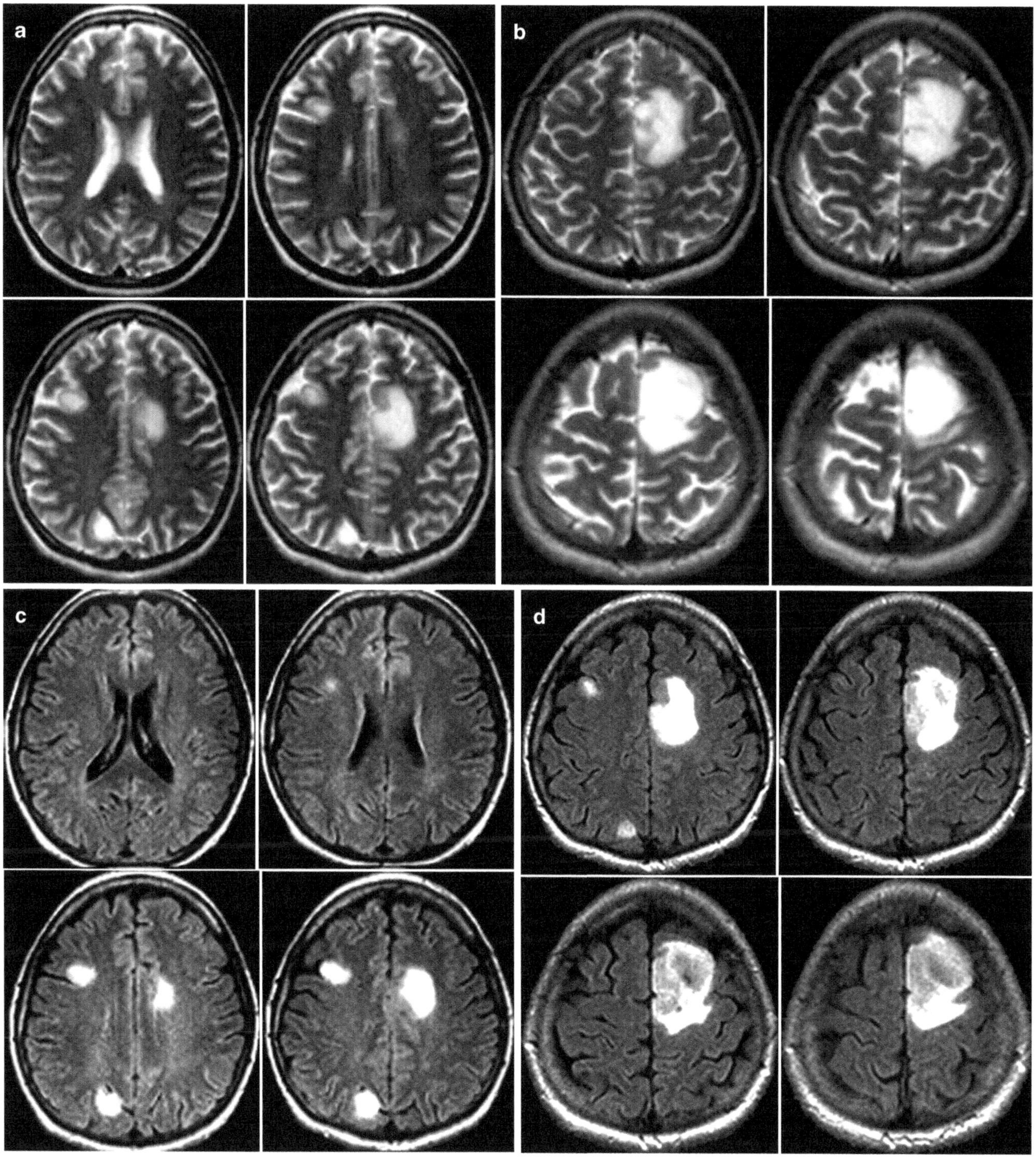

Fig. 28.3 Multiple astrocytomas. Studies at several levels. On T2-weighted (**a**, **b**) and T2-FLAIR MRI (**b**, **d**), there are multiple foci with an increased subcortical MR signal. On DWI MRI (**e**), these lesions are virtually undetectable. On all scanning sequences, the lesions have identical characteristics. On MR spectroscopy, the NAA peak is decreased; the Lip-Lac complex peak is visualized

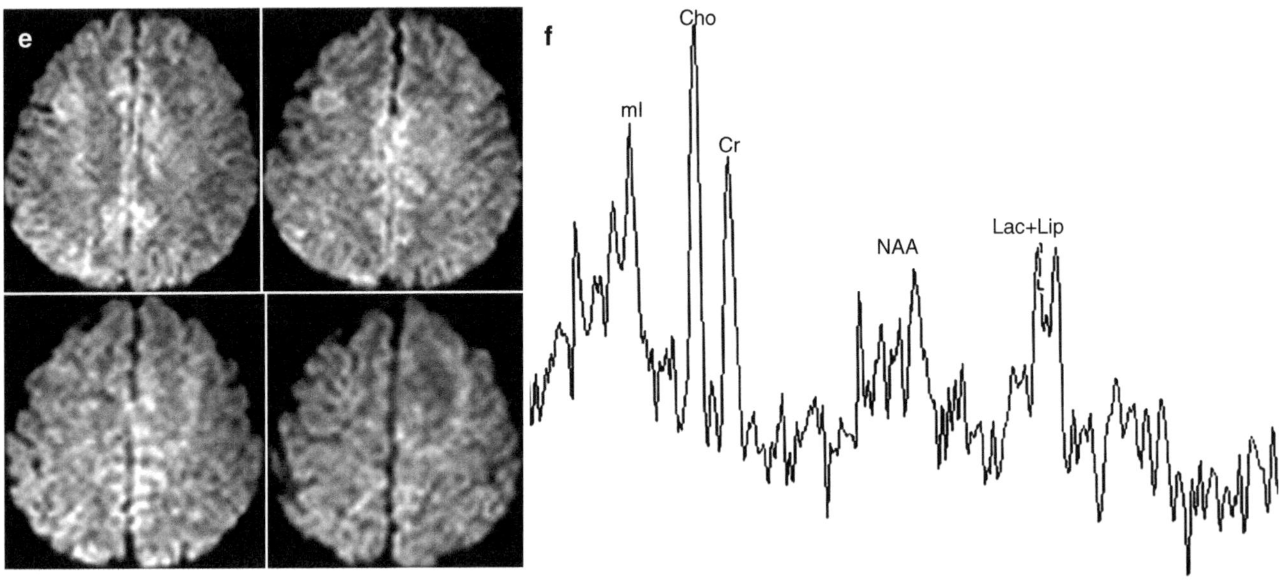

Fig. 28.3 (continued)

agent accumulation may characterize tumor portions with more aggressive growth. Although rare, a combination of several CNS disorders is a possible event, particularly, if the fact of long-term multiyear growth of LGASC is considered.

In such cases, it is important not only to recognize the lesions but also to establish their different origins or, on the contrary, to identify allegedly common histogenesis of tumors, which is especially important in multiple primary ASCs (Fig. 28.4).

On PET studies, benign intracerebral tumors are characterized by low RP accumulation. On PET with ^{18}F-FDG, tumor lesions may manifest as ametabolic areas, which is why the use of amino acids (^{11}C-methionine, ^{18}F-tyrosine) or ^{18}F-choline with low background accumulation allows to determine neoplastic origin of the disease, as well as suggest the prognostic factors for tumor growth (Fig. 28.5).

Anaplastic astrocytoma (*AnASC*) is an infiltrative tumor as a rule with well defined boundaries. In cystic degeneration, hemorrhages are often observed, but necrosis cannot be detected by a histological examination. AnASC amounts to up to one third of all astrocytomas and 25% of all gliomas. It develops in the majority of cases (75%) from LGASC. At a microscopic examination, AnASCs are characterized by aggregation of closely spaced astrocytes with polymorphism and nuclear hyperchromatism.

On CT, AnASCs are inhomogeneous tumors with mixed density. According to some researchers (Osborn 2004), AnASCs are characterized by inhomogeneous contrast enhancement on CT. The presence of annular contrast enhancement suggests the tumor transformation into glioblastoma. Around the tumor, there is usually an edema with varying severity, having a low density and typically growing into the white matter. Calcifications and hemorrhages are rare.

On MR images, AnASC often it looks like a poorly separated lesion with a heterogeneous signal on T1-weighted and T2-weighted MRI. On T1-weighted MRI, there are areas with a mixed iso- and hypointense signal; often hemorrhagic lesions with increased signal intensity can be detected. Most AnASCs are typically distinguished by the signal enhancement after administration of the contrast agent (Fig. 28.6).

On DWI MRI, there is an increase in the heterogeneity of the MR signal, appearance of high signal areas on DWI with factor of $b = 1000$ s/mm^2 is normally not observed in LGASCs. In this case, ADC values vary in tumor tissues accumulating and not accumulating the contrast agent. Mean ADC values in the tumor tissue, based on the results of our studies, varied within the range of about 1.18–1.23 ± 0.32 mm^2/s. With increasing anaplastic changes in the tumor, a decrease in the fractional anisotropy index is noted.

Infiltrative tumor growth results in a total destruction of the main structural elements of the white matter, in particular, conductive tracts. MR tractography becomes, under these conditions, one of the unique methods of in life and, most importantly, preoperative evaluation of the latter (Jellison et al. 2004). On MR spectroscopy, AnASCs are characterized by an increase in the Cho/Cr peak ratio and a decrease in the NAA peak height (Podoprigora et al. 2001a, b; Nelson et al. 2002). CT and MRI perfusion studies further contribute to the assessment of structural changes occurring in the tumor tissue in the course of anaplastic transformation. Anaplastic lesions are characterized by a typical inhomogeneous increase in hemodynamic parameters; this particularly concerns the local cerebral blood flow in the areas corresponding or not corresponding to the contrast agent accumulation. Anaplastic astrocytomas are characterized by high accumulation of radiopharmaceuticals, such as ^{11}C-methionine and ^{18}F- and ^{18}F-choline-tyrosine (Fig. 28.7).

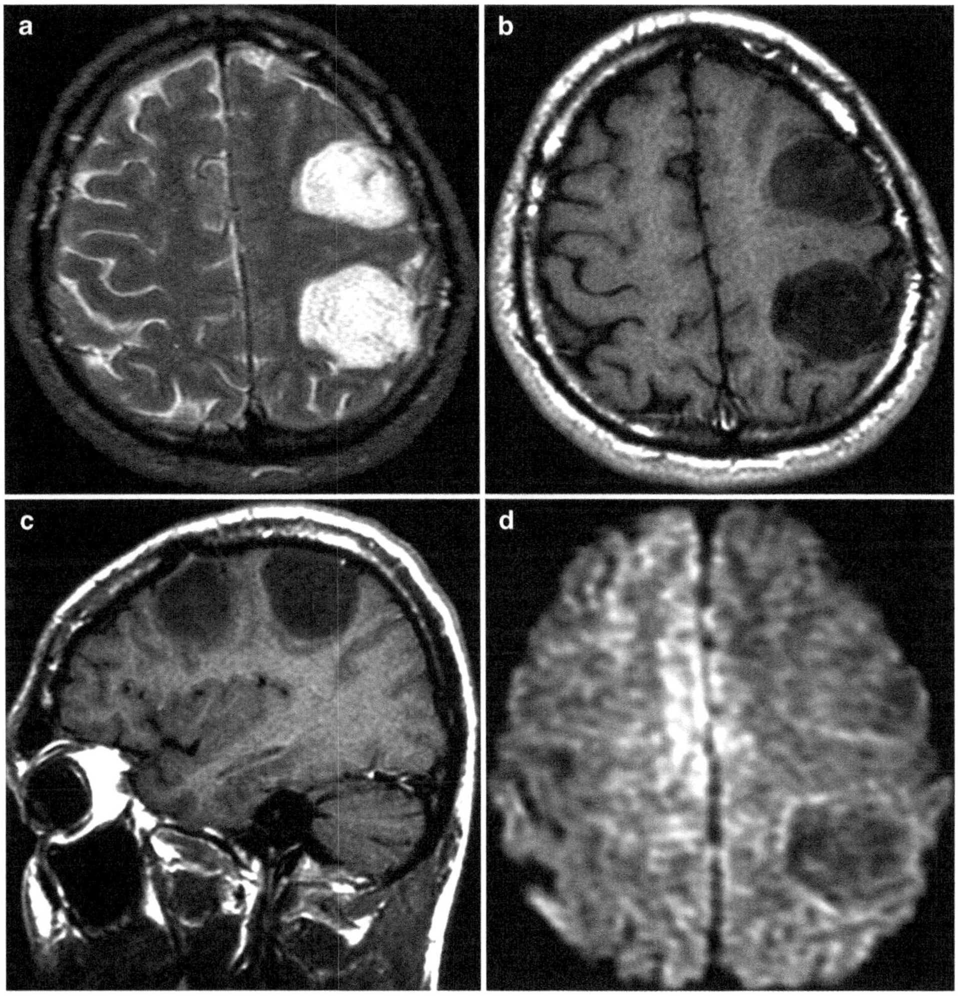

Fig. 28.4 Multiple astrocytomas of the left cerebral hemisphere. On T2-weighted (**a**) and T1-weighted MRI (**b**, **c**), two lesions are visualized, having an increased T2-weighted MR signal and a decreased T1-weighted MR signal. On DWI MRI (**d**), these lesions are iso-hypointense. Tumor lesions have similar MR characteristics on T1-weighted and T2-weighted MRI images, but they differ on DWI MRI

Glioblastoma (GB) is the most malignant of all glial tumors and occupies the extreme part of the spectrum of astrocytomas. It is the most common primary CNS tumor, which amounts to about 10–20% of all intracranial tumors (Orrison and Hart 2000; Osborn 2004). Approximately half of all gliomas belong to GBs. This is the most common supratentorial tumor in adults and is usually diagnosed in patients over 50 years of age and is rare before 30 years of age. A slight predominance of the male population is noted. Glioblastomas in particular account for the major set of differential diagnostic radiological errors with metastatic tumors.

Macroscopically, GBs are usually lesions with a heterogeneous structure with central necrosis and a richly vascularized stroma. Intratumoral hemorrhages are often observed. Histologically, GBs have pronounced tumor cell atypia and high mitotic activity. A characteristic feature of GBs are multiple foci of necrosis with the presence of so-called pseudopalisade formations that are presented by a multinucleated palisade of elongated hyperchromatic nuclei and marked proliferation of vascular endothelial cells (Matsko 1998). Like in other infiltrative gliomas, there is no clear boundary between the tumor, edema, and normal brain tissue; however, due to pronounced contrast enhancement, the solid part of the tumor on CT and MRI images looks quite localized.

On CT, the tumor density is heterogeneous. The central low-density area is presented by necrosis, which is observed in 95% of cases. Calcifications in GBs are very rare. Various hemorrhages can be identified. The tumor is usually surrounded by a pronounced perifocal edema merging visually with the infiltrative part of the tumor. After intravenous administration of the contrast agent, expressed, but inhomogeneous, contrast enhancement is observed, often in the form of a ring with jagged internal contours.

MR manifestations of GBs, in general, reflect abnormal changes, showing significant tumor heterogeneity. On T1-weighted images, there is a poorly localized, space-occupying lesion with a mixed (iso-hypointense) signal and central necrosis that usually has a reduced signal relative to the tumor mass. On T2-weighted and T2-FLAIR MRI, tumor manifestations are also diverse, with areas of a hypo-, iso-, and hyperintense signal from the GB stroma, necrosis, cysts, and hemorrhages. An extensive mass effect and edema of the white matter often also accompany small-sized tumors, which occurs in metastases (Figs. 28.8 and 28.9).

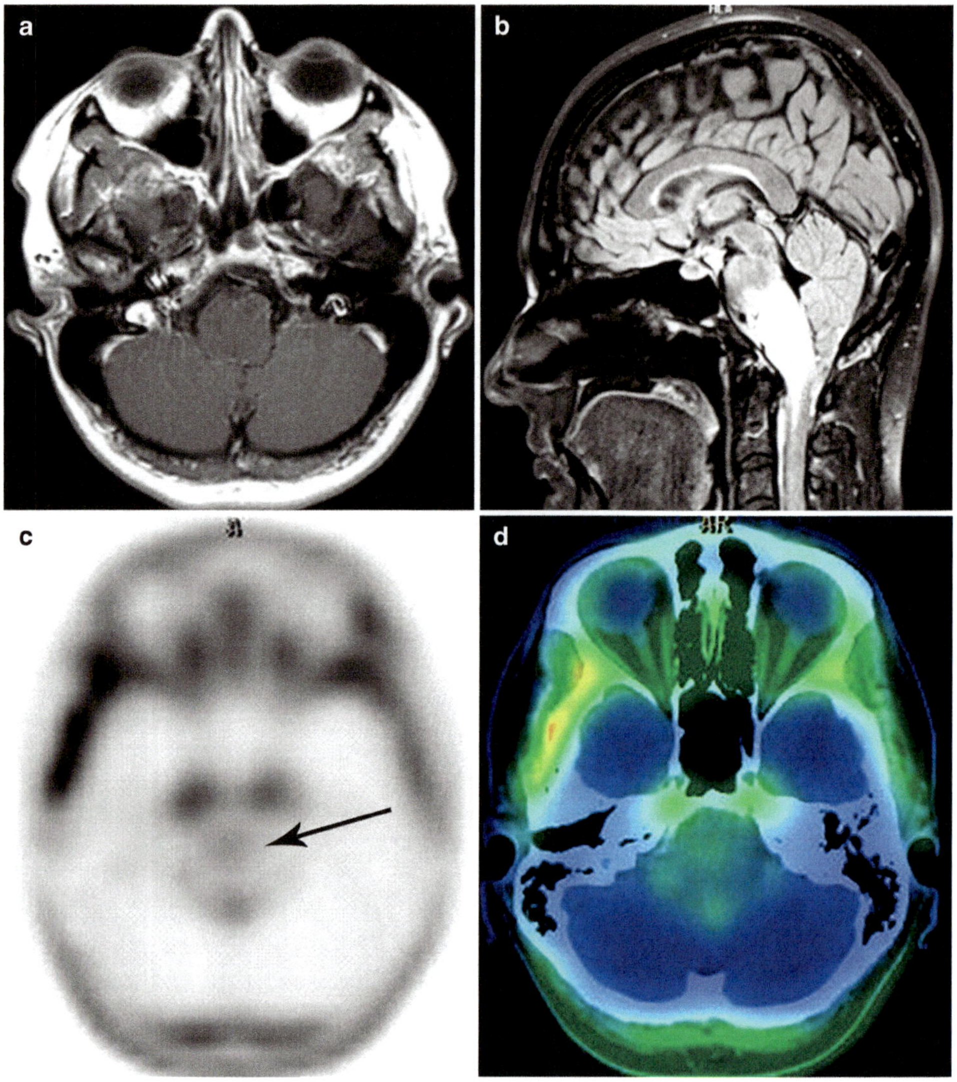

Fig. 28.5 Diffuse glioma of the brainstem. On T1-weighted MRI with contrast enhancement (**a**) and T2-FLAIR MRI (**b**) in the sagittal projection, in the region of the medulla oblongata, there is an extensive, diffusely spreading lesion with no signs of abnormal CA accumulation. On PET with ^{18}F-choline (**c**, **d**), there is low RP accumulation in the affected area (the *arrow*)

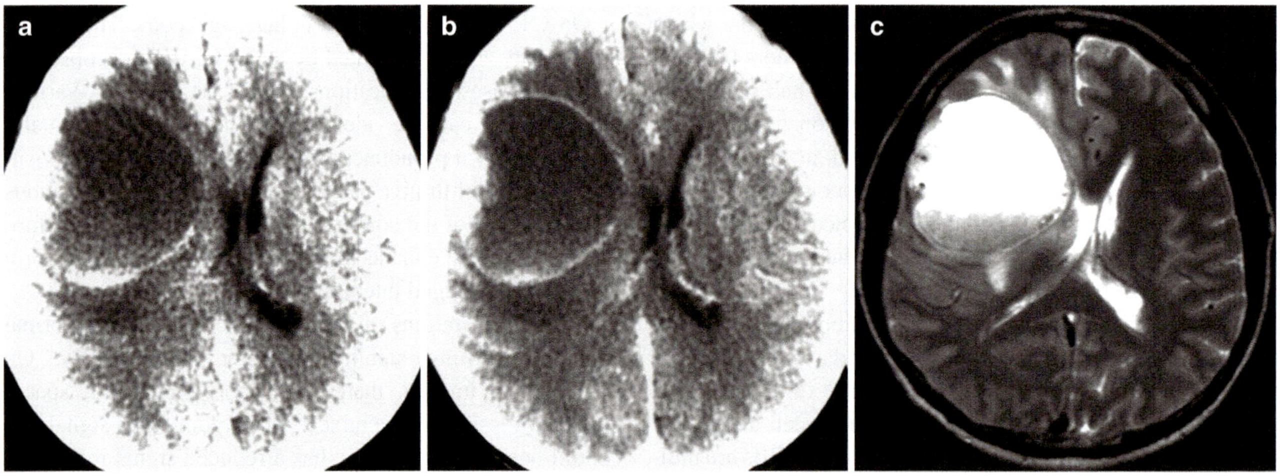

Fig. 28.6 Anaplastic astrocytoma. In the right frontotemporal region on CT with (**b**) and without (**a**) contrast enhancement, there is a large lesion that includes a small solid nodule on its lateral contour and a large tumor cyst. The brain ventricles are compressed. On T2-weighted (**c**), T2-FLAIR (**d**), and T1-weighted MRI, on the background of contrast enhancement (**e**, **f**), there is a nonhomogeneous tumor with expressed contrast enhancement and a hemorrhagic/protein intracystic component characterized by a heterogeneous signal and forming a hypointense signal along the lower contour (**d**, the *arrow*)

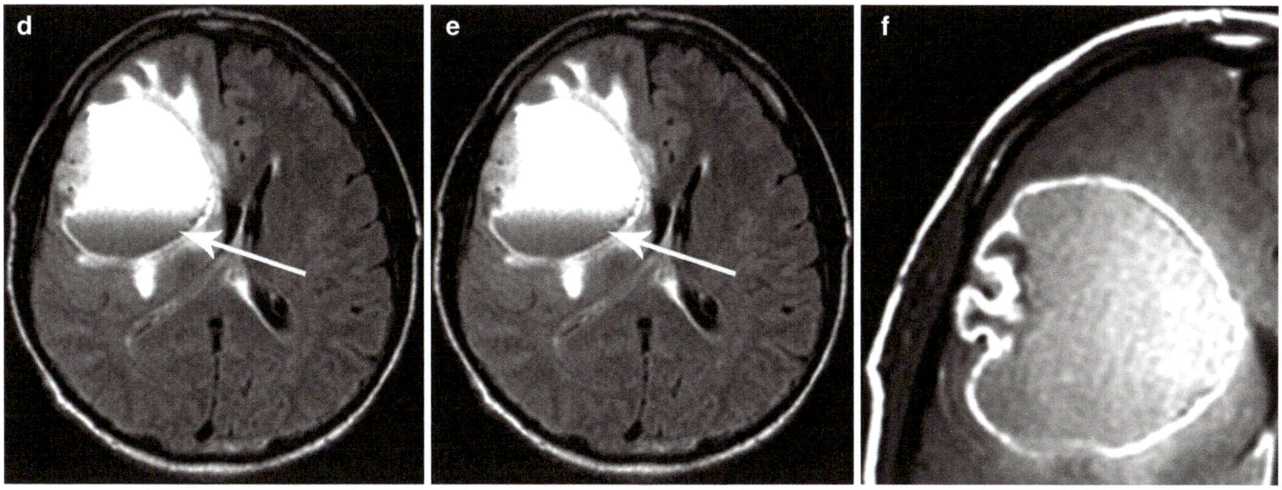

Fig. 28.6 (continued)

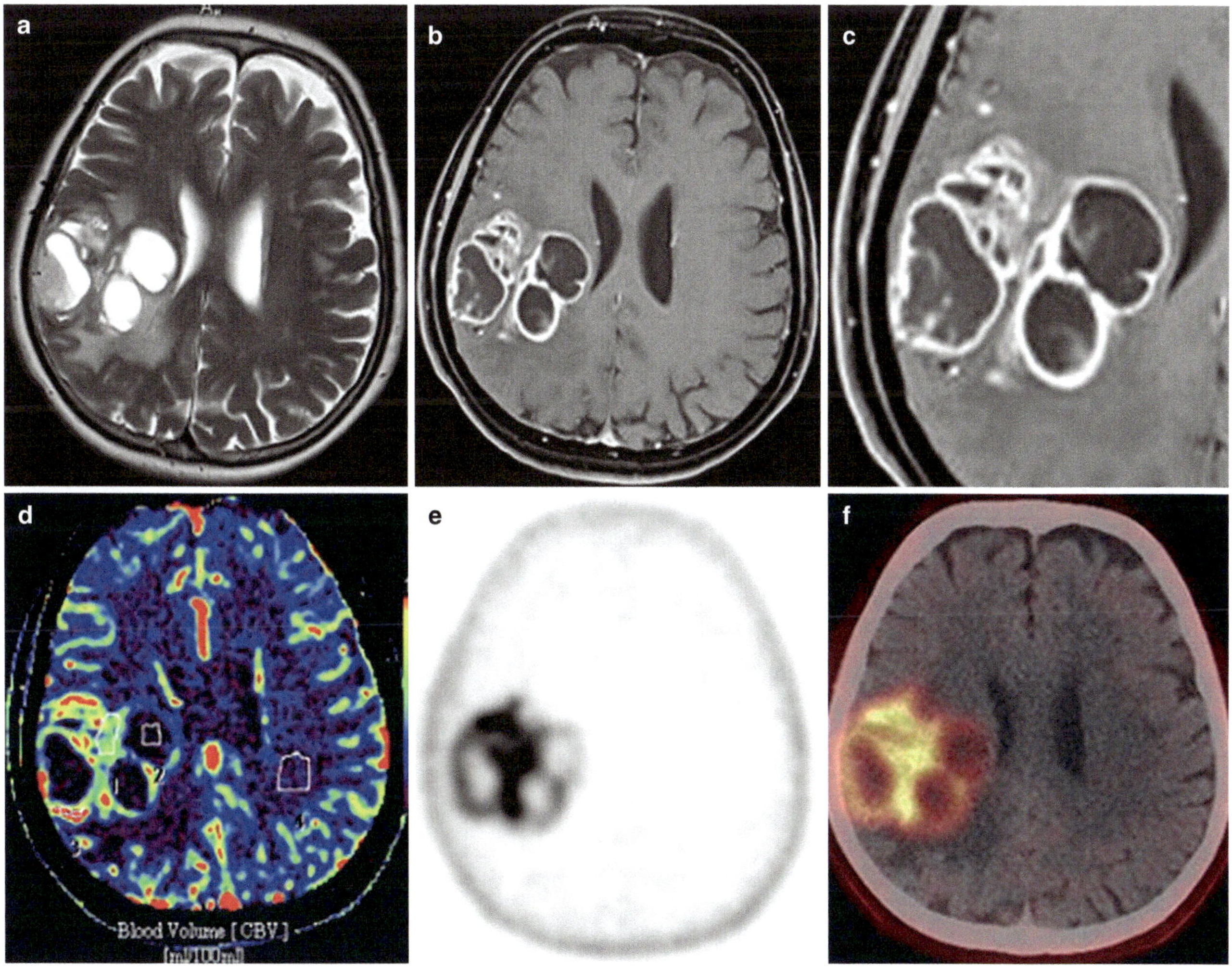

Fig. 28.7 Anaplastic astrocytoma. MRI in the right frontoparietal region visualizes a multicystic tumor with a hyperintense area of moderate perifocal edema on T2-weighted MRI (**a**). There is intense accumulation of the contrast agent on T1-weighted fat sat MRI with contrast enhancement (**b**, **c**), on the periphery and in the solid component of the lesion. On CT perfusion, CBV values (**d**) are high in the solid component of the tumor and low in cystic one. On PET CT with ^{18}F-choline (**e**, **f**), there is its intense accumulation in the solid component of the lesion

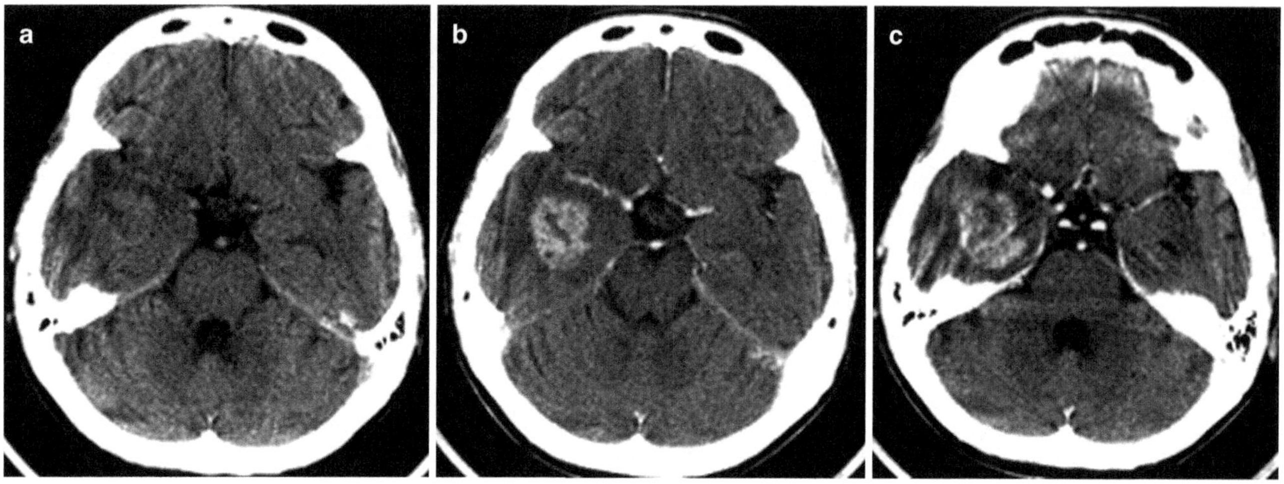

Fig. 28.8 Glioblastoma. In the right temporal lobe on axial CTs before (**a**) and after contrast enhancement (**b**, **c**), there is a tumor intensely accumulating the contrast agent. In the center of the tumor, there is a small area of necrosis. A hypodense area around the tumor is presented by edema

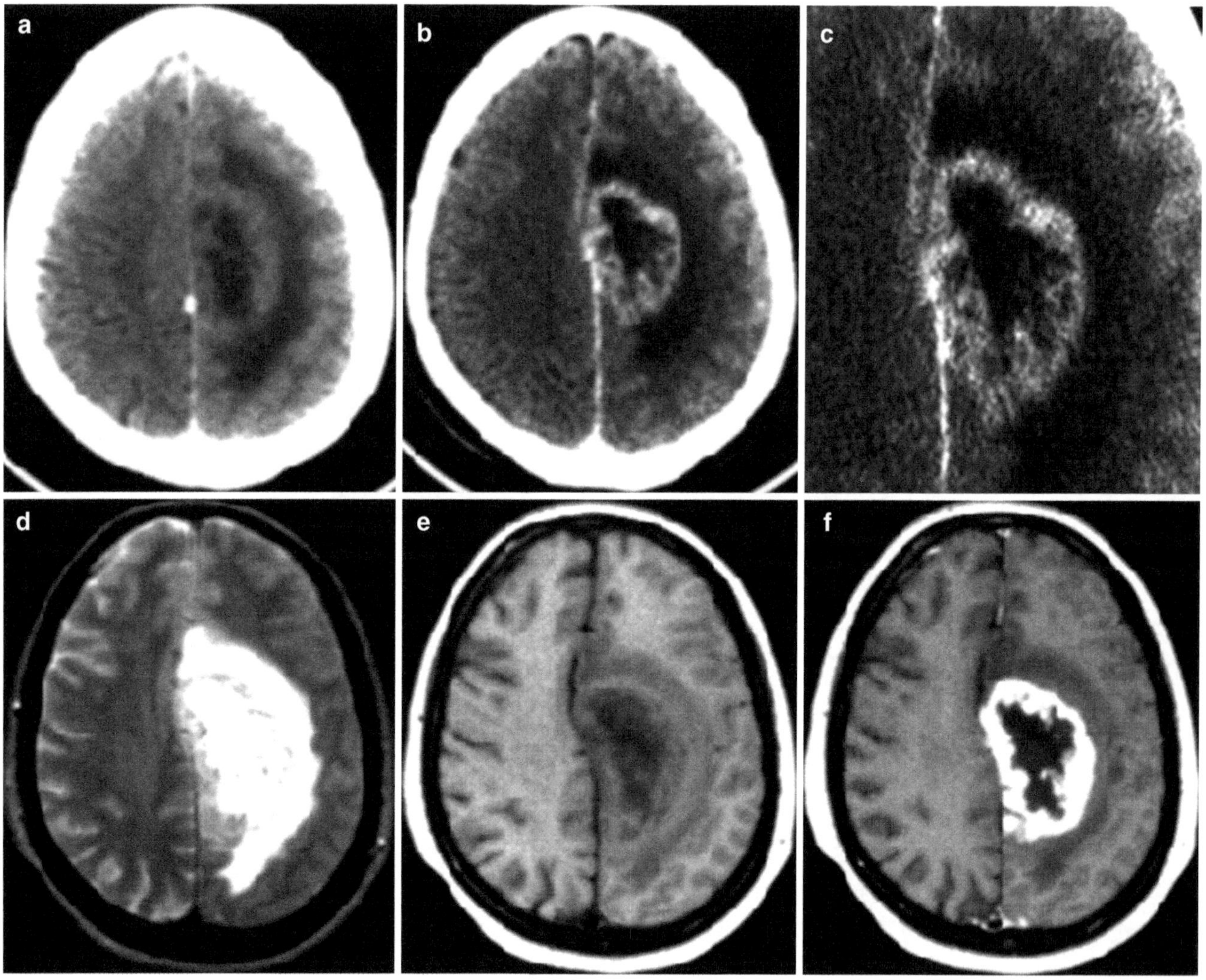

Fig. 28.9 Glioblastoma. On CT before (**a**) and after (**b**, **c**) contrast enhancement in the left postfrontal area, parasagittally, there is a tumor with marked peripheral contrast enhancement and perifocal edema. The central area of necrosis does not accumulate the contrast agent. On T2-weighted (**d**) and T1-weighted MRI (**e**) and after (**f**) contrast enhancement, a tumor with a heterogeneous structure is identified. Perifocal edema has an equally high MR signal as compared to the area of central decay. On T1-weighted MRI (**f**), there is intense, marginal contrast enhancement typical for glioblastoma. The inner and outer contours of the contrast-enhanced tumor are irregular

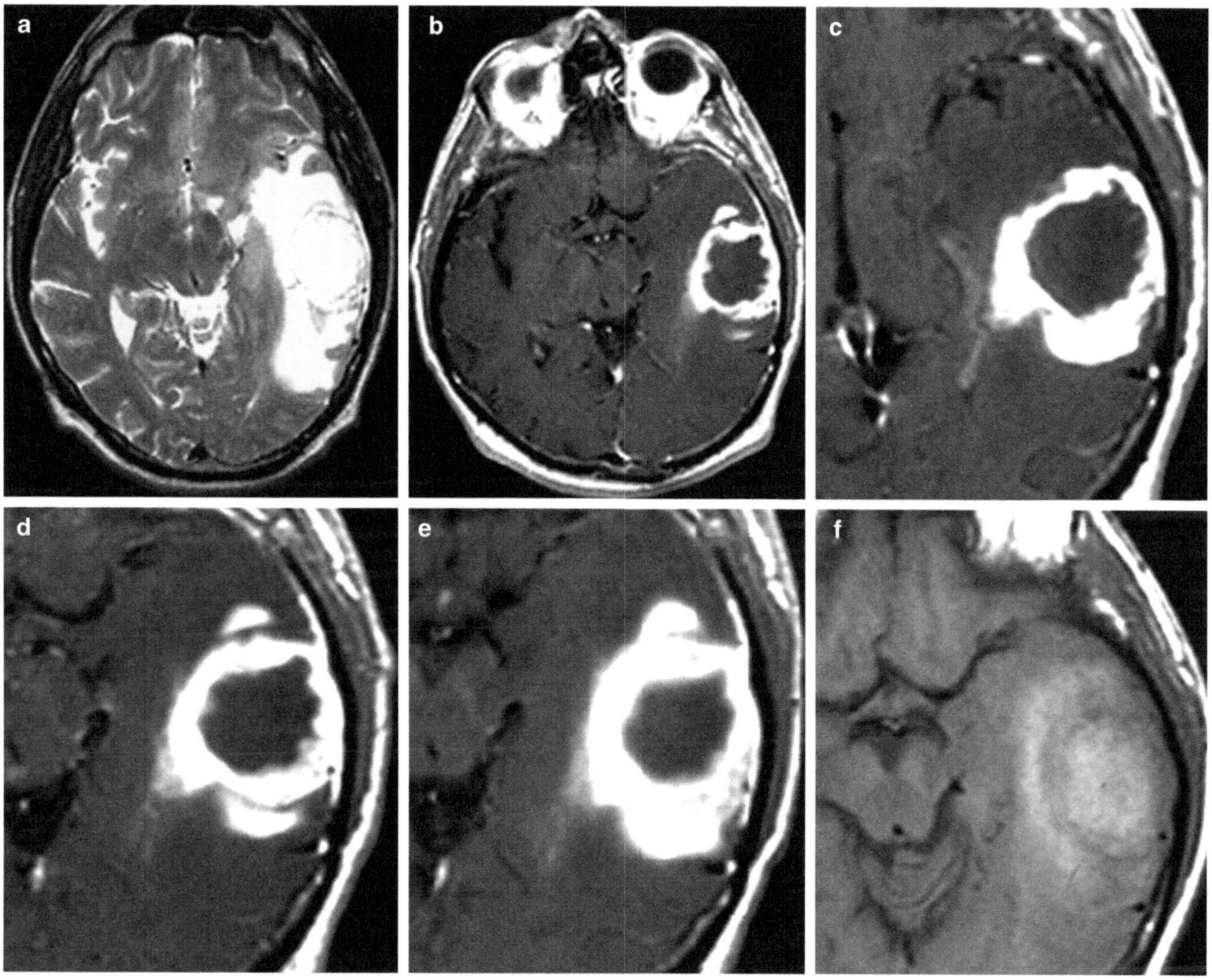

Fig. 28.10 Glioblastoma. Changes in the contrast enhancement. In the left temporal region on T2-weighted (**a**) and T1-weighted MRI (**b**, **c**) with the double dose of CA, performed 5 min after the intravenous injection, a heterogeneous structure of the tumor with central necrosis, annular contrast enhancement, and severe peritumoral edema are visualized. 20 minutes after the intravenous injection of CA, there is an increase in abnormal contrast enhancement area on MRI (**d**) due to the expansion of both external and internal borders; individual foci of contrast enhancement merging with the main mass of the tumor are also visualized. On dynamic MRI 1 hour later, the expansion of the contrast enhancement area (**e**) continues. On MRI at 24 h (**f**), there is residual contrast enhancement in the area of edema/tumor infiltration and in the central necrosis area. The original "ring" became hypointense as compared with edema and necrosis

As with AnASCs, tumor cells in GBs may be present outside the signal enhancement area and perifocal edema detected by MRI. GBs spread extensively and quickly along the tracts of the white matter, destroying the latter. In the structure of GBs, often hemorrhage with varying degrees of severity are visualized. In subacute hemorrhage, MR signal increases in T1-weighted images.

Most GBs significantly and heterogeneously accumulate the contrast agent on MRI; their borders cannot be differentiated on T1-weighted images in the absence of a pronounced hemorrhage in the glioblastoma stroma. The use of high doses of the contrast medium and delayed investigations increase the possibility of visualization of the infiltrative part of the tumor extensively invading the surrounding brain tissue (Fig. 28.10).

Multiple GBs occur in 5% of cases, when they are virtually indistinguishable from metastases without performing a biopsy. The fact of gradual transformation of LGASCs first into AnASCs and then into GBs is well known. In such cases, changes in CT density and MRI signal typical for individual nosological forms of gliomas within the same tumor, a combination of different forms of gliomas, or transformation of changes can be simultaneously visualized in follow-up studies.

Perfusion MRI or CT demonstrates a marked increase in the main hemodynamic parameters both in solid and infiltra-

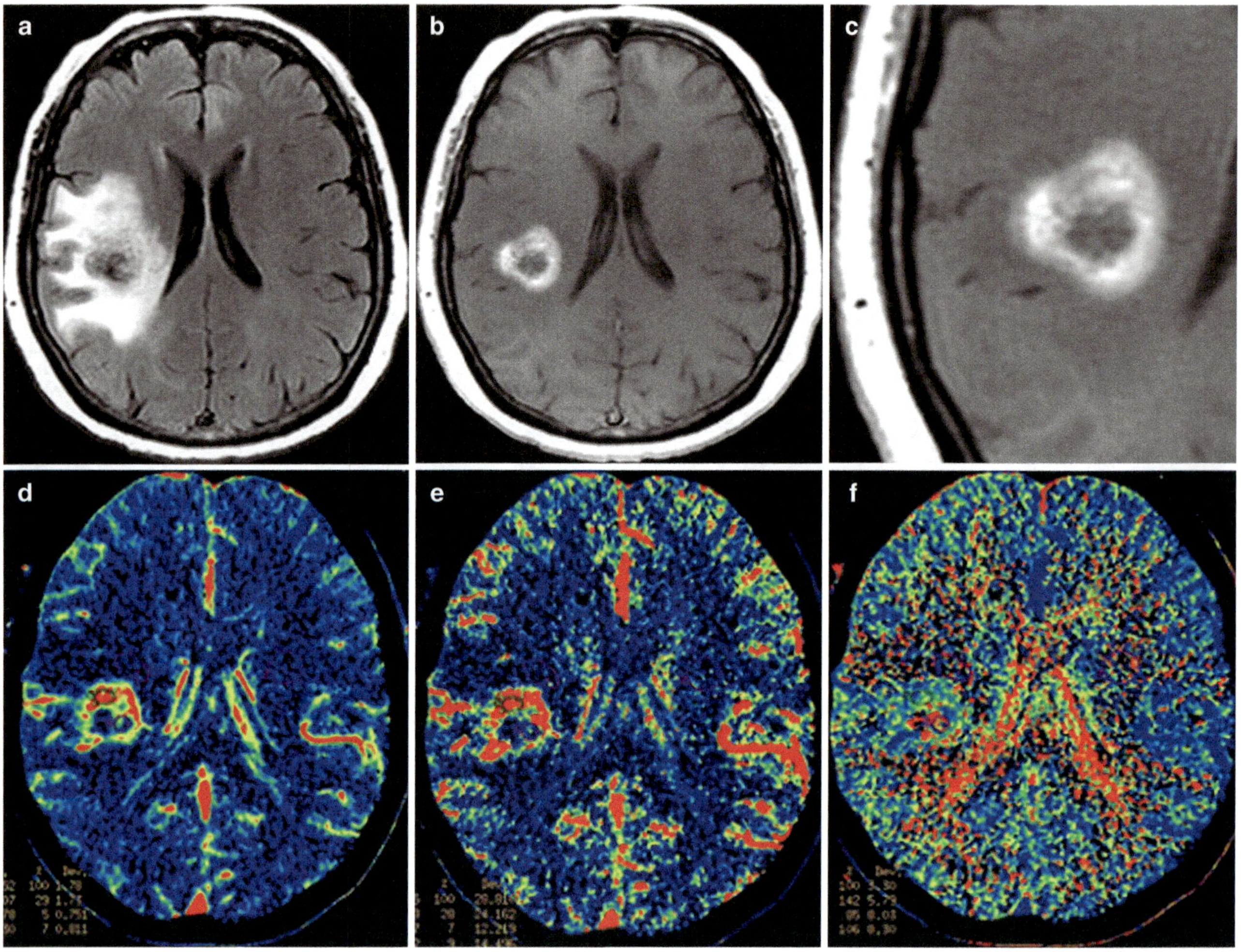

Fig. 28.11 Glioblastoma. On MRI in the deep parts of the right frontotemporal region on T2-FLAIR (**a**) and T1-weighted contrast-enhanced MRI (**b**, **c**), there is a space-occupying lesion with signs of central necrosis, intensely accumulating the contrast agent on the periphery, with a pronounced perifocal edema (ring enhancement). On CT perfusion maps, there is an increase in CBV (**d**) and CBF values (**e**) in the peripheral regions of the tumor, MTT values (**f**) are increased to a lesser extent

tive parts of GBs. In the central necrotic part of GB, regardless of the degree of necrosis, blood flow values are drastically reduced.

Our studies and data from publications strongly suggest that perfusion CT (or MRI) allows to differentiate brain gliomas with a high degree of reliability, depending on their degree of malignancy. With an increasing degree of malignancy in the tumor tissue, a clear trend to an increase in CBV and CBF values is observed. Thus, all malignant gliomas are characterized by higher values of CBV and, in particular, cerebral blood flow rate, CBF (Fig. 28.11). These changes are clearly visualized on the background of the surrounding brain substance.

The highest values of perfusion parameters we obtained in glioblastomas within the group of glial tumors (Fig. 28.12). Initially, their main histological feature is the presence of abundant blood supply with formation, in many cases, of arteriovenous shunts. On the perfusion maps, these tumors typically have a high volume (CBV) and a particularly high blood flow rate (CBF).

The central necrotic part of glioblastoma is characterized by low perfusion values and is clearly contoured on the maps with the infiltrative part of the tumor, which correlates with PET findings (Fig. 28.13). Most of metastases in the brain are also characterized by high perfusion values, and only in cases of relatively low values (ovarian, lung, prostate cancer), secondary nature of tumors can be assumed; however, in this case, an intense accumulation of the contrast agent on T1-weighted images is the mandatory parameter, which, to some extent, allows to eliminate grade 2 gliomas.

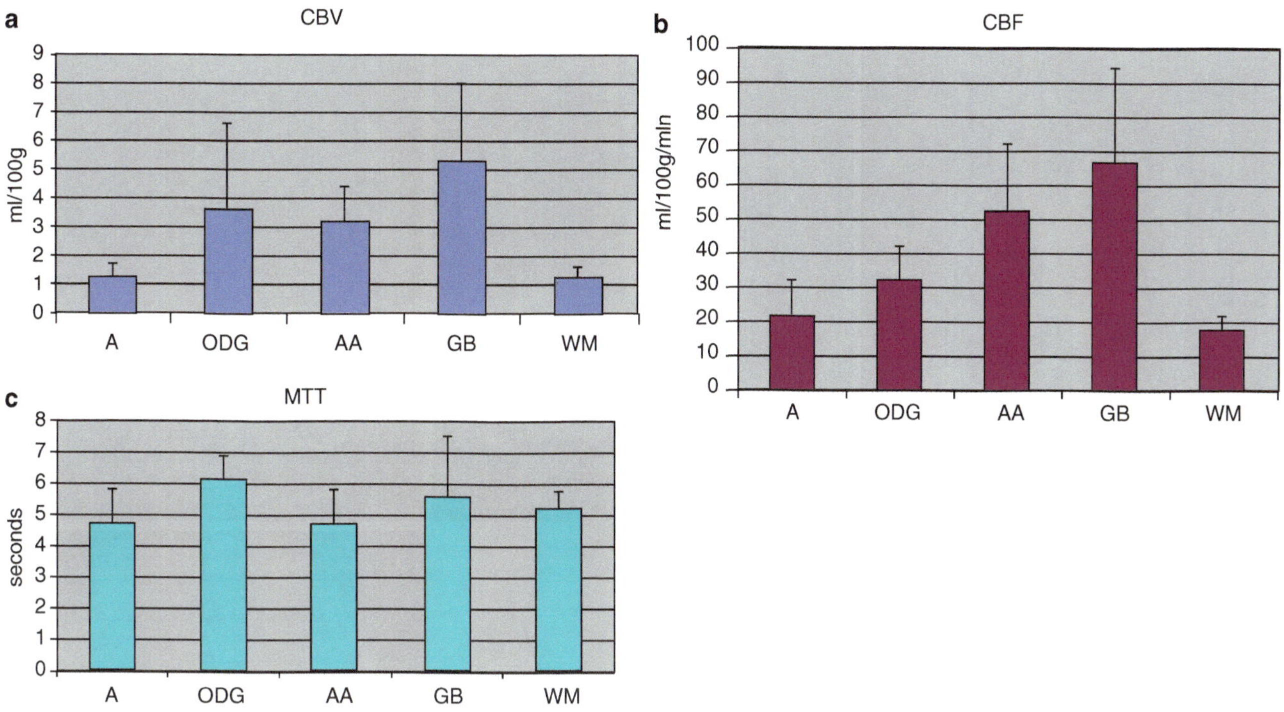

Fig. 28.12 Quantitative CT perfusion parameters in patients with glial tumors as compared to the white matter. (**a**) CBV, (**b**) CBF, (**c**) MTT. On the graphs, "A" refers to astrocytoma, "ODG" oligodendroglioma, "AA" anaplastic astrocytoma, "GB" glioblastoma, and "WM" white matter

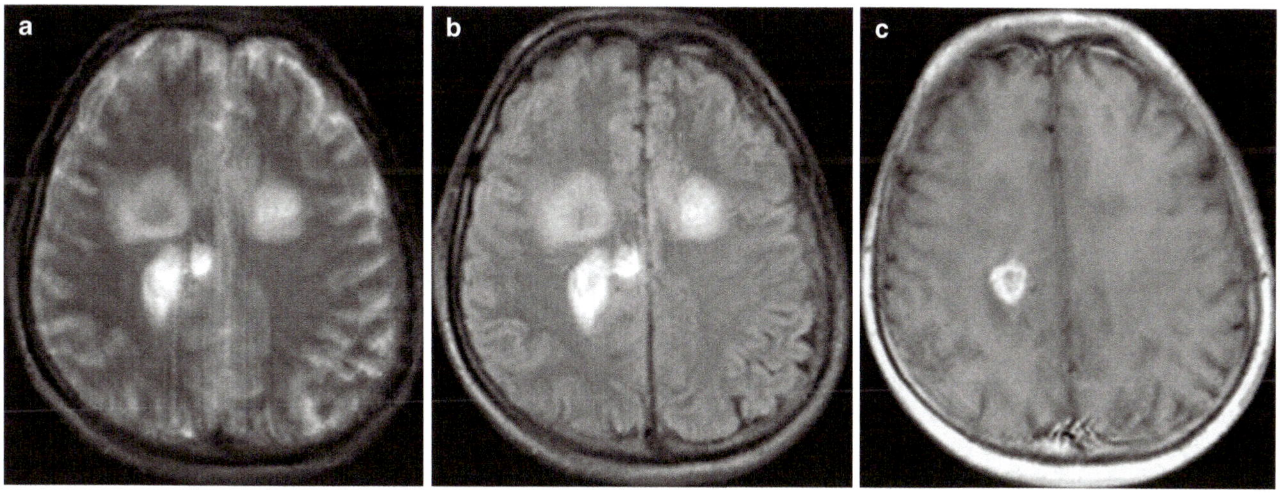

Fig. 28.13 Multifocal glioblastoma. A follow-up study. At the patient's first presentation, MRI visualizes multiple space-occupying lesions with indistinct contours and a hyperintense signal on T2-weighted and T2-FLAIR MRI (**a**, **b**) in the substance of both cerebral hemispheres. After CA administration, its accumulation is noted in only one of the lesions (**c**). Two weeks later, on the background of a sharp deterioration of health, a drastic increase in the size of lesions was noted with formation of a larger lesion consisting of two pieces in the right frontoparietal region: lateral (necrosis area) and medial (solid part of the tumor). In the central fragment, CT (**g**) shows an increase in the density due to the hemorrhagic component. On CT perfusion maps of CBV (**d**), CBF (**e**), and MTT (**f**), high values are observed in the medial tumor fragment and low in the necrotic area (lateral fragment). On PET/CT with ^{18}F-tyrosine (**h**, **i**), intense RP accumulation is observed by the solid component of the tumor in the right hemisphere and its weak accumulation in the left frontal area, indicative of a benign tumor (the *arrow*)

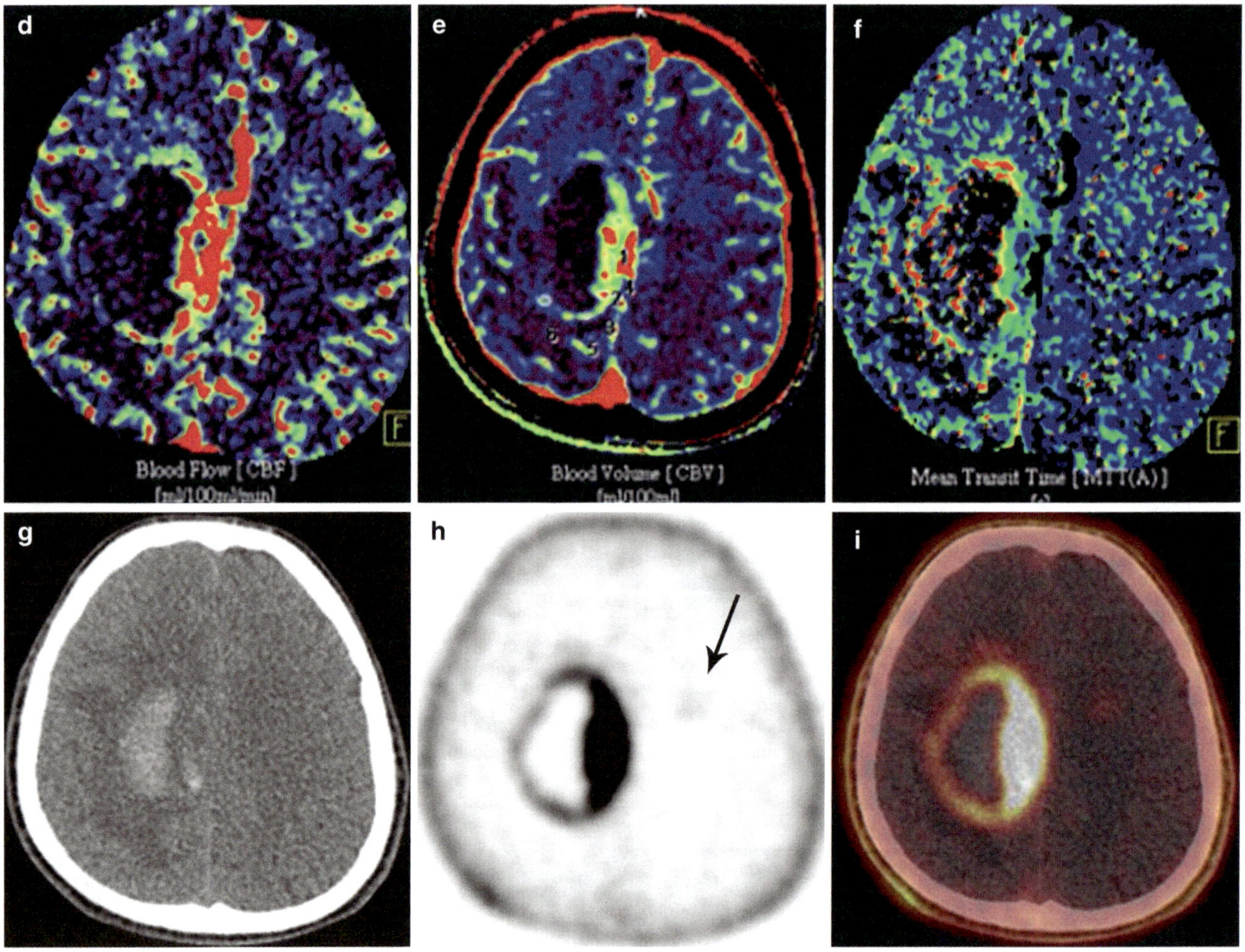

Fig. 28.13 (continued)

28.1 DWI

The degree of invasion by tumor cells on the tumor/normal tissue borderline is of fundamental importance for the radicality of treatment of primary and secondary brain tumors. Metastatic tumors are usually known to grow expansively and have only a mechanical effect on the brain tissue. They have a clear boundary with respect to the brain substance in contrast to primary glial tumors that diffuse into the normal brain tissue. Metastases, as previously shown, can be presented not only by various forms, but also change their imaging characteristics detected on CT and MRI with contrast enhancement during growth. From this viewpoint, the method of diffusion-weighted MRI (DWI) helps identify those regions of tumor tissue that have expressed qualitative differences, which is useful in the differential diagnosis of metastatic lesions of any origin. Studies of the tumor borderline area and comparison of images with contrast enhancement and ADC maps showed that qualitative values of the diffusion coefficient correlate with the presence of tumor cells on the tumor/normal tissue borderline: the more tumor cells in the border area, the greater probability of the presence of the primary tumor, not a metastasis in the brain. The big disadvantage of the diffusion-based methods is a marked dependence of the diagnostic results on the presence and severity of perifocal edema.

Metastases, unlike primary glial tumors, have a lower DWI signal in the edema area, which is likely due to a less dense structure of the brain tissue and more free movement of water molecules in the extracellular space. In case of a higher diffusion coefficient (ADC) on the periphery, metastases should be suspected. At lower ADC values in this area, glioblastoma can be suspected.

On the tumor/normal tissue borderline, ADC values in the group of cases of patients with brain metastases were higher ($p < 0.05$) than in patients with a primary tumor—glioblastoma. Thus, with a typical GB structure, its central part (necrosis area) generally has a reduced MR signal and high ADC values. The average ADC values in the GB stroma accumulating the contrast agent amounted to $1.19 \pm 0.29 \times 10^{-3}$. However, numerical ADC values determined in GB, as well as in solid, contrast-enhanced AnASC areas, quite widely overlap, which does not allow, based solely on DWI findings, to assume the

Table 28.1 Average ADC values in metastatic brain lesions (measured by DWI MRI)

Region of study	Tumor stroma	The nearest peritumoral area	Vasogenic edema area
Obtained ADC values (in 10^{-3}mm²/s)	1.15 ± 0.2	1.37 ± 0.2	1.56 ± 0.2

Table 28.2 Averages ADC values in glioblastomas (measured by DWI MRI)

Region of study	Tumor stroma	The nearest peritumoral area	Vasogenic edema area
Obtained ADC values (in 10^{-3} mm²/s)	1.19 ±0.2	1.29 ± 0.1	1.51 ± 0.3

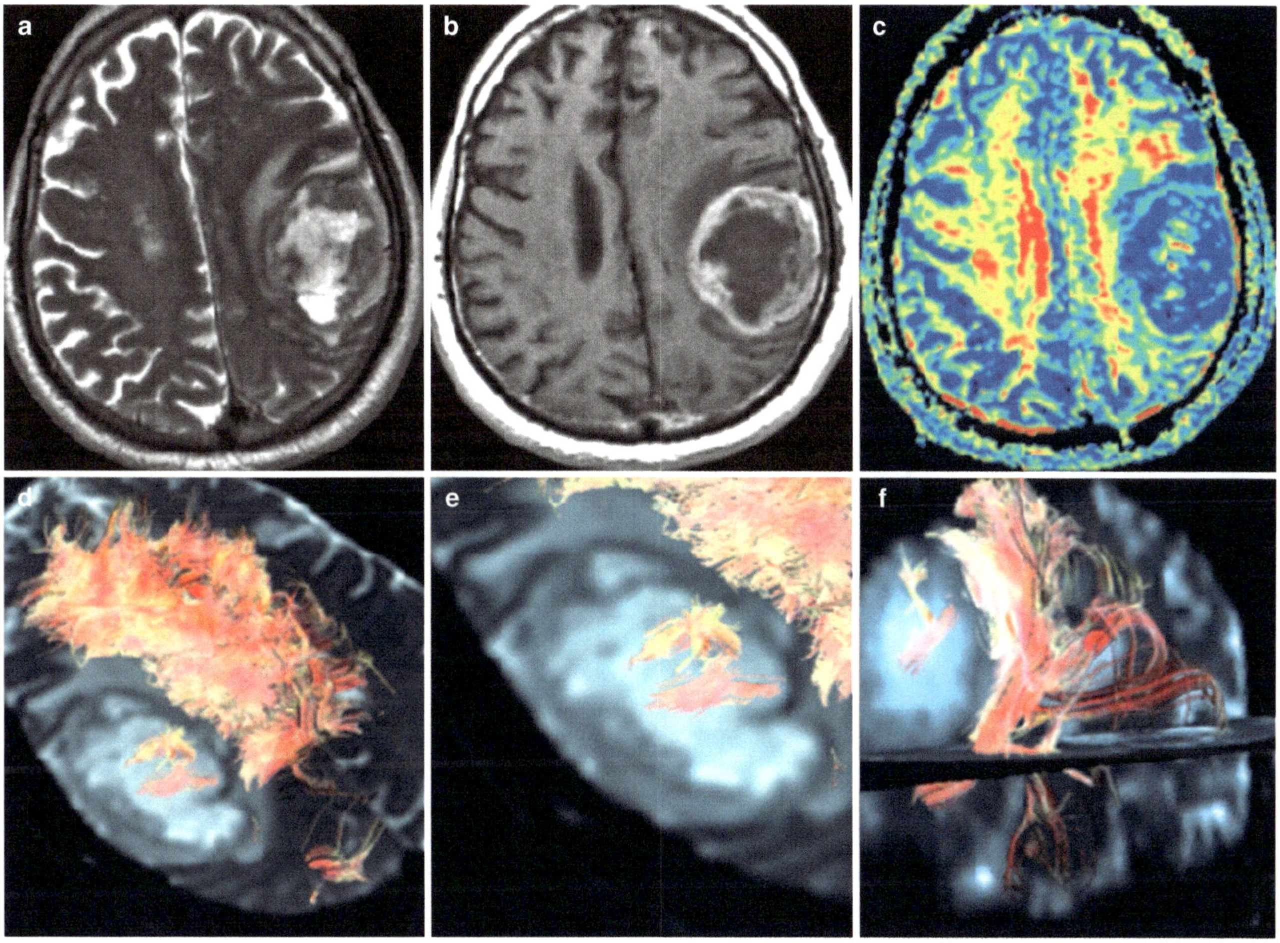

Fig. 28.14 Glioblastoma. On MRI in the left temporoparietal region on T2-weighted (**a**) and T1-weighted MRI, on the background of contrast enhancement (**b**), there is a tumor with a heterogeneous structure and signs of central necrosis and perifocal edema. Glioblastoma destroys conductive tracts of the white matter in the tumor infiltration area; a part of the conductive tracts in the center of the lesion is intact (a partial anisotropy map (**c**) and 3D MR tractography (**d–f**))

type of a neoplasm. In out material, average ADC values for metastases were, respectively, 1.15 ± 0.2 × 10^{-3} mm²/s in the tumor stroma, 1.37 ± 0.2 × 10^{-3} mm²/s in the near peritumoral area, and 1.56 ± 0.2 × 10^{-3} mm²/s in the vasogenic edema area. ADC values in the tumor itself were highly heterogeneous. In the control group of glioblastomas, the average ADC values in the solid part of the tumor were, respectively, 1.19 ± 0.2 × 10^{-3} mm²/s in the tumor stroma, 1.29 ± 0.1 × 10^{-3} mm²/s in the near peritumoral area, and 1.51 ± 0.3 × 10^{-3} mm²/s in the vasogenic edema area. DWI characteristics and average ADC values in different areas of metastatic lesions, glioblastomas, and peritumoral edema are presented in Tables 28.1 and 28.2.

As can be seen from the tables, ADC values on the tumor border in the group of patients with metastatic cancer were slightly lower ($p < 0.15$) than in patients with GBs. A comparative analysis of the perifocal area in the group of glioblastomas and metastases allowed us to suggest different variants of the tumor effect on the surrounding brain substance in 85% of cases.

On MR tractography, the destructive tumor growth in the brain substance results in disintegration and destruction of neural tracts of the white matter at the GB site, with islets of intact tracts observed in separate tumor fragments. This is an important distinction between GBs in the differential diagnosis with solitary metastases, which are characterized by displacement and dislocation of tracts (Fig. 28.14).

Proton MR spectroscopy in most cases demonstrates the prevalence of a large lipid-lactate complex on the background of a marked reduction in the peaks of all other cerebral tissue metabolites. Manifestations of GBs, according to MRS, are indistinguishable from manifestations of any other tumor, where there is an area of decay (Fig. 28.15). According to Fan et al. (2004), the method allows to perform the differential diagnosis between metastases and glioblastoma based on the ratio of choline and creatine peaks. However, in our studies, a high peak of the Lip-Lac complex and a high choline peak were determined in the majority of glioblastomas. When selecting the region of interest, it is extremely important not to capture the adjacent brain structures or necrosis area, which will immediately affect the occurrence of "brain" or "dead" peaks both in GB and a metastatic tumor.

The use of multi-voxel MRS with the possibility to position the region of interest in any area of the selected section provides new possibilities in the assessment of changes in the biochemical status of the tumor tissue, perifocal area, and surrounding cerebral edema (Fig. 28.16). Construction of color metabolite distribution maps complements the overall picture of changes in metabolites.

28.2 SWI (SWAN)

Unlike secondary tumors, glioblastoma does not necessarily pass a number of initial growth stages and, above all, does not need to "fight" with the defenses of the recipient organ. The tumor grows diffusely, involving and transforming normal tissues. Characteristics of the structure of the capillary wall of microvessels in glioblastomas very often result in the development of intratumoral micro- and even macroscopic hemorrhages and necrosis foci resulting from the oblitera-

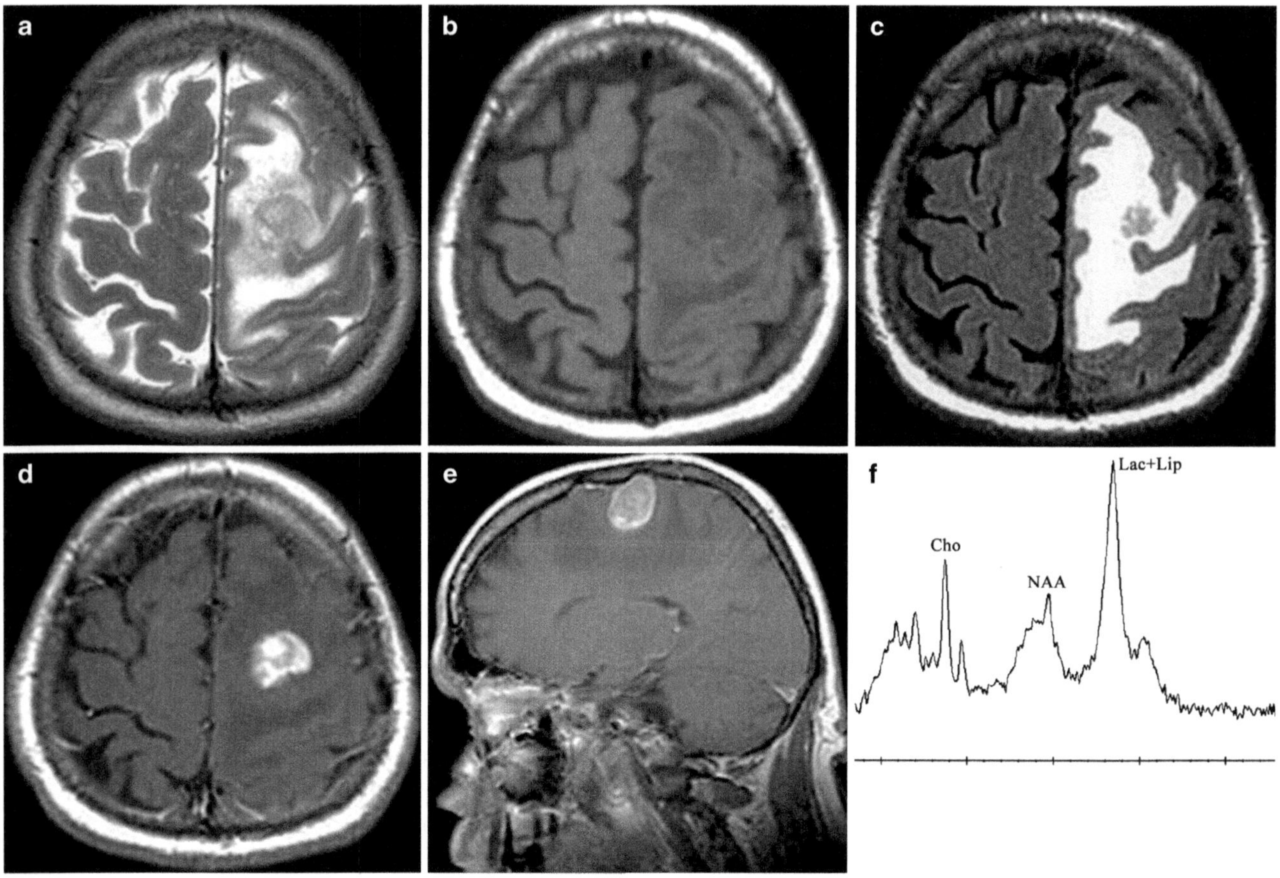

Fig. 28.15 Glioblastoma. In the left postfrontal region, there is a space-occupying, irregularly shaped lesion with sharp contours, an iso- and hyperintense signal on T2-weighted (**a**) and T2-FLAIR MRI (**c**) and an isointense signal on T1-weighted MRI (**b**), with a pronounced perifocal edema. Following intravenous CA administration on T1-weighted MRI in axial (**d**) and sagittal (**e**) projections, its intense and inhomogeneous accumulation is observed in the tumor. On the spectrum (**f**), the Lip-Lac complex is prevalent, but also Cho and NAA peaks are well differentiated

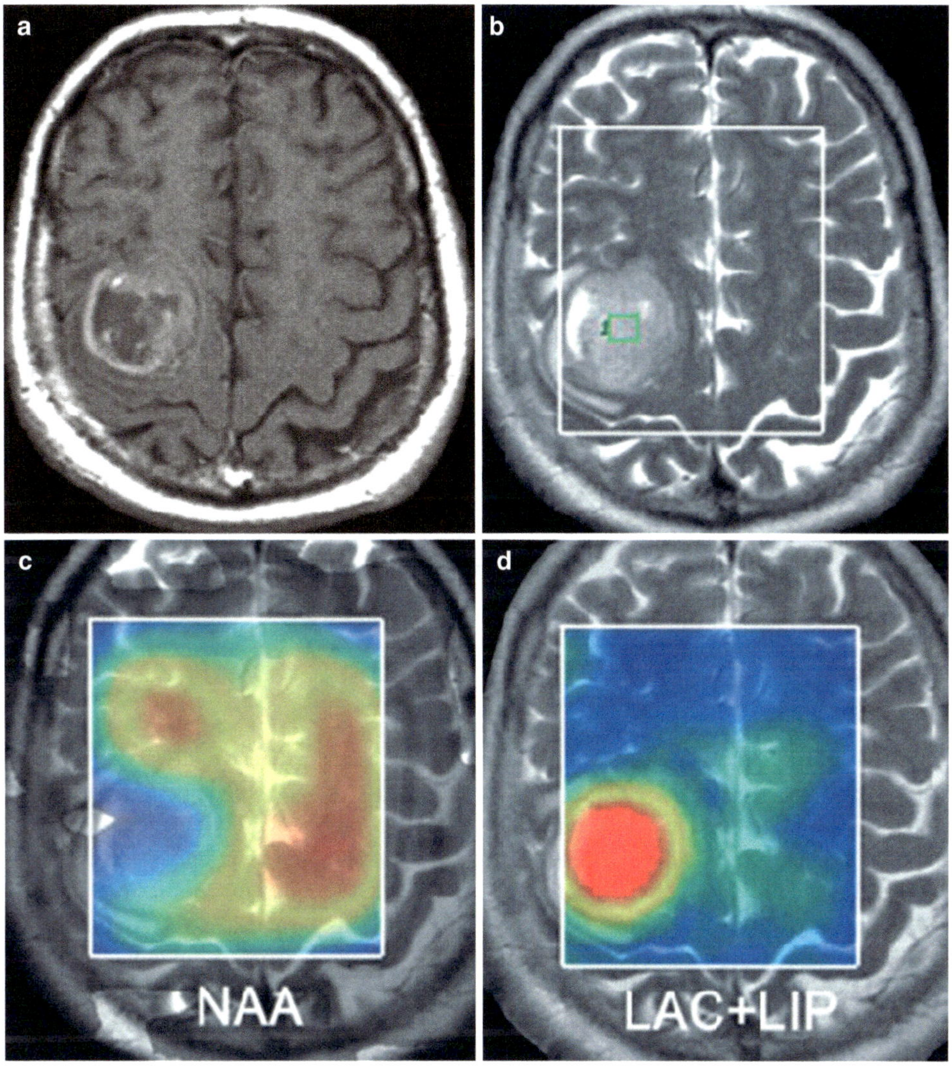

Fig. 28.16 Glioblastoma. T1-weighted MRI (**a**), on the background of contrast enhancement and T2-weighted MRI (**b**) with the display of the multi-voxel proton MR spectroscopy area with the local region of interest demonstrates an inhomogeneous structure of the neoplasm with peripheral contrast enhancement and a central necrotic part. Color metabolite maps (**c**, **d**) clearly demonstrate an NAA reduction and an expressed Lip-Lac complex in the tumor

tion of blood vessels. The tumor tissue contains a lot of small and large abnormal new vessels and the so-called arteriovenous shunts.

MR sequences weighted by magnetic susceptibility SWI (SWAN) allow to visualize these vascular changes. On axial sections on SWI (SWAN) MRI, abnormal vessels have a pinpoint or convoluted form. Microhemorrhages surpassing by their area abnormal vessels are visualized in the form micronodules or stains. It should be noted that these changes in the MR signal are not detected on standard T2-weighted MRI.

Findings obtained using the SWI (SWAN) method allowed to identify previously undetectable pathophysiological changes in the glioblastoma tissue, which certainly complements our knowledge of the structural organization of the tumor, allowing to identify some of the characteristics that were previously detected only histologically. A comparison of findings from the histological analysis of glioblastoma biopsy samples revealed a high degree of correlation with SWI (SWAN) findings in the identification of multiple arteriovenous shunts and hemorrhages. These findings were observed in 92% of cases, and, in 8% of cases, only abnormal blood vessels without hemorrhages were noted. We did not encounter a “homogeneous variant” of glioblastoma in our cases at all. Thus, the destruction of vascular walls and hemorrhages in the glioblastoma structure were observed twice as often as in metastatic tumors (Fig. 28.17).

We have noted high sensitivity of SP SWI to administration of paramagnetic materials (gadolinium-containing contrast agents) in the presence of a solid part of the tumor. Despite the fact that the relative degree of contrast enhancement in the tumor structure on SWI (SWAN) MRI was lower

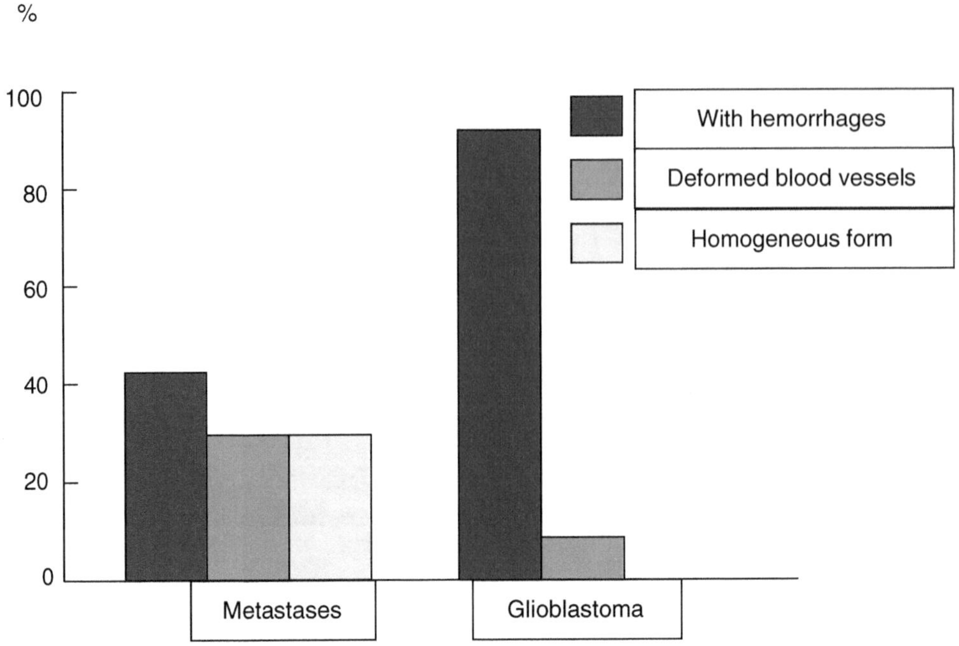

Fig. 28.17 The ratio of microhemorrhages and abnormal vessels in the structures of metastatic brain tumors (MTS) and glioblastomas (GB) obtained from the analysis of SWI findings (hypointense inclusions with various sizes)

than on routine T1-weighted MRI, in all cases, there was an increase in the MR signal on the post-contrast series of images from the infiltrative part of tumors and arteries. This allowed to clearly distinguish between the tumor tissue and perifocal edema that has a hyperintense MR signal in SWI (SWAN) images (as opposed to T1-weighted images). This undoubtedly provides additional information to assess the characteristics of intracerebral lesions.

The quantitative assessment of changes in the relative intensity of MR signal in the solid part of secondary tumors and glioblastomas on SWI (SWAN) MRI before and after intravenous administration of the contrast material conducted during the study using the software package FUNCTOOL enabled a detailed analysis of the character of CA accumulation in these tumors (Fig. 28.18). Thus, metastases were divided into two groups: with and without signs of hemorrhages.

The greatest difference in the values of relative signal intensity was found in the structure of secondary tumors without any signs of hemorrhages—a homogeneous form and a variant with tortuous vessels (from 0.56 to 1.09 and from 0.63 to 1.09, respectively), as well as in the solid part of glioblastomas (from 0.86 to 1.15). In a much lesser extent, the signal increased in the structure of metastatic tumors with signs of hemorrhages (from 0.69 to 0.76).

A further advantage of contrast-enhanced SWI (SWAN) MRI is the possibility to perform specific differentiation between tumor vessels that accumulated contrast agent and became brighter on MRI and hemorrhages that maintained their hypointensity (Fig. 28.19).

The analysis of the use of pulsed SWI (SWAN) sequence revealed specific pathophysiological changes in the tissues of growing metastases and glioblastoma. Lower perfusion rates in metastasis tissues, as opposed to the perfusion values in glioblastomas, despite the lack of multiple hemorrhages detected on SWI (SWAN) MRI, indicate a less pronounced blood supply to the tumor ($p < 0{,}05$) and suggest that these features are related to the blood supply of tumors due to vessels formed by tumors directly (which is more characteristic of metastases) and not due to the altered primary vessels of the brain (Fig. 28.20).

Infiltrative growth of glioblastoma with the development of related changes (deformation and tortuosity) in microvessels surrounding the "main" lesion in the brain tissue is accompanied by prolongation of the mean transit time (MTT). It can be assumed that vascular transformation precedes tumor growth, but this requires further investigation with inclusion of brain tumors with various histological structures into the analyzed sample. MTT values lower relative to the solid portion of the tumor around metastases suggest a greater degree of demarcation of the tumor tissue from the cerebral structures.

The availability of such valuable additional information on the tumor structure and configuration of its flow, especially when combined with the results of the methods quantitatively assessing hemodynamic changes (CT/MR perfusion, PET, etc.), without any doubt, becomes an important condition for improving the accuracy and specificity of the diagnosis of various brain tumors.

Fig. 28.18 Quantitative parameters of the signal changes in the structures of metastases (MTS) and glioblastomas (GB) before and after administration of the contrast medium on SWI MRI

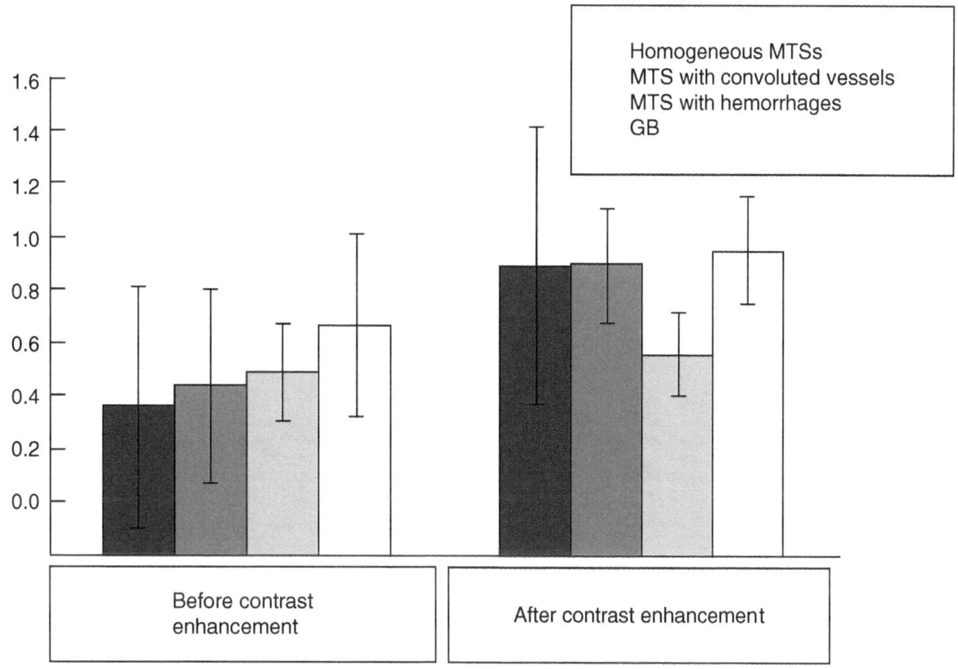

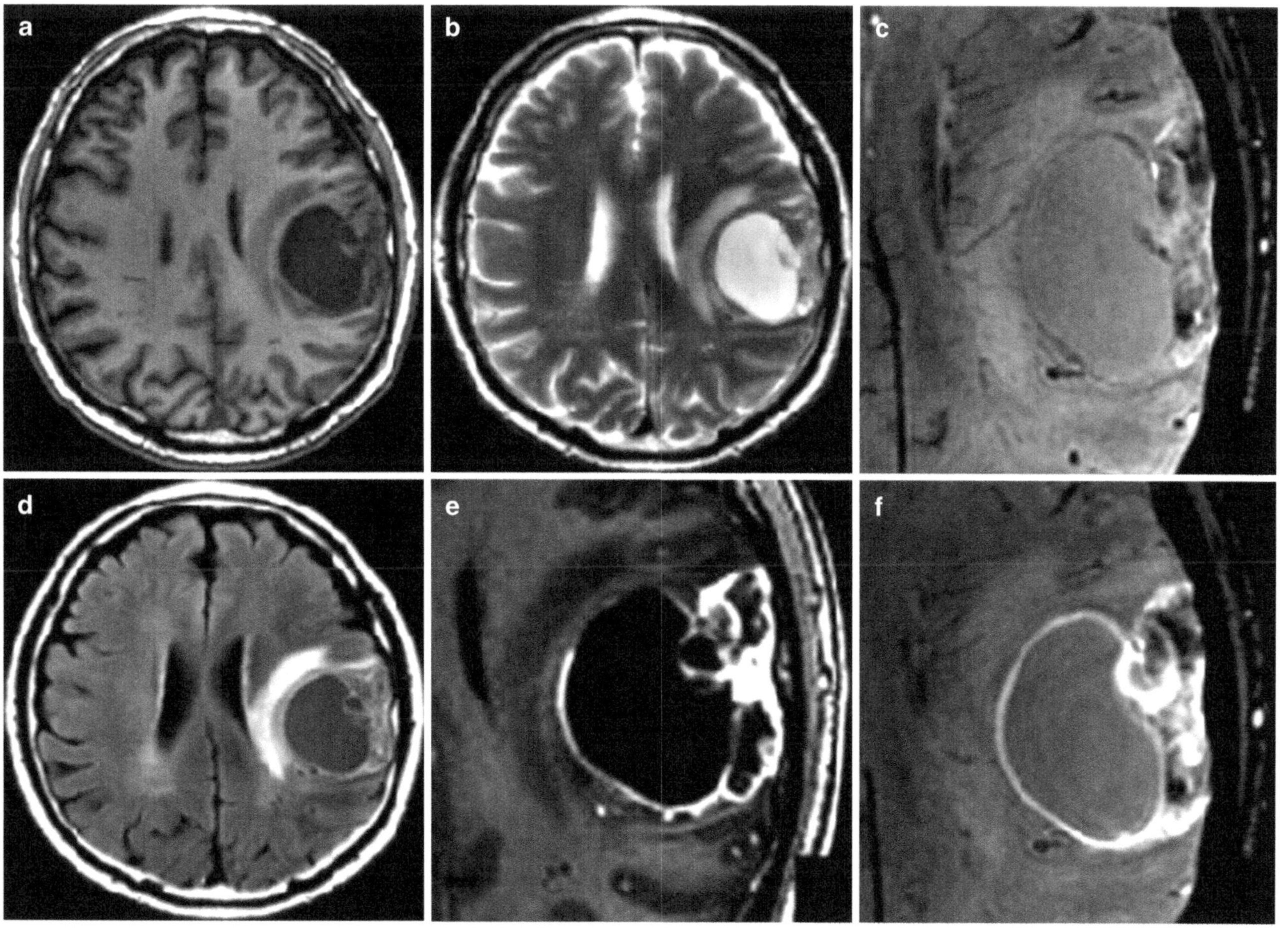

Fig. 28.19 Glioblastoma. In the left frontoparietal region on T1-weighted MRI (**a**), T2-weighted MRI (**b**), T2-FLAIR MRI (**d**), and T1-weighted contrast-enhanced MRI (**e**), there is a cystic tumor with a moderate perifocal edema. CA accumulation on T1-weighted MRI in the solid part of the tumor is inhomogeneous (**e**), which is associated with necrotic and hemorrhagic inclusions, although they are not clearly identified on routine MRI but are well visualized on SWI MRI—hemorrhagic hypointense areas on SWI MRI (**c**) also retain the low signal after the administration of contrast medium (**f**); vascular elements accumulate the contrast agent. The boundary between the cystic and solid portions of the tumor is well visualized on the background of perifocal edema with an increased signal in T2-weighted and SWI images

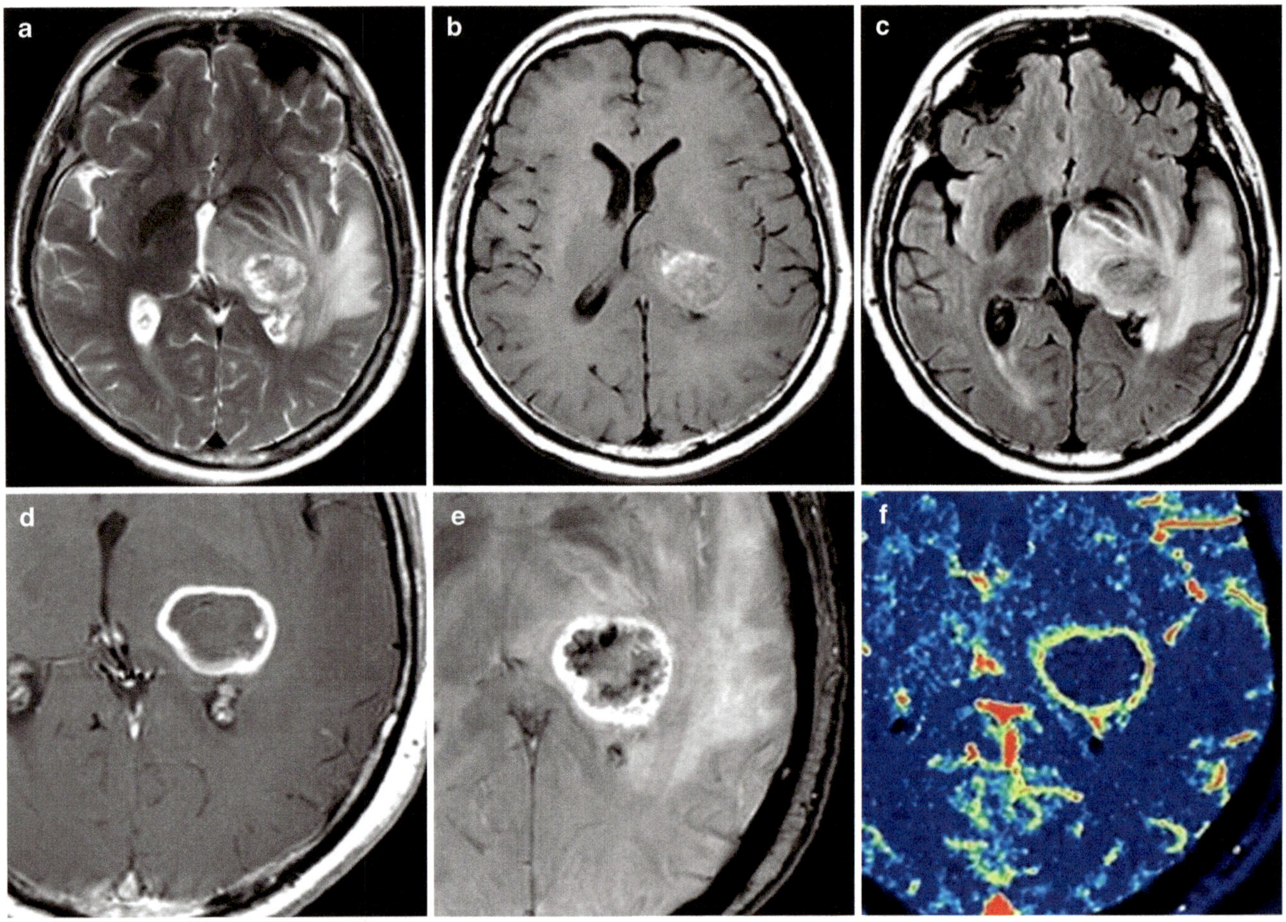

Fig. 28.20 Glioblastoma. In the posterior regions of the thalamus to the left, on T2-weighted MRI (**a**), there is a rounded, space-occupying lesion, with an iso- and hyperintense signal in T1-weighted MRI (**b**). On T2-FLAIR MRI (**c**), the signal from the lesion is heterogeneously increased; there is a pronounced perifocal edema. After CA administration (**d**), the lesion intensely accumulates it on the periphery. On SWI MRI (**e**) after CA administration, multiple hypointense inclusions are observed in the tumor structure. On a CT perfusion map of CBV (**f**), high values are observed in the peripheral regions of the tumor

Positron emission tomography (PET) with administration of a radiotracer based on amino acids, for example, ^{11}C-methionine, is the method of choice for assessing post-radiation changes and continued growth of intracranial tumors, including glioblastomas. PET is used much less frequently for the primary diagnosis of intracerebral lesions. Glioblastomas, as well as anaplastic astrocytomas and metastases, rapidly accumulate ^{11}C-methionine and other radiopharmaceuticals, for example, ^{18}F-tyrosine or ^{18}F-choline (Fig. 28.21).

The comparative analysis of the findings obtained by PET with the most common RP, such as ^{18}F-fluorodeoxyglucose([^{18}F]FDG) and ^{11}C-methionine in glial tumors, revealed that the sensitivity and specificity of the method using the above radiopharmaceuticals are 75–86% and 22–94%, respectively (Langleben and Segall 2000; Chao et al. 2001; Chang et al. 2002; Belohlavek et al. 2003). The accumulation index (AI) of methionine correlated with the degree of anaplasia of gliomas (Derlon et al. 1989), benign gliomas are characterized by "cold" lesions (AI within 1.5), while malignant ones are characterized by "hot" lesions (AI > 2) (Rudas et al. 2007, Skvortsova et al. 2014) (Fig. 28.22).

Fig. 28.21 Glioblastoma. On MRI in the right temporoparietal region, there is a lesion with a hyperintense signal on T2-weighted, T2-FLAIR, and DWI MRI (**a**, **c**, **f**) and heterogeneously hypointense on T1-weighted MRI (**b**), with a pronounced perifocal edema. After CA administration on T1-weighted fat sat MRI (**d**, **e**), there is intense and inhomogeneous accumulation in the solid structure of the tumor. On MR tractography (**g**), the conductive tract in the projection of the tumor cannot be traced. On PET-CT with ^{18}F-choline (**g**, **i**), there is a marked intense accumulation of the radiopharmaceutical in the vascularized part of the tumor and its absence in the necrosis area

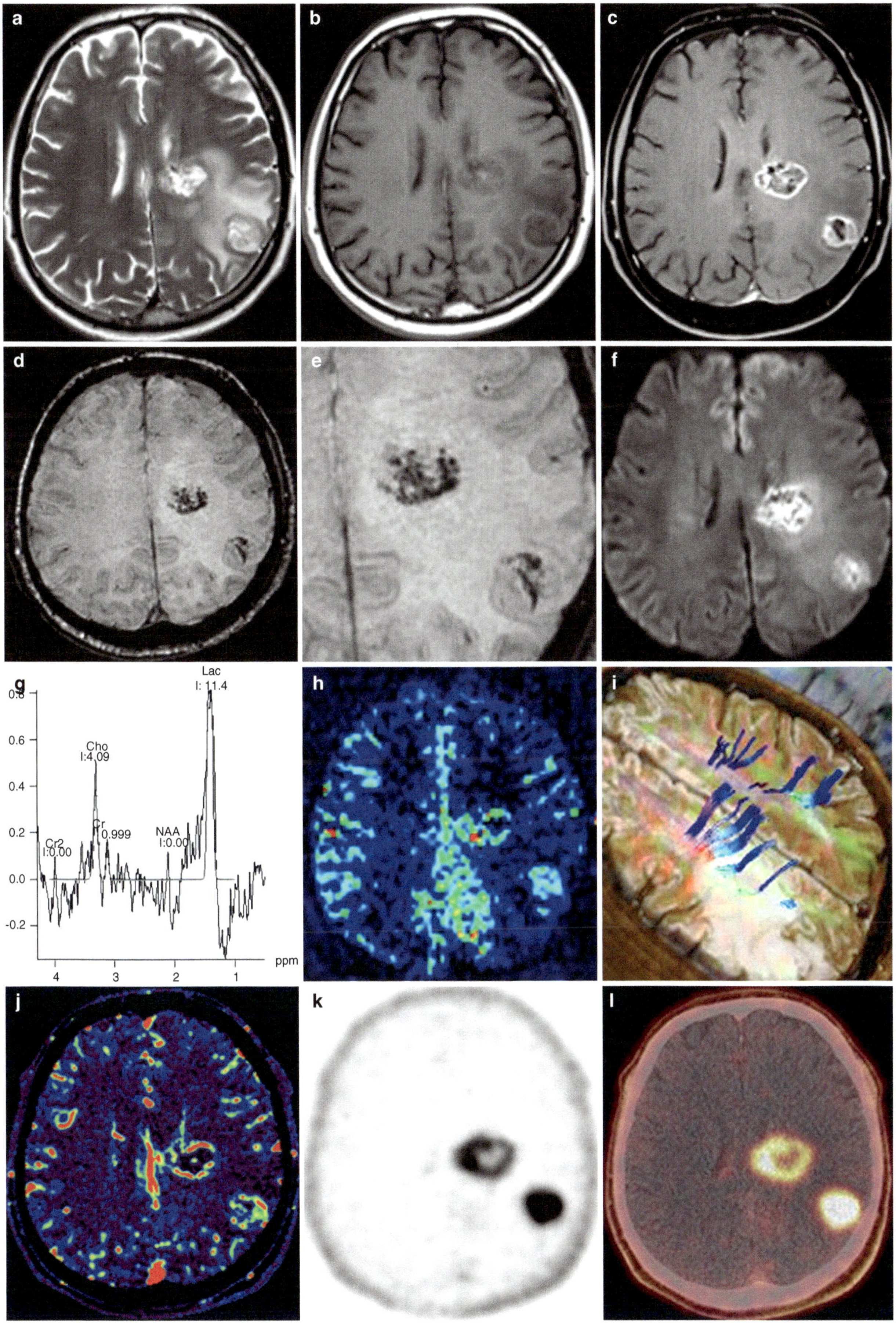
a
b
c
d
e
f
g
Lac
I: 11.4
Cho
I:4.09
Cr
0.999
Cr2
I:0.00
NAA
I:0.00
0.8
0.6
0.4
0.2
0.0
-0.2
4
3
2
1
ppm
h
i
j
k
l

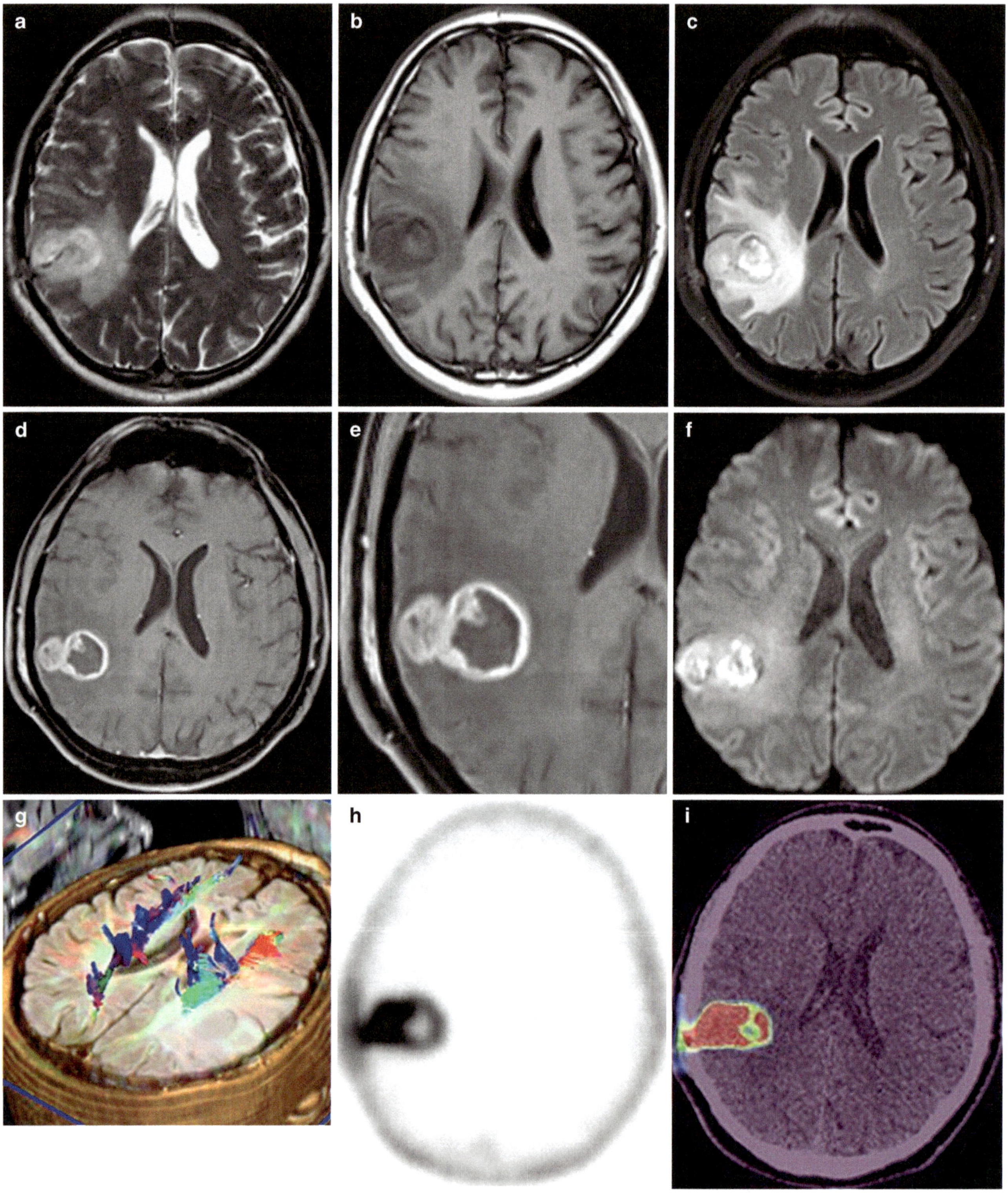

Fig. 28.22 Glioblastoma. On MRI in the right temporoparietal region, there is a lesion with a hyperintense signal on T2-weighted, T2-FLAIR, and DWI MRI (**a**, **c**, **f**) and heterogeneously hypointense on T1-weighted MRI (**b**), with a pronounced perifocal edema. After CA administration on T1-weighted fat sat MRI (**d**, **e**), there is intense and inhomogeneous accumulation in the solid structure of the tumor. On MR tractography (**g**), the conductive tract in the projection of the tumor cannot be traced. On PET-CT with ^{18}F-choline (**h**, **i**), there is a marked intense accumulation of the radiopharmaceutical in the vascularized part of the tumor and its absence in the necrosis area

In metastatic brain lesions, PET with ^{18}F-FDG can be used as a more affordable product, while in large solid metastases, RP accumulation values are always high before radiotherapy; their decrease is observed after the treatment (Maruyama et al. 1999), but in small (less than 1 cm) metastases and their cystic forms, as well as when tumors are located in the cortical and subcortical region, the diagnostic value of PET decreases (Rohren et al. 2003).

According to our data, glioblastomas, even with a relatively solid structure, are often characterized by high accumulation of ^{18}F-FDG and at the same time markedly accumulate ^{18}F-tyrosine and ^{18}F-choline (Figs. 28.23 and 28.24).

Gliosarcoma (GS) is the simultaneous combination of GB and angiosarcoma (or fibrosarcoma). Macroscopically, GS is a solid tumor with central necrosis. The sarcomatous part is clearly separated from the adjacent brain substance, while the astrocytic component has a soft structure and is poorly separated from the surrounding structures. Histological diagnosis of GS depends on the identification of the glial and mesenchymal tumor components. The infiltrative GS component is almost always glioblastoma.

In 15–30%, GSs produce extracranial metastases. They also metastasize via a hematogenous route to the visceral organs. GSs are characterized by superficial localization and spread with possible dural invasion. Most often the temporal lobe is affected. Manifestations of GS are variable. The tumor may resemble metastases, meningioma, or GB. GSs are usually less homogeneous than meningiomas, are widely attached to the dura mater, and are always surrounded by a

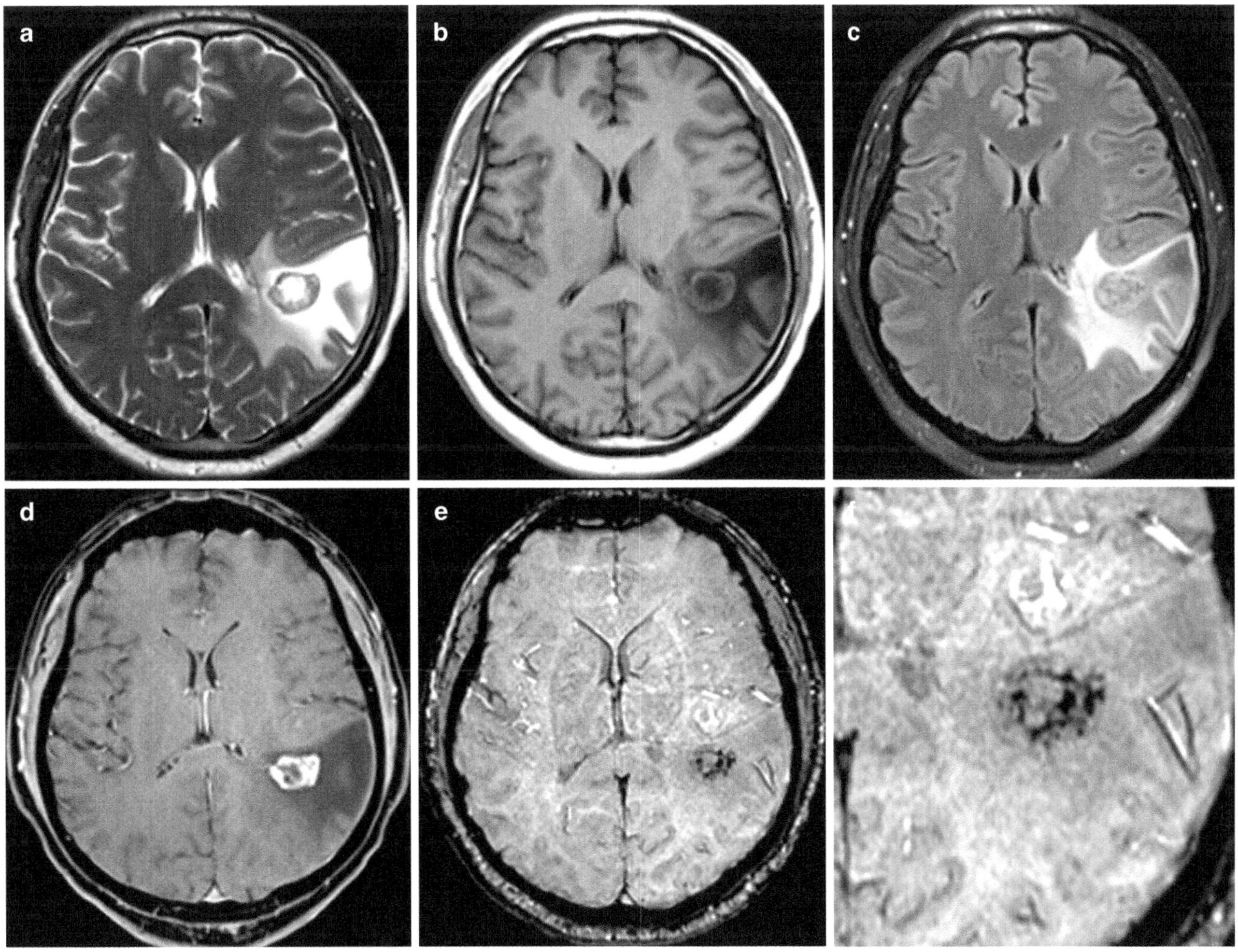

Fig. 28.23 Glioblastoma. On MRI, in the deep parts of the left frontoparietal region, the lesion is detected with signs of central necrosis and a moderately increased signal in the peripheral regions in T2-weighted, T1-weighted, and T2-FLAIR images (**a**–**c**). After CA administration on T1-weighted fat sat MRI (**d**), the tumor intensely and inhomogeneously accumulates CA. On SWI MRI (**e**, **f**), there are multiple hypointense areas in the lesion structure, preferably on the periphery. On MR spectroscopy (**g**), there is a pronounced increase in the Lip-Lac complex peak and a moderate Cho peak. On PET with ^{18}F-FDG (**h**), there is an ametabolic area; on PET with ^{18}F-choline (**i**), there is a significant increase in the RP accumulation. On CT perfusion maps of CBV (**j**), CBF (**k**), and MTT (**l**), there are high values for all parameters in peripheral tumor fragments

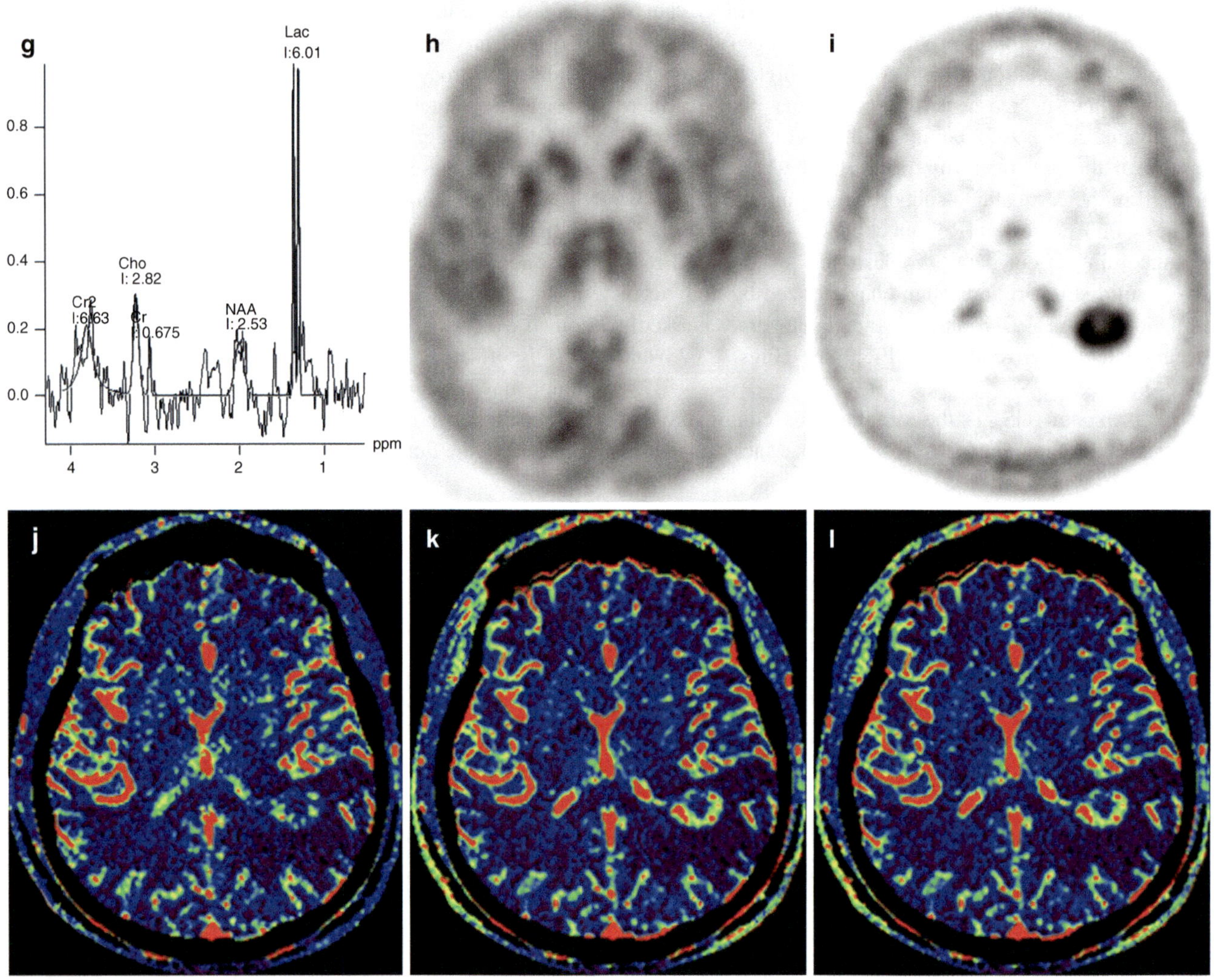

Fig. 28.23 (continued)

Fig. 28.24 Glioblastoma. A two-level study. On T2-weighted (**a**, **d**) and T1-weighted contrast-enhanced MRI (**b**, **e**) in the left frontal region, there is a space-occupying lesion consisting of three fragments: a rounded lesion with necrosis in the center, intensely accumulating the contrast agent on the periphery of the fragments and without clear outlines, and without any signs of contrast material accumulation, located, respectively, parasagittally and convexitally. On the spectra in the central fragment of the lesion (**c**), there is a pronounced increase in the Cho peak and a moderate increase in the Lip-Lac complex; the peaks of NAA and Cr are sharply decreased. In the parasagittal part of the lesion (**f**), there is a decrease in the NAA peak and an increase in the Cho and Lip-Lac peaks. On CT (**h**), there is an increase in the density from the rounded lesion and a decrease in the density in the parasagittal fragment. On CT perfusion maps, there is an increase in CBF (**h**) and MTT values (**i**) only in the rounded lesion. On PET images with ^{18}F-choline (**j**, **l**) in the fusion mode (**k**), the picture is similar to that in CT perfusion

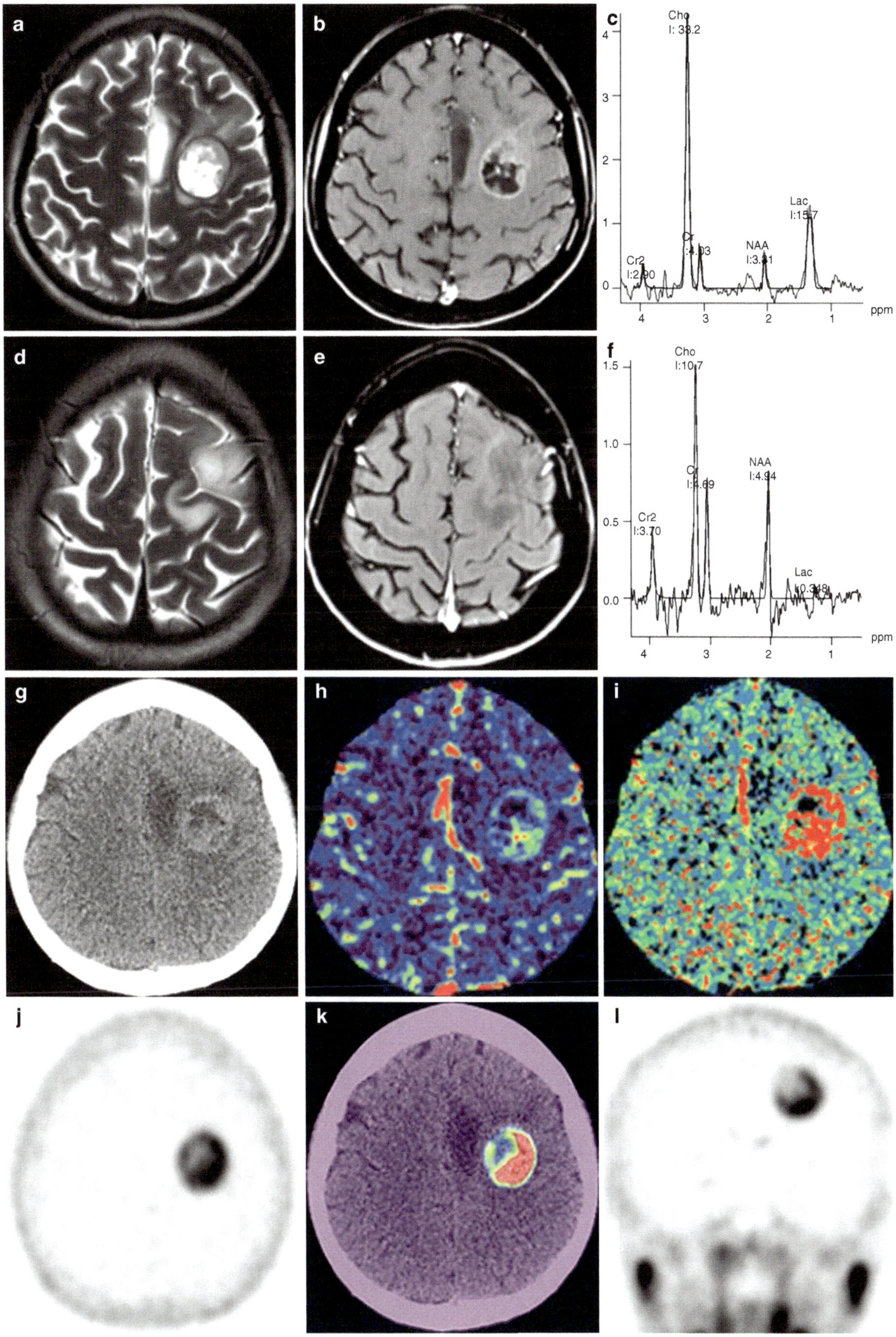
a
b
c
Cho
I: 38.2
Lac
I:15.7
Cr
I:4.03
NAA
I:3.31
Cr2
I:2.90
ppm
d
e
f
Cho
I:10.7
Cr
I:4.69
NAA
I:4.94
Cr2
I:3.70
Lac
I:0.348
ppm
g
h
i
j
k
l

perifocal edema. Significant heterogeneity or nonuniform annular enhancement after administration of the contrast medium is typical for GSs. Standard MRI demonstrates an inhomogeneous, quite localized tumor. This tumor is frequently accompanied by necrosis and hemorrhages. Following contrast enhancement, an increase in the signal from the tumor is observed; however, its structure in the MR image has heterogeneous character (Fig. 28.25). Nevertheless, based on the MR characteristics, GS cannot be differentiated from metastases, especially when it is small.

Pilocytic astrocytoma (PASC) is a subtype of ASC. Patients' age, site, and prognosis for PASCs differ significantly from those for diffuse infiltrative fibrous ASCs. PASCs represent only 5–10% of all cerebral gliomas but account for about one third of glial tumors in children. Of these, tumors most often occur in the supratentorial area, in the projection of the bottom of ventricle III and the optic chiasm, and, subtentorially, in the cerebellar hemispheres. Macroscopically, the appearance of PASCs varies depending on their site. Cerebellar PASCs are well-marginated lesions that can be a large cyst with a parietal nodule. Optochiasmal hypothalamic PASCs have a nodular shape and are well demarcated; thus, they may mimic metastases.

On CT, PASCs are visualized as round or oval lesions, well demarcated and having hypo- or isodense characteristics. Calcifications are observed in 10–20% of all PASCs (Osborn 2004). Contrast enhancement is variable in nature. Some tumors with solid structure have homogeneous and pronounced contrast enhancement; others have a mural nodule in the large cyst (Fig. 28.26).

On T1-weighted MRI, the solid part of PASC has usually a hypo- or isointense signal; on T2-weighted MRI, this part of the tumor appears hyperintense. The cystic part of the neoplasm has a high MR signal in T2-weighted and T2-FLAIR images. When using gadolinium-containing products, there is an intense signal enhancement from the solid portion of the tumors, mainly heterogeneous and quite pronounced (Arslanoglu et al. 2003). The walls of the cystic tumor in some cases can also accumulate the contrast agent. Cases of malignization of the tumor and/or dissemination along the meninges are exceptions, although described in publications and observed in our series.

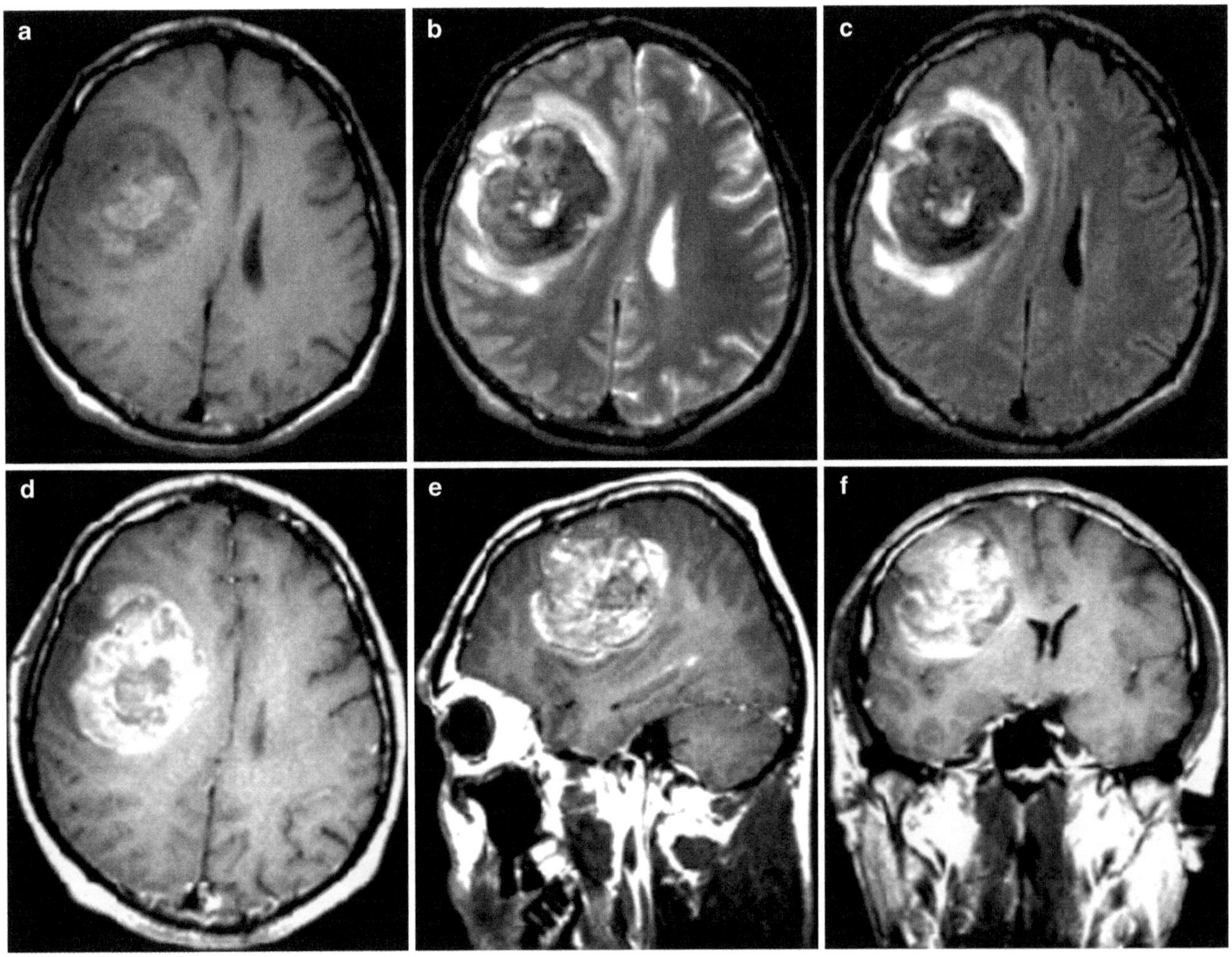

Fig. 28.25 Gliosarcoma. In the right frontal region, on T1-weighted (**a**), T2-weighted (**b**), and T1-weighted contrast-enhanced MRI in three projections (**d–f**), a large tumor is identified, having a low MR signal on T2-weighted (**b**) and T2-FLAIR (**c**) MRI. The tumor intensely and inhomogeneously accumulates the contrast agent. Perifocal edema is mild; the ventricular system is deformed

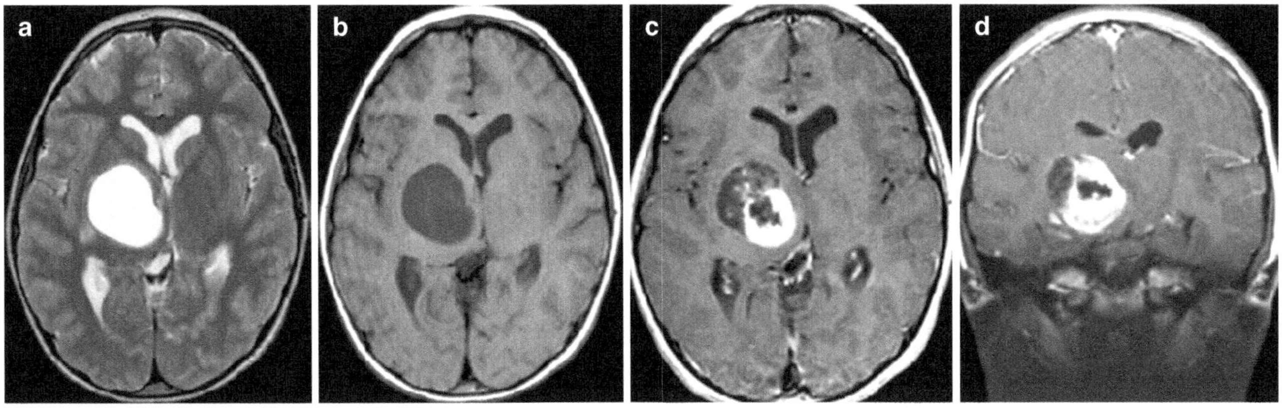

Fig. 28.26 Pilocytic astrocytoma. On T2-weighted MRI (**a**) and T1-weighted MRI (**b**) in the projection of the subcortical nuclei on the right, the tumor is visualized with a relatively homogeneous structure without a perifocal edema. The contrast agent accumulation in the tumor (**c**, **d**) is heterogeneous, showing a mostly solid structure of the neoplasm with central necrosis and a cyst on the anterior pole. The third ventricle is narrowed

29 Oligodendroglioma (ODG)

Oligodendroglioma (ODG) is a relatively rare glioma, also quite a demarcated tumor. Moreover, "pure" ODGs are even more rare; mostly mixed gliomas are observed (oligoastrocytomas). The tumor develops from a specific type of glial cells—oligodendrocytes—and accounts for 2–10% of all primary intracranial tumors and 5–25% of gliomas. Most of ODGs are slow-growing, benign, non-encapsulated infiltrative tumors of the white matter, which are usually located paraventricularly. 85% of tumors are supratentorial, affecting mostly the frontal lobe. The tumor is characterized by the formation of foci of cystic degeneration and calcifications. Malignization of ODGs manifests by cellular atypia, occurrence of mitoses in the tumor, and proliferation of vascular endothelium (Fig. 29.1).

Oligodendroglioma is a most common intracranial tumor that calcifies, which is clearly seen on CT. The neoplasm has a mixed density. 75% of ODGs do not accumulate contrast agent. MRI identifies a tumor with mixed hypo- and isointensity in T1-weighted images and hyperintense foci in T2-weighted images (Fig. 29.2).

Although MRI is less sensitive than CT in determining tumor calcifications, it is superior to CT in identification of the tumor spread. In addition to the above, it is better to use T2-weighted and T2-FLAIR MRI than T1-weighted MRI. MR contrast enhancement of ODGs is inhomogeneous. It is observed in up to 50% of cases and is more pronounced with malignization of the tumor.

MRI and CT perfusion studies demonstrate the presence of hyperperfusion foci in the structure of histologically benign ODGs, characteristic of high-grade astrocytomas (Lev 2004).

ODGs on PET with ^{18}F-fluorodeoxyglucose show RP accumulation parameters close to those in the white matter. The use of ^{11}C-methionine contributes to the differential diagnosis between benign and malignant forms of the tumor. ^{18}F-tyrosine and ^{18}F-choline are accumulated rapidly and allow to detect malignant fragments.

Anaplastic ODG can develop both primarily and directly from the benign tumor tissue. With increasing anaplasia, the tumor heterogeneity increases (cysts, necrosis, hemorrhages occur), perifocal edema becomes more severe, the brain dislocation worsen, and expressed contrast enhancement is observed (Fig. 29.3).

Thus, the main issue of the differential diagnosis of metastases with primary brain tumors occurs in the presence of intense contrast enhancement of the latter and formation of the demarcated contour. Diffuse forms of intracerebral tumors or heterogeneously contrast enhanced, with formation of "islands" of CA accumulation, usually do not cause any differential issues. The full range of MR sequences described above should be used for the differential diagnosis.

DWI MRI allows to suggest the intracerebral nature of the tumor based on slightly higher ADC values. A large dispersion of ADC values in our cases allows only to suggest the secondary nature of neoplasms. However, it should be remembered that patients with large space-occupying lesions may have been receiving hormones for some time to reduce the edema, which affects these parameters.

CT or MR perfusion, including non-contrasted options, definitely does not allow to perform the differential diagnosis due to heterogeneous manifestations of both primary and secondary tumors, especially in patients with a newly diagnosed brain lesion. In cases of metastases of ovarian, pancreatic, or parotid gland cancer, the secondary origin of tumors in the brain can be assumed by a slight increase in the perfusion values.

MR spectroscopy allows to suggest the primary origin of tumors in the brain by intact peaks from the brain matter (Cr, NAA). It is important to consider the choice of the area of voxel application in this study in order to avoid capturing the brain tissue surrounding the tumor lesion into the region of interest.

SWI (SWAN) MRI works well in practice, but only in cases of anaplastic variants of intracerebral tumors (anaplastic astrocytoma, glioblastoma), where a large number of modified vessels and microhemorrhages are identified. Metastases, except for those of melanoma and colon cancer, contain much less hypointense inclusions.

M. Dolgushin et al., *Brain Metastases*, DOI 10.1007/978-3-319-57760-9_29

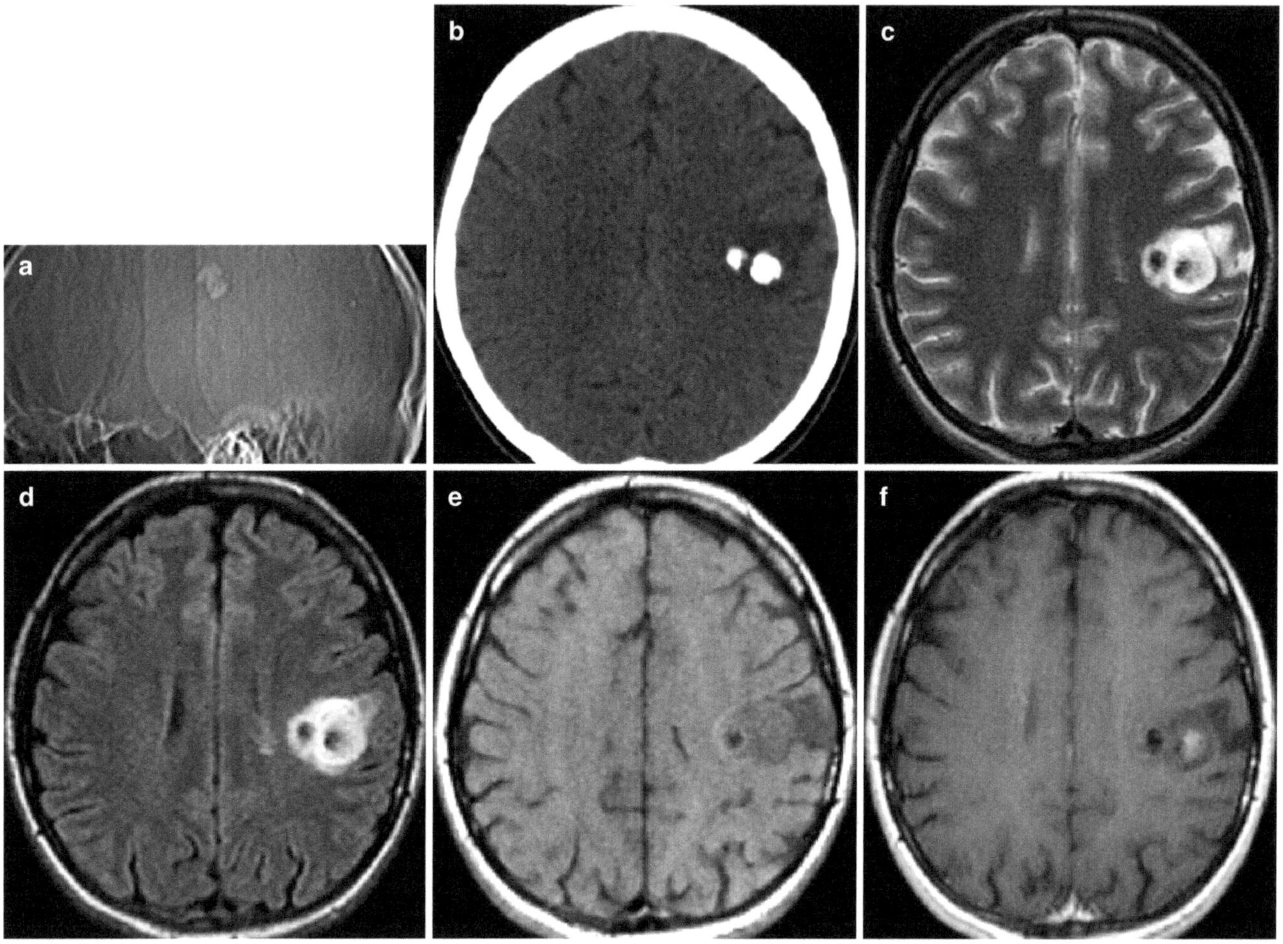

Fig. 29.1 Oligodendroglioma. In the left postfrontal area, on the lateral radiograph (**a**) and CT in the axial projection (**b**), two adjacent calcifications are visualized. On CT, there is additionally an area with decreased brain tissue density, surrounding calcifications. In a series of T2-weighted (**c**), T2-FLAIR (**d**), T1-weighted MRI before (**e**) and after intravenous contrast enhancement (**f**), a space-occupying lesion is determined, having mostly an increased MR signal (T2-weighted, T2-FLAIR MRI) with portions of the reduced signal (calcifications) and a local area of abnormal CA accumulation

Oligodendroglial tumors should be discussed separately; they can be characterized by insignificant accumulation of the contrast agent, even their anaplastic variants. Calcified inclusions may distort the picture on MR spectroscopy, SWI (SWAN), or ASL MRI. They are also characterized by a heterogeneous picture on CT perfusion imaging. However, they rarely manifest by total contrast enhancement on MRI. The presence of portions not accumulating the contrast agent allows to rule out metastases.

The use of PET with ^{18}F-FDG for the differentiation of malignant intracranial tumors and metastases does not make sense, although in some cases, according to our observations, glioblastoma do not accumulate ^{18}F-FDG, with intense accumulation of ^{18}F-Tyrosine and ^{18}F-Choline. Metastases, in turn, can blend with physiological ^{18}F-FDG accumulation in the brain tissue, which is particularly characteristic for a small solid part (cystic variants).

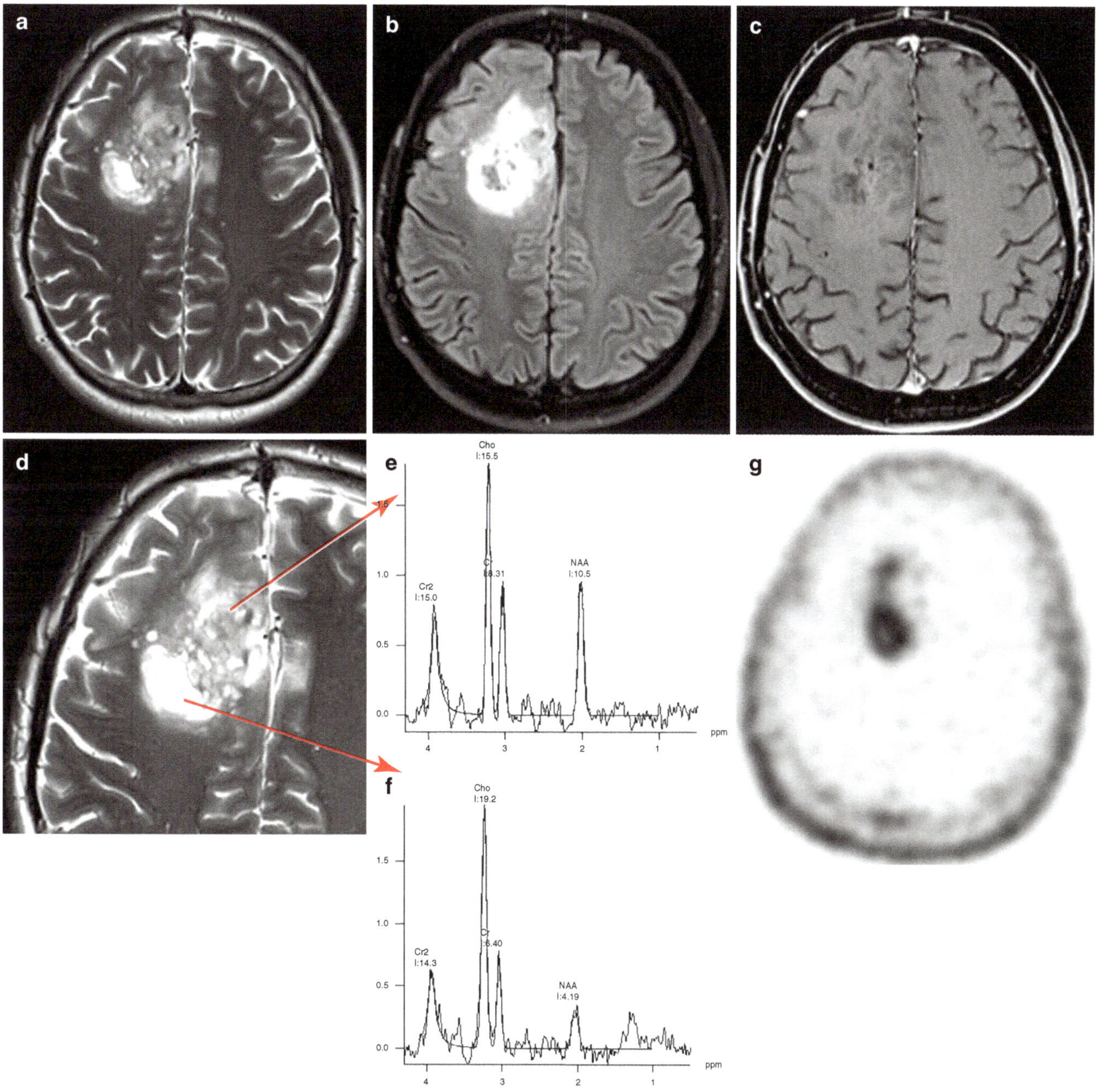

Fig. 29.2 Oligodendroglioma. In the right frontal region in T2-weighted (**a**, **d**) and T2-FLAIR MRI (**b**) images, there is a large space-occupying lesion with a heterogeneously high signal. After CA administration, on T1-weighted (**c**), there are no signs of its accumulation in the tumor. On the spectra from the anterior (**e**) and posterior poles (**f**) of the tumor, benign and malignant characteristics are observed, respectively (appearance of the Lip-Lac complex peak and a pronounced increase in the Cho peak). On PET with ^{18}F-tyrosine, tumor fragments are well differentiated with different RP accumulation, corresponding to various malignancy grades (**g**)

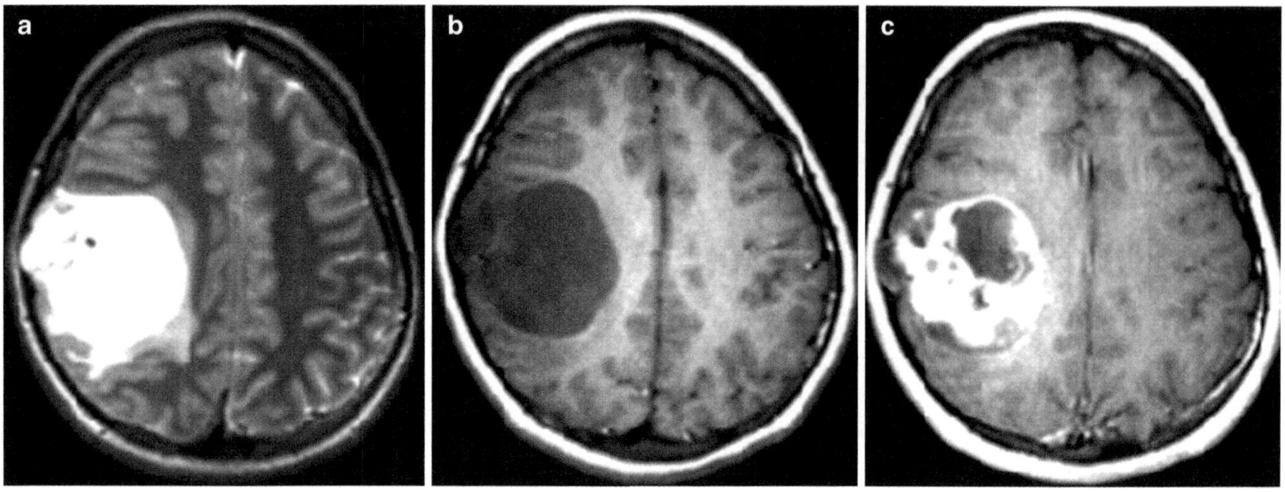

Fig. 29.3 Oligodendroglioma. In the right frontoparietal region on T2-weighted (**a**) and T1-weighted MRI before (**b**) and after (**c**) contrast enhancement, a well-demarcated, large tumor is observed with pronounced contrast enhancement. The central departments of the tumor are presented by a cyst. Perifocal edema is minimal

30 CNS Lymphoma

Primary lymphomas (PCNSL). Until recently, primary lymphoma of the central nervous system has been quite a rare disease and accounted for about 1% of all brain tumors. Among other diseases, in which the risk of primary CNS lymphoma increases, are systemic collagenoses (systemic lupus erythematosus, rheumatoid arthritis, etc.) and chronic viral infections, in particular, Epstein-Barr virus infection. By their histological structure, PCNSLs are virtually always represented by a non-Hodgkin's type and are mostly B-cell lymphomas (Bergmann and Edel 1991). Primary T-cell CNS lymphomas are also described but are rare. By their location, 90% of all lymphomas are supratentorial. Majority of all cases (73%) are presented with a solitary lesion; in other cases multiple brain lesions are determined. Leptomeningeal or dural distribution typically occurs in systemic lymphoma.

In order to verify the histological diagnosis and for subsequent chemotherapy and radiation therapy for suspected brain lymphoma, a stereotactic biopsy (STB) is advisable. Therefore, establishing the diagnosis of primary lymphoma at the preoperative stage is an extremely important task, which would significantly reduce the percentage of unjustified surgical interventions.

Tumor lesions look like quite clearly demarcated, space-occupying lesions with various sizes, often rounded, with clear contours, so they may mimic metastases or glioblastoma. At the same time, a solid, compact tumor structure is observed in some patients and the presence in the stroma of necrotic areas with different sizes in others (a smaller proportion). The latter is considered a typical manifestation of lymphomas in HIV-infected patients.

According to CT, the tumor in most cases has an increased density. An isodense tumor is diagnosed in only 20% of cases. A necrotic area in the center of the tumor has lower density relative to the stroma. Intense accumulation of the contrast medium in the stroma of lymphoma after intravenous injection is the characteristic CT manifestation of the tumor and occurs almost always. Edema of the surrounding brain substance, with varying severity, is identified as an area with decreased density around a hyperdense tumor lesion (Fig. 30.1).

The lymphoma stroma on standard MRI sequences has an isointense or slightly hypointense MR signal relative to the unaffected gray matter. In the presence of a necrotic decay cavity in the tumor (usually in the central sections of the tumor), this area is characterized by a high and low signal in T2-weighted and T1-weighted images, respectively. Perifocal edema with a high signal on T2-weighted MRI and a low signal on T1-weighted MRI was noted in 30–40% of cases. With intravenous administration of the contrast medium, intense homogeneous opacification of the tumor stroma is observed, in the absence of accumulation in the necrotic area (if any)—ring-shaped contrast enhancement (Figs. 30.2, 30.3, and 30.4).

Many authors reported both the absence and the presence of mild peritumoral edema in lymphomas (in our study, only 32% of lymphomas were accompanied by a perifocal edema). However, as is known, the use of hormones reduces the severity of cerebral edema. Furthermore, the use of steroids results in a significant reduction and even complete disappearance of lymphoma nodules, which is certainly not observed in metastases.

On diffusion-weighted MR images, lymphomas are characterized by a high signal and the values of the apparent diffusion coefficient (ADC) close to those of the normal gray matter or have slightly increased ADC. The analysis of DW MRI yielded the following findings (Table 30.1).

M. Dolgushin et al., *Brain Metastases*, DOI 10.1007/978-3-319-57760-9_30

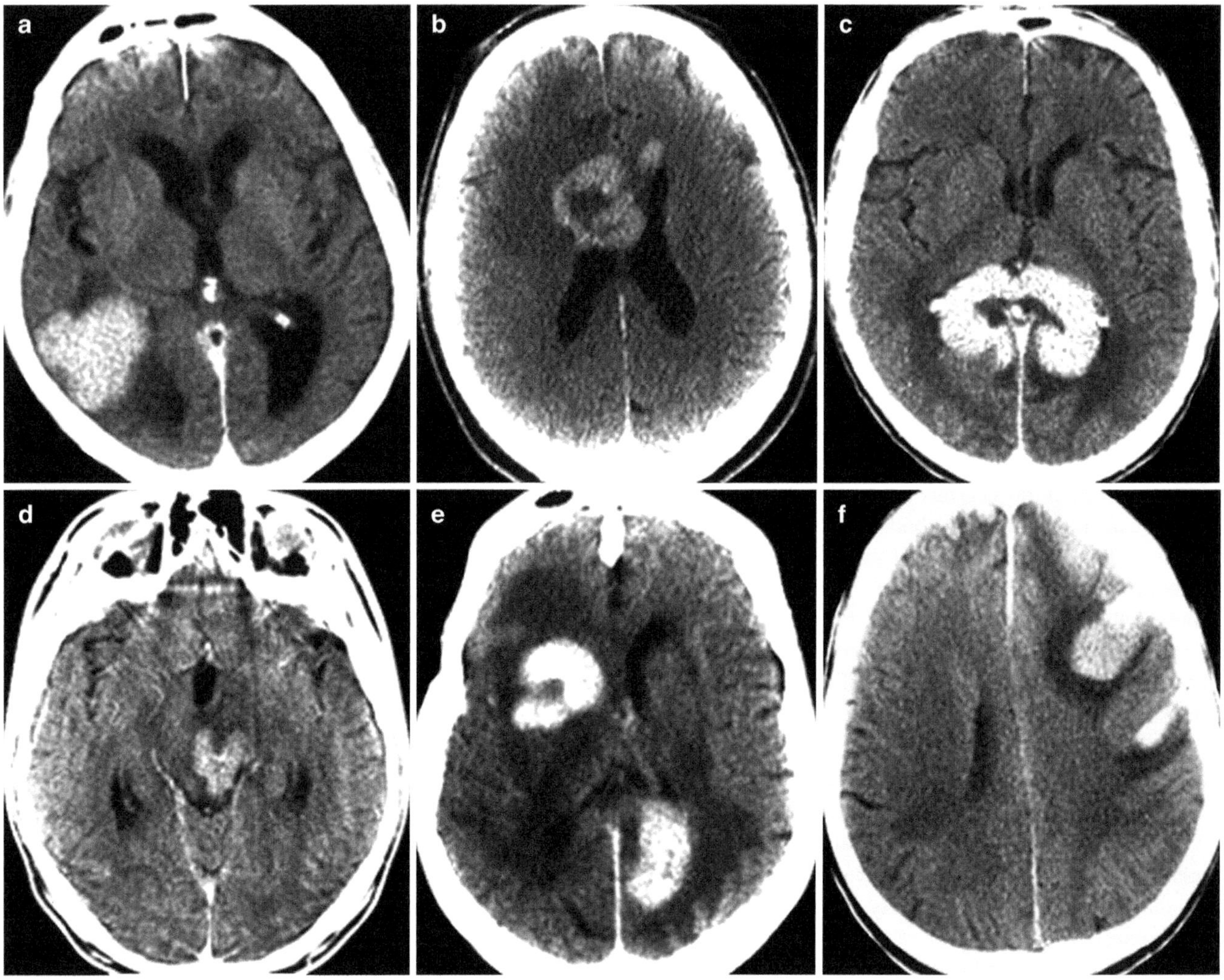

Fig. 30.1 Lymphoma. CT variants of lymphomas with different structure and location: (**a**) solid tumor in the right temporoparietal convexital area; (**b**) mixed lymphoma with central necrosis of the genus of corpus callosum; (**c**) solid tumor of the splenium of the corpus callosum; (**d**) nodular solid tumor of the midbrain; (**e**) mixed, multiple lymphoma; (**f**) multiple, convexital tumor with a hemorrhage

Proton MR spectroscopy (PMRS) determines in lymphomas a spectrum similar to that in malignant glial tumors. However, both metastases and lymphoma spectra show a significant increase in the lipid-lactate complex (which is also found in glioblastomas and, to a lesser extent, in anaplastic astrocytomas), but the reduction of the *N*-acetylaspartate peak is not sharply pronounced. Thus, the signs of spectra of brain lymphoma are the following: a moderate decrease in the NAA peak on the background of increased Cho peaks and Lac (+Lip) and a low mI peak. The analysis of results of our spectroscopic studies allowed us to determine the mean values of the metabolite ratio in the spectrum, characteristic of brain lymphoma (Table 30.2). The Lip-Lac complex usually prevails in strongly pronounced central necrosis, which does not allow to perform differentiation with a metastasis.

While MR spectroscopy parameters overlap to some extent with signs occurring in metastases, MR/CT perfusion studies show higher specificity of lymphomas. As it turned out in studies conducted by many authors, numerical values determined in the stroma of lymphomas were characterized by lower perfusion rates, not similar to those of metastases with an identical degree of contrast enhancement on contras-enhanced MR images. Table 30.3 presents mean values of perfusion parameters in the stroma of lymphomas.

Mortality after removal of lymphomas is higher than in surgery of all intracerebral tumors. The frequency of complications in stereotactic biopsy of lymphomas for the purpose of verification of the diagnosis appears to be also higher (up to 50%). Basically, this is hemorrhagic impregnation of the tumor stroma. In these circumstances, it becomes extremely important to diagnose CNS lymphomas using noninvasive methods, such as contrast-enhanced MRI and CT perfusion, capable to suggest the presence of lymphoma with a high degree of probability and allowing to avoid surgery.

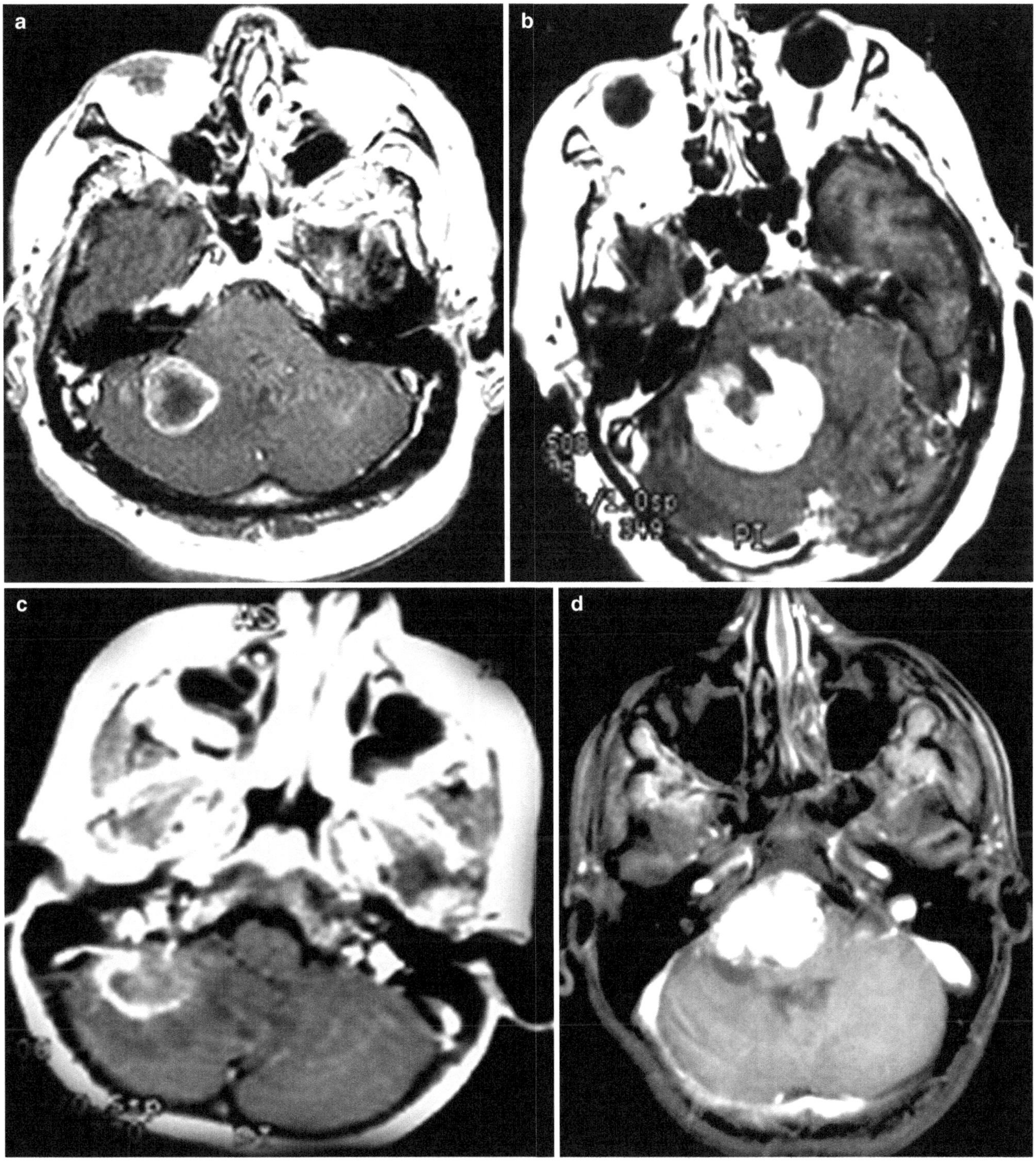

Fig. 30.2 Space-occupying lesions of the cerebellopontine angle. T1-weighted MRI with contrast enhancement. The differential diagnosis of a variety of lesions characterized by intense accumulation of the contrast agent and dislocation of the brainstem structures: lung cancer metastasis (**a**), lymphoma (**b**), ependymoma (**c**), hemangioblastoma (**d**)

Using PET with ^{18}F-FDG allows to quite accurately suggest CNS lymphoma, as it is characterized by high SUV values (up to 20 units), which may occur as well only in melanoma metastases and less likely in renal cell carcinoma metastases (Fig. 30.5).

High sensitivity of PET with ^{18}F-FDG to changes in the metabolic activity of lymphomas on the background of hormonal therapy or chemotherapy should also be noted, which is manifested in the reduction of SUV values immediately after the initiation of the treatment.

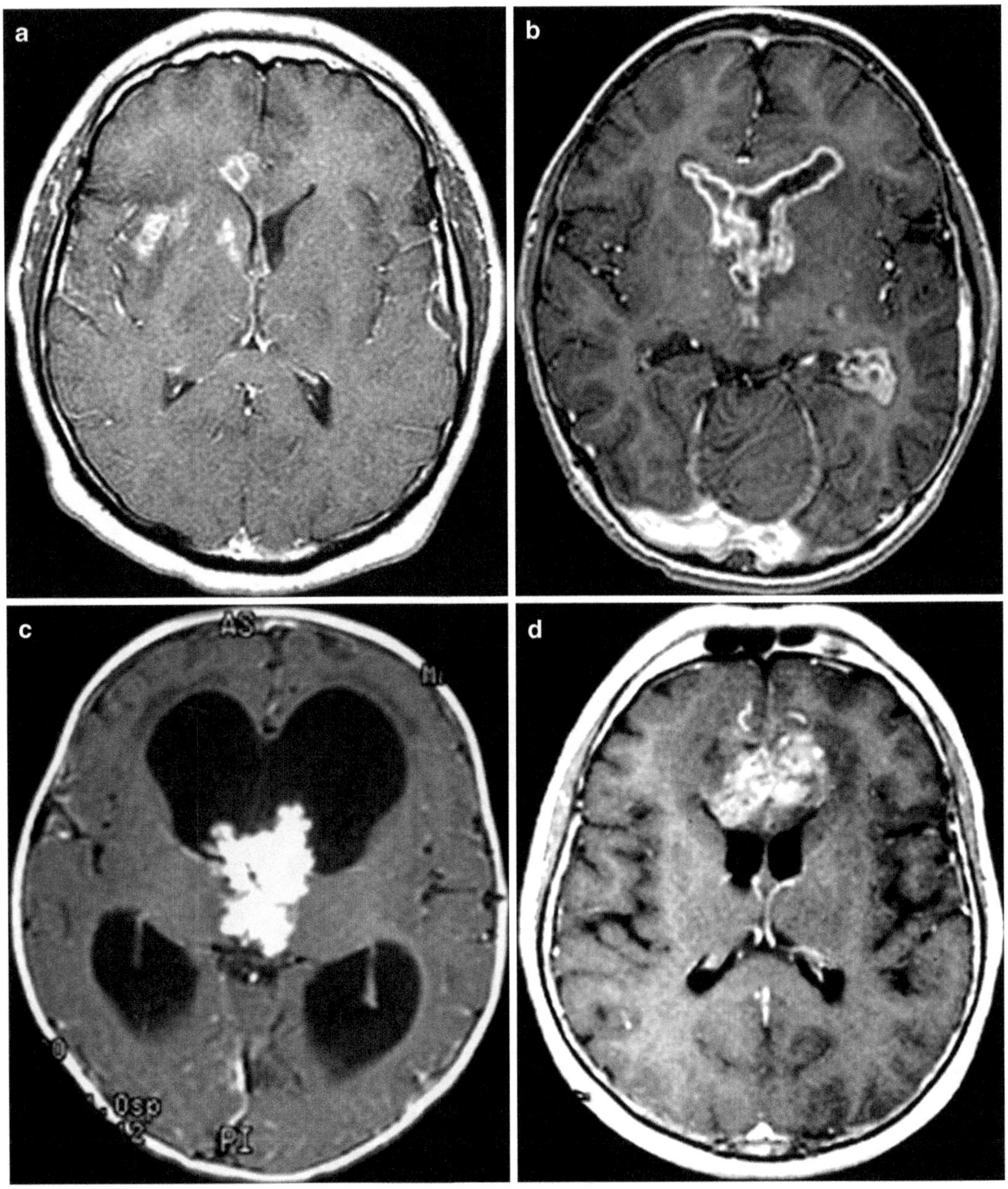

Fig. 30.3 T1-weighted MRI with contrast enhancement. Differential diagnosis. Different brain lesions characterized by intense accumulation of the contrast agent, extending to the ependyma of the lateral ventricles: glioblastoma (**a**), ependymoma (**b**), choroid plexus papilloma (**c**), lymphoma (**d**)

These positive changes with time on MRI, CT, and PET during the treatment are a convincing argument in favor of lymphoma.

Recently, conservative methods of treatment of lymphomas have been increasingly used—chemotherapy with or without boost irradiation, achieving a stable remission and regression of the tumor in many cases, even if it was initially large. However, there are structurally rare CNS lymphomas characterized by rapid growth and resistance to currently used standard regimens of chemotherapy and radiotherapy.

Thus, by their manifestations, lymphomas often mimic intracerebral tumors, especially when localized in the corpus callosum and subcortical nuclei. Lymphomas can be differentiated from metastases by low CBF values and a high signal on DWI images (b = 1000). Lymphomas are characterized by a pronounced accumulation of ^{18}F-FDG in a PET study, significantly greater than the physiological accumulation parameters. In this case, it is important to know whether the patient receives hormones at the time of the PET study, as lymphoma pretty quickly reacts to such treatment, and the picture may be distorted, showing low accumulation of radiopharmaceuticals.

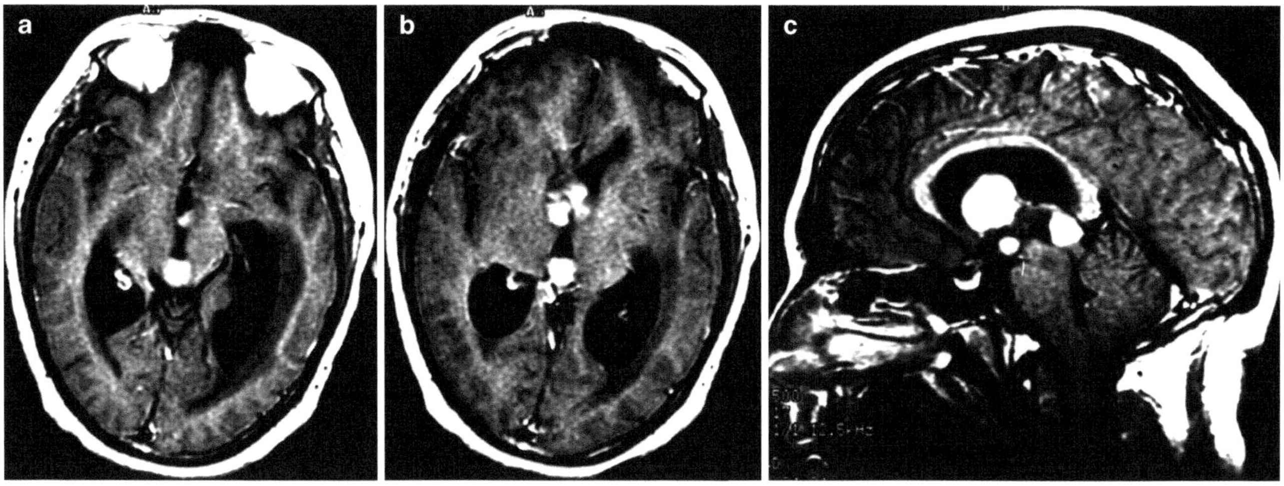

Fig. 30.4 Multiple lymphomas. On T1-weighted MRI after contrast enhancement, in the axial (**a**, **b**) and sagittal (**c**) projections, multiple tumor lesions are identified in the third ventricle of the brain, in the projection of foramina of Monro and mammillary bodies

Table 30.1 Mean ADC for brain lymphomas

Factor *b*	Tumor stroma	Necrosis area	Edema area	Intact white matter
b = 500	0.95 ± 0.23	1.81 ± 0.31	2.04 ± 0.19	0.83 ± 0.04
b = 1000	0.83 ± 0.20	1.73 ± 0.28	1.87 ± 0.11	0.78 ± 0.02

Table 30.2 The mean values of the ratio of major metabolites to the reference value of the creatine peak in the stroma of lymphomas

Ratios	NAA/Cr	Cho/Cr	mI/Cr	Lac/Cr	NAA/Cho
Mean, SD	1.75 ± 0.28	1.60 ± 0.20	0.72 ± 0.16	1.95 ± 0.77	1.09 ± 0.11

Table 30.3 Average values of major CT perfusion parameters in the stroma of lymphomas

Perfusion parameters	CBV (ml/100 g)	CBF (ml/100 g/min) g/min)	MTT (s)
Lymphoma	2.93 ± 0.91	16.38 ± 3.87	6.06 ± 3.70
Intact white matter	2.0 ± 1.1	25 ± 11.3	5 ± 2.1

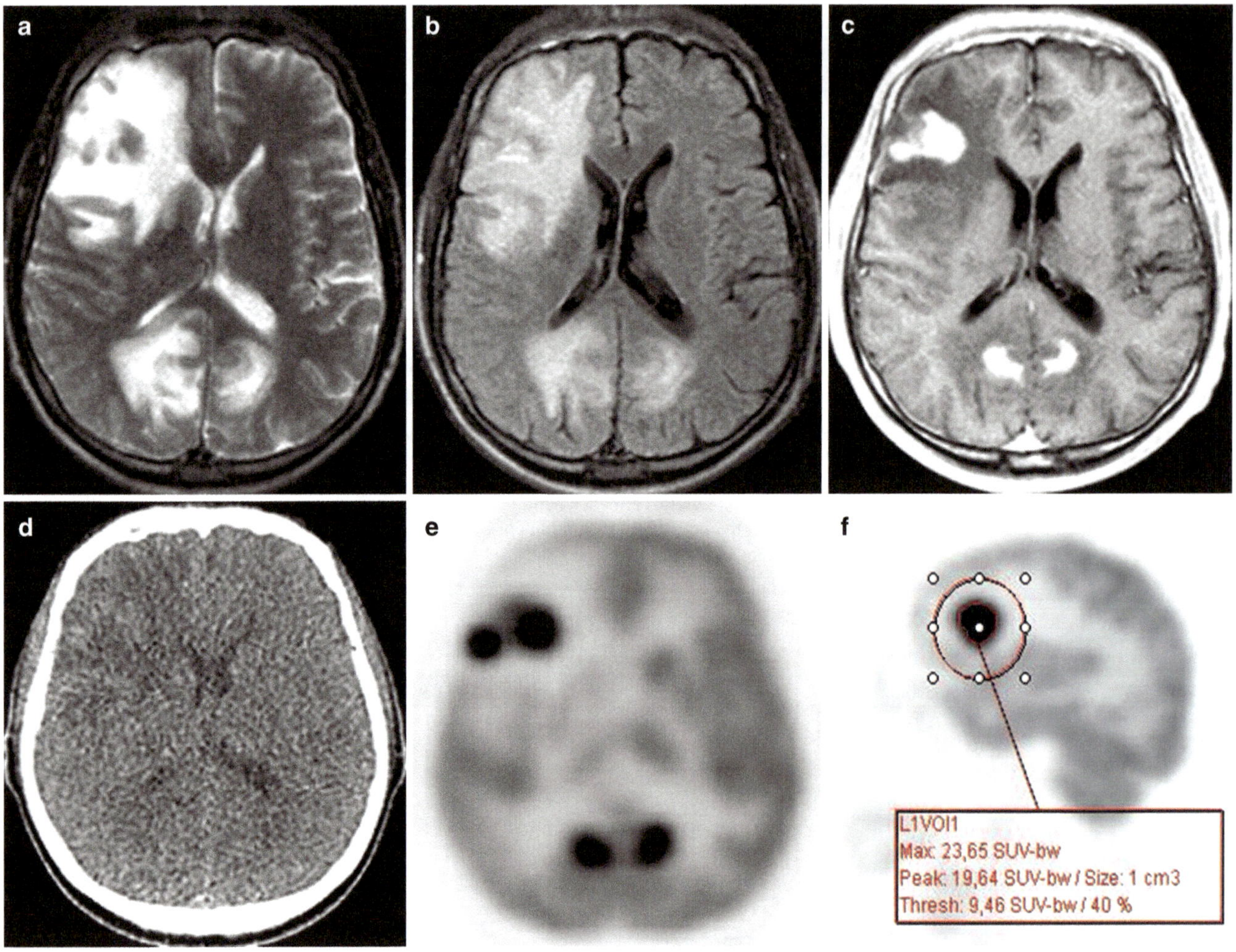

Fig. 30.5 Lymphoma. In the right frontal and parietal areas, there are multiple lesions with a heterogeneously high signal on T2-weighted (**a**) and T2-FLAIR (**b**) MRI, rapidly accumulating the contrast agent (**c**). On CT, the lesions cannot be differentiated; only the edema area is visualized in the right frontal region. There is a typical increase in ^{18}FFDG (**e**, **f**) accumulation in the lymphoma foci with high SUV values (more than 10.0)

Meningioma

31

Meningioma is the most common intracranial tumor among neoplasms of non-glial origin (Buetow et al. 1991; Osborn 2004). Benign forms of meningiomas are histologically characterized by a uniform arrangement of cells with moderate polymorphism of nuclei, lack of necrosis and mitoses. In this group, there are the following meningiomas: fibroblastic, meningotheliomatous, secretory, transitional, psammomatous and other meningiomas. Atypical (usually meningotheliomatous and mixed) meningiomas are characterized by pronounced polymorphism of cells and nuclei, presence of necrosis and mitotic figures, which results in the characteristic radiographic manifestations similar to those in metastases.

Meningiomas occur most frequently in the falx cerebelli and parasagittal area (up to 50%) and in the ACF base region (up to 10% of all intracranial meningiomas). The neoplasm grows from the dura mater covering the intracranial surface of the skull or dural sleeves extending to some cranial nerves. Classic bone hyperostosis is detected in about 5% of cases, however, the majority of patients are examined by MRI, and, therefore, many examinations do not clearly visualize and evaluate hyperostotic bone changes. Bone erosion can occur in all types of meningiomas; they can also cause bone destruction, but still hyperostoses are more frequently observed.

By their appearance, meningiomas are subdivided into two main forms. The first group includes tumors with a spherical, lobular shape. The second group is characterized by a flat form infiltrating the adjacent meninges and often the bone (Fig. 31.1).

Meningiomas are usually well separated from the adjacent brain substance. The surface of most tumors is smooth or lobular. There is often a pronounced arachnoid (CSF) cleft containing dislocated vessels and elements of the dura mater between the brain substance and the surface of the meningioma.

CT with contrast enhancement is one of the main methods of primary visualization for meningiomas, allowing to diagnose at least 95% of intracranial neoplasms (Konovalov and Kornienko 1985a, b). Meningiomas are most often identified as lesions with well-differentiated contours due to intense (40–45 HU) contrast agent accumulation. Therefore, the use of contrast enhancement is one of the principal constituent elements of CT diagnosis of meningiomas. In a quarter of cases, meningiomas weakly accumulate the contrast material. In general, in up to 75% of all cases, meningiomas have more or less hyperdense characteristics. Up to 25% of meningiomas contain calcifications in their structure, which can be individual or multiple, punctate and very large. 3D CT reconstructions are useful in hyperostotic meningiomas to estimate the extent of bone destruction (Fig. 31.2).

On perfusion-weighted CT images, meningiomas are divided into three main types based on their hemodynamic manifestations that correlate well with the results of direct cerebral angiography. We distinguished the following hemodynamic types of tumors:

Type 1—low CBV (2.5–5.0 ml/100 g) and CBF (25–30 ml/100 g/min) values with or without tumor vasculature minimally visualized on AG;

Type 2—a moderate increase in CBV, CBF (10–11 ml/100 g and 70–80 ml/100 g/min, respectively) with a moderately expressed vascular spot in the capillary phase of AG;

Type 3—a pronounced increase in meningioma hemodynamics (CBV—21–24 ml/100 g, CBF—110–125 ml/100 g/min) in the presence of a highly vascularized tumor on angiograms (Fig. 31.3).

The nature of MR signal changes in different histological forms of meningiomas is ambiguous. On T1-weighted MRI, most meningiomas, regardless of their histological type, appear as iso- or hypointense space-occupying lesions as compared to the cerebral cortex. Changes in MR signal on T2-weighted MRI can correlate with histologic subtypes of meningiomas. Thus, up to 90% of fibroblastic and transient subtypes, as well as psammomatous meningiomas have

M. Dolgushin et al., *Brain Metastases*, DOI 10.1007/978-3-319-57760-9_31

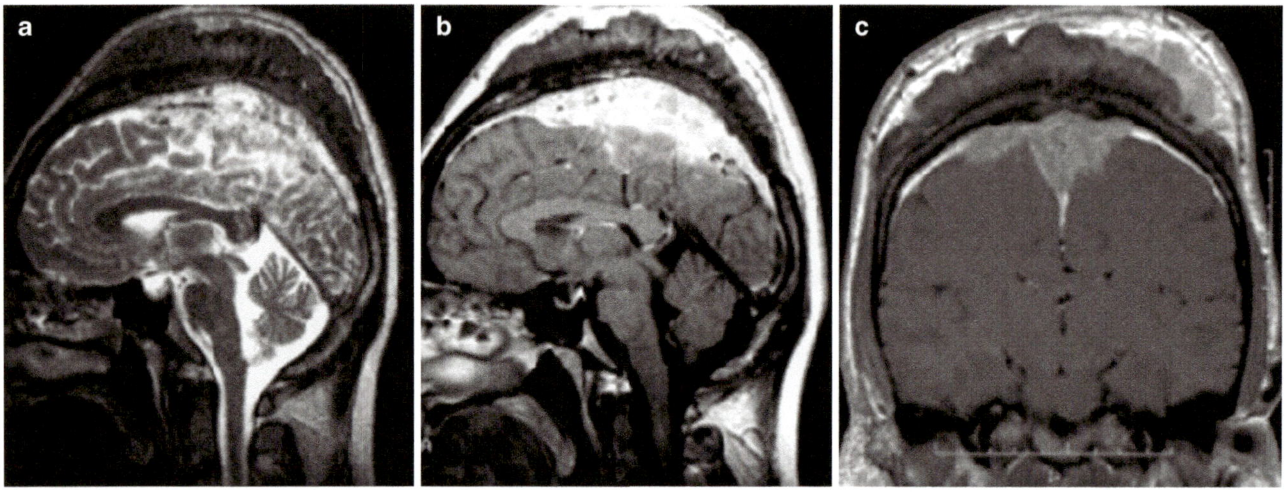

Fig. 31.1 Meningioma. In the fronto-parietal convexital area on T2-weighted (**a**) and T1-weighted MRI after intravenous CA administration (**b**, **c**), a flat space-occupying lesion is detected, intensely accumulating the contrast agent, infiltrating the adjacent bone, meninges and soft tissues of the fronto-parietal region. The tumor that has V-type spread along the falx completely invades the superior sagittal sinus

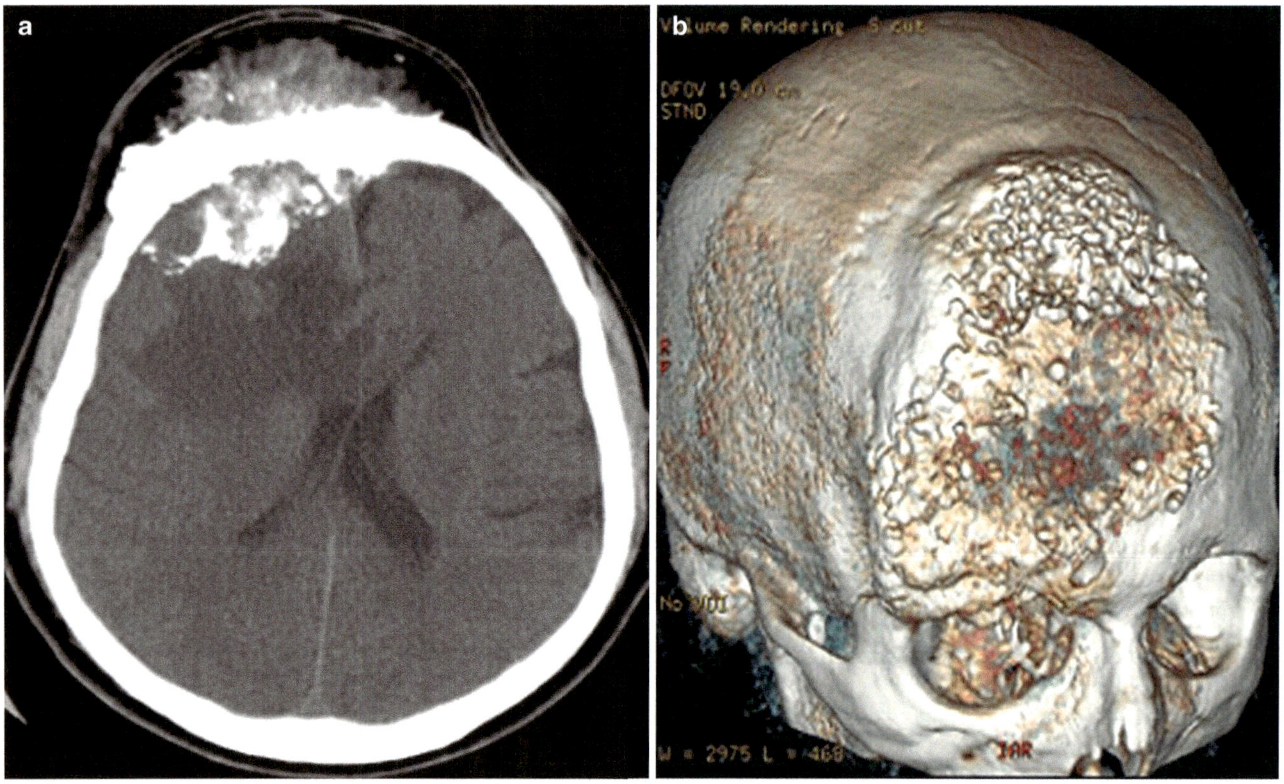

Fig. 31.2 Meningioma. On CT, in the area of the squama of the frontal bone (more on the right), there is a large lesion with hyperostotic inclusions. In the axial projection (**a**), there are tumor structures with increased density, extending both intra- and extracranially. On 3D-reconstruction (**b**) the extent of destruction of the bone tissue can be clearly determined

lower signal intensity in T1- and T2-weighted images as compared to the white matter of the brain, while two thirds of meningotheliomatous tumors are hyperintense in T2-weighted images.

Typical for olfactory fossa meningioma is the presence of a vascular tumor matrix that contains blood vessels running radially from the site of the primary meningioma growth. Vessels are clearly visualized on sagittal T1-weighted and T2-weighted MRI and can also be seen as hypointense structures with contrast enhancement (Fig. 31.4).

On MRI, most meningiomas intensely accumulate the contrast agent. Accumulation of the contrast material may extend beyond the main tumor nodule with formation of so-called dural "tails" or infiltrative changes in the dura mater on the periphery of the tumor. This symptom occurs in 50% of all cases and only suggests the probable diagnosis of

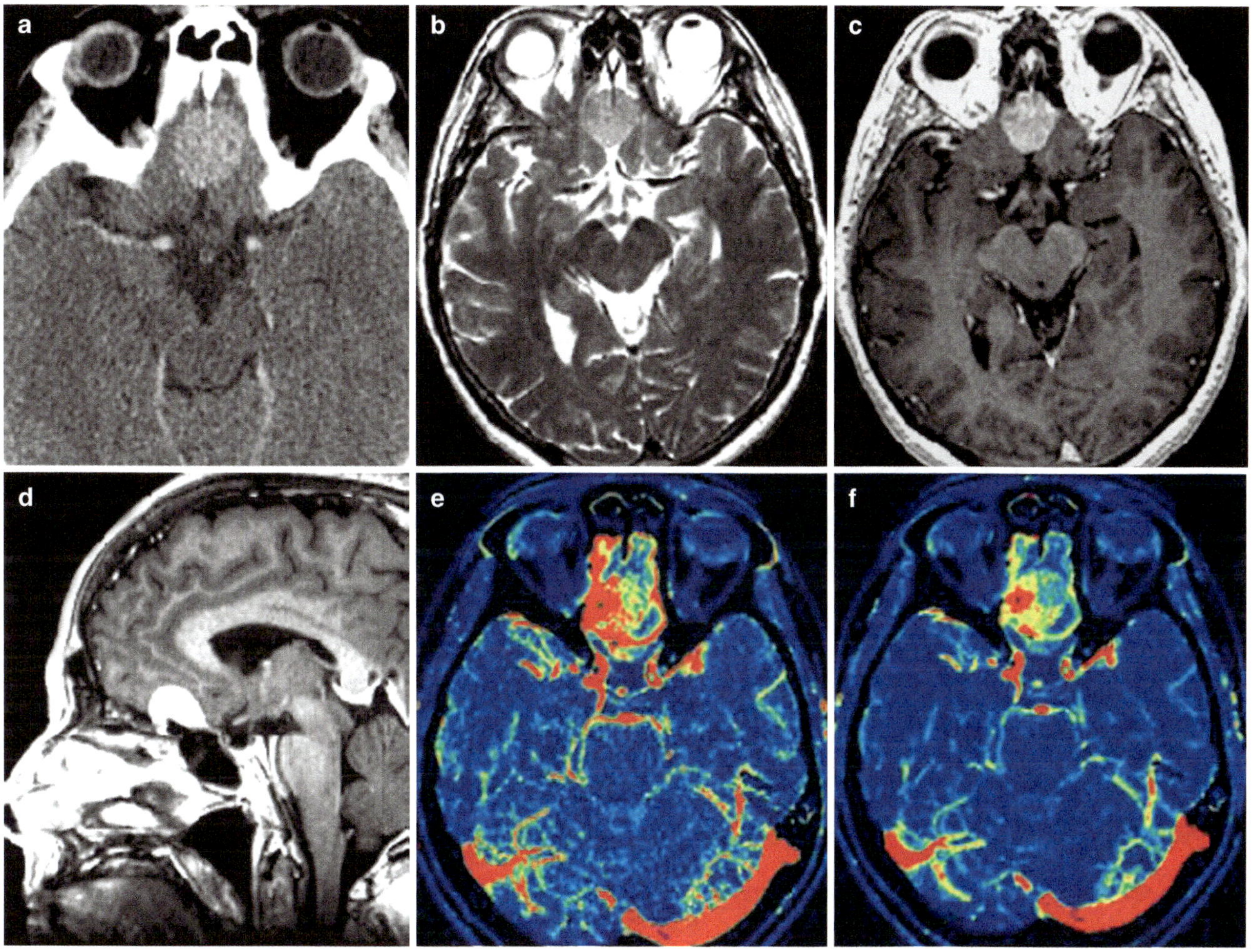

Fig. 31.3 Meningioma. In the projection on the olfactory fossa, on axial CT (**a**) with contrast enhancement, on T2-weighted (**b**) and T1-weighted MRI after CA administration (**c**, **d**), a lenticular tumor lesion is determined with homogeneous contrast accumulation. On CT perfusion of CBF (**e**) and CBV (**f**), there are areas with both high and average blood flow values

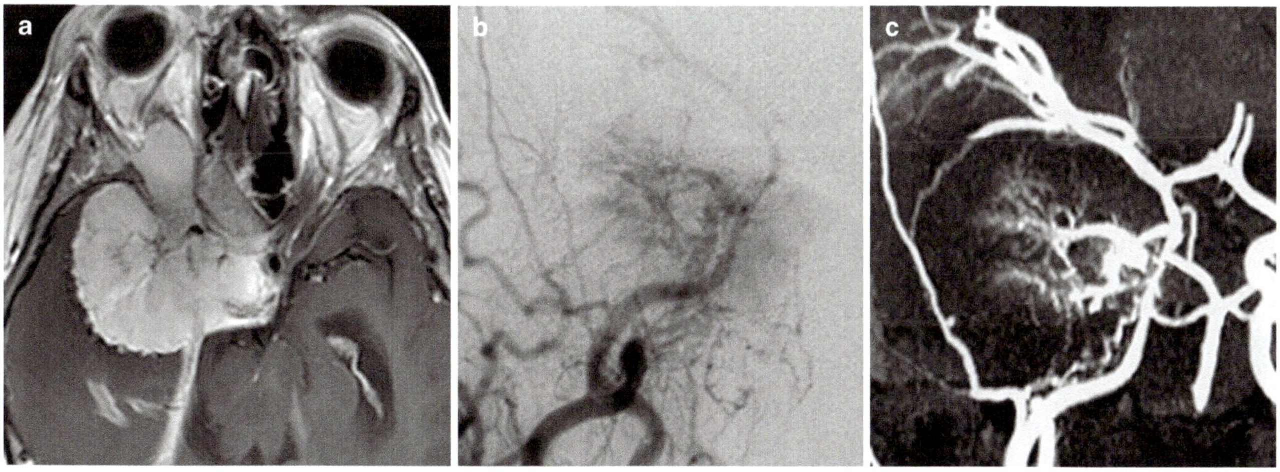

Fig. 31.4 Meningioma. On T1-weighted MRI with contrast-enhanced (**a**), there is a large tumor of the wings of the sphenoid bone on the right with the spread into the orbit on the cavernous sinus, sella cavity and the right temporal area. On direct angiograms (**b**) and MR angiograms (**c**), the tumor vasculature and its main supplying vascular trunk from the maxillary artery are well visualized

meningioma, not being an absolute pathognomonic symptom (Tokumaru et al. 1990). A dural tail can also occur in reactive changes in the meninges of other genesis.

Rarely, meningiomas can acquire unusual multicystic CT or MRI manifestations. Calcifications are determined as areas with low signal intensity on T1- and T2-weighted images. Completely calcified meningiomas occur in 10% of cases, they have a hypointense MR signal on all sequences, being more evident in T2-weighted and T2*-weighted images (Figs. 31.5, 31.6, and 31.7).

A CSF cleft on the surface of the tumor is identified in the majority of cases (up to 70–80%) along the outer contour of the tumor with high signal intensity on T2-weighted MRI and a decreased signal on T1-weighted MRI, with no differ-

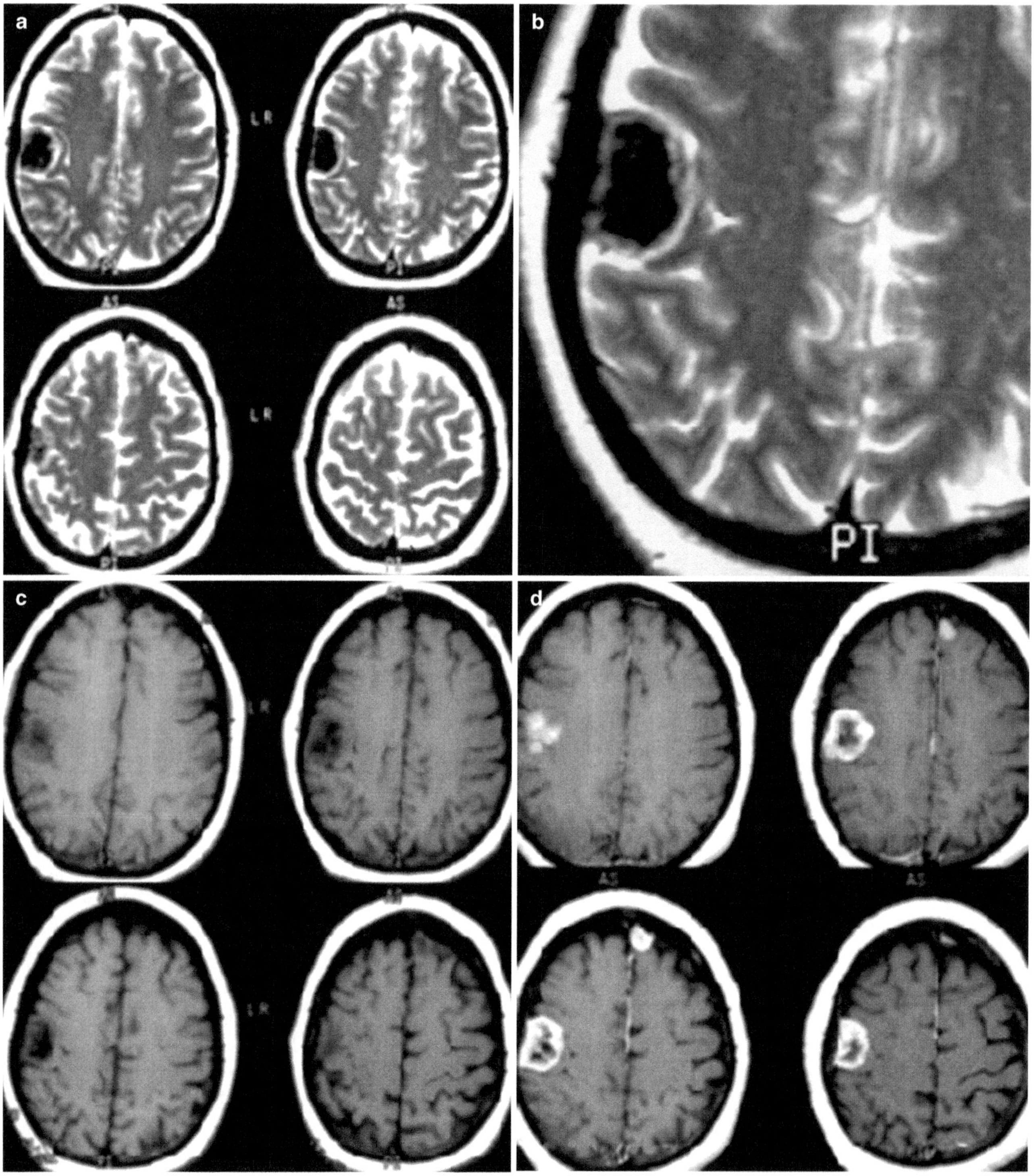

Fig. 31.5 Calcified (psammomatous) meningioma. In the right post-frontal convexital area on T2-weighted (**a, b**) and T1-weighted MRI (**c**), a tumor is identified with a hypointense MR signal in all sequences. Following contrast enhancement (**d**), intense CA accumulation in the tumor tissue located around the calcificate periphery. Additionally, the second, smaller meningioma nodule is clearly visualized in the left frontal parasagittal region. The T2-weighted MR image shows a marked decrease in the signal from the calcified part of meningioma

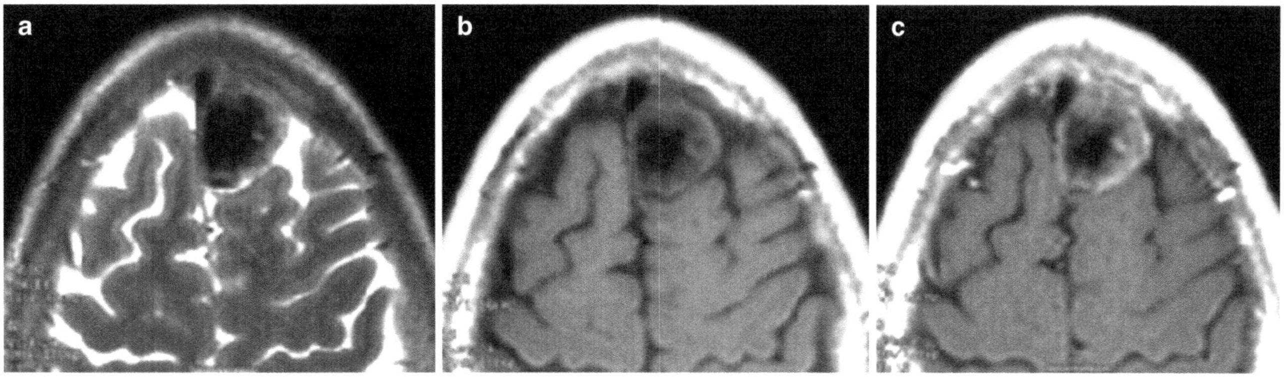

Fig. 31.6 Calcified meningioma. On T2-weighted (**a**) and T1-weighted MRI (**b**) in the left frontal parasagittal region, there is a tumor with a hypointense MR signal in all sequences. With contrast enhancement (**c**), there is CA accumulation in the solid part of the tumor, located on the periphery of the calcificate

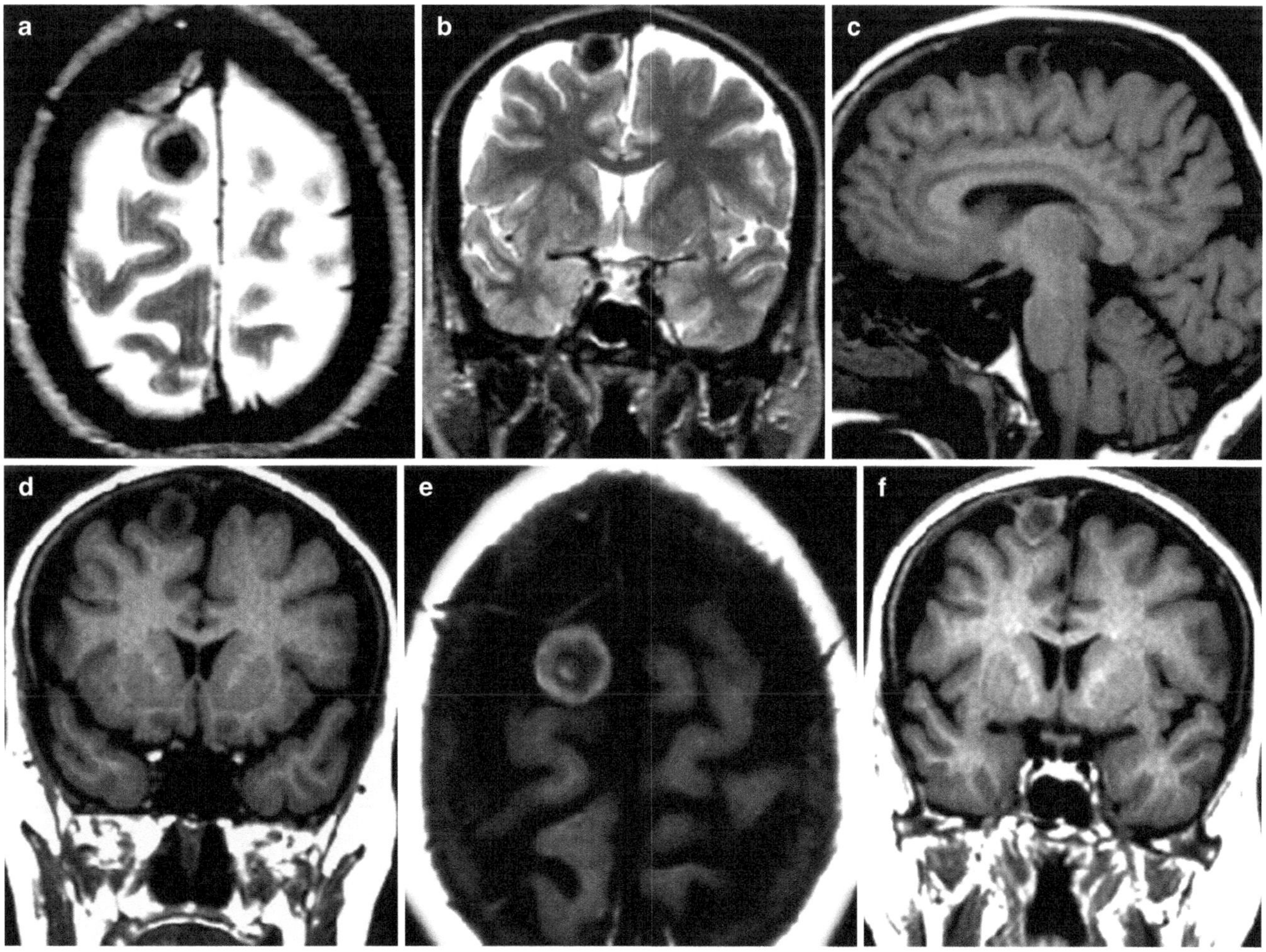

Fig. 31.7 Calcified meningioma. On T2-weighted (**a**, **b**) and T1-weighted MRI before (**c**, **d**) and after (**e**, **f**) intravenous CA administration, a small tumor with a hypointense MR signal (better visualized on T2-weighted MRI) is identified in all sequences in the convexital departments of the right postfrontal area. With contrast enhancement, poor accumulation of contrast agent is observed in the solid part of the tumor, located on the periphery of the calcificate

ences in the signal intensity from CSF clefts located at some distance (Fig. 31.8). A CSF cleft around the tumor can be undetectable in atypical and anaplastic meningiomas. Usually, this is not observed over the entire contour of the tumor, but in separate portion of contact with the brain. It is there, where the perifocal edema is most pronounced. This may indicate (although not in 100% of cases) a high probability of invasive tumor growth.

Metastatic tumors can also grow exophytically and cause infiltration of the dura mater, but the above CSF and vascular formations are never located between the tumor and the brain.

More than half of patients with meningiomas experience a perifocal edema of the brain substance. In cases where meningiomas have isointense characteristics relative to the brain on T2-weighted MRI, they are generally well visualized on the background of the brain edema. Only in rare cases, especially in small meningiomas of the anterior and middle cranial fossae and the falx, the tumor contours can be poorly visualized due to a pronounced perifocal edema. Isointense, small meningiomas can be easily missed in standard MR images. Contrast enhancement is the method of choice in the visualization of meningiomas.

On DWI, meningiomas are distinguished by certain heterogeneity of MR signal changes and ADC with a tendency to the presence of distinctions between benign, atypical and anaplastic forms (ADC values—0.83 ± 0.11; 0.91 ± 0.16 and

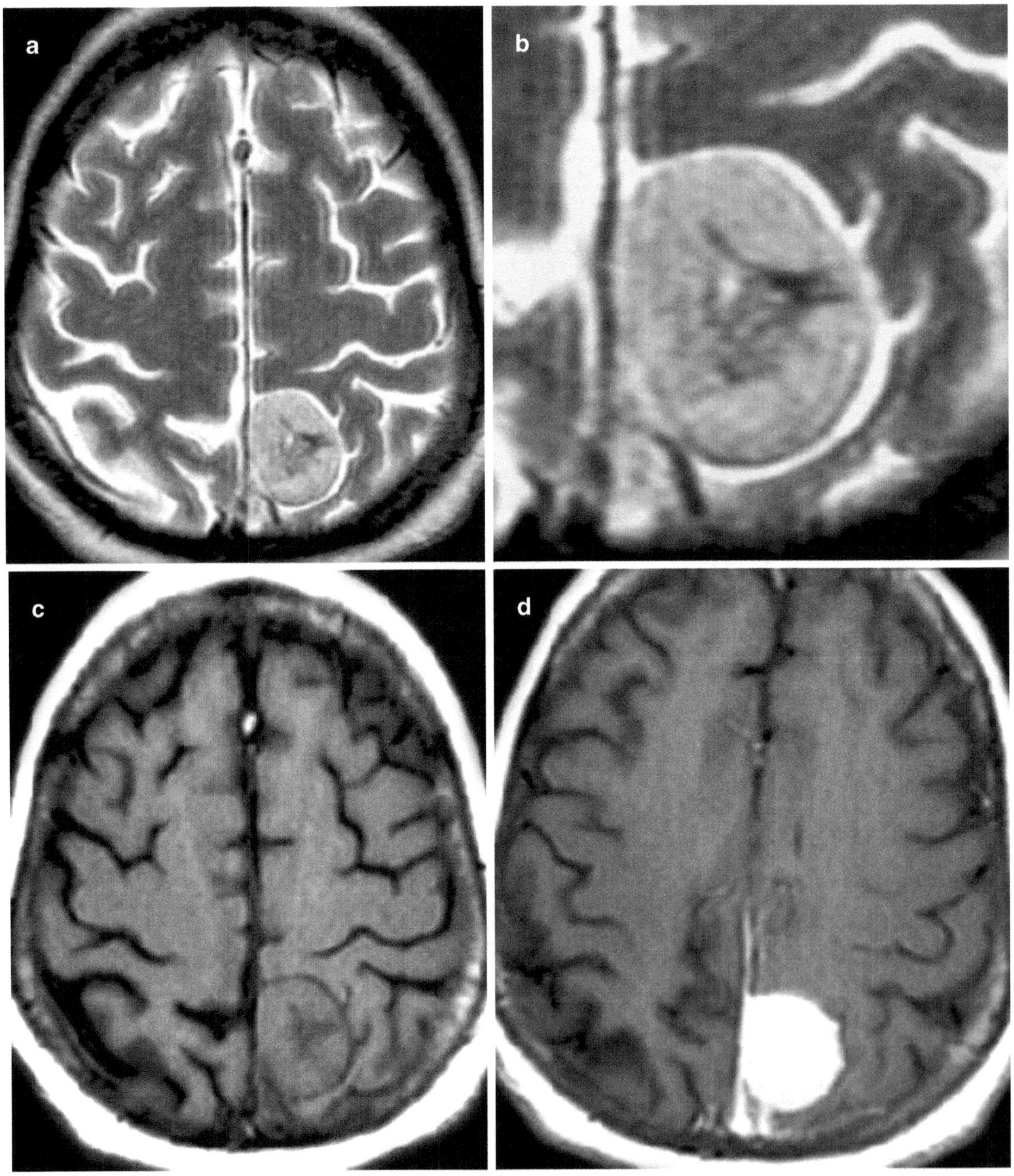

Fig. 31.8 Meningioma. On T2-weighted (**a, b**) and T1-weighted MRI (**c**), in the left parietal-parasagittal region, there is a relatively small lesion adjacent by its medial contour to the falx and partly to the wall of the superior sagittal sinus; a CSF cleft symptom around it (**b**) and contrast enhancement of surrounding falx departments (**d**)—a "tail sign"—are observed

0.97 ± 0.19, respectively). Benign meningiomas have a homogenous, slightly increased or isointense signal relative to the unaffected brain substance on DWI b = 1000 s/mm². While edema surrounding the tumor usually has a higher signal than the tumor on DWI b = 500 c/mm² and becomes invisible on DWI b = 1000 s/mm². On ADC maps, meningiomas visually did not differ from the white matter, but in the presence of a peritumoral edema they clearly stood out on its background. In some cases, ADC maps clearly identified "the CSF cleft symptom" in the form of a thin band with high intensity on the map between the meningioma capsule and the surrounding structures. In the stroma of benign meningiomas, average ADC values were $0.89 \pm 0.13 \times 10^{-3}$ mm²/s.

MR spectroscopic characteristics of supratentorial meningiomas are identical to those for tumors with subratentorial location—there is a flattened and broad Glu-NAA peak and a high choline peak. Meningiomas are characterized by occurrence of an alanine peak (Ala). In combination with this peak, there is a marked increase in the choline peak (Cho), the presence of lactate (Lac) and lipid (Lip) peaks. Lactate and lipid content can have different proportions. A decreased NAA (*N*-acetylaspartate) peak and a high Glx peak (glutamine/glutamate) form a so-called single trapezoid complex. Some researchers have noted a decrease in the creatine peak (Cr) in meningiomas. In general, in comparison with other tumors, meningioma spectrum is distinguished by the combination of high Cho, Glx, Lac + Lip peaks, a low NAA peak and the presence of an Ala peak (1.5 ppm) that is not detected in the spectrum of other neoplastic lesions. In non-neoplastic lesions, the Ala peak occurs, for example, in the spectrum of a bacterial abscess.

Multiple meningiomas (meningotheliomatosis) is a rare phenomenon. They develop in neurofibromatosis type II in children and adolescents in combination with other manifestations of the underlying disease or as an independent condition in adults (Sheehy and Crockard, 1983), accounting for 1–10% of all meningiomas (Figs. 31.9 and 31.10).

Thus, isolated typical meningiomas, due to intense accumulation of the contrast agent, are usually well differentiated

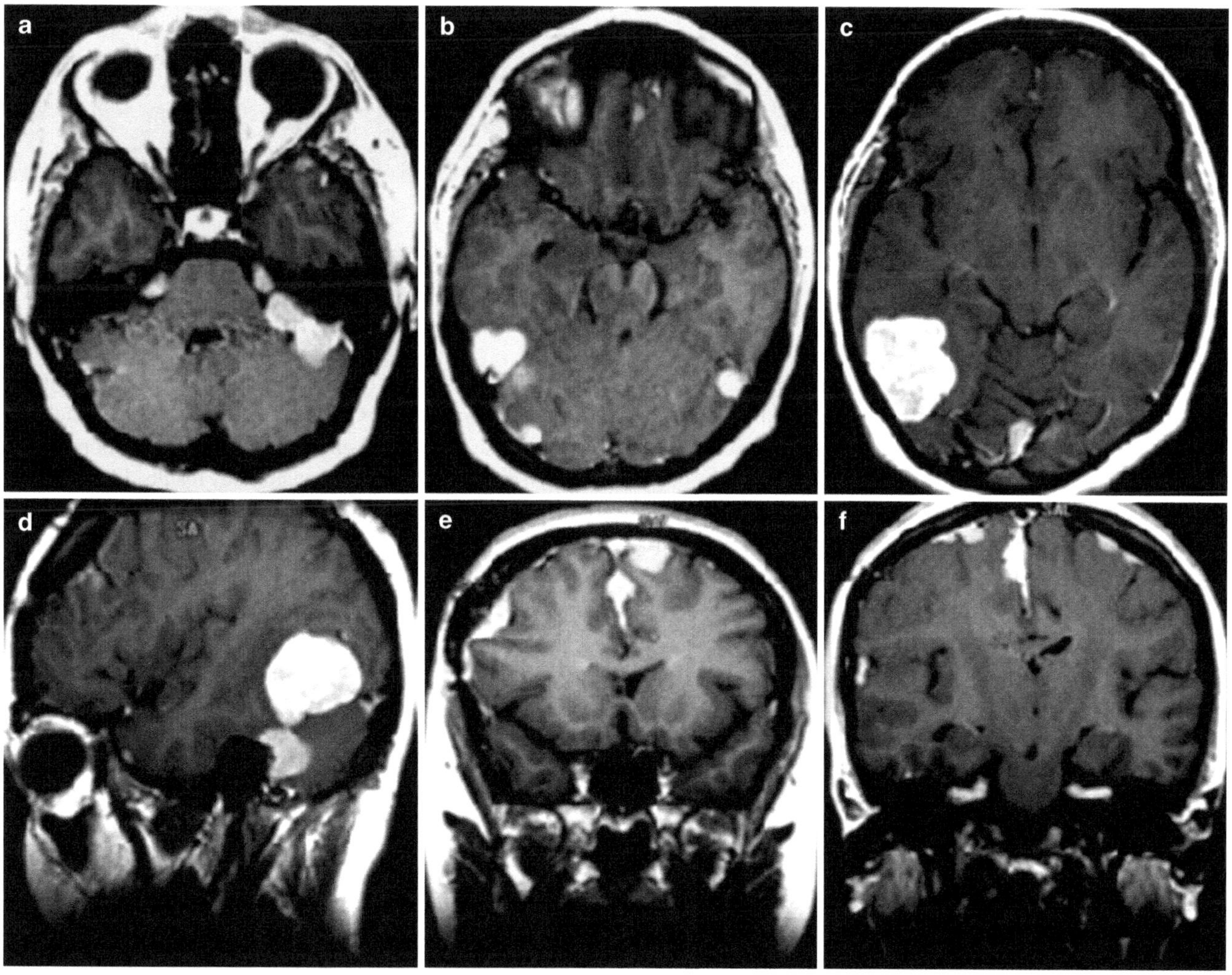

Fig. 31.9 Multiple meningiomas. Neurofibromatosis type II. On a MRI series with contrast enhancement, in the axial (**a–c**), sagittal (**d**) and frontal (**e, f**) projections, multiple sub- and supratentorial tumor nodules are determined with distinct and homogeneous contrast enhancement

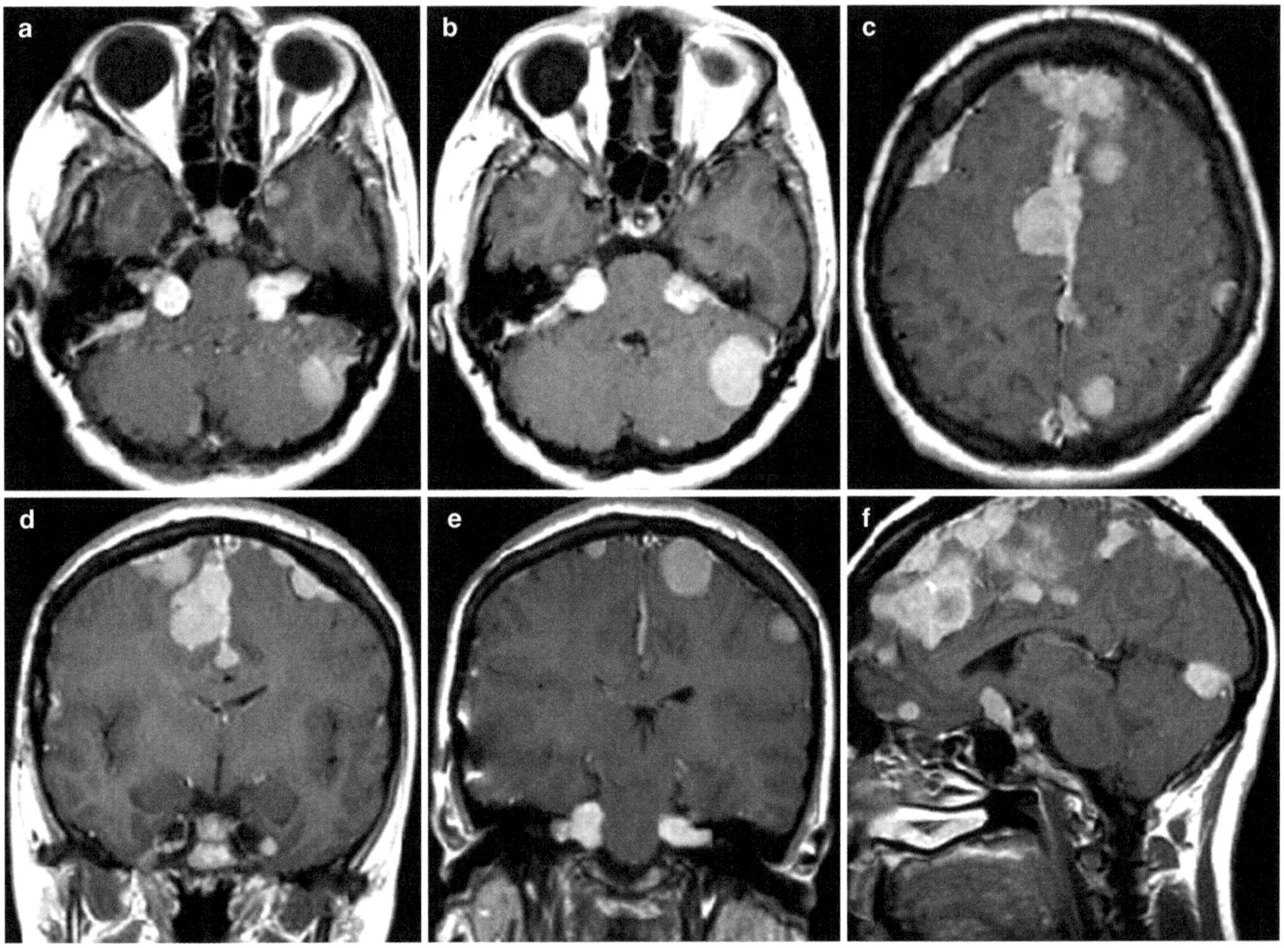

Fig. 31.10 Neurofibromatosis type II. On T1-weighted MRI after administration of the contrast agent, in the axial (**a**–**c**), frontal (**d**, **e**) and sagittal (**f**) projections, there are bilateral vestibular schwannomas and multiple meningiomas of the brain both sub- and supratentorially (mainly parasagittal location)

on the background of the brain, and their diagnosis is rarely difficult. When solitary meningiomas causing perifocal edema are located in the ventricular system or when they have multiple manifestations, diagnostic difficulties occur, especially if the patient has a history of cancer. Such radiographic symptoms as "tail" or presence of calcificates in the tumor may have a diagnostic value. Meningiomas are usually characterized by high perfusion values both in CT and MRI studies, which is typical for the majority of metastases. In spectroscopy, a high Cho peak allows to rule out metastases, but close location of small tumors to the skull bones often makes it difficult to obtain adequate study results. Identification of the meningioma matrix with contrast enhancement or angiography is a pathognomonic sign; this type of blood supply is not typical for metastases. Malignant meningiomas with signs of decay can fully simulate metastases.

32 Hemangiopericytoma

Hemangiopericytoma is a rare (up to 1%) primary intracranial neoplasm. According to the WHO classification, hemangiopericytoma belongs to tumors of unknown origin, although some consider them to be histologically similar to angioblastic meningiomas. There is a hypothesis that they come from pericytes—cells surrounding capillaries (Casentino et al. 1993; Parker et al. 1999). Macroscopically hemangiopericytomas resemble meningiomas. Mostly these are dense tumors with a lumpy surface, often well demarcated, infiltrating the brain tissue, and attached to the dura mater with their wide base and are exceptionally well vascularized (Konovalov et al. 2005).

On CT, hemangiopericytomas have heterogeneously increased density without contrast enhancement and are characterized by marked contrast enhancement that further highlights the heterogeneity of the tumor structure, mainly due to the presence of cysts and areas of necrosis. A CT perfusion study demonstrates exceptionally high flow rates in the tumor stroma, with the heterogeneity of its distribution, more pronounced than that in meningiomas. Distinctive features of metastases are rather hyperostotic than destructive changes in the adjacent bone structures.

MR signs of hemangiopericytoma are variable. The heterogeneity of the tumor structure is best demonstrated on T2-weighted MRI, while on T1-weighted MRI, they may look almost isointense. The accumulation of the contrast agent has also pronounced and heterogeneous character. Very often large abnormal blood vessels can be detected in the tumor stroma (Fig. 32.1).

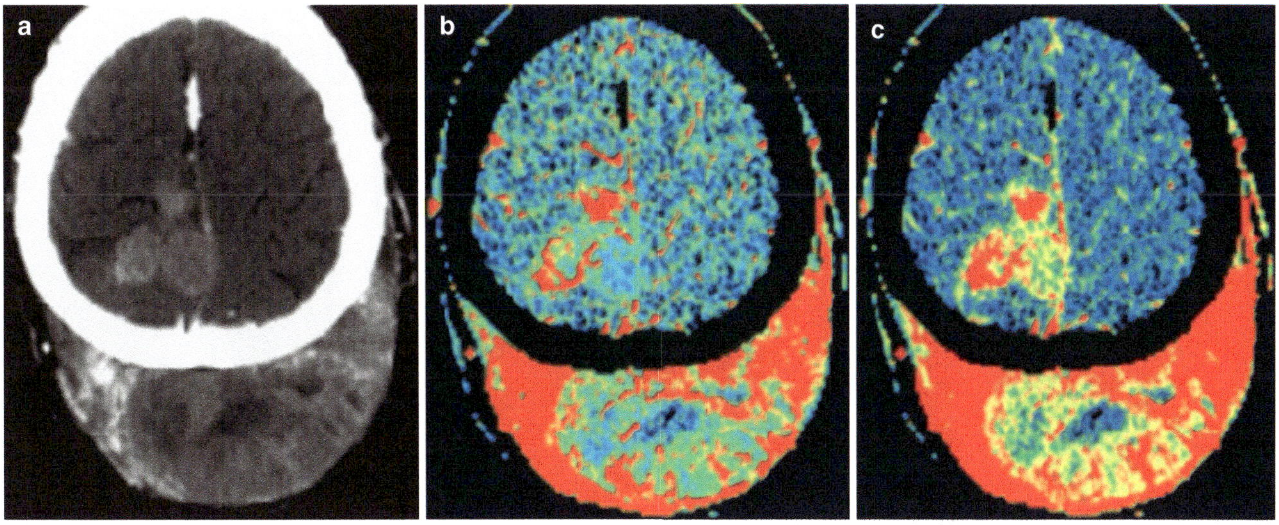

Fig. 32.1 Hemangiopericytoma. On contrast-enhanced CT (**a**), in the parietal region, there is an extensive intra-extracranial tumor, as well as a multinodular lesion in the right parietal region without a significant perifocal edema. On perfusion maps of CBV (**b**) and CBF (**c**), the tumor is characterized by a sharp increase in the blood flow

M. Dolgushin et al., *Brain Metastases*, DOI 10.1007/978-3-319-57760-9_32

Hemangioblastoma

33

Hemangioblastoma belong to rare, benign tumors, whose histological origin is still debated. It is believed that hemangioblastoma (HMB) occurs in 1–2.5% of all intracranial tumors. The proportion of childhood tumors accounts for about 20% of all Hemangioblastoma. The tumor is detected as one of the manifestations of von Hippel-Lindau disease in up to 10% of cases.

The tumor is detected on non-contrast-enhanced CT as a lesion with similar and higher density as compared to that of the brain substance. It is located on one of the cystic walls, entering into its lumen, and intensely accumulates the contrast material (up to 60–85 HU). In the solid form, the whole tumor mass becomes hyperdense after contrast enhancement. In the cystic form, MRI well visualizes the cystic component, which is characterized by a low MR signal on T1- and high signal on T2-weighted images. On this background, a mural solid nodule of hemangioblastoma is visualized, intensely accumulating the contrast agent (Figs. 33.1 and 33.2).

Solid HMB forms have rounded and convoluted areas of a signal loss from the blood in large neoplasm vessels in the tumor stroma. The presence of a large number of such vessels better visualized by T2-weighted MR sequences in the HMB structure is highly pathognomonic for this type of tumors. In all such cases, especially in craniospinal location, direct angiography should be carried out in order to clarify the location of multiple large vessels and determine surgical tactics. It should be remembered that in case of von Hippel-Lindau disease, there may be multiple HMBs with both intracranial and intravertebral location. This makes it advisable to conduct a comprehensive MRI study of the CNS with the mandatory use of intravenous contrast enhancement, since small tumor nodules can remain undetected on conventional MR images.

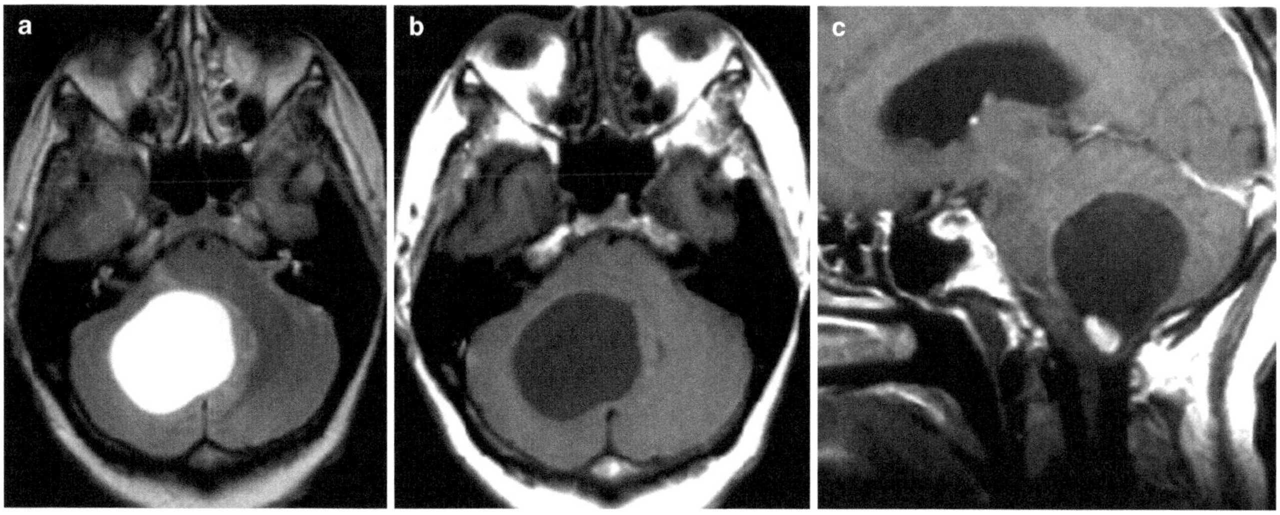

Fig. 33.1 Hemangioblastoma. On T2-weighted (**a**) and T1-weighted MRI (**b**), in the projection of the medial portions of the right cerebellar hemisphere, there is a cystic lesion with a mural nodule, which is located at the level of the foramen magnum and well visualized on T1-weighted MRI with contrast enhancement (**c**)

M. Dolgushin et al., *Brain Metastases*, DOI 10.1007/978-3-319-57760-9_33

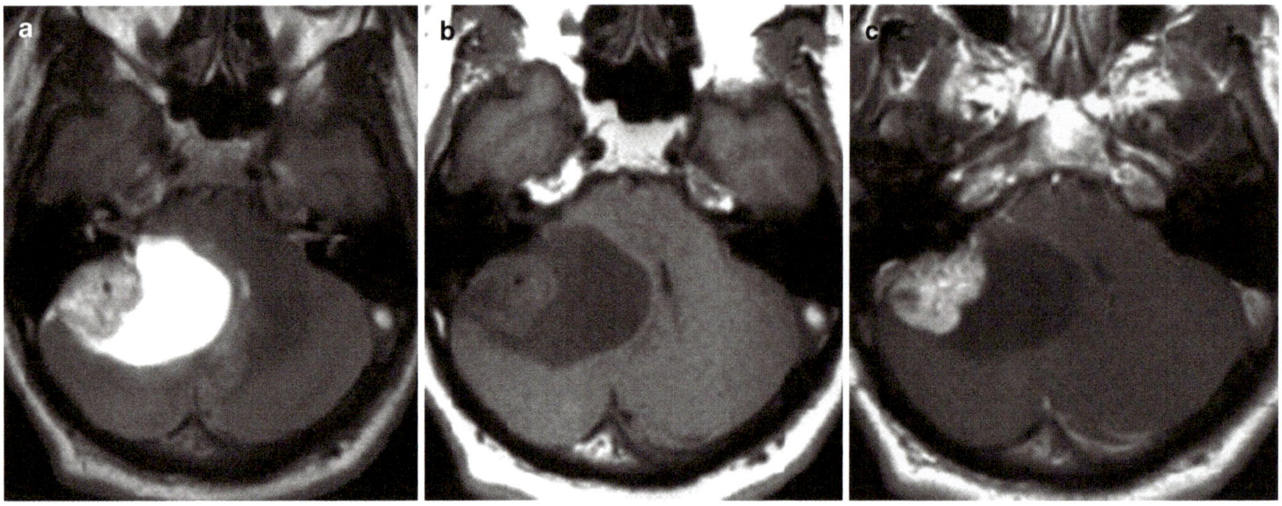

Fig. 33.2 Hemangioblastoma. On MRI, in the projection of the lateral parts of the right cerebellar hemisphere, there is a large, space-occupying lesion with a mixed structure and a cystic component that is located medially to the solid fragment of the tumor; the latter is quite clearly visualized on axial T2-weighted (**a**) and T1-weighted images (**b**). After contrast enhancement, there is an increase in the MR signal from the tumor; cystic walls do not accumulate the contrast agent (**c**), which is not typical for metastatic tumors

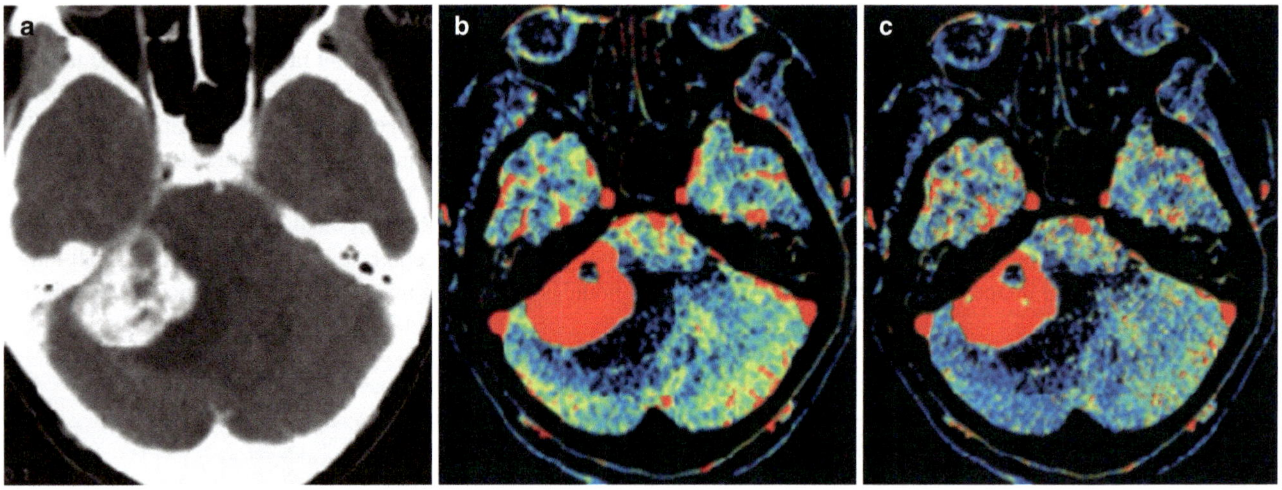

Fig. 33.3 Hemangioblastoma. CT. On axial CT (**a**), on the background of contrast enhancement in the projection of the right cerebellopontine angle, a space-occupying lesion with high density and a heterogeneous structure is visualized. CT perfusion maps (**b**, CBV; **c**, CBF) demonstrate high blood flow levels in the tumor tissue

The use of a perfusion CT study helps improve the preoperative differential diagnosis of HMBs, especially in cases of a predominantly solid tumor structure. CBV and CBF values of the tumor are the highest among intra- and extracerebral tumors with the subtentorial location (Fig. 33.3).

Thus, despite the fact that hemangiopericytoma and hemangioblastoma are rare tumors, their X-ray picture with accompanying intense accumulation of the contrast agent causes a number of diagnostic difficulties. In this case, the use of CT perfusion imaging allows to reliably confirm hemangiopericytoma by very high CBV and CBF values; the possible exceptions can be melanomas characterized by similar values of perfusion. In cases of cystic Hemangioblastoma, the solid component is usually small. Weak or completely absent contrast enhancement of the cystic cavity walls is typical.

34 Cavernous Angiomas, Cavernous Malformations

Cavernous angiomas, cavernous malformations, were allocated into the group of true malformations in the international histological classification of tumors of the central nervous system only in 1979. Before this, cavernous angiomas (CAs) were regarded as tumors. CAs represent the system of communicating vascular cavities with various sizes and sinusoid shapes, filled with blood. Vascular cavities are separated by connective partitions with different thicknesses, which are common to several adjacent microcavities. The walls of the cavities are lined with the endothelium forming papillary excrescences. Each cavity is characterized by an independent argyrophil framework, lack of muscle, and elastic fibers; capillaries or intertwined bands of endothelial cells can be located between them. There is no brain tissue in the CA structure; however, there can be cysts, areas of thrombosed masses, sclerosis, and calcificates. The origin of sclerotic changes in the majority of cases is unequivocal—development of clots characteristic of CA. Microhemorrhages within the malformation, as well as beyond its borders, are considered a typical feature of CAs. The perifocal area is characterized by reactive changes in the glia with its yellow discoloration due to imbibition of the brain substance with hemosiderin accumulated in macrophages. The size of CAs varies from several microns to several centimeters. In a hemorrhage inside the cavernoma, a rupture of the inter-cavity walls and formation of larger cavities are possible. This results in the fact that in some cases cavernous angioma consists of only a few cavities filled with blood, i.e., they are essentially a one- or multi-chamber hematoma.

Diagnosis of cavernous angioma on the background of hematoma on CT and MRI is very difficult, which is due to several factors—a small size of the malformation and a possible self-destruction of the malformation in case of the hemorrhage.

MR manifestations of hematomas are more specific. In the early stages, contrast enhancement of hematomas is determined primarily by the presence of water molecules—they look isointense in T1-weighted images and hyperintense in T2-weighted images. In the following hours, oxyhemoglobin transforms to deoxyhemoglobin, which substantially shortens the relaxation time T2 in the hematoma area. The latter becomes very dark in T2-weighted images but is still isointense on T1-weighted MRI. Further oxidation results in the formation of methemoglobin, which significantly increases the signal from hematoma in T1-weighted and T2-weighted images. An increase in the MR signal (especially on T1-weighted MRI) extends from the periphery to the center, indicating lysis of erythrocytes and "release" of methemoglobin—intracellular methemoglobin has a high MR signal in T1-weighted images and a low signal in T2-weighted images, and "free" methemoglobin is characterized by a high MR signal in all sequences (Figs. 34.1 and 34.2). At the late subacute phase and early chronic phase, on the periphery of the hematoma, a narrow area of a low signal, visible in T2-weighted images, begins to form, represented by the deposition of hemosiderin in macrophages of the hematoma capsule. By this time, the hematoma has an increased signal from the center and a low signal as a thin rim from the periphery in all sequences (Fig. 34.3).

Of great importance for determining the surgical treatment and a follow-up scheme is the determination of the form of mixed vascular malformations underlying the hematoma. It should be borne in mind that visualization of small malformations on the background of a hematoma is impossible, since the latter "covers" all other effects. The type of malformation can be determined only in the absence of a hematoma or its small size.

On CT, cavernous angiomas (if they are large enough) are visualized as foci with a regular, round, or irregular shape and high density, virtually not accumulating the contrast agent. With long-term (more than 1.5 months) persistence of a CT focus with increased density without undergoing any substantial transformation, a cavernous angioma can be suspected, *as the hematoma density will certainly change with time*. This "classic" picture is detected maximum in half of suspected cavernous angiomas located supratentorially.

M. Dolgushin et al., *Brain Metastases*, DOI 10.1007/978-3-319-57760-9_34

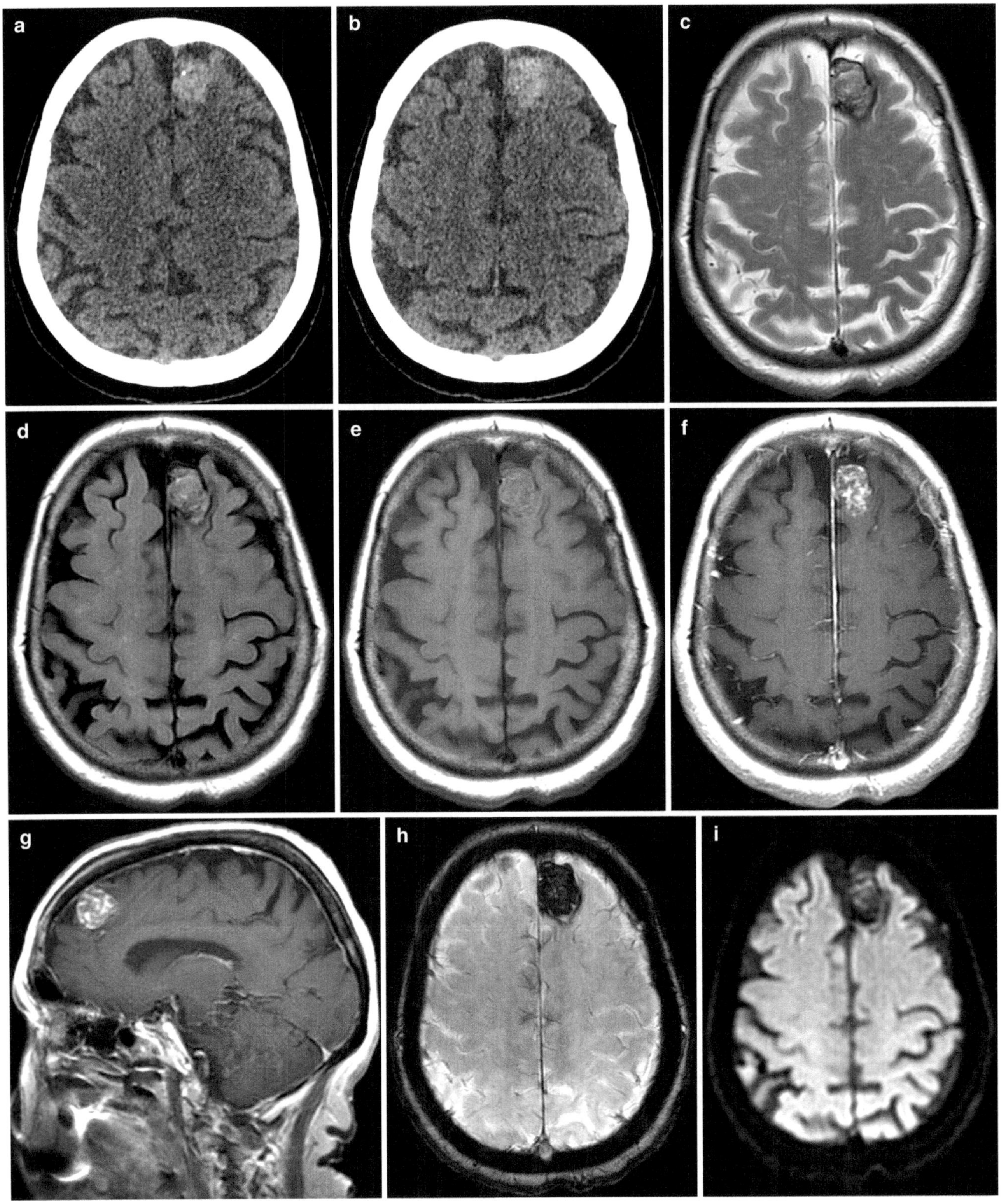

Fig. 34.1 Cavernous angioma. In native axial CT sections (**a**, **b**), there is a hyperdense lesion with microcalcifications in the structure in the left frontal region. On a series of brain MRIs performed in T2-weighted (**c**), T2-FLAIR (**d**), and T1-weighted sequences before (**e**) and after (**f**, **g**) intravenous contrast enhancement, the lesion has a heterogeneous MR signal with a hypointense peripheral rim in the left frontal lobe. A speckled nature of the contrast enhancement of this lesion is noted. On SWI (**h**) and DWI (**i**) MRI, a marked reduction of MRI signal from the whole structure of the lesion is noted

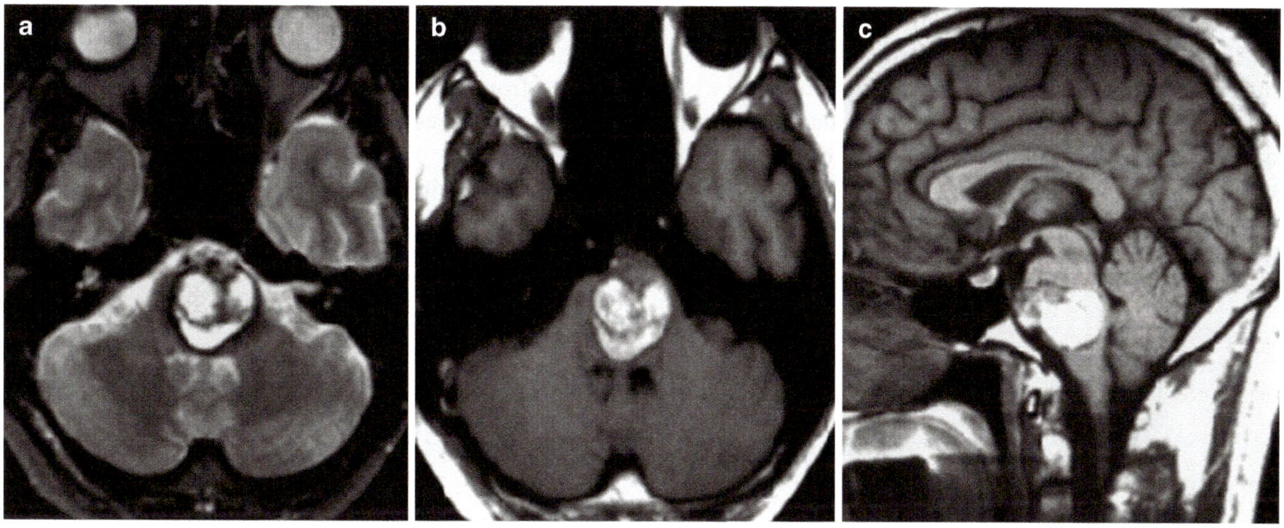

Fig. 34.2 Cavernous angioma. On T2-weighted (**a**) and T1-weighted MRI (**b**, **c**), an area of nonuniform signal change is identified in the projection of the pons. On T2-weighted images, peripheral parts of this area have a marked hypointense signal. On T1-weighted MRI in the axial (**b**) and sagittal (**c**) projections, along with areas of an increased signal represented by the hemorrhagic component, there is an additional area of signal changes that has access to the ventral surface of the pons—a solid portion of cavernous angioma

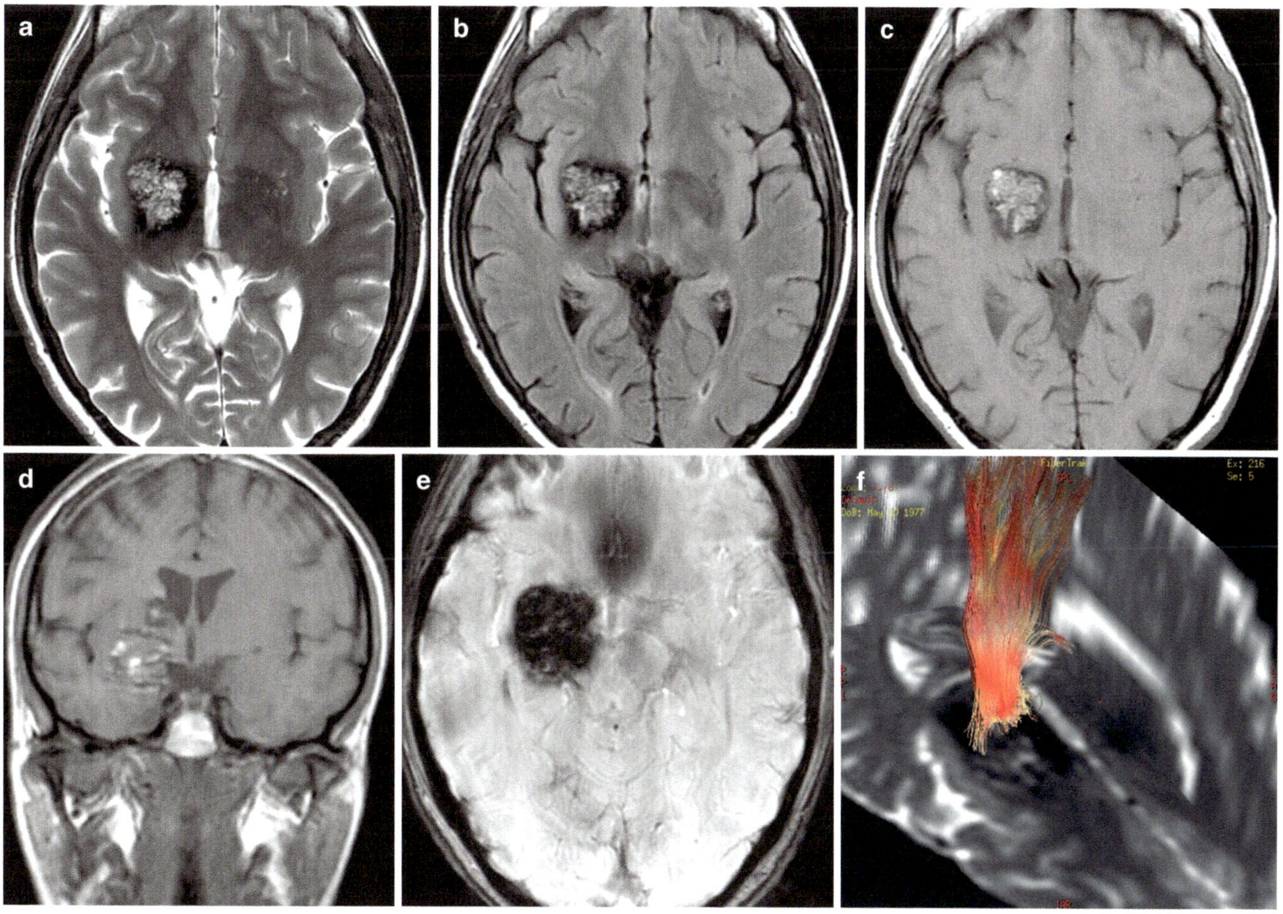

Fig. 34.3 Cavernous angioma. At the level of the right basal ganglia, there is a hypointense lesion on T2-weighted MRI (**a**) and T2-FLAIR MRI (**b**) and a space-occupying lesion on SWI MRI (**e**). A cellular structure is clearly visualized in the central parts of the lesion. On T1-weighted MRI (**c**, **d**), the lesion has "mottled" appearance due to the presence of small subacute hemorrhages (an increased MR signal). There is no perifocal edema, which is not typical for a metastatic lesion with a hemorrhage. On MR tractography, the corticospinal tract runs along the posterior contour of the hypointense area, with no signs of damage (**f**)

Thus, standard CT or MRI allows to suspect CA based on the heterogeneity of the hemorrhagic content (bleedings differentiated by time), especially in prolonged cases; CT can visualize calcifications that are the most significant signs of cavernomas. Calcifications in metastases can only be observed on long-term chemotherapy (primarily with Avastin). Uneven, "lumpy" accumulation of the contrast agent in the CA structure is also a characteristic feature. Using applications such as MR spectroscopy, DWI, or ASL is not reasonable because of pronounced artifacts from hemosiderin. CT and MR perfusion imaging is characterized by low values, reflecting a very poor blood flow, or its complete absence, allowing to rule out the metastatic tumor origin. SWI (SWAN) MRI is highly sensitive, and its use in some cases allows to identify additional small CAs.

35 Tumors of Sellar and Parasellar Region

The sellar region usually consists of the Turkish saddle with adjacent structures located near the CSF cisterns with the hypothalamus, the bottom of third ventricle, and the cavernous sinus. Metastases to this area do not occur often, and in our cases, we observed this process more often in breast cancer. The main issue of the differential diagnosis is the clinical picture, including hormonal changes in the anterior pituitary, which may be characteristic of a number of primary tumors of the sellar region (Fig. 35.1).

35.1 Pituitary Adenoma

Pituitary tumors occupy the third place among the central nervous system neoplasms and, according to different authors, range from 4% to 17% (Kadashev 1992). Based on their size, pituitary adenomas are classified as *microadenomas* (10 mm) and *macroadenomas* (over 10 mm).

Visualization of macroadenomas with modern CT and MRI does not present too much difficulty (Kornienko 1993; Konovalov 1997; Dedov 1997; Kornienko 2012). More difficult in this case becomes the differential diagnosis with other space-occupying lesions of the optic chiasm and sellar region (Asa 2008). Thus, in most of our cases, the tumor had extrasellar growth at the time of initial diagnosis. In these cases, it is important to determine the extent of the process and its association with the lesions in the parasellar region, such as the optic chiasm, optic nerves, internal carotid artery, cavernous sinus, etc.

In the study using CT, the destruction of the sellar walls is identified. Pituitary tumors can spread parasellarly into the middle cranial fossa and anteriorly to the bottom of the anterior cranial fossa and into the main cavity of the sphenoid sinus and ethmoid cells.

On spiral CT, adenoma in the absence of an intratumoral hemorrhage is usually iso- or weakly hyperdense relative to the brain substance. Hemorrhage areas have higher density in the acute phase.

On T1-weighted MR images, macroadenomas typically look like space-occupying lesions coming from the cavity of the dilated and deepened Turkish saddle and are characterized by an iso- or hypointense MR signal. The intact anterior pituitary can be traced along the adenoma contour as a brighter fragment. In T2-weighted and T2-FLAIR images, macroadenomas are characterized by a high signal more often than microadenomas. Following intravenous contrast enhancement, there is quite pronounced accumulation of the contrast material by adenoma, making it hyperintense relative to the brain, in most cases.

On MR spectroscopy, we found a marked increase in the choline peak and an increase in the lipid-lactate complex peak on the background of a decrease in the N-acetylaspartate peak in pituitary adenomas.

The study of tumor hemodynamics has become an important part of a comprehensive evaluation of pituitary adenomas, especially those that are accompanied with hemorrhages. The method of CT perfusion imaging in the diagnosis of skull base tumors and, in particular, in the differential diagnosis of pituitary adenomas showed high sensitivity and high specificity in verification of histology of neoplasms. Low values of blood flow velocity (sometimes comparable to those of the brain), a moderately pronounced CBV increase, and very high values of the transit time MTT are typical for pituitary adenomas, no matter what size they reach. These properties help perform a differential diagnosis of pituitary adenomas from other lesions, including parasellar metastases in most cases (Figs. 35.2 and 35.3).

Thus, it is extremely difficult to differentiate pituitary adenomas from metastases on routine CT and MRI; the most appropriate is the use of CT perfusion imaging that identifies the characteristics of pituitary adenomas, described above. Moreover, the secondary nature of a sellar tumor can be suggested only in case of a patient with a previous history of cancer.

M. Dolgushin et al., *Brain Metastases*, DOI 10.1007/978-3-319-57760-9_35

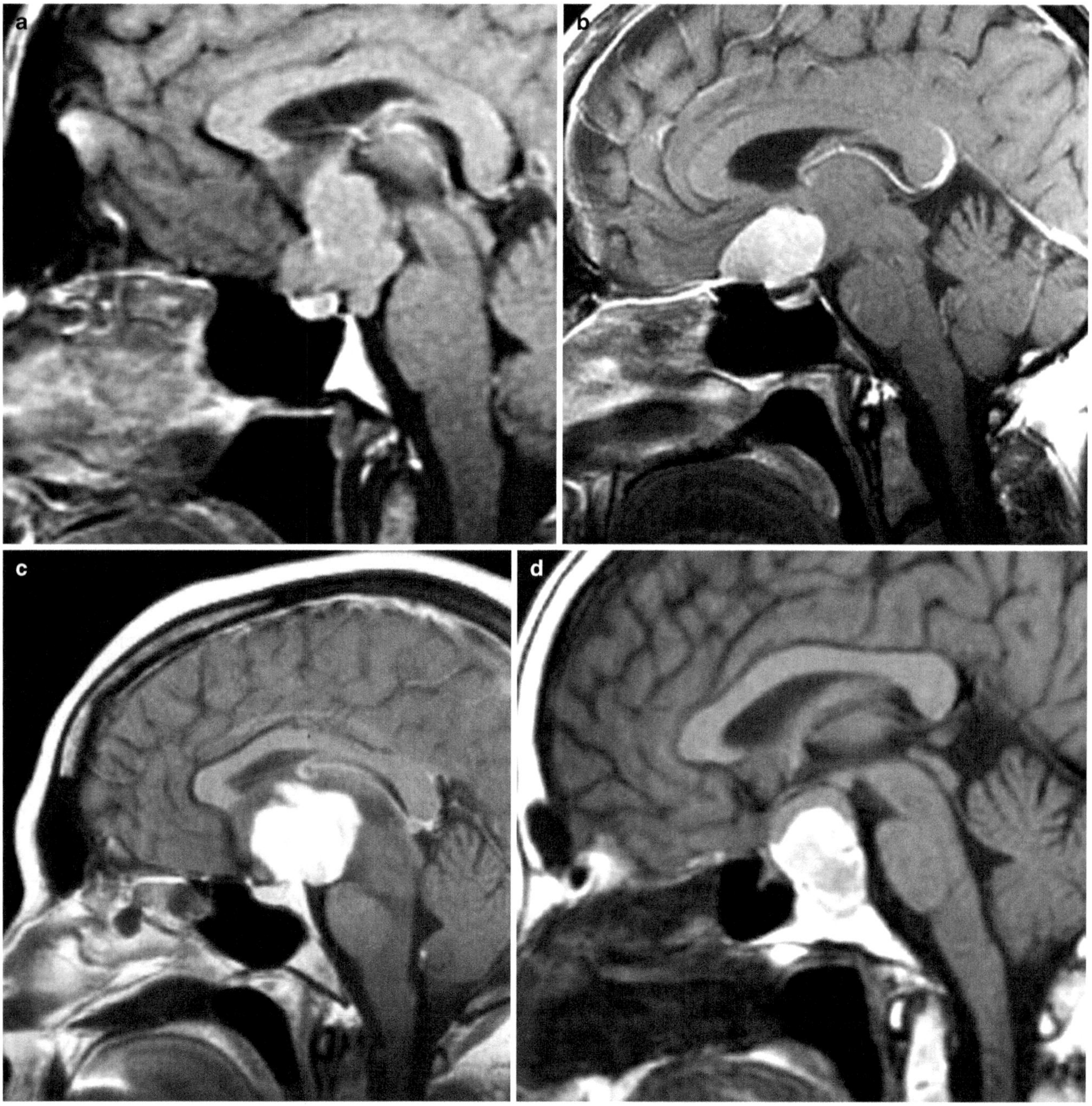

Fig. 35.1 MRI with contrast enhancement. Metastasis (**a**), meningioma (**b**), astrocytoma (**c**), adenoma (**d**). Differential diagnosis: all lesions are characterized by intense accumulation of the contrast agent and the suprasellar spread

35.2 Meningiomas (Parasellar, Sphenoid Wing Meningioma, Pterional)

Meningiomas (parasellar, sphenoid wing meningioma, pterional) constitute about 12% of all intracranial meningiomas. The site of their initial growth may be the tuberculum sellae, anterior clinoid process, medial portions of the large wing, cavernous sinus, rarely dorsum sellae, and diaphragm. Meningiomas initially growing from the optic nerve sheath may also grow into the cavernous sinus. Olfactory fossa meningiomas often grow into the tuberculum sellae region and directly into the sella. The tumor border is more difficult to differentiate if it is located in the projection of the cavernous sinus. Tumors of the wings of the sphenoid bone, even small ones, can cause the development of an extensive perifocal edema of the temporal lobe of the brain.

Based on CT findings, bone changes can be detected that occur both in metastases and in meningiomas, in particular bone destruction, bone marrow invasion, and, last but not least, hyperostosis. The latter changes are frequently diagnosed in meningiomas of the wings of the sphenoid bone and tuberculum sellae.

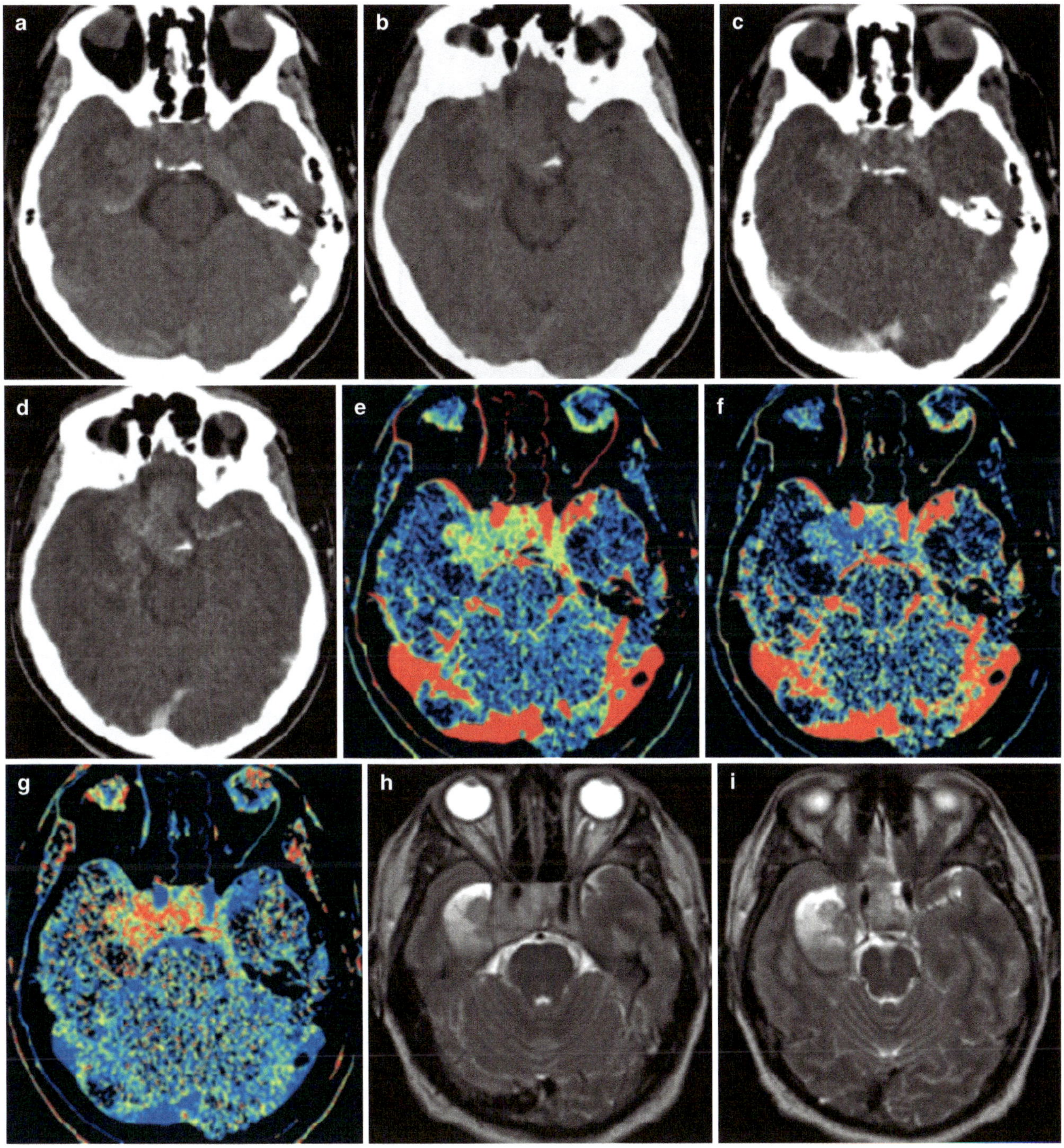

Fig. 35.2 Pituitary adenoma. On a CT series before (**a**, **b**) and after (**c**, **d**) contrast enhancement, there is a large pituitary tumor with predominantly laterosellar growth to the right, where a cystic part of the tumor is further visualized (a hypodense area). The tumor rapidly accumulates CA. CT perfusion of CBV (**e**), CBF (**f**), and MTT (**g**) shows an increase in the blood flow volume and prolongation of the contrast agent transit time. Changes in the blood flow velocity in adenoma are characterized by a minimal increase in comparison to the brain tissue. On T2-weighted MRI (**h**, **i**), the tumor structure, spread, and enveloping of carotid siphons are clearly visualized

In T1-weighted MR images, the majority of meningiomas are characterized by an iso- or hypointense, relatively homogeneous MR signal. The symptom of the dura matter enhancement at the MCF floor (as well as along the clivus of the sphenoid bone) can be identified only by MRI. Sometimes after contrast enhancement, the outer wall of the cavernous sinus can be visualized, if the tumor mass pushes it outwards; lateral contours of the tumor are usually smooth and oval (meningioma grows within the sinus from the inner layer of the dura mater). If a dark MR signal band from the sinus wall is included in the tumor stroma and the outer contour appears lumpy on MRI, these are typical manifestations of the

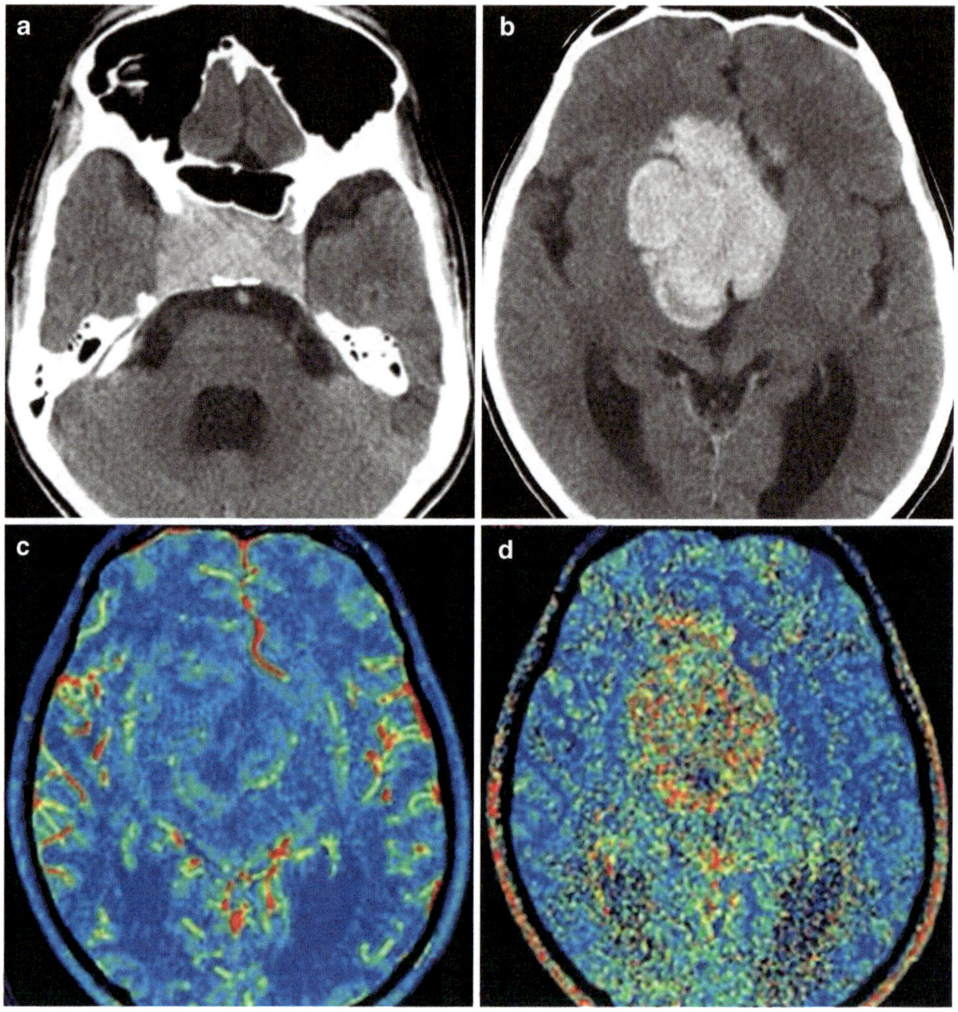

Fig. 35.3 Pituitary adenoma. On CT with contrast enhancement, there is an intra-suprasellar tumor intensely accumulating the contrast agent (**a**, **b**). Perfusion maps show low CBF values (**c**) and prolongation of the transit time (**d**)

cavernous sinus wall invasion with involvement of both dura mater layers. Rarely, meningiomas of the anterior cranial fossa and tuberculum sellae can grow toward the sphenoid sinus and ethmoid bone cells.

Spiral CT perfusion imaging may be useful for a differential diagnosis of parasellar pituitary adenomas and cavernous sinus meningiomas, as CBF and CBV values are significantly higher in meningiomas, while pituitary adenomas are mostly characterized by a prolongation of MTT values (Fig. 35.4). Differentiation of metastases from meningioma is quite difficult, as both are characterized by high perfusion values.

35.3 Glioma of the Optic Nerves, Chiasm, and Hypothalamus

Glioma of the optic nerves, chiasm, and hypothalamus comprises 3–5% of all intracranial tumors and 25–30 % of tumors of the optic chiasm and sellar region in children. Tumors of the optic chiasm often involve the hypothalamus and third ventricle in the process. Largely, these are benign piloid astrocytomas (75%), but, despite their benignity, they are characterized by an unfavorable prognosis depending on their site and spread. Tumors of the optic nerve cause an enlargement of the optic canal on the affected side; in case of the involvement of both optic nerves, the enlargement of the optic canals occurs on both sides (symmetric or asymmetric); in case of the chiasmal involvement, changes in the sella turcica appear; in case of giant tumors, changes in the sella turcica and hypertensive hydrocephalic changes develop.

In case of the involvement of the optic chiasm, optic tracts, and hypothalamus, CT shows an iso- or hypodense space-occupying lesion moderately accumulating the contrast material. In case of advanced tumors, accumulation of the contrast material along the optic tracts up to the lateral geniculate bodies and often around the third ventricle is observed.

Most informative in the differential diagnosis for all lesions at this site are CT and MRI, while cerebral angiography is additionally preferred for vascular lesions. The degree

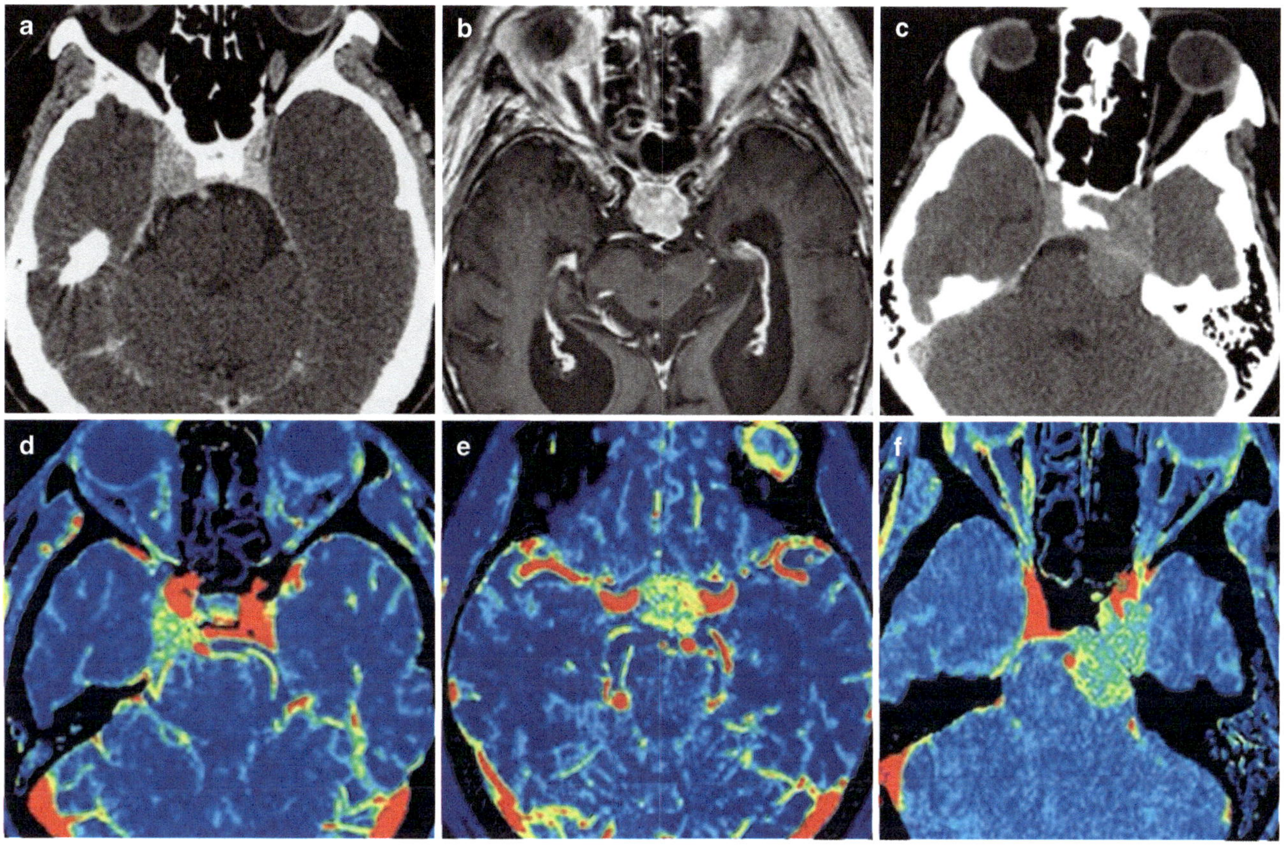

Fig. 35.4 Meningioma. Cases of several patients. Case No. 1. Meningioma of the right cavernous sinus (**a**, **d**). Post-contrast SKT (**a**) and perfusion CBV map (**d**) show a small tumor with a high blood flow volume. Case No. 2. Meningioma of the tuberculum sellae. MRI with contrast (**b**) and CBV map (**e**) show an intensely contrast-enhanced tumor of the suprasellar region with a high CBV value. Case No. 3. Meningioma of the left cavernous sinus with the spread into the posterior cranial fossa. On a CT (**c**) and CBV map (**f**), there is a lesion intensely accumulating the contrast agent and characterized by high perfusion values throughout the tumor stroma

of blood supply to optic chiasm gliomas can be estimated using CT perfusion: low or moderately increased CBV and CBF values are typical, and MTT values are variable (Fig. 35.5).

An MRI signal from the tumor is equal to the signal from the brain tissue or is hypointense in T1-weighted images and moderately hyperintense in T2-weighted images. Often, cystic cavities are formed in the tumors or are adjacent to them, which is most typical for giant gliomas. Density of cystic components on CT and their signal on MRI are equal to the density and signal from the cerebrospinal fluid. T2-weighted imaging successfully detects tumor growth along the optic tract, even in cases where CT with contrast enhancement fails to detect these changes. Intravenous enhancement shows accumulation of the contrast material in the tumor from minor to homogeneously intense (Fig. 35.6). Most often piloid astrocytomas are intensely contrasted. A high degree of contrast enhancement also distinguishes anaplastic gliomas located at this site.

Thus, benign gliomas, poorly accumulating or not accumulating the contrast agent on MRI, do not cause any difficulties in the differential diagnosis. In other cases, differentiation of chiasmosellar glioma is difficult, since edema that accompanies active growth of a metastasis can also simulate the diffuse distribution of glioma, for example, along the optic tracts.

35.4 Sellar Germinoma

Only 20% of them develop in the suprasellar cistern and very rarely in the pituitary fossa. Germinomas contain large polygonal fetal cells, agglomerates of lymphocytes, and dense connective tissue stroma. Suprasellar germinomas are non-encapsulated tumors with infiltrative growth; they can metastasize to the ventricular walls and basal cisterns.

On a CT study without contrast enhancement, germinomas have moderately increased density, which homogeneously

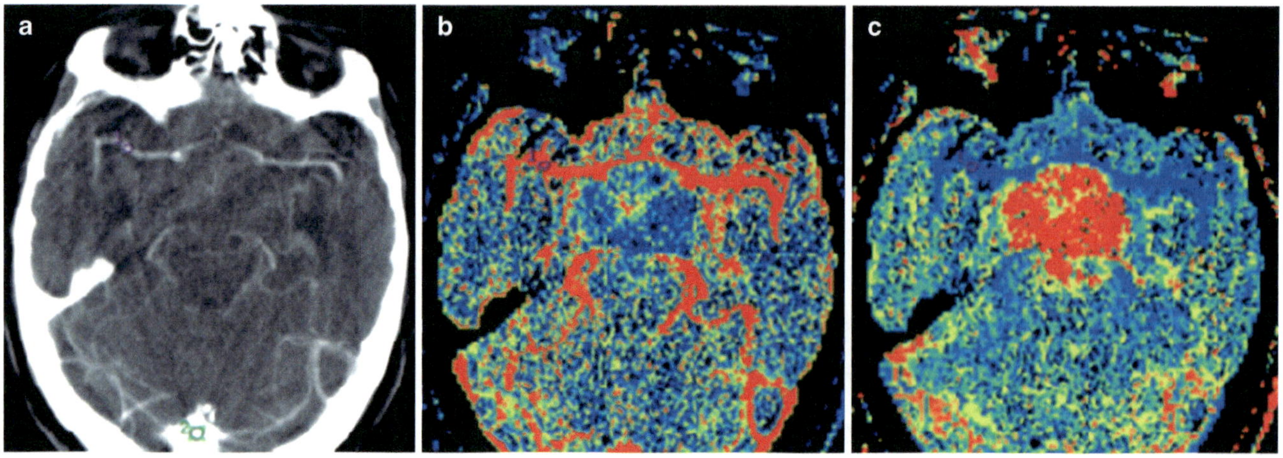

Fig. 35.5 Glioma chiasma. On CT after intravenous CA administration (**a**), there is a large tumor in the chiasmosellar area with isodense characteristics and minimally marked contrast enhancement in the central parts of the tumor. CT perfusion of CBF (**b**) shows low levels of blood flow velocity in the tumor tissue as compared to the brain substance on the background of a marked prolongation of the contrast agent transit time MTT (**c**)

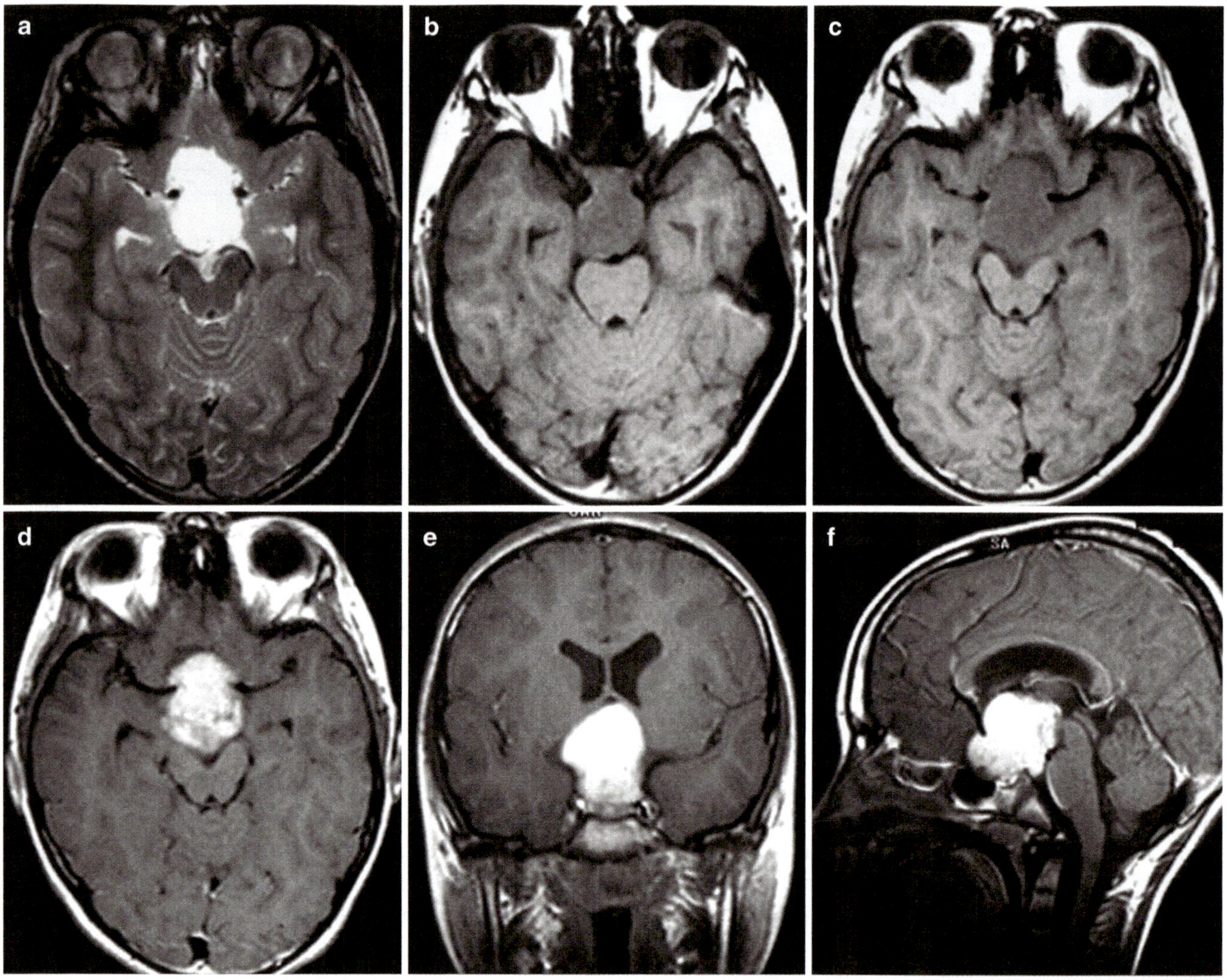

Fig. 35.6 Gliomas of the chiasm and third ventricle bottom (piloid astrocytoma). On MRI, a space-occupying lesion is detected endosuprasellarly, characterized by an increased signal in T2-weighted images (**a**) and slightly decreased in T1-weighted images (**b**, **c**). On post-contrast T1-weighted MRI, in the axial (**d**), frontal (**e**), and sagittal (**f**) projections, there is uneven, but intense, accumulation of the contrast agent by the tumor

increases after administering the contrast agent. The tumor contains no calcifications. Primary germinoma pineal region can be detected in this case. The described characteristics are similar to those of lymphoma, and differences can include age, patient history, and presence of a tumor in the pineal region.

Most suprasellar germinomas are well determined by MRI, as their size by the time of clinical manifestations is already significant. Typically, they are located along the midline at the floor of the third ventricle. The germinoma structure is homogeneous, and only in rare cases the tumor stroma contains small cysts, usually located on the periphery. The signal from germinomas moderately differs from the signal of the brain tissue. Germinomas are iso- or slightly hypointense in T1-weighted images and iso- or slightly hyperintense in T2-weighted images. Typically, germinomas intensely accumulate the contrast agent, and metastatic tumor foci can be detected along the lateral ventricle ependyma and in the subarachnoid space (Fig. 35.7). In general, in case of a primary tumor in the pineal region, neoplasms always have a certain similarity in their structures, which is better visualized on MRI.

35.5 Fibrosarcoma (FS)

Fibrosarcoma (FS) is one of the most common malignant soft tissue tumors that is formed from immature fibrous connective tissue. It is often located in the muscles of the extremities (hip, shoulder) or torso. There are infantile fibrosarcoma (in children under 10 years of age) and adult fibrosarcoma (common in children older than 10 years of age and in adults, more often at the age of 40–55 years old) (Toro 2006).

CT and MRI manifestations of craniofacial fibrosarcoma are generally indistinguishable from those of other malignancies growing in this area. By the time of primary diagnosis, the tumor is usually advanced. On CT, this is a soft tissue space-occupying lesion, causing the destruction of the bone structures in the anterior cranial fossa and craniofacial region. Presence of calcifications in the tumor stroma is uncharacteristic.

An MRI pattern depends on the predominant histological structure. On T1-weighted images, this is usually an isodense lesion as compared to the brain; on T2-weighted images, the MR signal is variable from hypo- to slightly hyperintense (Fig. 35.8).

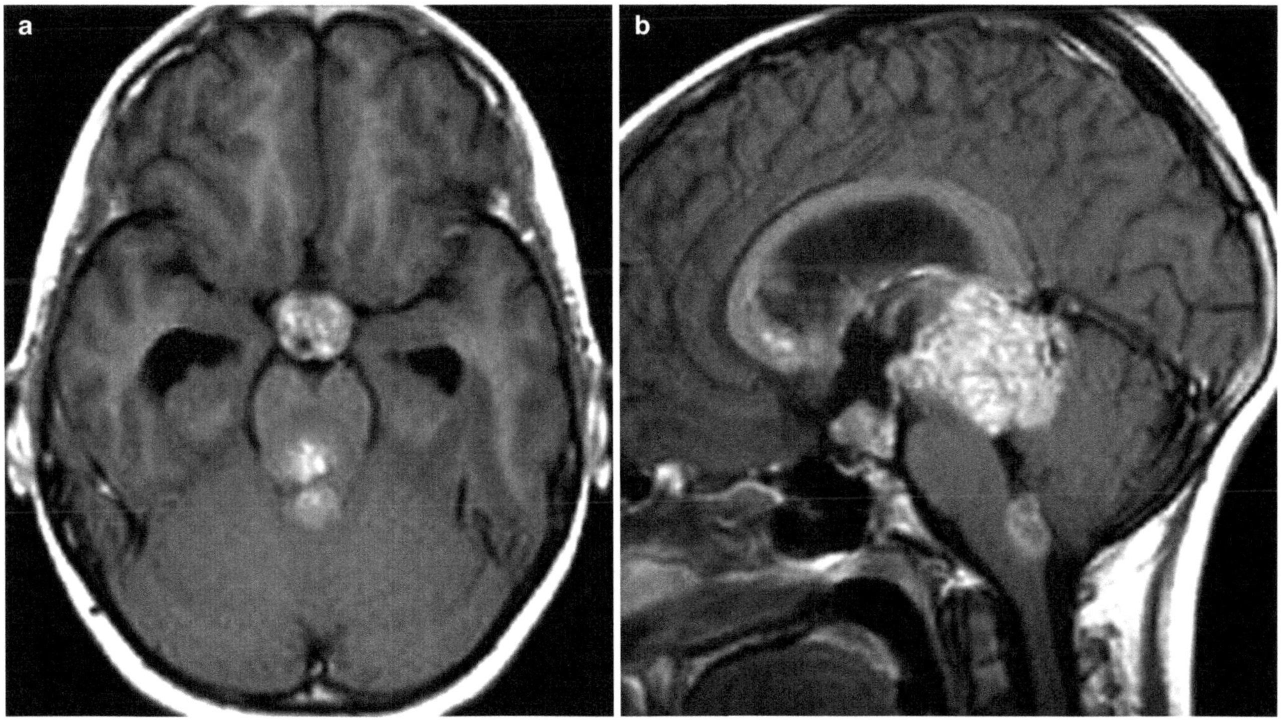

Fig. 35.7 Germinoma. On T1-weighted MRI, in the axial (**a**) and sagittal (**b**) projections after CA administration, there is a large space-occupying lesion in the projection of the pineal region, intensely accumulating the contrast agent, as well as metastases in the chiasmo-sellar area, subependymal in the anterior horns of the lateral ventricles and in caudal portions of the fourth ventricle

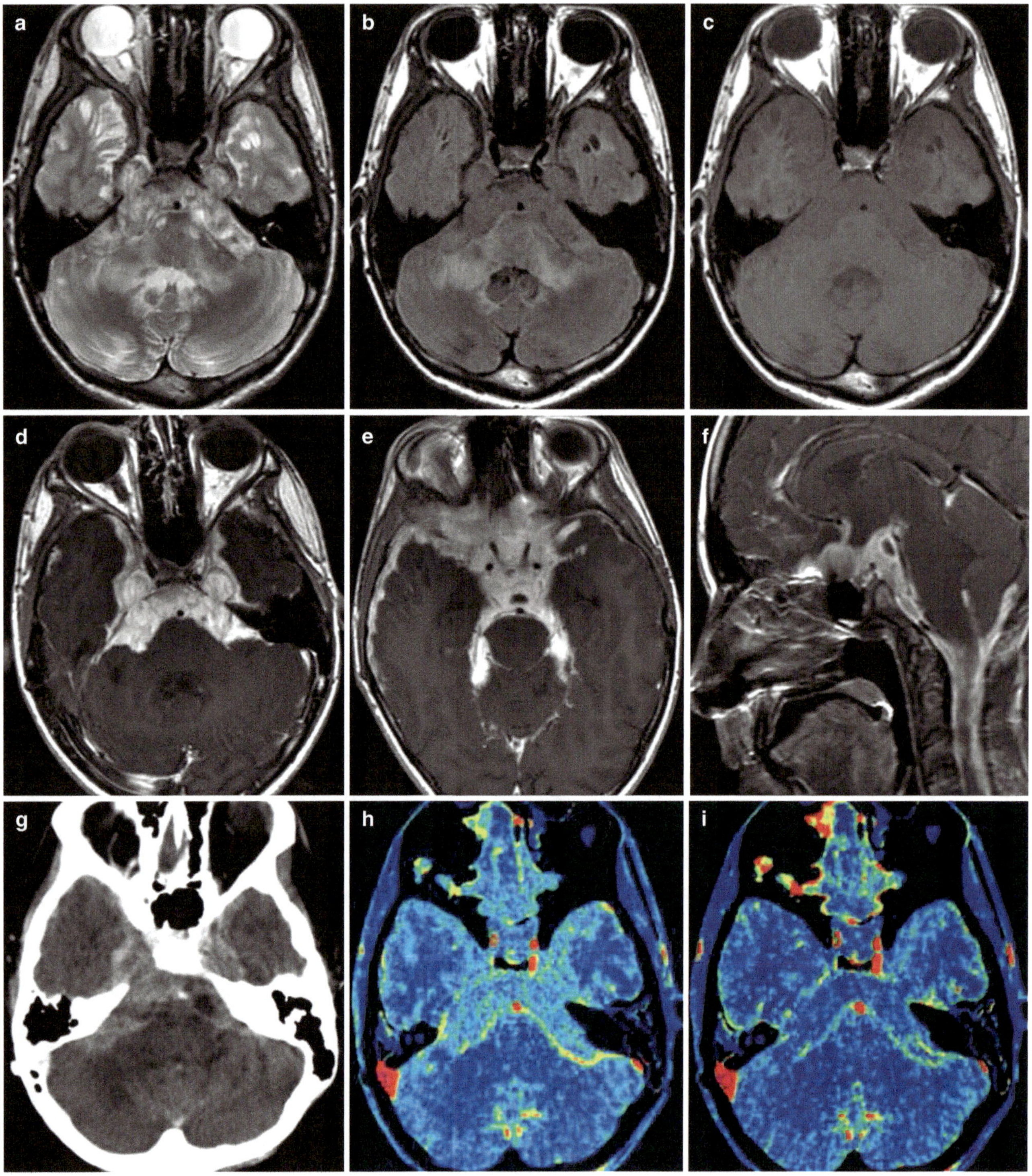

Fig. 35.8 Fibrosarcoma. On T2-weighted (**a**), T2-FLAIR (**b**), and T1-weighted MRI before (**c**) and after (**d–f**) intravenous contrast enhancement, in the subarachnoid spaces of the skull base, and, to a lesser extent, supratentorially, there is an abnormal soft tissue structure which fills the specified spaces, including the cerebrospinal fluid cisterns of the skull base. The tumor mass is better visualized after contrast enhancement. The degree of tumor enhancement is also quite pronounced on CT (**g**). The perfusion study shows a moderate increase in CBF values (**h**) and low CBV values (**i**) in the tumor structure

36 Tumors of the Pineal Region

Metastases to the pineal region of malignant tumors are quite rare, occurring not more than in 1%. Primary tumors of the pineal region are also relatively rare, accounting for 0.5–1% of all intracranial tumors; in children, their proportion in the structure (3–8%) is slightly higher. Both benign and malignant (75%) tumors develop in the pineal region (Jooma et al. 1983; Bruce et al. 1993; Allen et al. 1996; Konovalov and Pitskhelauri 2004). According to the modern histological classification (2016), tumors of the pineal region are presented by four major groups: (a) *pineocytoma*, (b) *parenchymal tumor*, (c) *pineoblastoma*, and (d) *papillary tumor*. Four main syndromes prevail in the clinical picture of the pineal region lesions: (a) intracranial hypertension due to compression of the cerebral aqueduct and hydrocephalus, (b) Parinaud syndrome (midbrain involvement), (c) cerebellar disorders, and (d) endocrine disorders (premature sexual development, diabetes insipidus).

36.1 Glial Tumors

Glial tumors spread to the pineal region from the neighboring structures and brain structures—the midbrain, thalamus, optic thalamus, quadrigeminal plate, and splenium of the corpus callosum. This series of tumors are mainly represented by astrocytomas and ependymomas. As a rule, in the group of astrocytic gliomas of the pineal region, benign forms are more common—diffusely growing gliomas of the optic thalamus or quadrigeminal plate; malignant ones (glioblastoma) are much rarer. CT and MRI characteristics of malignant astrocytomas, including glioblastoma, are characterized by various structures and types of accumulation of the contrast agent (Fig. 36.1).

36.2 Germ-Cell Tumors

Germ-cell tumors are dysembryogenetic tumors that mostly affect the reproductive organs but can also be identified within the CNS, while being usually located medially. In the central nervous system, they are more likely to occur in the pineal region, followed by the suprasellar region, and they are rarely diagnosed in the optic thalami and basal ganglia, ventricular system, cerebellum, etc. According to their histological structure, germ-cell tumors can be divided into several subtypes: germinoma, embryonal carcinoma, endodermal sinus tumor, choriocarcinoma, teratoma, and mixed tumors. Embryonal carcinoma, endodermal sinus tumor, and choriocarcinoma are regarded as non-germinal germ-cell tumors.

36.2.1 Germinomas

Germinomas are observed in up to 67% of cases among germ-cell tumors, and their typical site is the pineal region; thus, they make up about 40% of all tumors in this area, though they may also be observed in other brain regions: suprasellarly—from 25% to 35%, in the projection of the basal ganglia—up to 10% of cases. Germinomas are non-encapsulated lesions, grow usually expansively, but may have infiltrative growth. They often become calcified and have hemorrhages. Histologically, testicular germinomas are identical to seminomas and consist of cords or meshes of glycogen-containing large tumor cells with large vesicular nuclei, surrounded by a fibrous connective tissue with lymphocyte accumulations located in-between (Macko 1998).

M. Dolgushin et al., *Brain Metastases*, DOI 10.1007/978-3-319-57760-9_36

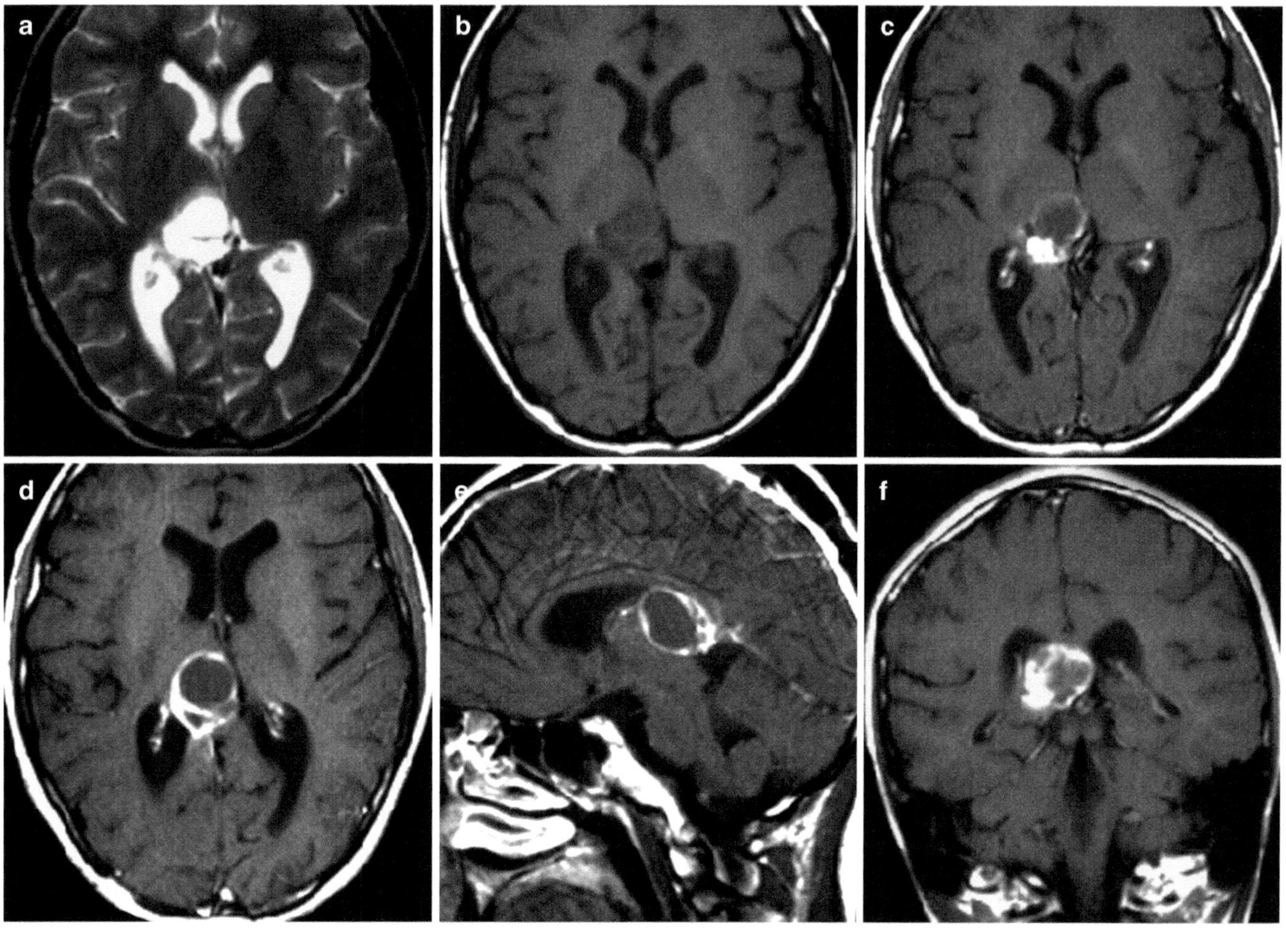

Fig. 36.1 Glioblastoma. On T2-weighted MRI (**a**) and T1-weighted MRI before (**b**) and after (**c–f**) intravenous contrast enhancement, in the projection of the right optic thalamus, there is a space-occupying lesion with a necrotic center and an intensely contrast-enhanced infiltrative peripheral part. There is no perifocal edema. The posterior sections of the third ventricle and quadrigeminal plate are deformed

On CT, germinomas have a typical location in the projection of posterior regions of the III ventricle, often with tamponade of the cisterna ambiens, and usually occlude the CSF tracts at this level by the time of the study. As a rule, germinomas look like a homogeneous (save for calcifications) and isodense lesion in relation to the brain, whose density after intravenous CA administration increases up to 50–65 HU.

MRI reveals a relatively homogeneous iso- or hypointense lesion relative to the brain in T1-weighted images and an iso- or hyperintense lesion in T2-weighted images. Around the tumor in T2-weighted images, an area with an increased signal is often visualized, presented with a reactive edema of the brain substance due to the tumor invasion. Contrast enhancement is usually pronounced, specifying the location and the extent of the tumor. MRI better than CT visualizes the quadrigeminal plate and internal cerebral veins. Germinomas tend to metastasize along the subarachnoid space, to the subependymal zone along the ventricular system and the spinal cord. At the same time, due to an unusual pattern of metastasizing of germinomas along the anterior regions of the lateral ventricles, it has a characteristic manifestation, sometimes referred to as the “ear sign” (Figs. 36.2 and 36.3).

When the tumor spreads along the spinal subarachnoid space, tumor lesions with an atypical form and structure may be formed that do not have certain differences, for example, from metastases in other organs.

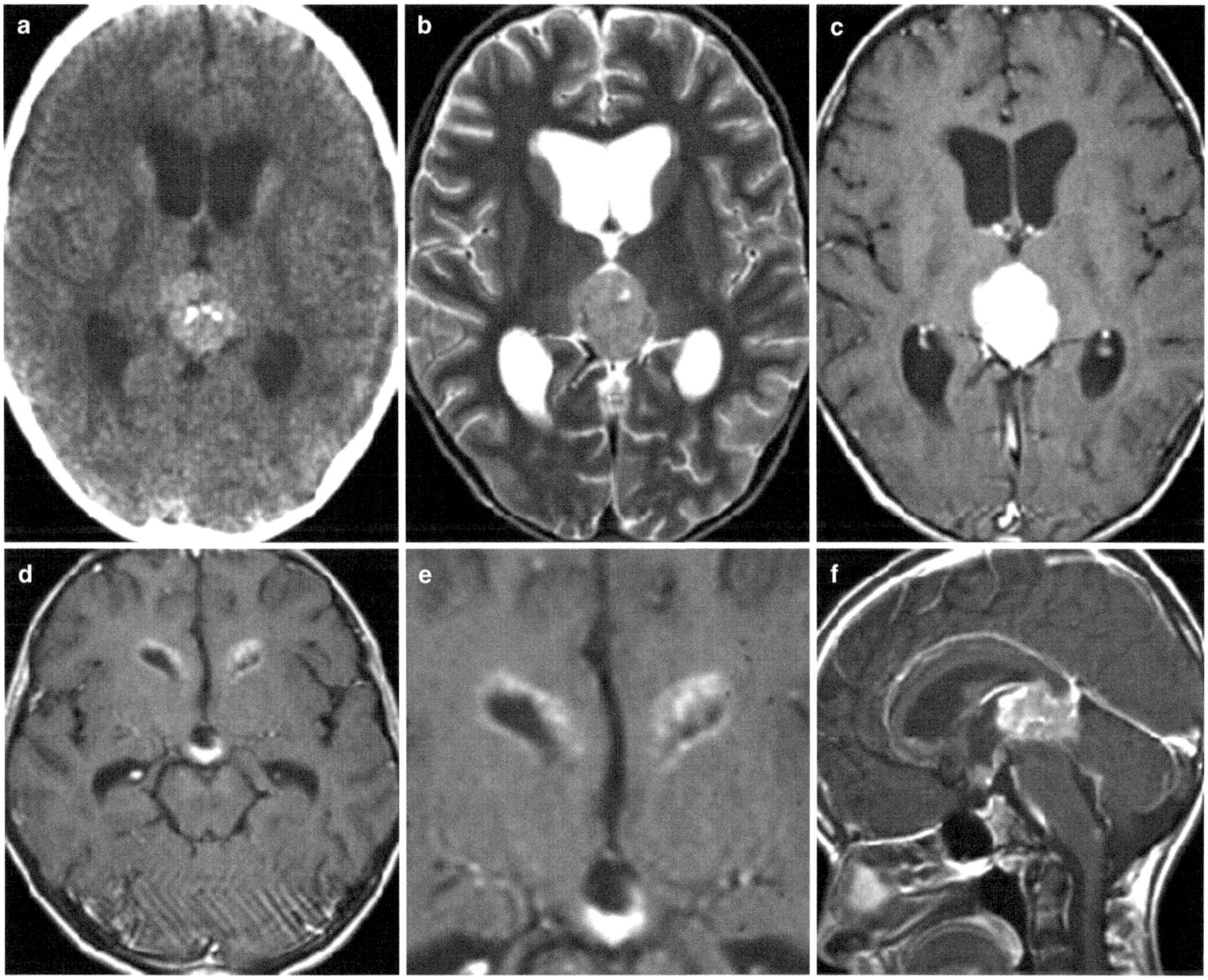

Fig. 36.2 Germinoma. On axial CT with contrast enhancement (**a**), there is a tumor with moderately high density in the pineal region with pinpoint calcified inclusions. On T2-weighted MRI (**b**), the tumor has a compact structure with a hyper-isointense signal with respect to the gray matter of the brain. On the background of contrast enhancement (**c–f**), a pronounced contrast enhancement of the tumors is observed with signs of its metastasizing along the ependyma of the ventricular system (the "ear sign" in the anterior horn of the lateral ventricles)

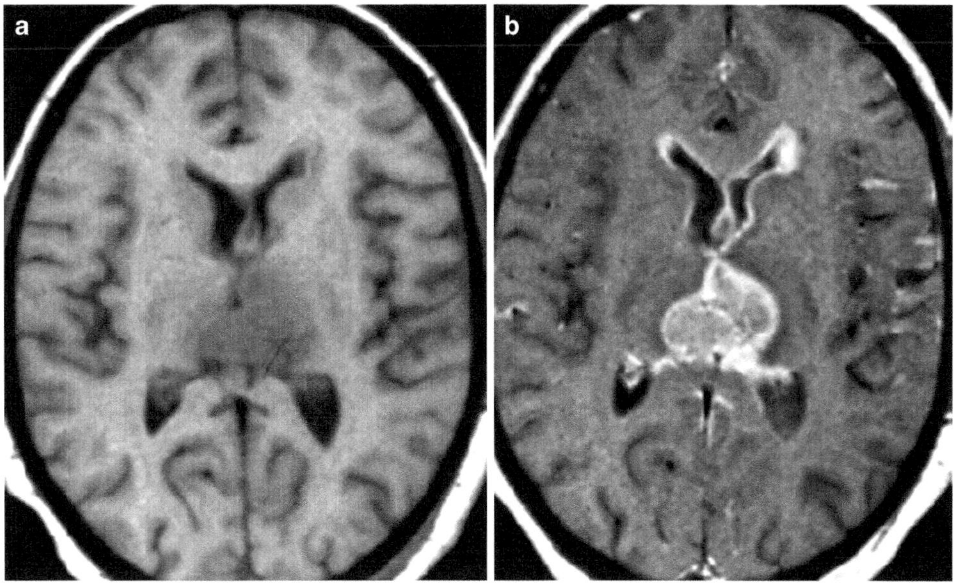

Fig. 36.3 Germinoma. On T1-weighted MRI in the axial projection (**a**), there is a space-occupying lesion with a decreased signal and with signs of infiltration of the adjacent sections of the optic thalamus in the pineal gland. After intravenous CA administration (**b**), in addition to enhancement of the signal from the pineal region tumor itself, there is widespread metastasizing along the ependyma of the ventricular system and subarachnoid spaces of the brain

36.3 Non-Germinal Germ-Cell Brain Tumors

Non-germinal germ-cell brain tumors are relatively rare malignancies of the brain. Their characteristic feature is production of specific tumor markers — alpha-fetoprotein and human chorionic gonadotropin.

36.3.1 Choriocarcinoma

Choriocarcinoma is the most rare among germ-cell tumors of the pineal region. Distinguished by high malignancy and invasive growth, they have a less favorable prognosis.

CT and MRI manifestations of the tumor are nonspecific. There is only their high vascularization with typical MR characteristics for subacute hemorrhages (Fig. 36.4). Increasing the level of human chorionic gonadotropin in the serum and cerebrospinal fluid is an important additional differential diagnostic criterion.

36.4 Mixed Germ-Cell Tumors

Mixed germ-cell tumors occur more frequently than the group of malignancies mentioned above and contain elements of these tumors. CT and MRI manifestations are nonspecific and are indistinguishable within this histological category of brain tumors. Areas of cystic degeneration, calcificates, and hemorrhages are identified. Contrast enhancement is expressed and heterogeneous. Typical signs are rapid growth, extensive invasion of the surrounding brain structures, and metastasizing (up to 30%) along the ependyma, lateral ventricles, and subarachnoid space (Fig. 36.5). However, in the early stages of the disease, tumors may be small.

As noted above, the differential diagnosis between different histological types of tumors of the pineal region is difficult. The MRI signal characteristics and CT density of tumors often overlap. The only exceptions are dermoids, lipomas, and teratomas that have manifestations differing from those of other lesions. Quadrigeminal plate gliomas cause its thickening and deformation with sings of obstruction of the cerebral aqueduct; contrast enhancement is not typical for them. Gliomas, growing into the pineal region, have a tendency to displacement of formations of posterior portions of the third ventricle and asymmetrical positioning with respect to the midline. The presence of a calcification in the pineal gland does not allow to perform the differential diagnosis, as it can occur both in germ-cell and parenchymal tumors of the pineal region.

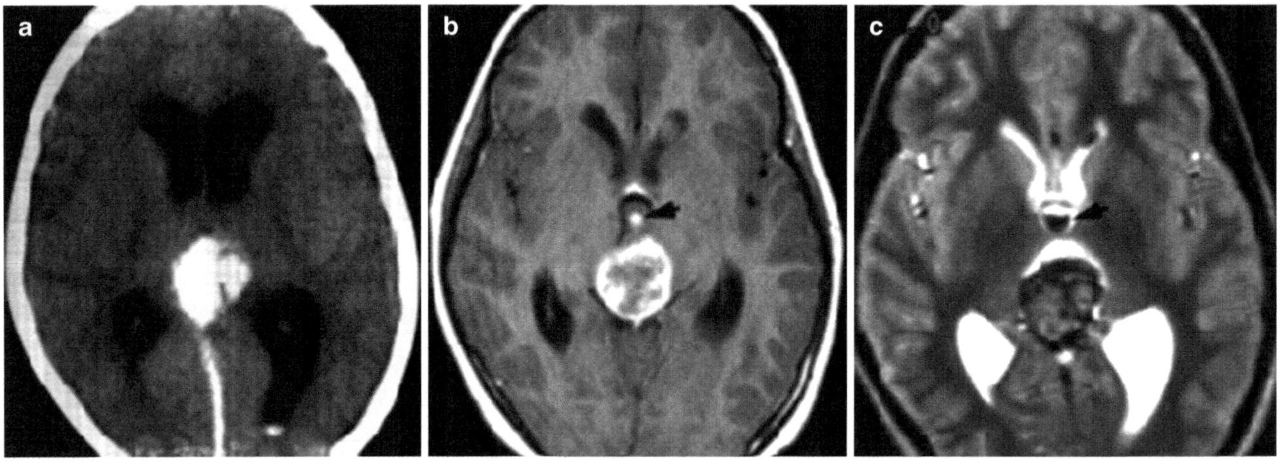

Fig. 36.4 Choriocarcinoma. On axial CT (**a**) without contrast enhancement, there is a tumor lesion with high density in the projection of posterior portions of the third ventricle. The lateral ventricles are dilated along the falx cerebri, and accumulation of fresh blood is visualized in the dorsal horn of the left lateral ventricle. On T1- (**b**) and T2-weighted MRI (**c**), there is a rounded lesion with traces of a fresh and subacute hemorrhage

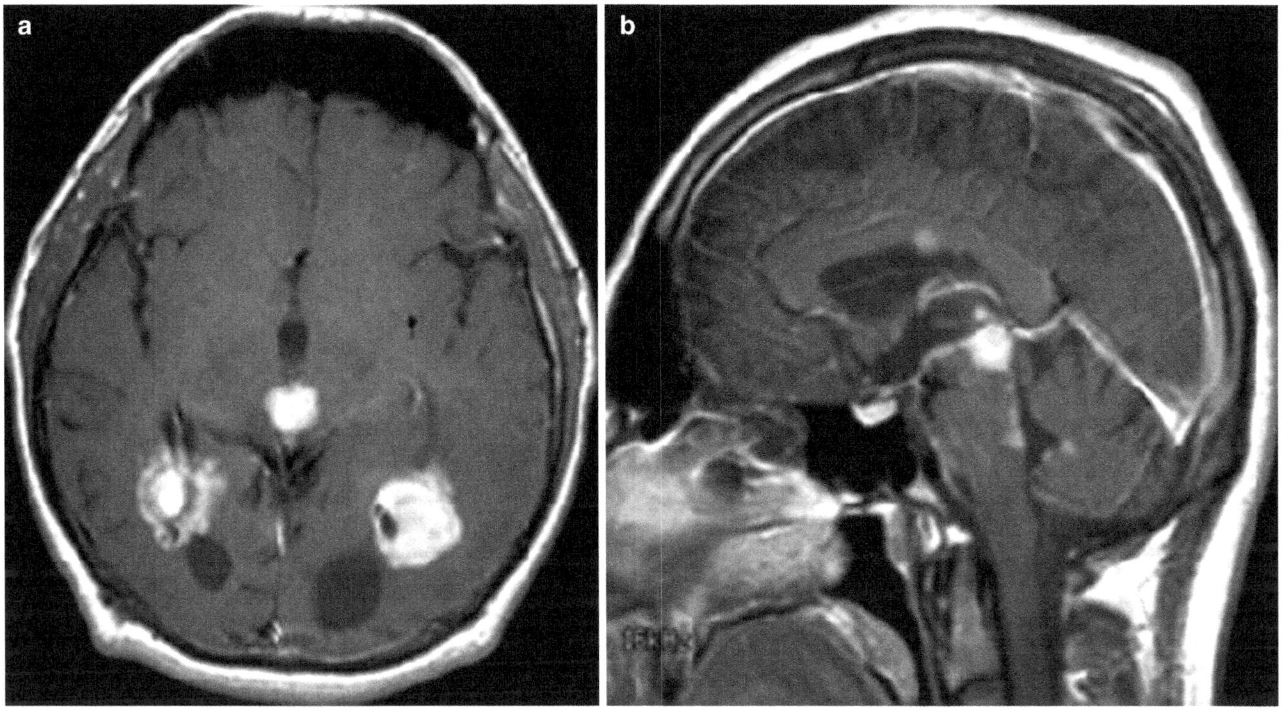

Fig. 36.5 A malignant mixed germ-cell tumor. On T1-weighted MRI, there are multiple tumor lesions (**a**) intensely accumulating the contrast agent in the projection of the lateral ventricles and the pineal region. On sagittal images, signs of metastasizing along the ependyma of the lateral and fourth ventricles are further visualized (**b**)

Orbital Tumors

37

According to publications, more than 100 different types of lesions can develop in the orbit (Rootman 1988; Baert 2006). The main role in the diagnosis of orbital lesions plays the analysis of history and clinical symptoms, and only a small proportion of cases requires neuroradiological studies to clarify the diagnosis. CT examinations of the orbit use mainly thin-slice helical scanning with reformations in the plane of interest. The use of CT perfusion imaging became a new approach in the diagnosis of orbital lesions, which opened a new era in the evaluation of hemodynamics of orbital tumors. MRI studies of the orbit are distinguished by the mandatory use of fat suppression techniques, both before and after intravenous contrast enhancement. Preference is given to T2- and T1-weighted sequences with thin 3-millimeter slices, directed along the course of the optic nerves in the axial, sagittal, and oblique views. Frontal projections should be oriented perpendicularly to the optic nerve; therefore, they are performed at least twice. Metastasizing of malignant tumors to the orbit is an uncommon event; however, attention should be paid to this area in melanoma and breast cancer.

37.1 Neurofibromas (NF)

Neurofibromas (NF) can be solitary, plexiform, and diffuse. Solitary NF usually develops in adults, while plexiform NF (typical for type I neurofibromatosis) develops within the first 5 years of life (Brovkina 1993). Plexiform (or reticular) neurofibromas are the most frequent in the orbit.

On CT, a single NF looks like a rounded, oblong, or oval encapsulated formation with the density close to that of the brain tissue, but this pattern, in general, is nonspecific; it has a medium degree of contrast enhancement.

On MR, NF has a homogeneous structure with irregular outlines: the tumor is usually represented by an infiltrative mass with irregular contours, which sometimes infiltrate the orbital adipose tissue. It is homogeneous and iso- or hypointense relative to the muscle tissue in T1-weighted images. On T2-weighted images, it can be homogeneously hyperintense or show a so-called target sign—a hypointense signal from the central area of the tumor, surrounded by a hyperintense rim. The contrast agent is accumulated heterogeneously in NF, and tumors can be indistinguishable from neuromas by the contrast enhancement pattern (Fig. 37.1).

Neurofibroma malignizes less often than neuroma. Malignization usually occurs in patients with type I neurofibromatosis. In the case of malignization, they become more aggressive and may grow intracranially.

37.2 Glioma of the Optic Nerve

Glioma of the optic nerve is often a benign, slow-growing tumor, amounting to 66% of all primary tumors of the optic nerve. In 65% of cases, glioma develops within the first decade of life, but only 5% of gliomas are detected before 2 years of age. According to Shields (1998), gliomas account for 1–2% of all orbital tumors, while according to Baert (2006), up to 4%. Women are affected more often than men (3:2). 30–40% of patients with gliomas have manifestations of NF I, and 15% of patients with NF I have an optic nerve glioma.

On CT, glioma of the optic nerve is usually visualized as a spherical, spindle-shaped, or lobular space-occupying lesion growing along the optic nerve. Its lobulation is caused by convolutions of the dilating optic nerve. The tumor spreads to the optic canal and into the cranial cavity, causing the dilation of the optic canal, and is easily detected by CT. Typically, the density of optic nerve gliomas on CT ranges from 25 to 60 HU.

Pilocytic astrocytomas, compared to other gliomas, are characterized by higher CBV and CBF values (Fig. 37.2). Fibrillary astrocytomas have basic hemodynamic parameters similar to those of the white matter of the brain.

According to MRI, the tumor has an isointense or slightly hypointense signal in T1-weighted images, as compared to the brain tissue, and a combination of an isointense signal in

M. Dolgushin et al., *Brain Metastases*, DOI 10.1007/978-3-319-57760-9_37

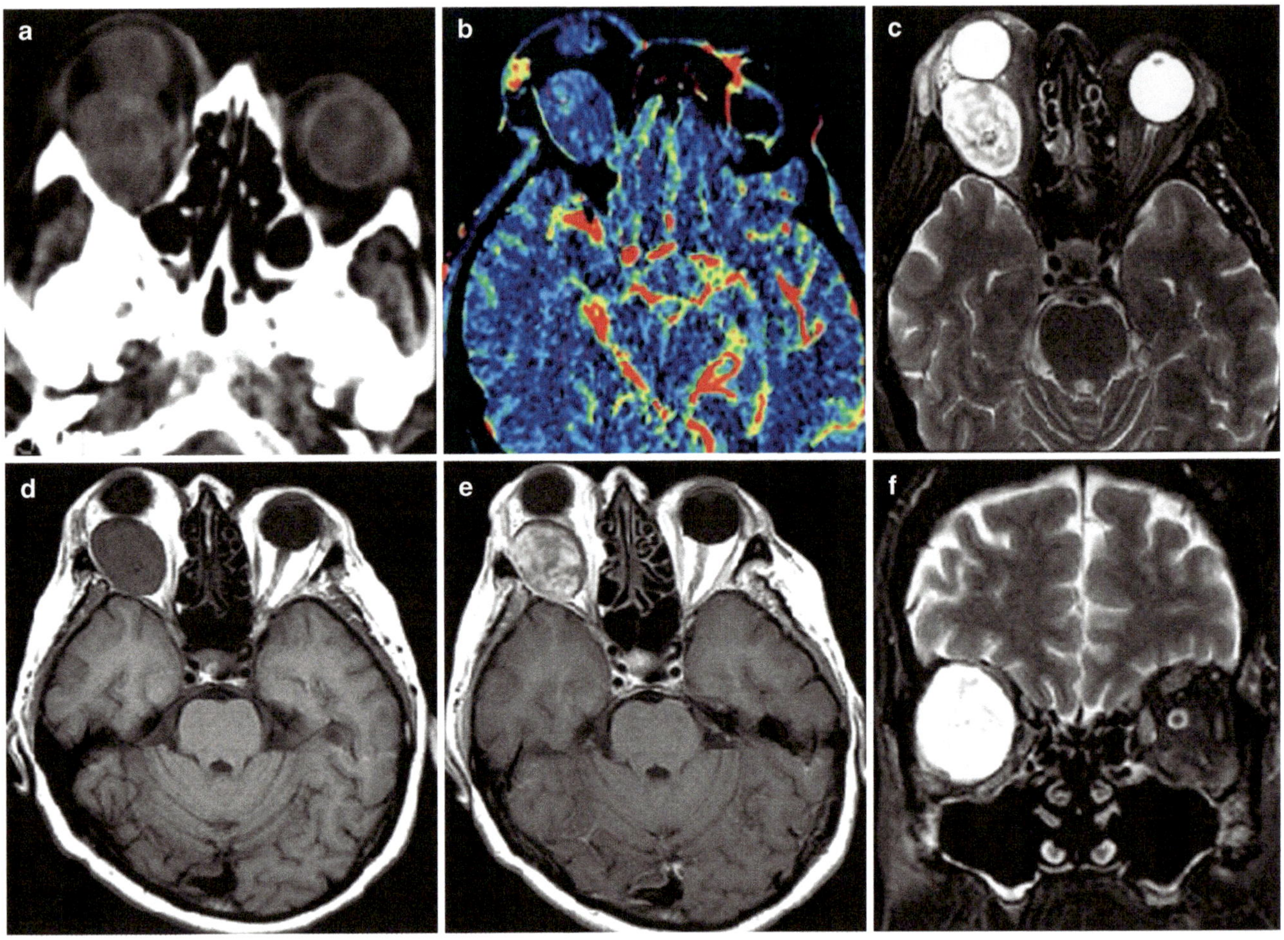

Fig. 37.1 Neurofibroma. On CT (**a**) in the right orbit, there is a large isodense tumor causing severe exophthalmos. Based on CT perfusion findings (**b**), hemodynamic parameters in the tumor (CBV) are not increased as compared to the white substance. On T2-weighted (**c**, **f**) and T1-weighted MRI (**d**), an encapsulated tumor is detected with a heterogeneous structure of the MR signal (hyperintense in T2-weighted images and a decreased signal in T1-weighted images). On T1-weighted MRI with contrast enhancement, there is intense, uneven accumulation of the contrast agent in the tumor (**e**)

the center and a hyperintense signal in the peripheral regions in T2-weighted images. There are hyperintense foci in the glioma structure due to small cysts. T2-weighted imaging successfully detects the tumor spread along the optic tracts, even in cases where CT with contrast enhancement fails to detect these changes. T1-weighted fat sat sequence achieves a clearer visualization of tumors, especially if they accumulate a contrast agent. Contrast enhancement varies from mild to intense; however, its use is advisable in all cases.

37.3 Sheath Meningioma

Sheath meningioma makes up about 1/3 of the primary tumors of the optic nerve and about 5% of primary tumors of the orbit. The source of growth for meningiomas at this site is arachnoid villi between the solid and arachnoid sheaths.

CT shows a thickened optic nerve (up to a four- to sixfold increase in the diameter); eccentric tumor growth is possible with local thickening along the optic nerve. There may be both single and multiple calcifications. Intense contrast enhancement (40–45 HU) of the tumor is a typical characteristic of meningiomas.

The MR picture may vary depending on the histological subtype of the tumor. Meningioma may be isointense as compared to muscles in T1-weighted images and isointense or hyperintense in T2-weighted images. The use of fat suppression techniques and contrast enhancement is most effective for detecting optic nerve meningiomas. In most cases meningiomas are intensely contrast-enhanced, and only in one quarter of cases contrast material accumulation is weak (Fig. 37.3).

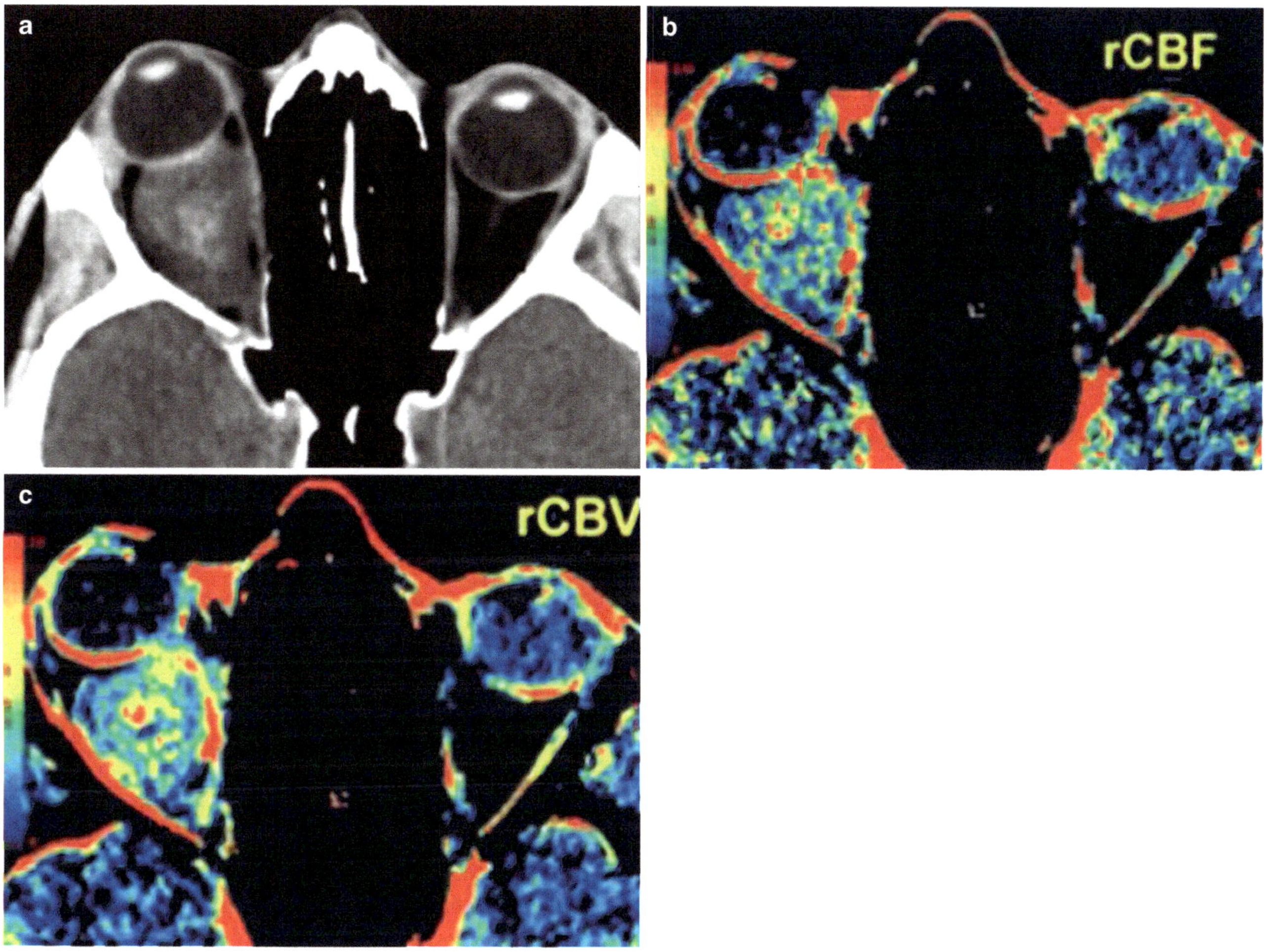

Fig. 37.2 Right-sided optic nerve glioma. On the CT scan in axial projection (**a**), there is a large heterogeneous tumor with a hyperdense site in the center. CT perfusion parameters are heterogeneous. An increase in the blood flow velocity (**b**) and volume (**c**) is observed primarily in the central parts of the tumor

37.4 Orbital Cancer

Among malignant orbital tumors, the most common are orbital sarcomas and lacrimal gland cancer, which constitute 13–16% of all tumors of the orbit. Lacrimal gland cancer occurs mainly at the age of 40–50 years. Its main morphological forms are adenoid cystic carcinoma (50–60%), malignant mixed tumor (34–48%), and adenocarcinoma (less than 20%). Primary orbital cancer also occurs. A tumor can be regarded as a result of the transformation of dystopic epithelial cells during embryogenesis. The tumor grows without a capsule, has a stringy structure, and is dense and whitish. Primary orbital cancer occurs twice less frequently than sarcomas (Brovkina 2008). Sarcomas are located intra- and extraconally in 47% of cases.

Primary orbital cancer and sarcoma have clear boundaries, irregular shape, and bone destruction on CT. Sarcomas are isointense in relation to muscles in T1-weighted MR images, while in T2-weighted images, they are hypointense and rarely have a heterogeneous signal. The eyeball is often affected. Contrast enhancement is moderate; the recommended sequence is one with fat suppression and contrast enhancement (Fig. 37.4).

37.5 Primary Orbital Melanoma

Primary malignant melanomas of the ciliary body (10%), choroid (85%), and iris (5%) are relatively rare. The majority of patients with secondary tumors underwent an enucleation or evisceration of one eye. The tumor recurred within one year in 50% of cases. The prognosis is generally poor due to frequent metastases (Atlas 1987). Tumor development is possible from the blue nevus, ectopic melanocytes, and congenital peridermal melanosis (Brovkina 2008). Eye melanoma can metastasize to the liver, lungs, kidneys, and brain. Elderly people suffer more often, with the average age of 53 years. The disease is diagnosed in men and

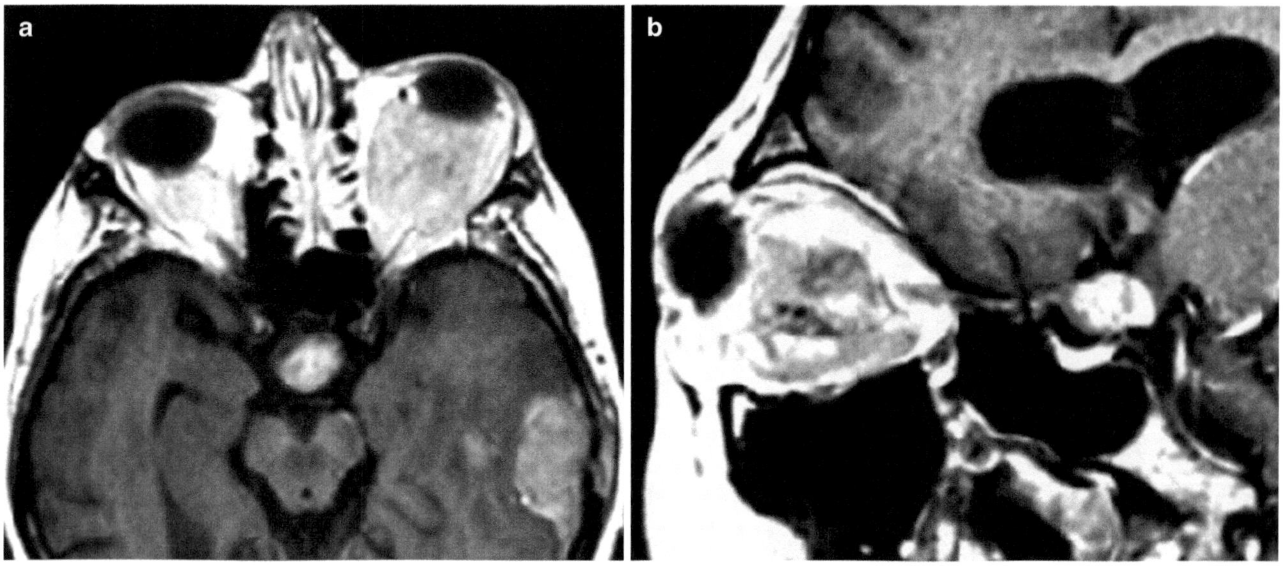

Fig. 37.3 Multiple meningiomas. On MRI in the axial (**a**) and oblique sagittal (**b**) projections on the background of intravenous contrast enhancement on T1-weighted MRI, there are bilateral intraorbital tumor lesions with formation of exophthalmos on the left, in the lesion depth; the optic nerve is tight. In addition, space-occupying lesions are detected in the tuberculum sellae and convexital departments of the left temporal region

women with an equal frequency. Northern Europeans are more prone to the disease, the disease being extremely rare in Africans.

In general, eye melanoma has similar CT and MRI characteristics with secondary metastatic melanomas in the brain. On CT, melanoma is hyperdense and sharply demarcated. The tumor diffusely accumulates the contrast agent (Fig. 37.5). The tumor is moderately to significantly hyperintense in T1-weighted images. Melanomas are hypointense in T2-weighted images. The tumor diffusely accumulates the contrast agent in T1-weighted images with contrast enhancement (Motoyama 2011).

On a PET study, melanoma is always characterized by an intense accumulation of radiopharmaceuticals, including expressed accumulation of ^{18}F-FDG. It is important to remember that whole-body PET scans should be performed in melanoma, including the extremities, since it allows to detect distant metastases (Fig. 37.6).

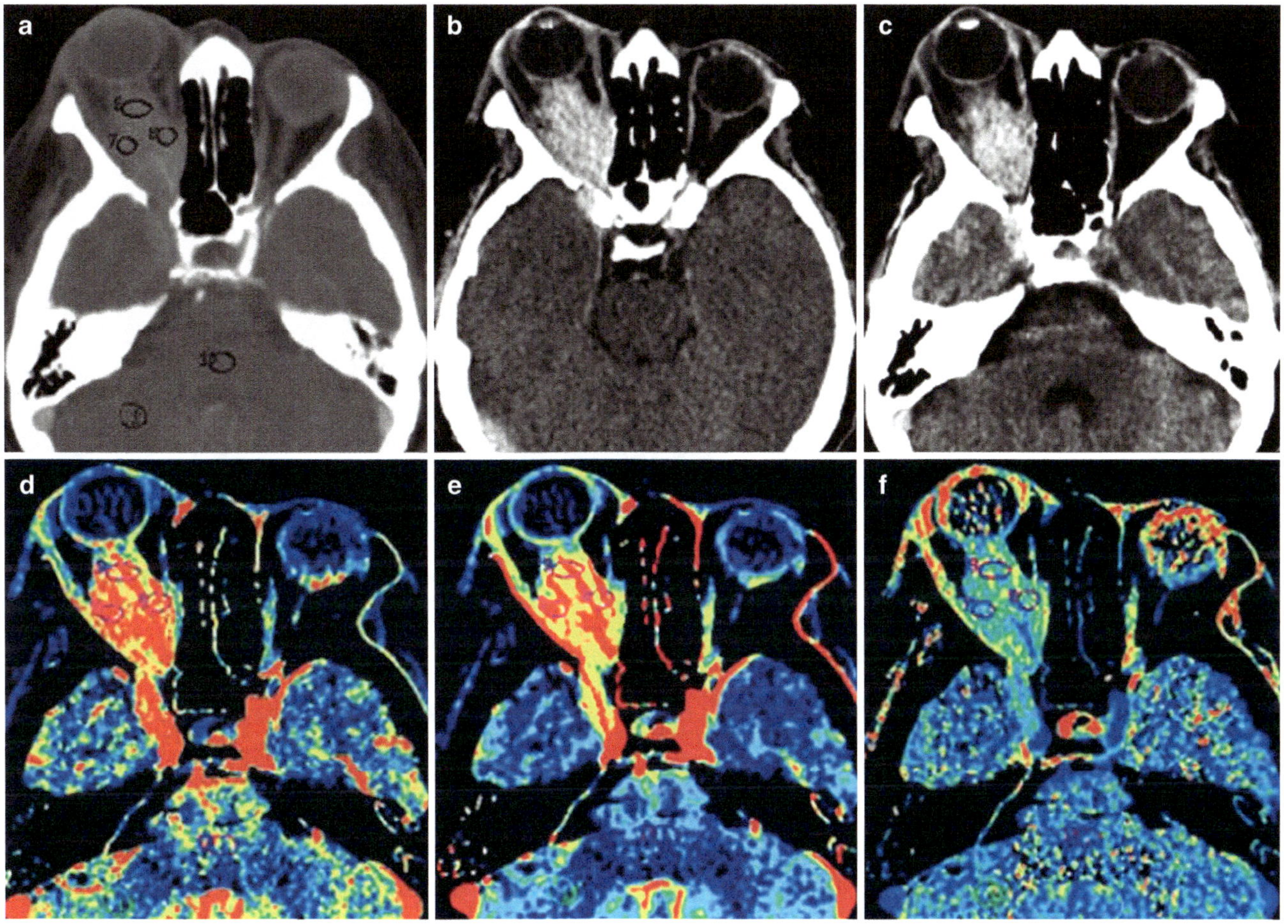

Fig. 37.4 Right-sided orbital cancer. On CT scan in axial projection with contrast enhancement at two levels (**a–c**) in the bone (**a**) and brain modes (**b**, **c**), a local destruction of the medial orbital wall with tumor invasion, which intensely accumulates the contrast agent, has high hemodynamic parameters during CT perfusion studies of CBF (**d**) and CBV (**e**) and an increase in MTT values (**f**)

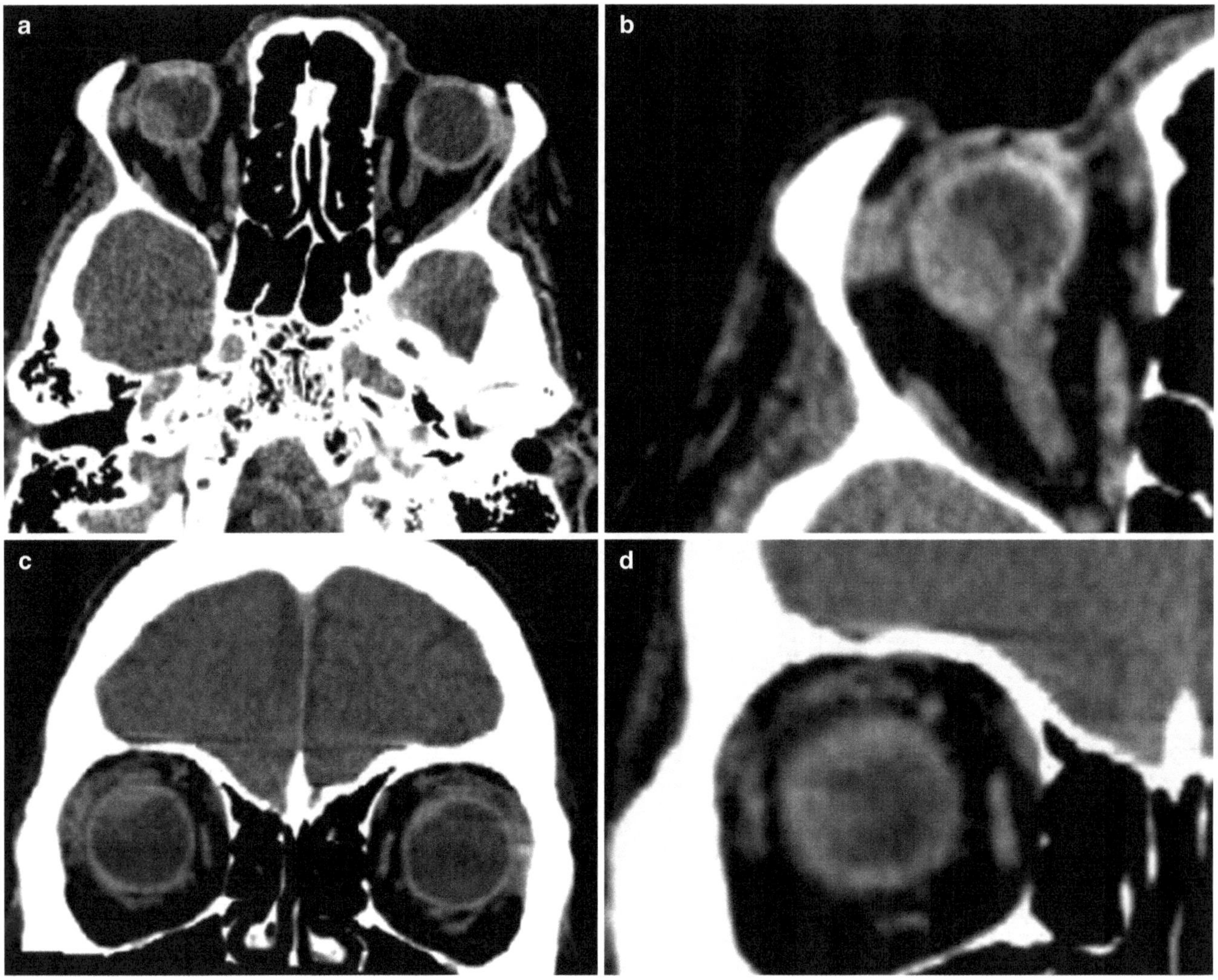

Fig. 37.5 Primary eye melanoma. On the axial (**a**, **b**) and frontal (**c**, **d**) CT in the projection of the eyeballs, there are well-visualized lenticular hyperdense lesions with clear contours. The eyeballs are not enlarged. There is no exophthalmos

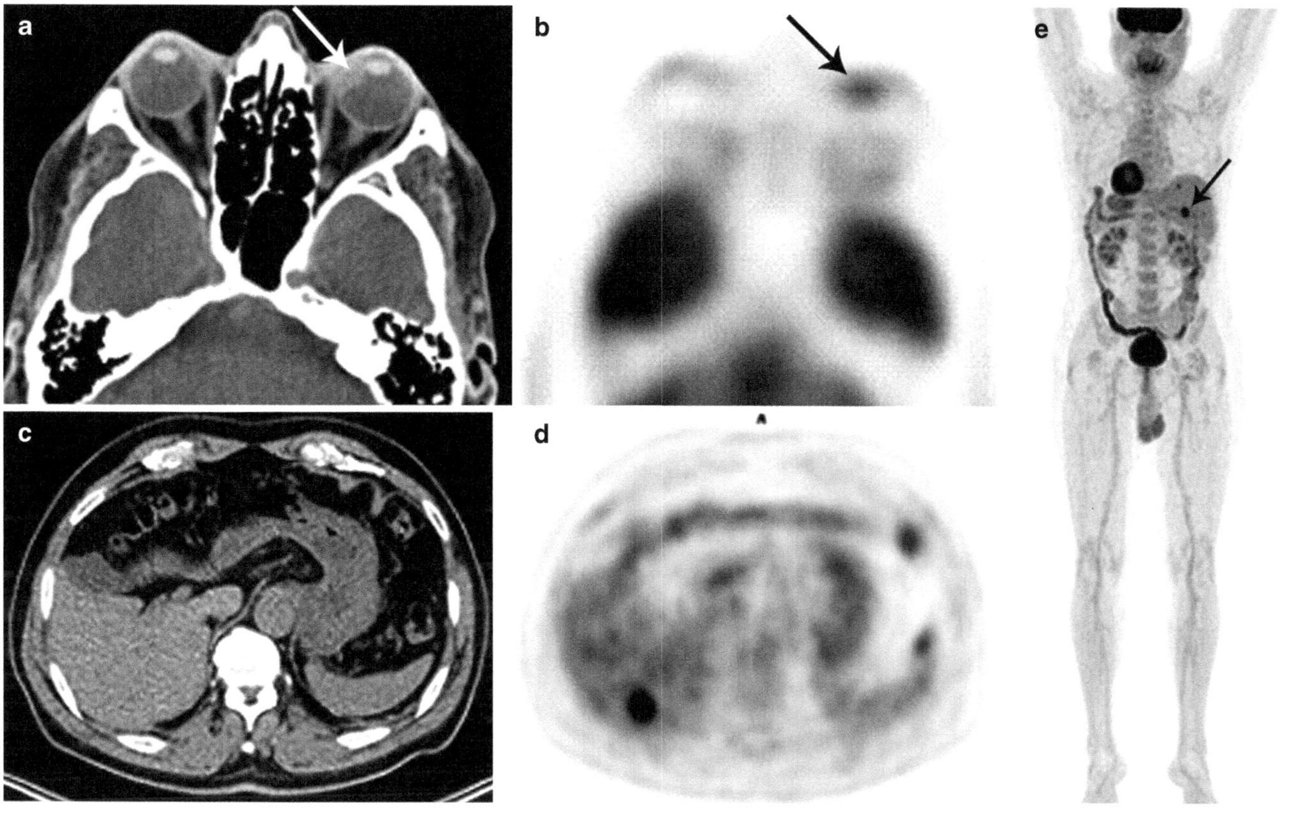

Fig. 37.6 Primary eye melanoma. On brain CT in the axial projection (**a**), along the medial contour of the eyeball, there is a lesion with high density (the *arrow*). On whole-body PET/CT with 18F-FDG in the projection of the medial contour of the left eyeball (**b**) and the liver (**c**, **d**, **e**), there are space-occupying lesions intensely accumulating RP (the *arrows*)

38 Orbital Sarcoidosis

Orbital sarcoidosis is a chronic multisystem granulomatous disease involving all organ systems. In case of systemic involvement, clinical manifestations of sarcoidosis occur in the CNS in 10% of cases (Mafee and Dorodi 1999). Typical features of the lacrimal gland involvement include an increase in its size, painless at palpation, and dry eyes. In case of involvement of the anterior chamber of the eye, symptoms include soreness, conjunctivitis, and uveitis; and involvement of the posterior chamber results to perivasculitis, infiltrates in the vitreous body and retinal changes, eyeball movement limitation, and diplopia. The optic nerve involvement manifests by perineuritis, papillitis, and loss of vision (Kellinghaus et al. 2004). Sarcoidosis more often occurs in adults aged from 30 to 50 years old, predominantly in women. It is ten times more frequently diagnosed among aborigines of the African deserts. Also, the disease is common in Puerto Ricans, Irish, and Scandinavians (Brovkina 2008).

An isodense increase in the nerve diameter is observed on CT before administration of the contrast material. After contrast enhancement, abnormal accumulation of the contrast agent by the optic nerve and other intraorbital structures is identified. In addition, IV contrast enhancement shows an increase of the lacrimal gland and diffuse irregular thickening of the extraocular muscles.

T1-weighted MRI sequences reveal an isointense enlargement of intraorbital structures. On T2-weighted images, hypointense (relative to normal muscle) or slightly hyperintense abnormal intraorbital masses can be visualized. T2 -FLAIR sequence can demonstrate sarcoidal parenchymal lesions in the brain. The optic nerve affected by orbital sarcoidosis and intraorbital granulomatous masses intensely accumulates the contrast agent. Contrast enhancement of the lacrimal gland and orbital muscles is also more pronounced than normal. In case of the CNS involvement, MRI shows contrast-enhanced intracranial cisternal and parenchymal lesions. Optimal scanning: study with contrast enhancement and suppression of fat MR signal. Not only the orbit should be examined but also the whole brain in order to identify other foci of sarcoidosis (Figs. 38.1 and 38.2).

Thus, the most informative method of differential diagnosis of tumors in the orbital area is CT perfusion, which allows to exclude a range of tumors characterized by relatively low flow rates. Also, metastatic involvement is characterized by the formation of nodular forms, while infiltrative spread of metastases to the oculomotor muscles is rare.

M. Dolgushin et al., *Brain Metastases*, DOI 10.1007/978-3-319-57760-9_38

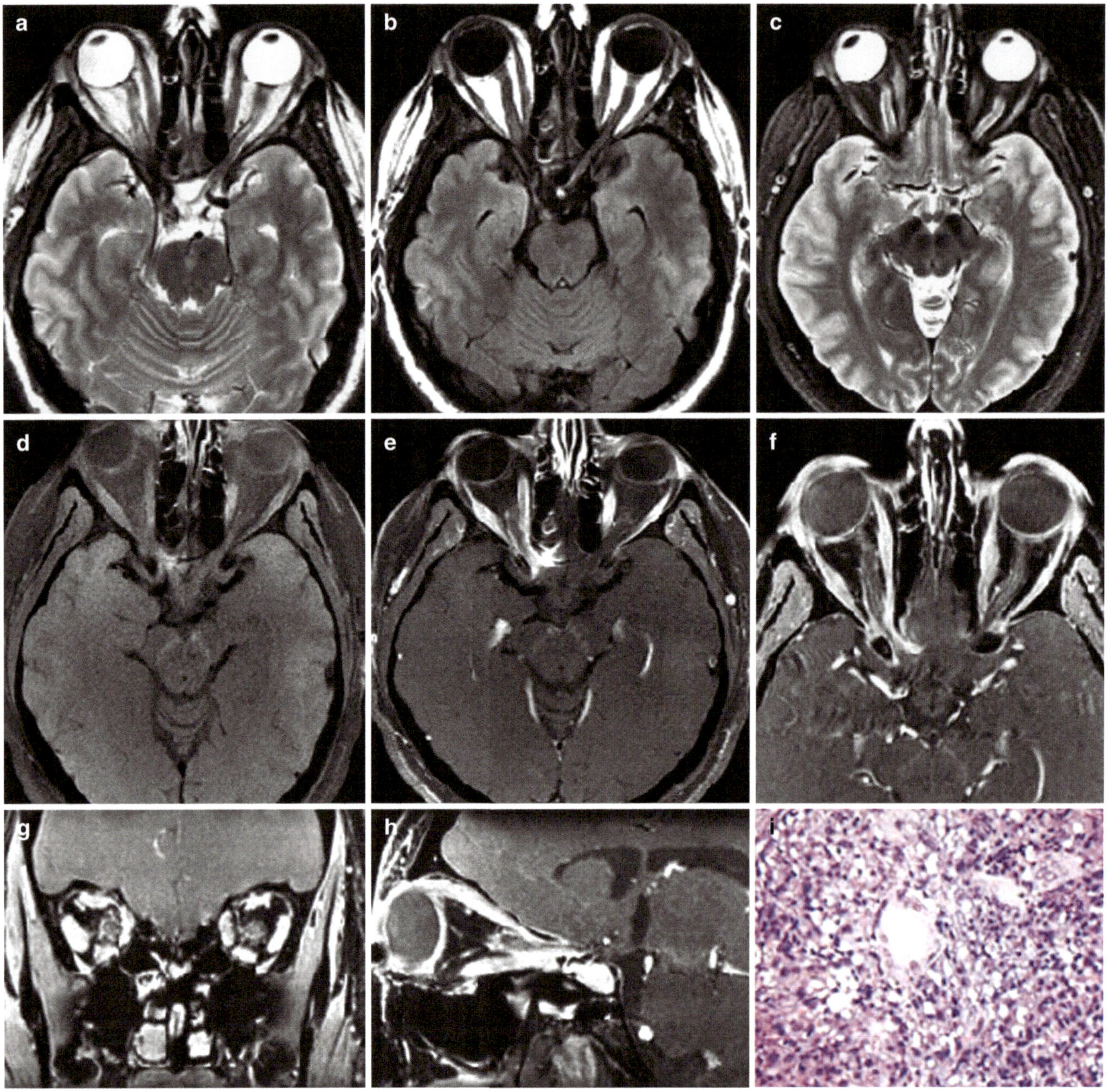

Fig. 38.1 Sarcoidosis. MRI of the orbits in T2-weighted (**a**), T2-FLAIR (**b**), T2 fat sat (**c**), and T1 fat sat (**d**) sequences shows uneven thickening of the medial and lateral rectus muscles of the right orbit. Following intravenous CA administration, abnormal contrast enhancement of the optic nerve membranes is observed with the spread to the optic nerve and the right optic canal and the spread along the meninges in the area of the frontal clinoid and the body of the sphenoid bone (**e–h**). Histological specimen (**i**)

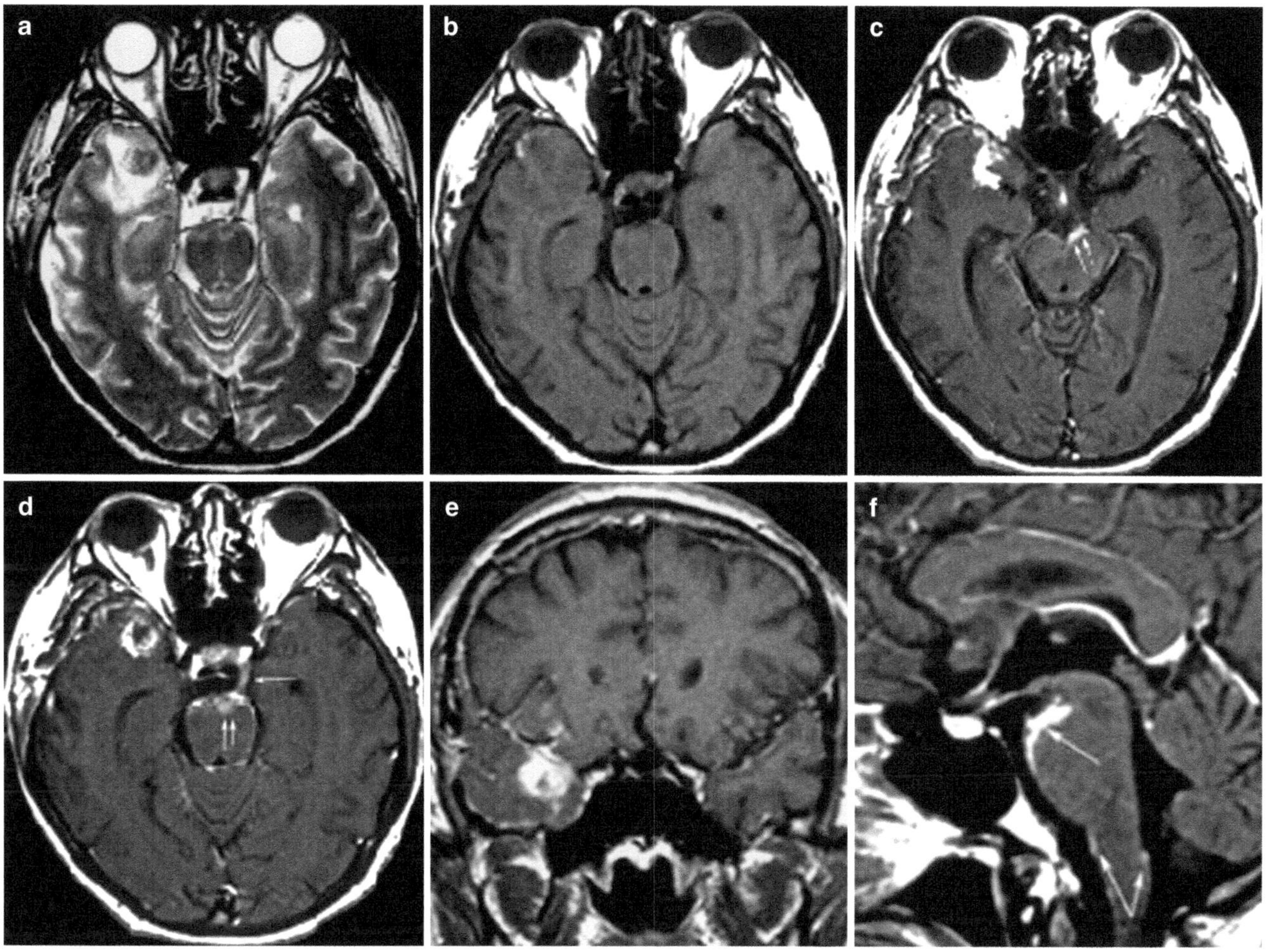

Fig. 38.2 Sarcoidosis. On T2-weighted (**a**) and T1-weighted MRI (**b**), an area with a nonuniform signal change is identified in the right temporal basal area with the sings of perifocal edema. After intravenous CA administration in T1-weighted MRI, in the axial (**c**, **d**), frontal (**e**), and sagittal (**f**) scans, sites of the contrast agent accumulation are visualized in the right temporal region and a contrast-enhanced site along the meninges of the brainstem and cranial nerves (*arrows*)

Intracranial Infection

39

According to many researchers, an increase of infectious and parasitic diseases of the central nervous system has been noted worldwide, despite the emergence of new therapies and the establishment of antimicrobial and anti-inflammatory pharmaceuticals (Yakhno and Shtulman 2001; Whiteman et al. 2002). This increase is partly attributed to the spread of acquired immunodeficiency syndrome (AIDS), as well as the use of immune-suppressing drugs to treat cancer and to perform organ transplants. Emergence of life-threatening infectious diseases of the central nervous system may be associated with a number of adverse factors, such as staying in the focus of infection, presence of an open head injury, cerebrospinal fluid leakage, sinusitis, otitis media, etc., especially in a compromised immune system. In these cases of decisive importance is early diagnosis of the disease. Such imaging methods as CT and MRI are particularly important for a comprehensive neurologic and laboratory (CSF analysis) investigation.

39.1 Bacterial Infection

A variety of pathogenic agents (bacterial, viral, fungal, and parasitic) may penetrate into the brain tissue through the blood or via a direct contact with the source of infection. Characteristics of the brain structure—absence of lymphocytes, a small number of capillaries in the subarachnoid space, and the presence of perivascular cerebrospinal fluid spaces—may result in an inflammatory reaction caused by pathogens entering the intracranial or intravertebral spaces. CSF, in particular, is an excellent medium for dissemination of an infectious process. Pathogens can penetrate the brain tissue and induce focal (abscesses, cysts) or diffuse (encephalitis) lesions and inflammation of the meninges (meningitis, ependymitis, arachnoiditis) or cerebrospinal fluid spaces (subdural and epidural empyema).

Inflammation of the brain and its membranes is usually accompanied by intense abnormal accumulation of the contrast agent in CT and MRI images. In cases of encysted and multiple lesions, the X-ray picture is similar to that in metastases.

Brain abscesses are a relatively rare intracranial pathology accounting for, according to different sources, 1–8% depending on the level of economic development of the country, where the study was carried out (Bhatia et al. 1973; Osenbach and Loftus 1992). The growing number of patients with HIV infection resulted in an increased incidence of brain abscesses. The male to female ratio is 2:1, while the average age of onset is 35–45 years. In 25% of cases, brain abscesses develop in children and adolescents younger than 15 years of age. Until 2 years of age, brain abscess is rarely diagnosed, mainly after meningitis caused by *Citrobacter diversus* or other gram-negative bacteria.

In adults, brain abscesses developing due to hematogenous metastasizing most often are caused by anaerobic bacteria or a mixture of aerobic and anaerobic bacteria. In children, the most common pathogens are staphylococci, streptococci, and pneumococci. In patients with head trauma or those undergoing surgery, abscesses are typically caused by *Staphylococcus aureus*.

Predisposing factors for the development of brain abscesses are chronic lung infections, osteomyelitis, cholecystitis, gastrointestinal infection, and purulent skin diseases (furunculosis, etc.). Therefore, inflammatory emboli carried over from the extracranial structures may be called "infectious metastases."

Standard CT and MRI methods used in the differential diagnosis of cerebral space-occupying lesions have high sensitivity (95%) but low specificity (50–60%); it is not always possible to give a definite answer about the origin of an abnormal intracranial lesion. The use of additional CT-MRI perfusion and MR-diffusion methods, as well as MR spectroscopy increases the specificity and provides the possibility to avoid diagnostic errors in the diagnosis (Chang et al. 2002; Fertikh et al. 2007; Kastrup et al. 2008; Chiang et al. 2009; Shetty et al. 2010; Pal et al. 2010; Hsu et al. 2013; Ozbayrak et al. 2015).

M. Dolgushin et al., *Brain Metastases*, DOI 10.1007/978-3-319-57760-9_39

On T2-weighted MRI, early cerebrosides are visualized as areas of increased signal intensity, weakly or virtually indistinguishable from the surrounding edema. Proton density-weighted MR images and T2-weighted and T2-FLAIR MR images allow to detect cerebritis earlier than CT, visualizing initial changes in the brain. On T1-weighted MRI, cerebritis appears isointense or hypointense relative to the intact brain tissue, with a possible mass effect, which manifests in the compression of gyri and/or the adjacent ventricle. On T1-weighted MRI, lesions with subacute microhemorrhages in the affected area as hyperintense areas relative to the normal or edematous brain substance. Contrast enhancement is usually slightly pronounced and inhomogeneous in the earliest stage. On CT, the affected area can be either undetected or visualized as the area with decreased density without clear boundaries with the brain.

A cerebritis focus eventually transforms into an abscess in its central portion of the liquid necrosis areas, which is well visualized on CT and particularly on MRI and is limited by a collagenous capsule (Fig. 39.1).

The most characteristic CT and MRI feature of a formed abscess is a rounded lesion with a thin-walled capsule, intensely accumulating the contrast agent (a "ring" phenomenon), with clear and smooth inner contours (Fig. 39.2).

In typical cases, the central part of the abscess has a reduced density on CT and a heterogeneously modified MR signal on MRI, increased on T2-weighted MRI and decreased on T1-weighted MRI relative to the brain. Thus, on T1-weighted MRI, the signal from the abscess center is always higher than that from the cerebrospinal fluid in the lateral ventricles. On T2-weighted MRI, the signal intensity varies depending on the choice of the echo time (TE) in the spin echo pulse sequence, protein composition, and viscosity of the central cavity contents.

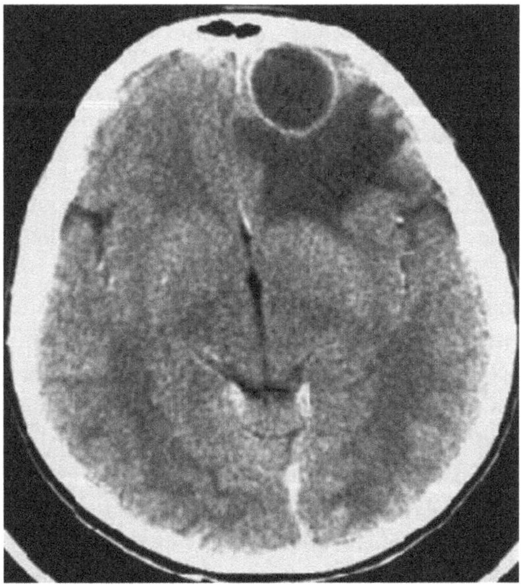

Fig. 39.1 An abscess. On CT with contrast enhancement, in the left frontal area, there is a rounded space-occupying lesion with a thin capsule and a pronounced perifocal edema

On non-contrast enhanced MRI, a mature abscess often has a distinctive rim around its edge. The signal on the edge of an abscess is isointense or slightly hyperintense than the signal of the white matter on T1-weighted MRI and hyperintense on T2-weighted MRI. Properties of the MR signal on the abscess edge are associated with collagen, products of hemorrhages, and the presence of paramagnetic free radicals in macrophages involved in the phagocytosis and heterogeneously distributed along the abscess periphery (Lai et al. 2005). With successful surgical or therapeutic treatment of the abscess and a decrease in the activity of phagocytes, the hyperintensive rim on T1-weighted MRI degrades. Thus, the presence of the rim may serve as a better indicator of the treatment course than the residual contrast enhancement that can be observed on MRI with contrast enhancement for several months after the treatment.

Multiple abscesses are rare (Fig. 39.3). A supratentorial location is typical for brain abscesses. In practice, however, abscesses in the posterior fossa also can be encountered.

DWI MRI usually reveals a marked increase in the MR signal from the central parts of the abscess (purulent-necrotic area), indicating a decrease in the diffusion of water molecules in the specified area. ADC values in the central zone and capsule of the abscess are significantly lower ($p < 0.005$) than in the white matter of the brain (Table. 39.1) with diffusion factor of $b = 500$ and $b = 1000$ s/mm^2.

Table 39.1 compares the ADC values inside the annular contrast-enhancement area of abscesses and glioblastomas. In patients with glioblastomas, the necrotic area in the center of the tumor had higher ADC values than in abscesses.

The reason for limited movement of the water molecules in the central portion of the abscess is primarily attributed to the presence of pus, having a high viscosity and containing large amounts of cellular components and debris. Ebisu et al. (1996), studying in vitro the pus aspirated from the abscess, found an increase in MR signal on DWI and low ADC values on ADC maps.

At the same time, it should be noted that not every abscess content has low values on ADC maps. According to our study, in approximately 25% of cases, ADC parameters from pus may be greater than those from the white matter. The explanation for this may be the effect of high T2 value from purulent masses on ADC values when constructing the maps (Fig. 39.4).

Proton MR spectroscopy is another method of increasing the MRI specificity in the differential diagnosis of brain abscesses (Dev et al. 1998; Burtscher and Holtas 2001). MR spectra obtained from the central part of the abscess have quite specific characteristics. In the spectra of untreated abscesses, there are peaks of acetate (1.92 ppm), lactate (1.3 ppm), alanine (1.5 ppm), succinate (2.4 ppm), and a pyruvate complex (0.9 ppm), which includes amino acids

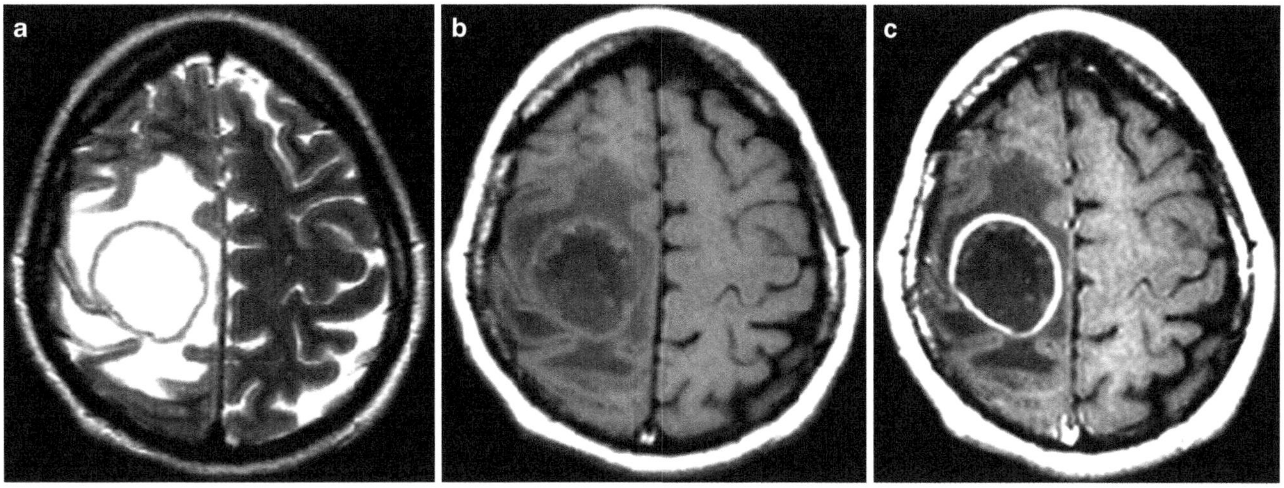

Fig. 39.2 An abscess. On T2-weighted (**a**), T1-weighted (**b**), and T1-weighted MRI after intravenous contrast enhancement (**c**), in the deep parts of the right frontoparietal region, there is a rounded space-occupying lesion with a thin capsule intensely accumulating the contrast agent and a pronounced perifocal edema

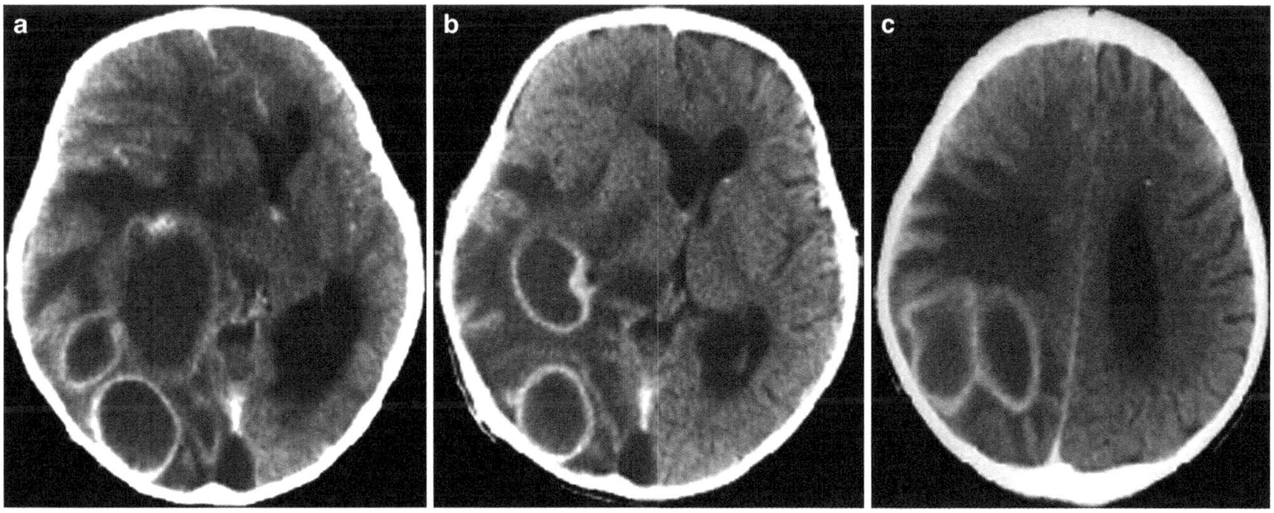

Fig. 39.3 Multiple abscesses. A three-level study. On CT scans in the axial projection with contrast enhancement (**a–c**) on the background of a pronounced cerebral edema, there is ring-shaped accumulation of the contrast material in the walls of multiple abscesses in the temporo-parietal-occipital region. The right lateral ventricle is drastically compressed, and the ventricular system is severely displaced to the left

Table 39.1 The apparent diffusion coefficient (ADC) of water molecules in abnormal brain tissues

ADC × 10^{-3} (mm^2/s)	Abscess ($b = 500$ s/mm^2)	Abscess ($b = 1000$ s/mm^2)	Glioblastoma ($b = 1000$ s/mm^2)
Abscess capsule/tumor	1.01 ± 0.16	0.997 ± 0.09	1.18 ± 0.09
Edema	1.83 ± 0.31	1.65 ± 0.25	1.59 ± 0.16
Pus/necrosis	0.58 ± 0.14	0.65 ± 0.15	2.15 ± 0.34
White matter	0.84 ± 0.07	0.80 ± 0.04	0.82 ± 0.04

valine, leucine, and isoleucine. Acetate, lactate, pyruvate, and succinate are metabolic end products associated with microbial activity. Acetate and succinate are never found in necrotic tumors and, therefore, are specific markers of pyogenic abscesses (Fig. 39.5).

A new approach in the study of abscesses and surrounding brain tissue is the use of perfusion methods in the diagnosis, especially those based on SKT. The capsule of the abscess in most cases is characterized by moderately elevated or decreased CBV and CBF values and high MTT values (Figs. 39.6 and 39.7).

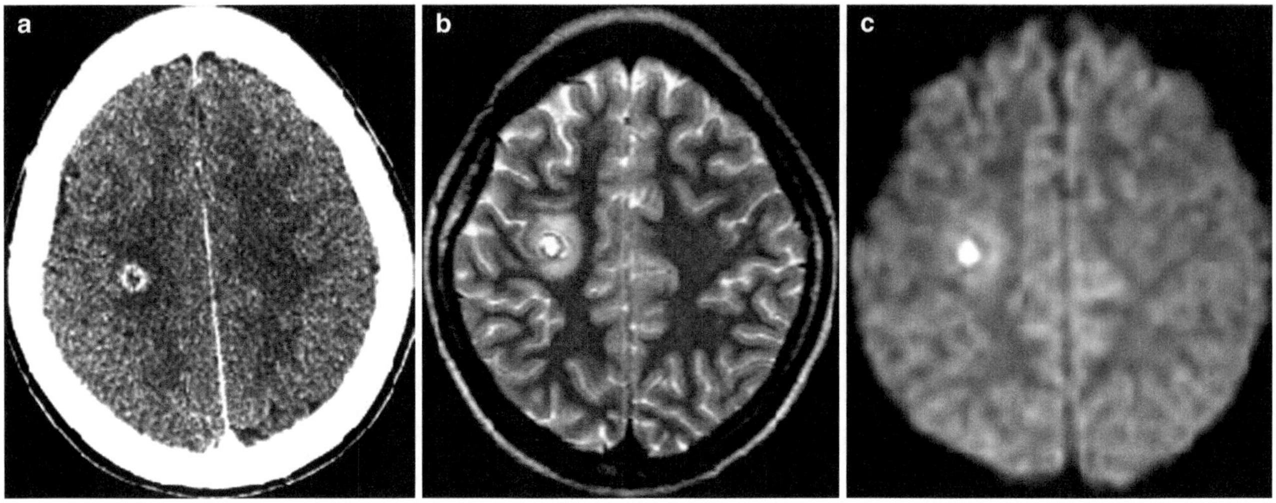

Fig. 39.4 Brain abscess. On CT (**a**) in the right frontal lobe of the brain, there is a microannular lesion. On T2-weighted MRI (**b**), a small-sized rounded lesion with a perifocal edema is detected. An MR signal is typically high on DWI sequences (**c**)

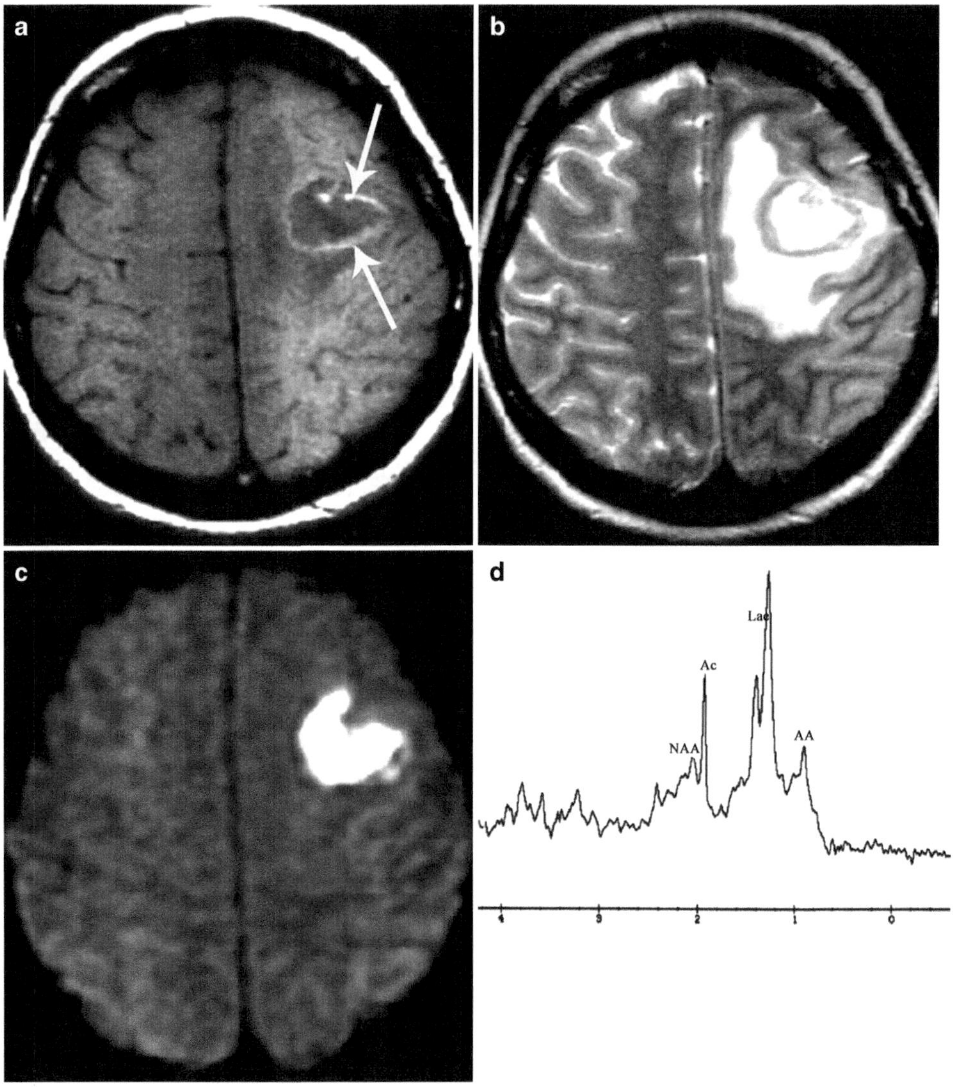

Fig. 39.5 Brain abscess. On T1-weighted (**a**) and T2-weighted MRI (**b**), in the left frontal region, there is a rounded space-occupying lesion with a fairly thick capsule and a perifocal edema. The abscess capsule has an increased signal on T1-weighted MRI (*arrows*) and a hypointense signal on T2-weighted MRI. On diffusion MRI (**c**), there is typically a high MR signal; the presence of acetate (Ac), lactate (Lac), and amino acid peaks (AA) is detected by MR spectroscopy (**d**). The NAA peak is reduced

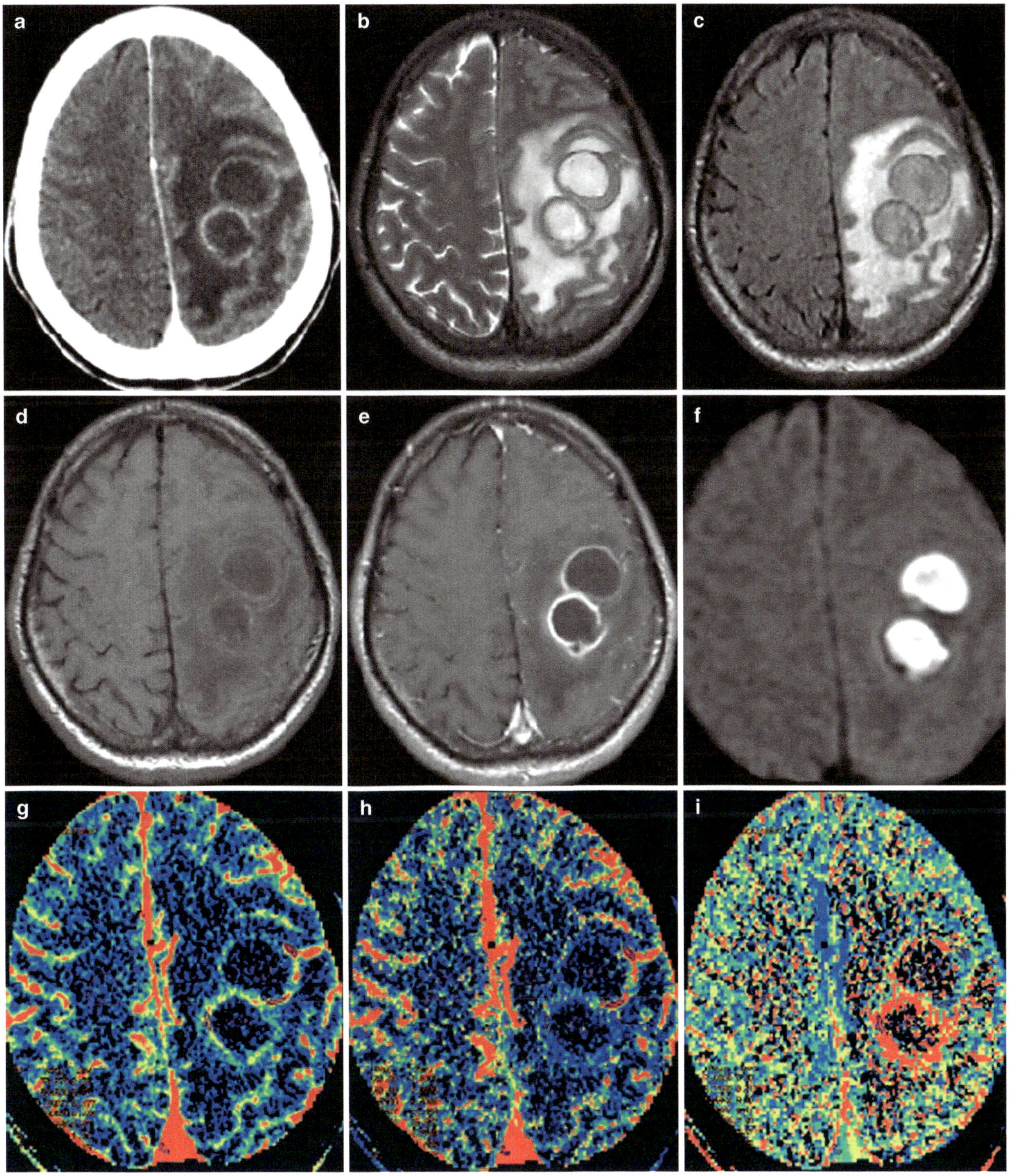

Fig. 39.6 Brain abscess. On contrast-enhanced CT (**a**), T2-weighted (**b**), T2-FLAIR (**c**), and T1-weighted MRI before (**d**) and after contrast enhancement (**e**), there are two ring-shaped lesions adjacent to each other, surrounded by a perifocal edema in the left frontoparietal region. On DW-MRI (**f**), a pronounced increase in the MR signal is observed. On CBV (**g**), CBF (**h**), and MTT (**i**) perfusion maps, there are characteristic changes in the blood flow in the capsule of the "growing" abscess

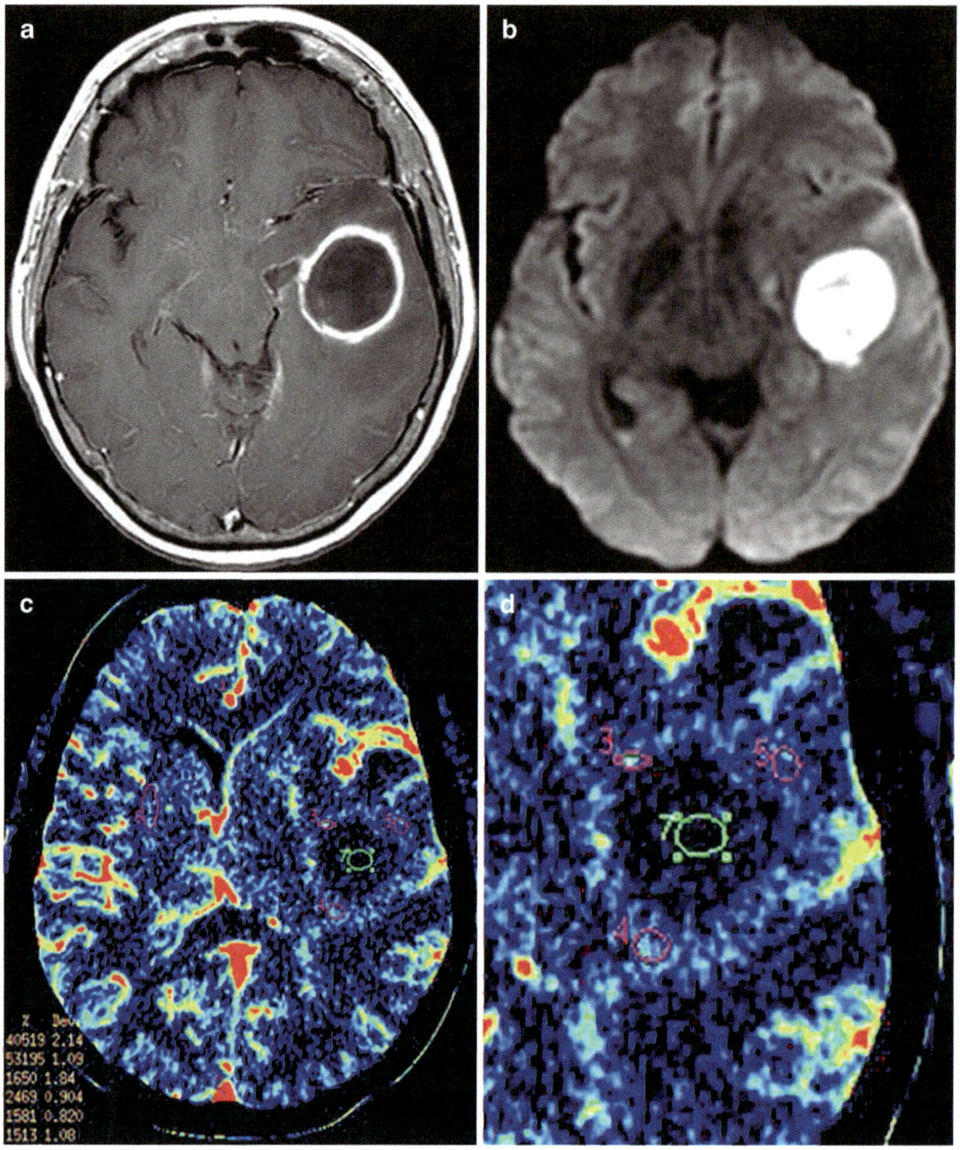

Fig. 39.7 Brain abscess. On MRI in the left temporal region, there is a rounded space-occupying lesion that intensely accumulates contrast agent on the periphery in T1-weighted images (**a**) with contrast enhancement, has a sharply increased signal in DWI (**b**), and decreased CBV values (**c**, **d**) on a CT-perfusion map

Thus, a sharp increase in the signal in DWI images (b = 1000), low perfusion values, and the presence of typical AA, Ac, or Succ peaks facilitate the correct diagnosis of a brain abscess.

39.2 Tuberculosis

One-third of the world's population are carriers of tuberculosis mycobacteria (Lonnroth et al. 2010); however, the disease only occurs in 10% of patients and generally develops in the pulmonary form (Russell 2007). Brain tuberculosis is still common in many developed countries. Tuberculomas may have a similar radiological picture with metastases, as they also manifest in the form of restricted lesions. The clinical picture is also similar and manifests by headaches, convulsions, paresis of cranial nerves. The active migration of the population, as well as the main provocative factor—human immunodeficiency virus may contribute to the development of tuberculosis in recent years (Idris et al. 2007). Tuberculosis of the central nervous system can manifest in different forms or their combinations—meningitis, abscesses, and much less frequently in the form of an isolated tuberculoma of the brain parenchyma. Keep in mind that chest radiography can give a positive result only in 30% of patients (Kaufmann 2006).

Tuberculoma consists of a central area of solid necrosis surrounded by a capsule of collagen tissue and epithelioid, polynuclear giant, and mononuclear inflammatory cells. TB bacilli can be detected both in the necrotic center and the capsule. There is an edema and proliferation of astrocytes outside the capsule. Tuberculomas may be located in the cerebral cortex; cerebellum; subarachnoid, subdural, and epidural spaces; and in the spinal cord and can be single and multiple (Bernaerts et al. 2003; Helmy et al. 2011). In most cases, these neoplasms are detected supratentorially, but, according to Kumar et al. (2000), in children, they are more often located subtentorially. In rare cases, tuberculomas are also rarely located in the Turkish saddle, cerebellopontine cistern, pineal, and intraventricular regions. The combination with involvement of meninges does not always occur. Most tuberculomas are diagnosed in patients with miliary pulmonary tuberculosis.

CT with contrast enhancement visualizes small lesions with annular opacification. One-third of patients have a special sign in the form of a centrally located calcification or pinpoint contrast enhancement, surrounded by a hypointense area with a rim with increased density. However, this sign is not pathognomonic.

Tuberculomas are isointense relative to the gray matter on T1-weighted MRI without contrast enhancement and may have a slightly hyperintensive rim (because of the possible accumulation of paramagnetic substances shortening T1, e.g., free radicals, etc.). On T2-weighted MRI, the signal from tuberculoma varies. They are often more iso- or hypointense than the brain matter, which is related to T2 shortening due to the presence of free paramagnetic radicals in macrophages heterogeneously dispersed within the tuberculoma. Thicker in structure than the brain substance, a mature tuberculoma has a decreased MRI signal on T2-weighted MRI. In case of the fluid contents in the center (necrosis), tuberculoma may be hyperintense on T2-weighted MRI (Figs. 39.8, 39.9, and 39.10). The surrounding edema is minimal around small lesions, and, as shown by CT studies, is always smaller than edema around a bacterial abscess with an appropriate size. The edema is significantly expressed at early stages of the lesion formation.

CT and PT characteristics in standard sequences do not have any differential diagnostic features—these are ring-

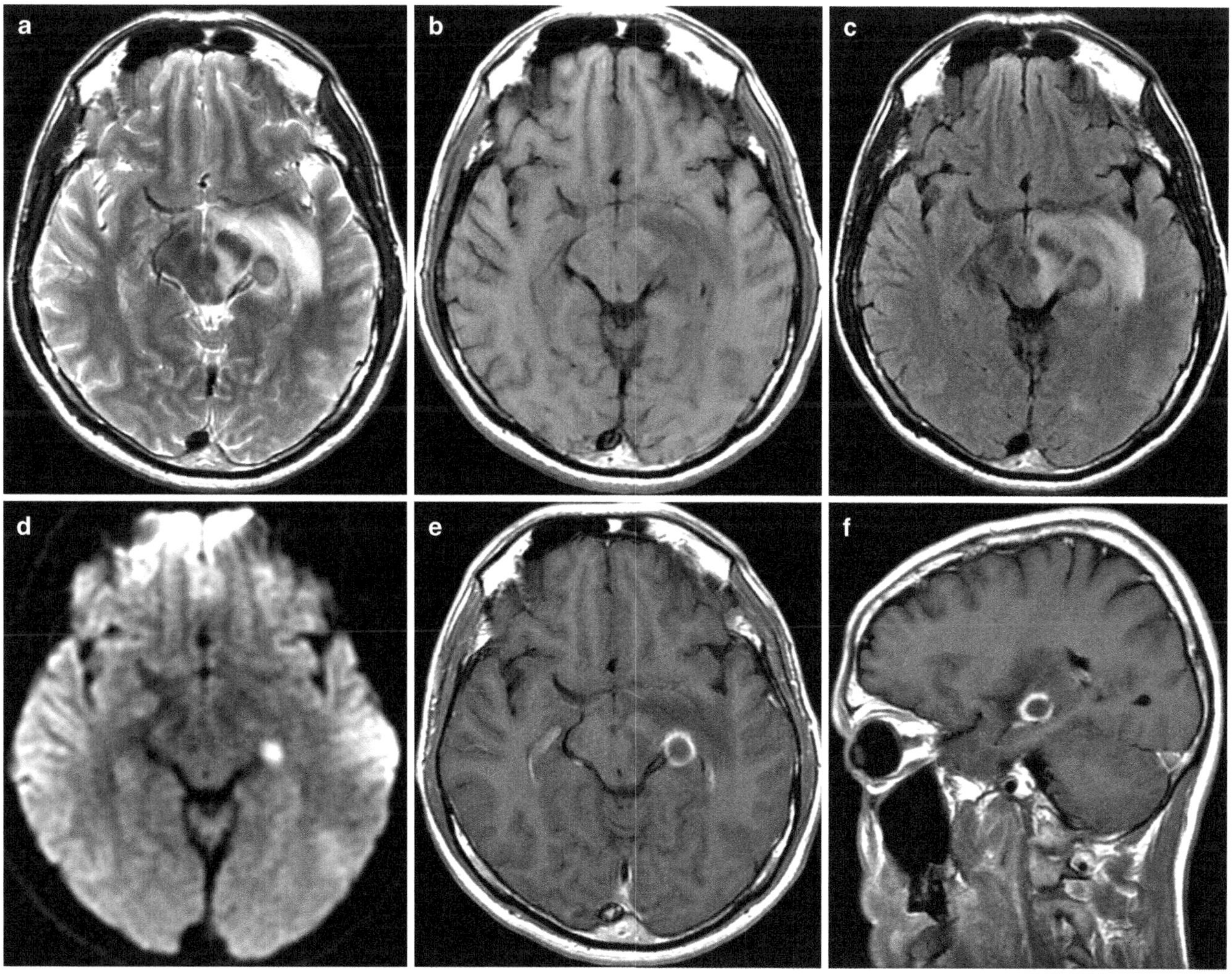

Fig. 39.8 Tuberculoma. On T2-weighted MRI (**a**) in the projection of the medial portions of the left temporal region, there is a hypointense rounded lesion with a pronounced perifocal edema; in T1-weighted images (**b**), the lesion is not differentiated on the background of edema. On T2-FLAIR MRI (**c**), the lesion is also hypointense. On DWI MRI (**d**), there is an increase of the signal from the lesion. After the administration of the contrast agent on T1-weighted MRI (**e**, **f**), its intensive accumulation along the contour of tuberculoma is noted

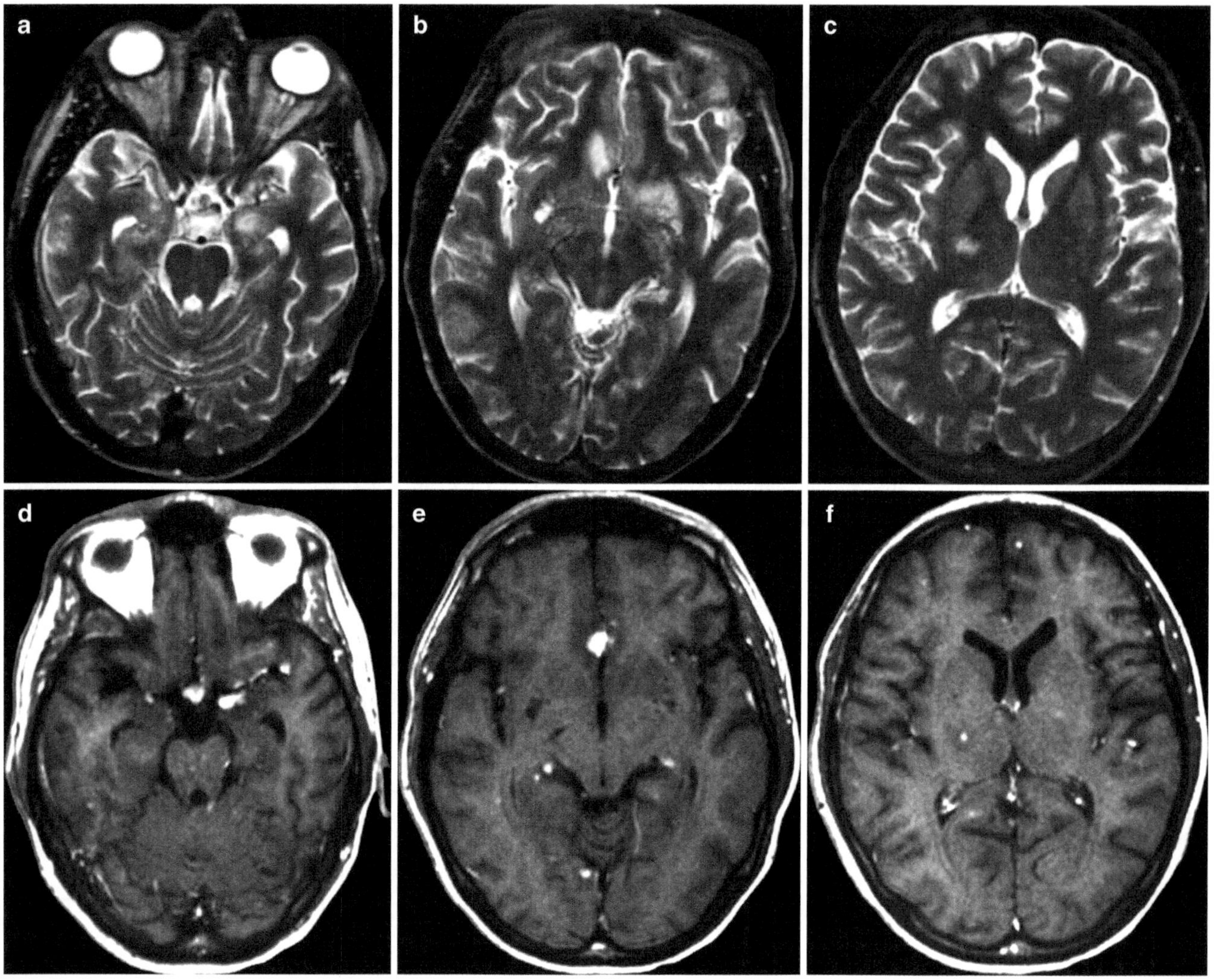

Fig. 39.9 Multiple brain tuberculomas. Three-level study. On T2-weighted MRI (**a**, **b**, **c**), there are multiple lesions with an increased MR signal in the cerebral hemispheres; on T1-weighted contrast-enhanced MRI (**d**, **e**, **f**), there are lesions with an increased MR signal in the chiasmatic cistern and cisterna ambiens, in the anterior portion of the great longitudinal fissure and lateral fissures, the lenticular nucleus on the right and the left frontal lobe

shaped cystic lesions with marked accumulation of the contrast agent along the contour. Calcifications are best determined by CT. On MRI, calcifications are best visualized by gradient echo sequence.

MR spectroscopy of tuberculomas in some cases allows to perform differential diagnosis, but not with metastases, as both are manifested by an increased Lip-Lac complex (Santy et al. 2011). Diagnosis is generally based on the study of cerebrospinal fluid. In case of involvement of the meninges, there are inhomogeneous conglomerates accumulating the contrast agent and fragments distributed along the arachnoid meninges in the form of "branches."

39.2.1 Meningitis (Bacterial, Tuberculous)

The causes and predisposing factors of bacterial meningitis can include a common infection (pneumonia, parameningeal infection), head injury, a defect in the brain meninges, prior surgery, cancer, alcoholism, immunodeficiency, etc. The agent type depends on the patient's age and predisposing factors.

Prior to entry into the CNS, bacteria usually colonize the nasal mucosa, subsequently entering the subarachnoid space by local tissue invasion or via a hematogenous route. Bacteria can penetrate the meninges directly through anatomical defects in the skull or from the parameningeal

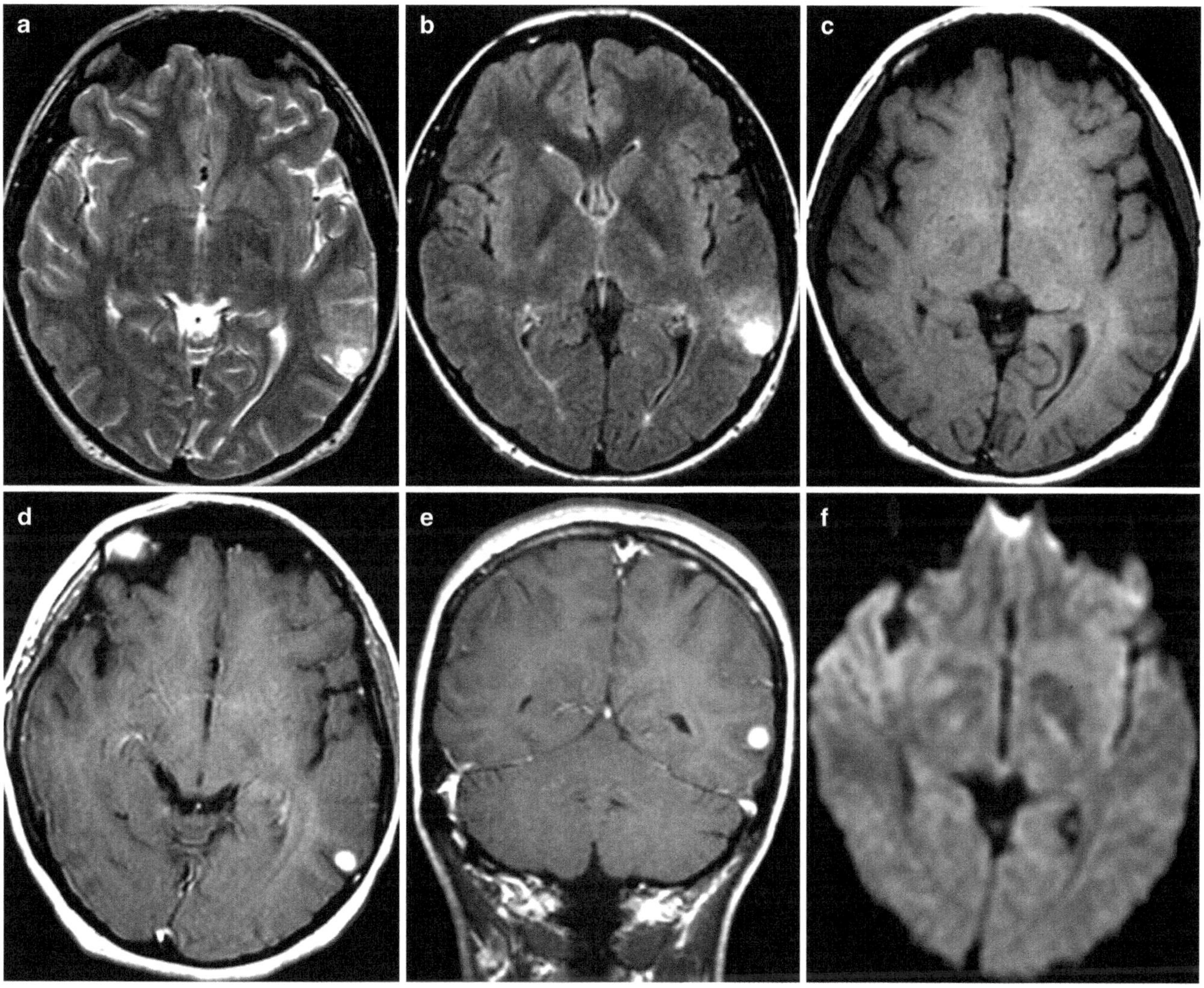

Fig. 39.10 Brain tuberculoma. On T2-weighted (**a**) and T2-FLAIR MRI (**b**), in the convexital parts of the left temporal lobe of the brain, there is a lesion with an increased MR signal; on T1-weighted MRI before (**c**) and after (**d**, **e**) contrast enhancement, expressed and homogeneous opacification is observed in the form of a circular lesion with clear contours. On diffusion MRI (**f**), an increase in the MR signal is undetectable

spaces, such as sinuses or middle ear. The resulting inflammatory response causes release of inflammatory cytokines, interleukin-1 and interleukin-6, and tumor necrosis factor, which increase the permeability of the blood-brain barrier, resulting in the development of a vasogenic brain edema and changes in the cerebral blood flow and may have a direct neurotoxic effect.

Cerebral edema, hydrocephalus, and cerebrovascular accident can occur as complications of bacterial meningitis, but infection of the brain tissue per se is rare. Complications may develop within a few days or weeks and are diagnosed in nearly 50% of adults with bacterial meningitis. Involvement of the brain parenchyma with edema and mass effect can be both diffuse and focal. Subdural fluid accumulation formed in case of infectious involvement of the arachnoid membrane and its necrosis become limited infectious foci—empyemas. Inflammatory occlusion of CSF pathways causes hydrocephalus. Ventriculitis is a relatively rare complication of leptomeningitis.

MRI without contrast enhancement in patients with uncomplicated bacterial meningitis has no specific features. Post-contrast MRI usually visualizes opacification of the thickened meningeal membranes surrounding the cerebral hemispheres (Fig. 39.11). Although symptoms of opacification of the meninges can also be identified by CT, however, the accuracy of MRI diagnosis is higher.

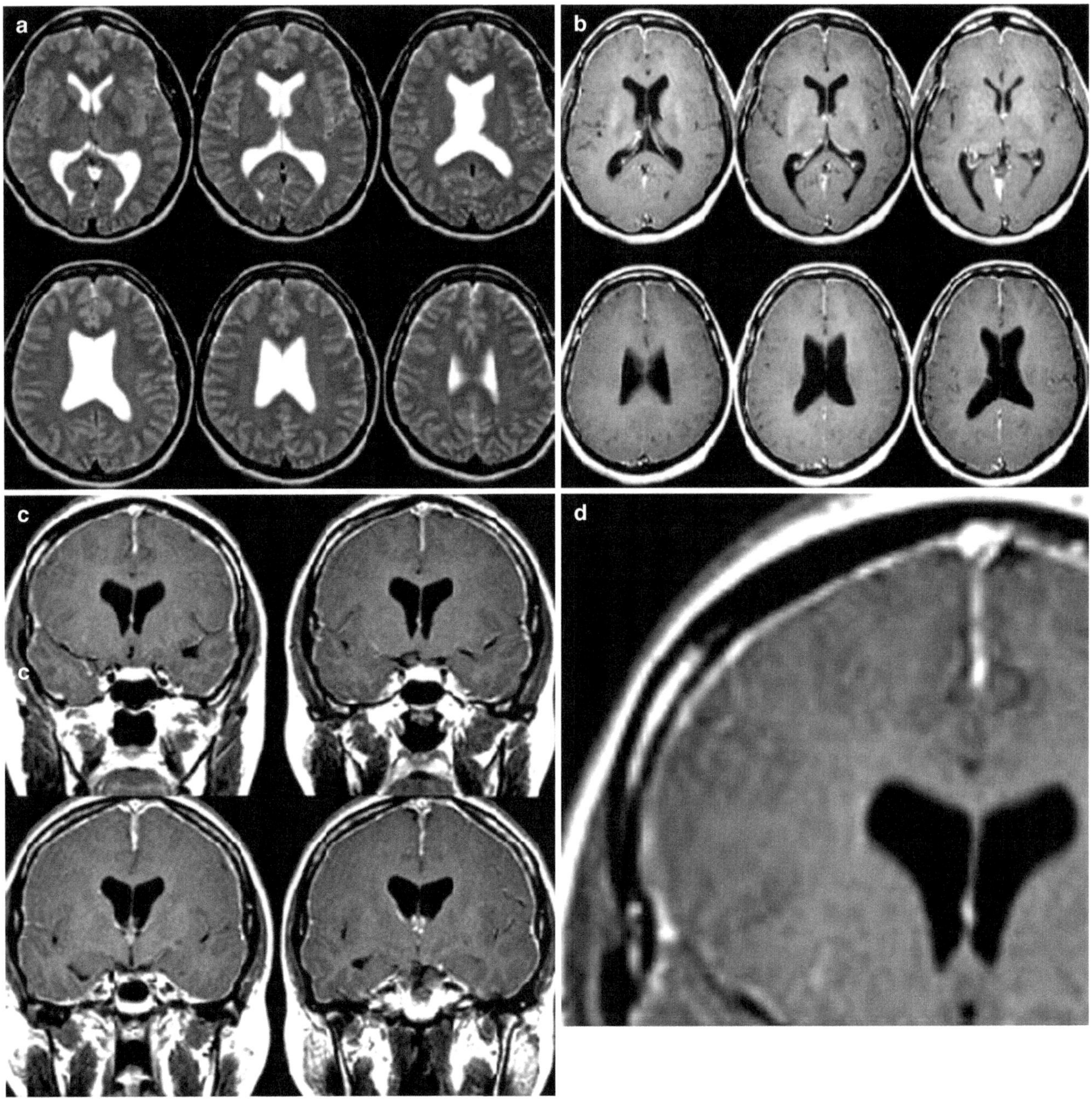

Fig. 39.11 Bacterial meningitis. On T2-weighted (**a**) and T1-weighted MRI in the axial (**b**) and frontal (**c**, **d**) projections, on the background of contrast enhancement, thickening and opacification of the dura mater are observed

Multiplanar MRI better visualizes the loss of elasticity of the subarachnoid space with dilation of the great longitudinal fissure, which, according to some researchers, is an early sign of acute meningitis. In general, standard MRI and MRI with contrast enhancement identify more manifestations of meningitis per se and its subsequent complications, including heart attack, cerebritis/abscess, subdural empyema, and ventriculitis, than CT.

39.2.2 Viral Infection

Early detection and accurate diagnosis of a viral causative agent in the CNS are extremely important, because most of these diseases can be treated. Viruses can affect the central nervous system in three ways: (1) by penetrating hematogenically (viruses carried by arthropods), (2) spreading along axons via axonal transport (herpes simplex virus), and (3) causing an autoimmune reaction resulting in demyelination of the nerve fibers (chicken pox or influenza virus).

Intracranial viral infections are manifested by focal or diffuse inflammatory processes in the brain tissue (encephalitis) and meninges (meningitis). The incidence of viral meningitis and encephalitis is particularly high in children and adolescents. The cause of the disease may be an acute or chronic CNS infection. Viral encephalitis is most often caused by pathogens of childhood exanthematous viral infections, viruses carried by arthropods, as well as herpes simplex virus type 1.

On MRI, abnormal changes caused by viral encephalitis manifest in the form of individual or interrelated hyperintense areas in T2-weighted images, iso- or hypointense on T1-weighted MRI, with a variety of mass effect signs. Foci of subacute hemorrhage (extracellular hemoglobin) show an increase in the MR signal intensity in T1-weighted images. Localized or generalized brain atrophy is best visualized on T2-FLAIR MRI. These main characteristics are observed in the majority of cases of viral encephalitis; however, some infections have specific manifestations that are characteristics of this infection and help perform the differential diagnosis.

Herpes simplex virus 1 (HSV-1) is a causative agent of 95% cases of herpesviral encephalitis. In adults, the infection occurs in persons with preexisting antibodies and, thus, represents the virus reactivation. In immunocompetent patients (without AIDS), HSV-1 virus can cause necrotizing encephalitis of the temporal lobes and the orbital surface of the frontal lobes. It may also affect the surface of the insular cortex, cerebral hemispheres, and posterior portions of the occipital cortex. The involvement is usually bilateral, with the spread to the basal ganglia (Schroth et al. 1987). Later, with the development of the disease, the affected area may also include the cingulate gyrus. Infections of the brainstem may occur, which are caused by the retrograde spread of the virus along the cisternal portion of nerve V to the brainstem.

CT imaging shows areas with reduced density in the temporal lobes, sometimes with involvement of the frontal or occipital lobes. Opacification and hemorrhages are rarely visualized. In herpesviral encephalitis, MRI shows early signs of a brain edema with an increase in the signal intensity in the temporal and anterior parts of the frontal lobes in T2-weighted and T2-FLAIR images.

In complicated cases, perfusion CT helps to perform the differential diagnosis of intracerebral malignant tumors. Despite abnormal contrast enhancement in the affected brain area, low blood flow values are registered in encephalitis. MR spectroscopy clearly visualizes the emergence of a Lac/Lip peak, especially in the acute phase, with its gradual decrease during the transition to the chronic phase. The NAA peak undergoes reverse changes: decreases in early disease and gradually increases as the brain structure recovers. The degree of NAA peak recovery depends on the severity of the primary brain involvement and the beginning of antiviral therapy. In a CT perfusion study, viral inflammatory changes are characterized by low blood flow values (CBV, CBF) and increased MTT values (Fig. 39.12).

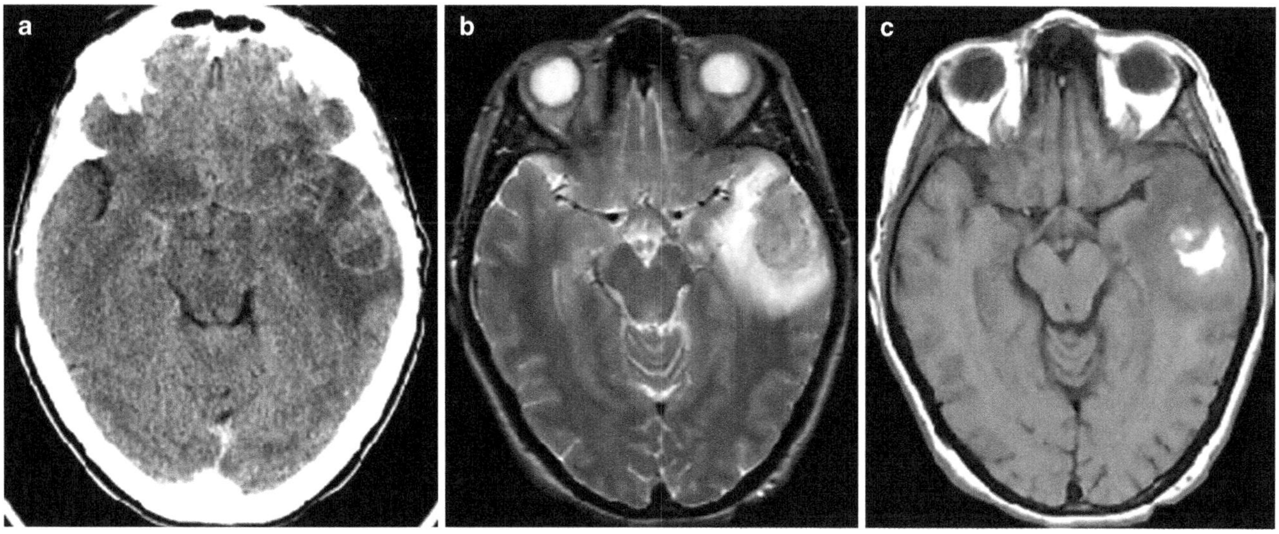

Fig. 39.12 The subacute phase of herpes encephalitis. On contrast-enhanced CT (**a**) and T2-weighted (**b**) and T1-weighted MRI (**c**), in the left temporal lobe, there is an extensive area with heterogeneous density and a high signal in T1-weighted images, typical of the subacute phase of a hemorrhage. After the contrast agent administration (**d**), its weakly expressed accumulation is observed on the periphery of the hematoma. CBV (**e**) and MTT (**f**) values are decreased

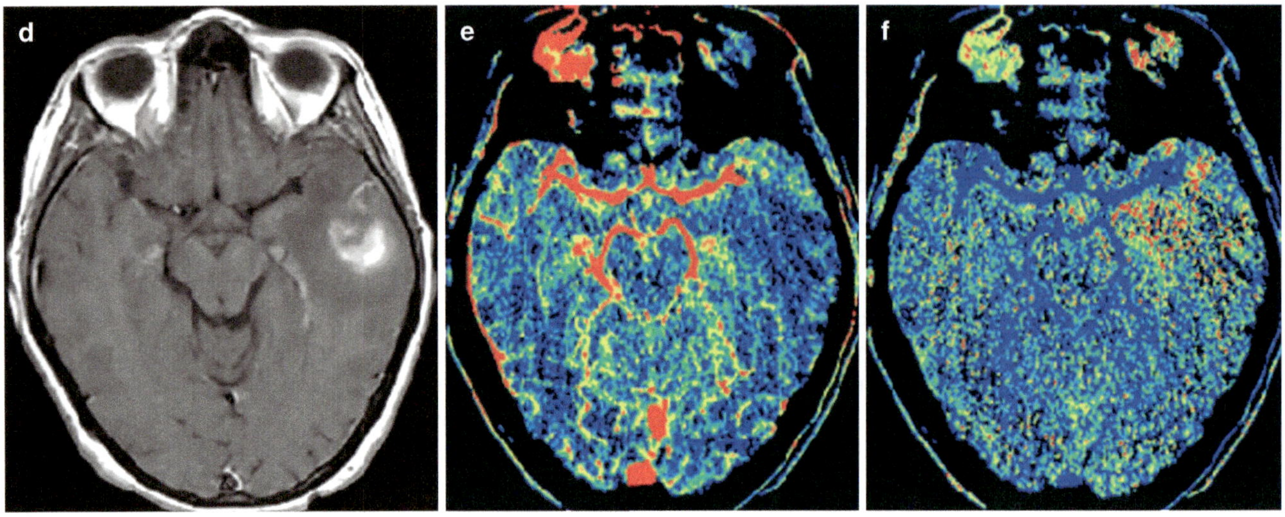

Fig. 39.12 (continued)

40 Parasitic Infestations

Toxoplasmosis is a parasitic disease caused by cysts of *Toxoplasma gondii*, contained in the raw meat. The infection in humans is possible not only as a result of consumption of such meat but also through animal's excrements, raw milk, blood transfusion, organ transplant, the use of non-sterile needles, cat litter, as well as via an intrauterine route. The causative agent of the disease is widespread. From 6 to 90% of people in different regions have anti-Toxoplasma antibodies, with up to 30% of the world population being infested on average. Toxoplasma much more commonly affects the internal organs (brain, lungs) in patients with AIDS.

On CT without contrast enhancement, toxoplasmic encephalitis has characteristic manifestations in the form of multiple iso- or hypodense areas located predominantly in the basal ganglia (76 to 88%) and corticosubcortical layer. The disease can affect the posterior cranial fossa. Hemorrhages are very rare. Dimensions of lesions range from ≤1 to ≥3 cm. (Osborn 2004). Post-contrast CT images demonstrate annular or nodular opacification. Annular opacification with the central region with decreased density is a common manifestation of toxoplasmosis. The rim of contrast enhancement is usually thin and smooth, but thick and uneven rims are encountered in large lesions (Post et al. 1983). The ring accumulating the contrast medium corresponds to an area of an intense inflammatory reaction, and an edema surrounds the periphery of the ring.

MRI with and without contrast enhancement is more sensitive to both new and chronic lesions of toxoplasmic encephalitis than pre- and post-contrast CT. On T2-weighted MRI, active lesions have a variable MRI signal. They can be more hyperintense than the brain substance and indistinguishable from the high-intensity edema area. There may be an iso- or hypointense lesion in the center, surrounded by a high-intensity edema area. On T1-weighted MRI, the signal from the affected area can be isointense or hypointense (Figs. 40.1 and 40.2). After administration of gadolinium, there is its annular or nodular accumulation in the active area, well distinguished from the surrounding hypointense edema. Typical is the uneven accumulation of the contrast agent with formation of a local thickening along the contour or at the center of the lesion. At the same time, some fragments of the rest of the cyst surface can remain non-contrast enhanced. MRI and CT patterns of contrast enhancement are generally similar. Hemorrhages in toxoplasmosis are rare.

If there are calcifications, the latter can be pinpoint or quite large and dense. An encephalomalacia area may be formed. On MRI, calcified lesions appear as areas with a hypointense signal in T1- and T2-weighted images and are better visible in the gradient echo sequence.

Cysticercosis is a quite frequent invasion of the central nervous system, observed worldwide. In endemic regions, it occurs both in immunodeficient and immunocompetent patients. The causative agent of the disease is the larval form of pork tapeworm (*Taenia solium*). The infection occurs by ingestion of food contaminated with larvae. A person infected by larvae becomes the main host of parasites during their entire life cycle. In the intestine, larvae develop into adult tapeworms of 1–8 m long. Tapeworms do not cause any symptoms by themselves, but they produce a large number of eggs found in the intestines and feces. In the digestive tract, a thick outer membrane of the egg dissolves, releasing an enclosed oncosphere. These oncospheres or primary larvae penetrate through the digestive tract walls into the blood, and 60–95% of cases affect the brain via hematogenous dissemination. Intracranially, oncospheres are located in the brain, meninges, choroidal plexus, and ependyma.

M. Dolgushin et al., *Brain Metastases*, DOI 10.1007/978-3-319-57760-9_40

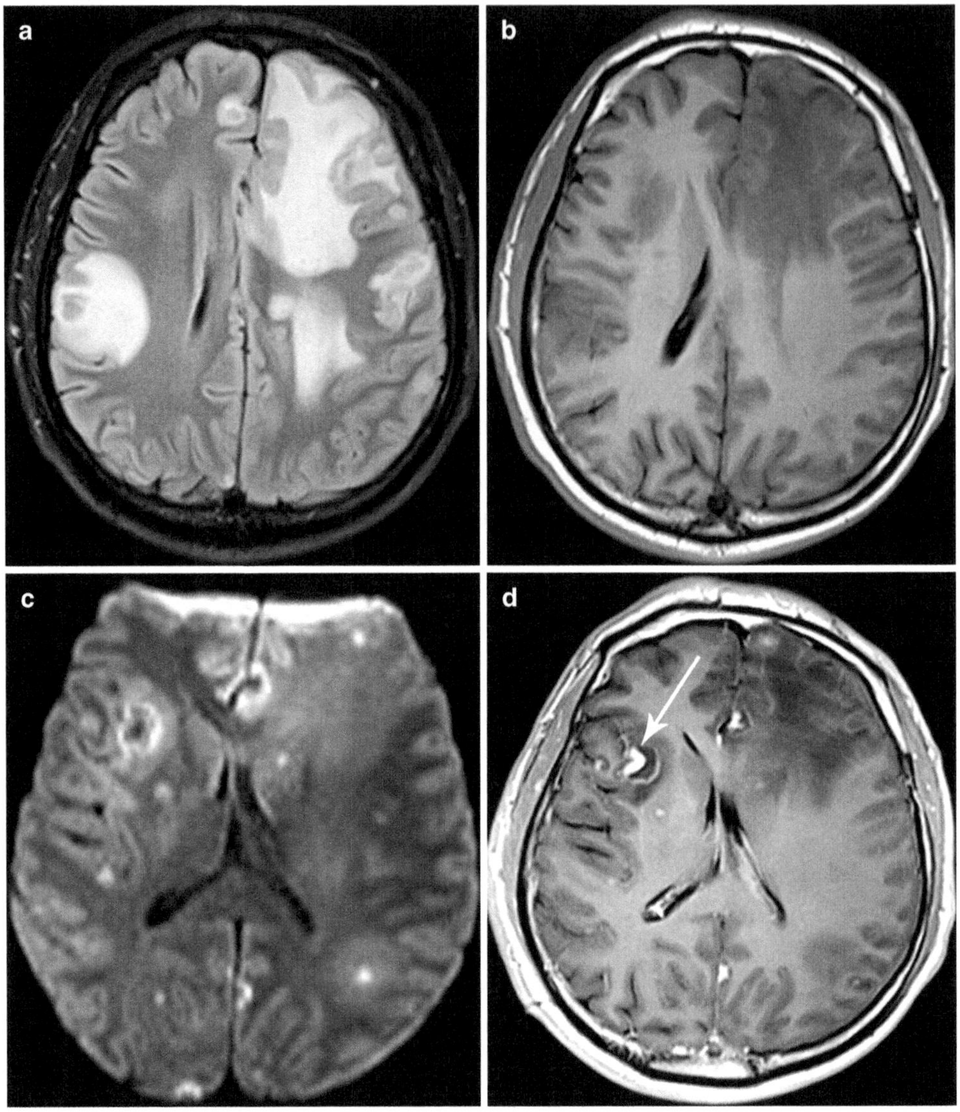

Fig. 40.1 Toxoplasmosis. On T2-FLAIR (**a**) and T1-weighted MRI (**b**), there are multiple foci with an increased MR signal in T2-FLAIR images and a decreased signal in T1-weighted images. On DWI MRI (**c**), there are multiple pinpoint areas with an increased signal; larger lesions are characterized by a heterogeneous signal. After CA administration, its intense accumulation in these areas is noted (**d**), with a clearly visualized, irregular thickening of the lateral wall in the largest lesion in the right frontotemporal area (the *arrow*)

At the initial stage called vesicular, the disease manifests as small foci that are hypodense on CT, hyperintense on T2-weighted MRI, and hypointense on T1-weighted MRI. These structures usually do not accumulate the contrast agent, do not have a cystic component, and may be undetectable at all (Hawk et al. 2005). Subsequently, a 1–2 cm cyst is formed within the next few weeks, which is well visualized by CT and MRI. Cysts can be seen at the boundary of the gray and white matter, as well as in the basal ganglia, cerebellum, and brainstem. An edema around the cyst is small and is often absent altogether. The cyst walls are thin and smooth. Protoscolex is visualized as a lesion or a nodule inside the cyst, which can be seen better on MRI than on CT (Fig. 40.3). A bright signal from CSF on T2-weighted MRI may disguise scolex; therefore, it is better seen in proton density-weighted or T2-FLAIR images. At this stage, cystic walls can sometimes accumulate the contrast agent. Cysts are isointense relative to CSF in MRI images obtained in all pulsed sequences and have the same CT density as that of CSF. MRI often reveals a larger number of viable cysts than CT.

In 5–7 years, a cysticercus larva begins to produce and dies (the colloidal vesicular stage), and an inflammatory

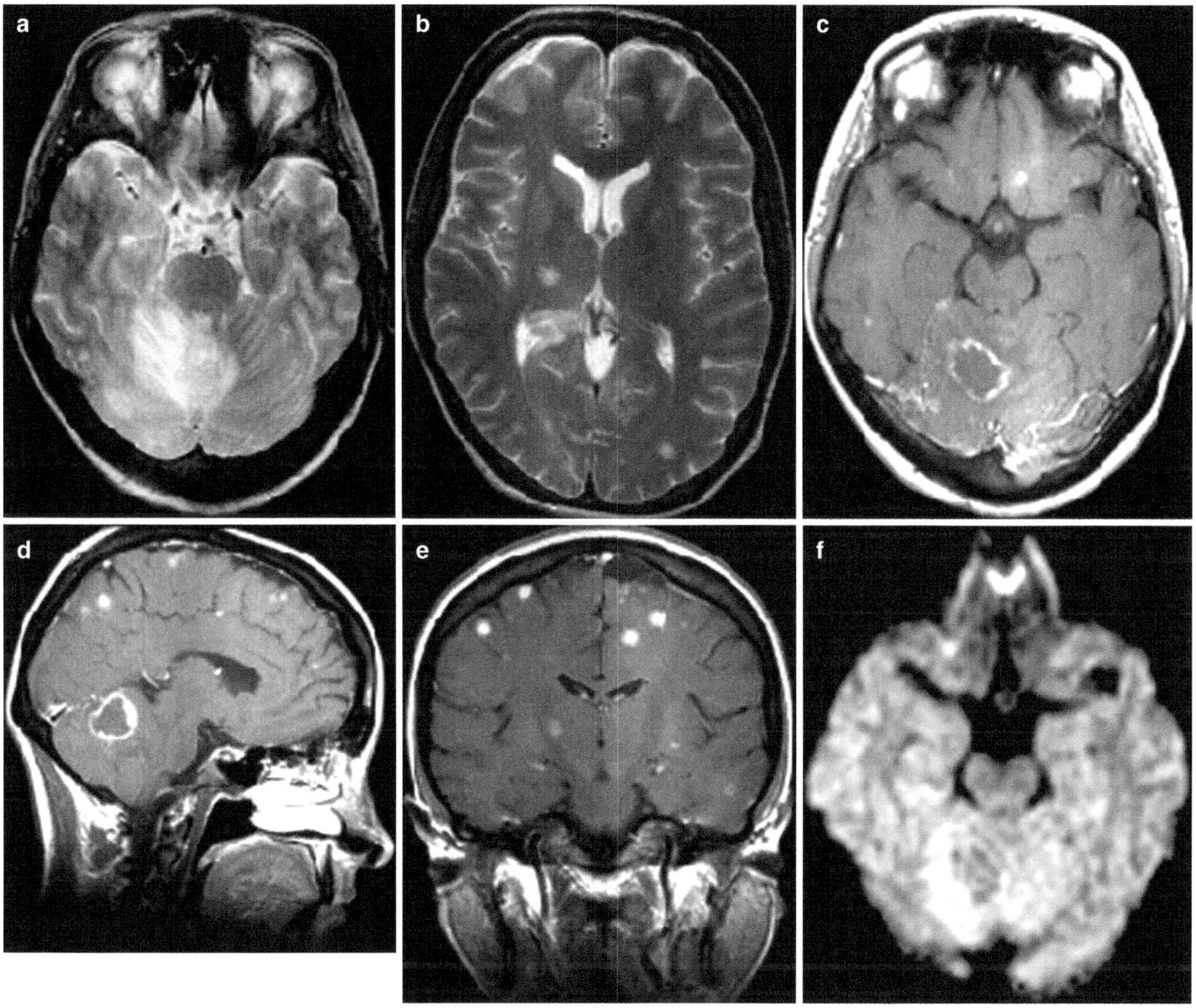

Fig. 40.2 Toxoplasmosis. On T2-weighted (**a**, **b**) and T1-weighted MRI on the background of contrast enhancement (**c–e**), there are multiple foci of an increased MR signal and signs of intense accumulation of the contrast agent. On DWI (**f**), the signal is increased at the periphery of the largest lesion in the right hemisphere of the cerebellum

reaction develops around the parasite with formation of a fibrous capsule. The protein concentration in the cystic fluid increases. As a result, cysts become slightly hyperintense on T1-weighted MRI and bright on T2-weighted MRI. A scolex inside the cyst is well visualized in the background of a high signal from the cystic contents on T2-weighted MRI. In the granular and nodular stage, the fluid resorption from the cyst occurs (moribund parasite), the capsule thickens, and a granulomatous nodule forms that has annular or homogenous contrast enhancement. At the final stage, the nodule becomes mineralized (calcified). Granulomatous nodules are replaced by gliosis with subsequent calcification, which is visualized on CT but can be also seen on T2-weighted MRI as a small section of a hypointense signal and even better in the gradient echo pulsed sequence.

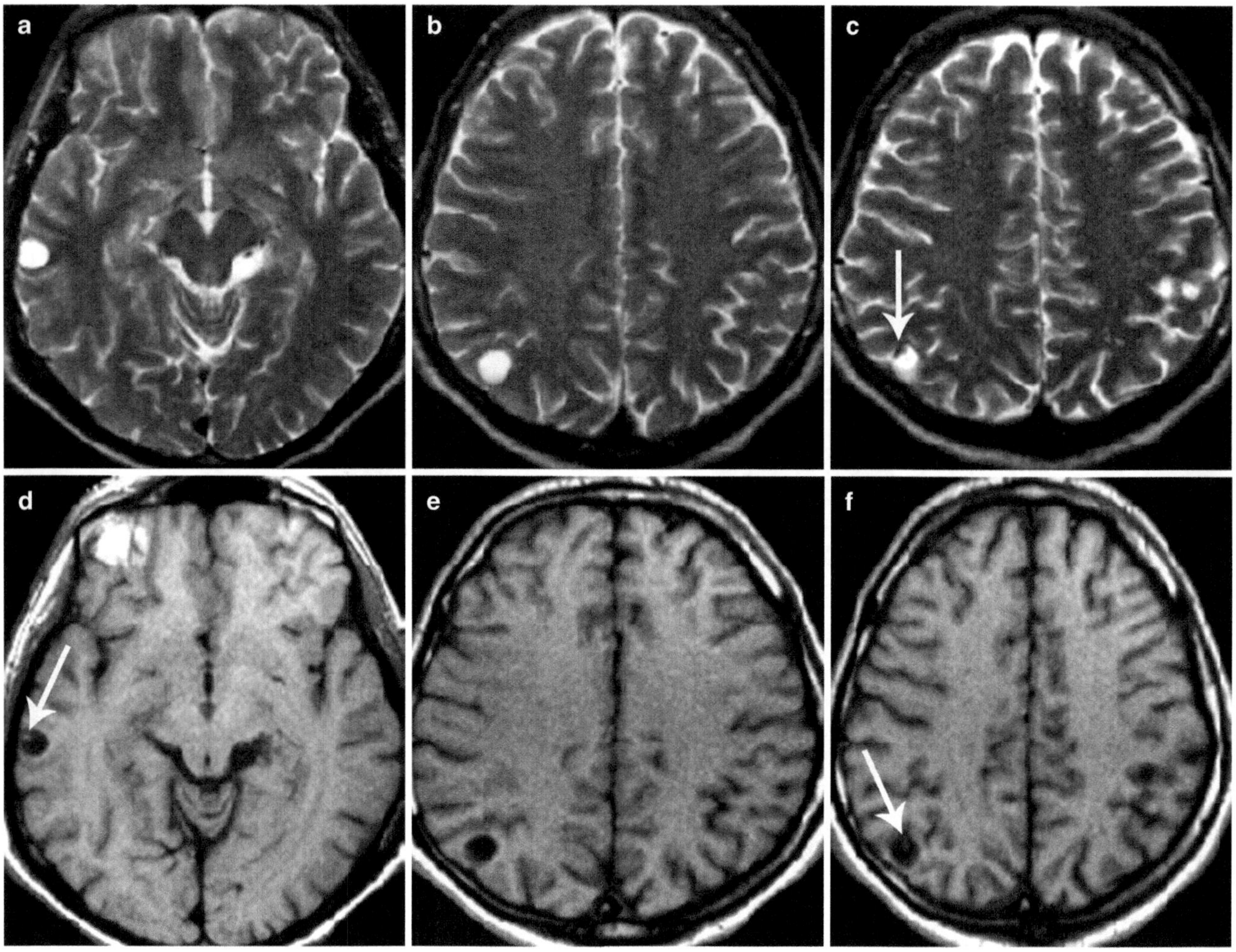

Fig. 40.3 Cysticercosis. A three-level study. On a series of T2-weighted MRI (**a–c**) and T1-weighted MRI (**d–f**), there are multiple small cysts located on the convexital surface of the cerebral hemispheres. Arrows show a parietal scolex of the parasite

40.1 Brain Echinococcosis

It is caused by a slowly growing cysticercus *Echinococcus granulosus*. Inside the bladder, daughter bladders are produced that cannot grow inward but outward from the main bladder, increasing its volume. *Echinococcus* is a tapeworm that lives in the digestive tract of the vertebrates. The life cycle of the parasite begins with excretion of its eggs with feces of a host, which can enter the digestive tract of an intermediate host. This parasite penetrates the intestinal wall and spreads in the body via venous and lymphatic routes (Zayats et al. 2002). This parasitic agent is often accumulated in the liver or lungs, while the brain may be the end organ. Intracranial parasites form gradually increasing cysts. *E. multilocularis* can also infect the brain, forming small clusters of cysts called alveoli.

CT detects *Echinococcus* as a clearly delimited, rounded, low-density area (equal to the density of CSF). Intravenous administration of a contrast material does not change the CT picture. The degree of displacement and deformation of the ventricular system depends on the *Echinococcus* size. Multiple cysts tend to be small sized and are combined in a single formation, extending sometimes quite widely along the subarachnoid space and the ventricular system (Fig. 40.4). Calcification of hooklets or walls of dead parasites is detected mainly in adult parasites and is related with the deposition of lime salts in the cyst capsule (extremely rare in immature parasites).

On MR studies, hydatid cysts are slightly more hyperintense than the gray matter (proton density-weighted MRI) and isointense in relation to the CSF on T2-weighted images.

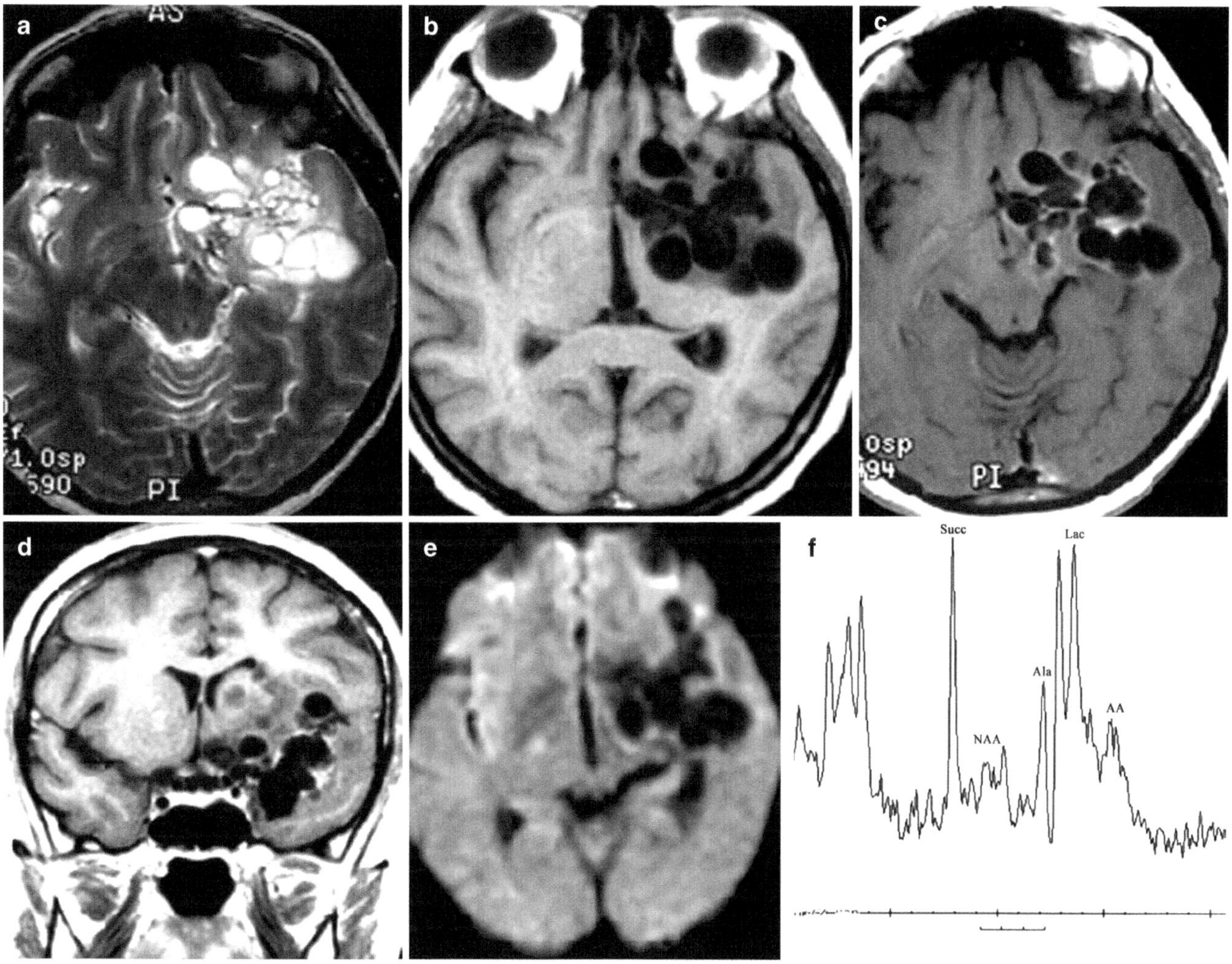

Fig. 40.4 *Echinococcus*. On T2-weighted (**a**) and T1-weighted MRI before (**b**) and after (**c, d**) contrast enhancement, a lesion is visualized in the left temporal region, consisting of a large number of cysts (a cluster). The walls of individual cysts accumulate contrast agents. On diffusion MRI (**e**), cysts have a low MR signal. Proton spectroscopy (**f**) of the central portions of the lesion with the cystic and capsular portions of the *Echinococcus* demonstrates the presence of high peaks of succinate (Succ), alanine (Ala), and lipid-lactate complex (Lac). The NAA peak is significantly reduced

Cysts typically have a slightly higher MR signal as compared to CSF on T1-weighted images. There is usually no edema. The accumulation of the contrast agent is observed in rare cases along the cyst periphery, probably due to a local inflammatory granulomatous process around the capsule. A slight mass effect can be noted. Hemorrhages into the cavity of hydatid cysts are rare, but possible. A distinctive feature is a low signal on DWI MRI (b = 1000), weak accumulation of the contrast medium, and the presence of amino acid peaks on MR spectroscopy.

Demyelinating Diseases

41

The term "demyelinating disease" (DD) of the central nervous system refers to primary, usually idiopathic, abnormal processes that cause the destruction of the normal myelin development. Such diseases currently include multiple sclerosis in the classical form, its atypical variants (Marburg disease, Balo sclerosis, Schilder's disease), and inflammatory demyelinating pseudotumor (IDP). In addition, demyelinating diseases include diseases with secondary demyelination and destruction of myelin, such as acute disseminated encephalomyelitis (ADEM), progressive multifocal leukoencephalopathy (PML), HIV leukoencephalopathy, and some slowly demyelinating leukoencephalitis of viral etiology. It must be emphasized that demyelinating diseases are characterized by *focal, multiple, and asymmetric* white matter lesions, due to which it can often acquire an MRI picture similar to that with secondary tumor lesions.

Demyelinating diseases are characterized by specific MR signal changes on T1-weighted, T2-weighted, and T2-FLAIR MRI. The entire group of demyelinating diseases, in contrast to other processes accompanied by contrast enhancement, is characterized by a specific and often unique sign allowing to make the correct diagnosis: a so-called "partial" type of contrast enhancement observed in some lesions, in the form of "half-rings" or "incomplete rings."

41.1 Multiple Sclerosis

It is a chronic, progressive autoimmune disease of the central nervous system, manifested by diffuse neurological symptoms and having a relapsing-remitting course in its initial stages in typical cases (Adams and Victor 1993). The history of the disease study begins in 1835, when the French pathologist J. Kruvelie described "spotted" or "insular" sclerosis. MS is considered the best understood in the group of demyelinating diseases, but its etiology is still unclear. Etiological hypotheses consider an infection, autoimmunity to normal myelin, a combination of infectious and autoimmune processes, and toxic and metabolic causes of MS. Currently, the most common is the hypothesis of multifactorial etiology of MS, according to which the disease develops, when a certain combination of external factors affects genetically susceptible individuals, causing chronic inflammation, autoimmunity, and demyelination of the white matter in the CNS. The genetic predisposition to MS remains unproven; however, the development of MS has been established to be most strongly associated with HLA class II DR2 haplotype. The role of other genes in the etiology of MS, as well as the possibility of a combination of different genetic factors, is still discussed.

In the majority of cases, these lesions have a relatively homogeneous MR signal and clear limits with the white matter. The form of MS plaques may be the most diverse, varying from round to irregular one. However, rounded lesions are encountered more often; they are identified mainly in the periventricular region and semioval centers and less frequently in the corpus callosum and subcortical structures. Individual plaques can be located in the projection of the brainstem and cerebellar hemispheres. On T1-weighted MRI, in relapsing-remitting MS, the plaques are not visible in most cases and only individual lesions are identified, which are characterized by a slightly hypointense MR signal. This group is also characterized by the absence of visualization of subtentorial plaques in T1-weighted images.

MS plaques may accumulate the contrast agent, reflecting transient BBB disorders. Contrast enhancement is used in MS to identify more or less specific features in the hyperintensity picture of multiple foci in T2-weighted images. It is known that the simultaneous detection of both contrast-enhanced and non-contrast-enhanced lesions is a characteristic of MS and puts in question other diagnoses (Fig. 41.1).

The diffuse type of contrast enhancement is characterized by opacification of an entire plaque. This type of contrast enhancement is a characteristic for multiple, small demyelination foci (a few millimeters in size). The annular type of contrast enhancement is observed with the accumulation of

M. Dolgushin et al., *Brain Metastases*, DOI 10.1007/978-3-319-57760-9_41

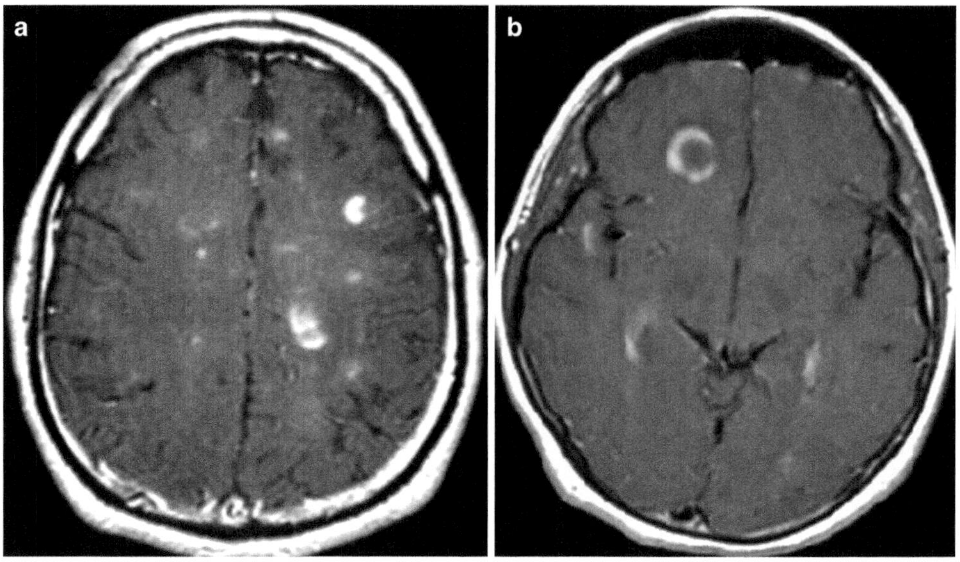

Fig. 41.1 Multiple sclerosis. **a, b** On T1-weighted MRI with contrast enhancement, multiple areas of its abnormal accumulation are observed. In "active" MS lesions, diffuse and annular types of contrast enhancement (**a**, **b**), as well as the partial type, half-ring accumulation, are observed

contrast agent in peripheral portions of larger foci—in the form of a ring. The dimensions of these lesions usually approach 1 cm or more. This type of contrast enhancement is a characteristic for plaques with the presence of a perifocal edema detectable in T2-weighted and DW images. This partial type of contrast enhancement, from our point of view, is the most pathognomonic for demyelination foci in MS, in general, and is manifested in the form of partial CA accumulation within the area of abnormal changes in the intensity of an MR signal detected by T2-weighted MRI. At the same time, the attention should be drawn to contrast enhancement of MS plaques in the form of a "half-ring" or a "half-moon," when an increase in the MR signal intensity on post-contrast T1-weighted images is observed only in a limited area on the plaque periphery, not confined to annular opacification (Fig. 41.2).

This semiannular or partial type of contrast enhancement should be used as one of the differential diagnostic criteria and pathognomonic symptoms of MS in the differential diagnosis with space-occupying brain lesions characterized by ring enhancement (full annular opacification), such as a metastasis, abscess, parasitic infestation, tumor cysts, and tuberculomas.

Proton MR spectroscopy (MRS) was conducted by many authors in MS and allows to accurately assess biochemical disturbances occurring in the lesions, to distinguish an edema from areas of demyelination and/or incomplete remyelination (Miller 1998). In MS, decreased NAA levels are noted in chronic MS plaques, as well as in the normal-looking white matter. A decrease in the NAA peak in MS is regarded as a sign of secondary neuronal death after primary demyelination. Consequently, this is a potential marker of irreversible damage to the brain tissue. The data obtained by H1-MR spectroscopy in patients with MS are dependent on the time of the study (Loevner and Grossman 1995). An early stage of demyelinating process is characterized by a relative increase in the choline (Cho) peak, the emergence of the lactate peak (Lac), a decrease in the N-acetylaspartate (NAA) peak, and the corresponding changes in the ratio of these peaks to the reference creatine peak (Cr). An increase in the Cho peak is due to the impaired integrity of cell membranes and destruction of axons in the area of active demyelination. An increase in the Lac peak also indicates destructive processes, cytotoxic edema, and anaerobic glycolysis processes with accumulation of lactic acid. A decrease in the NAA peak is due to the decrease in the neuronal mass in the affected area. An increase in the myoinositol (mI) peak is not a characteristic for an acute demyelination process and only occurs in chronic demyelinating diseases as a result of developing gliosis. However, taken separately, MR spectroscopy findings are insufficient for the differential diagnosis between a demyelinating process and glial brain tumors (e.g., anaplastic astrocytomas) having a similar spectral picture (Podoprigora 2001). Overall, the findings suggest that MR spectroscopy is able to reflect stages of histopathological changes in MS, allowing to track the history of disease and monitor the effectiveness of treatment.

MR/CT perfusion studies are also promising directions in the study of MS, identifying characteristics of tissue perfusion in the "seemingly normal" and affected white and gray matter. This study revealed differences in perfusion of acute (active) and chronic (inactive) MS plaques (Fig. 41.3).

It should be noted that there is no involvement of the meninges and ependymal layer of the ventricular system in MS. Furthermore, MTSs are characterized by an annular type of uniform contrast enhancement with simultaneous opacification of all the lesions, and there is no contrast enhancement in the form of "half-rings."

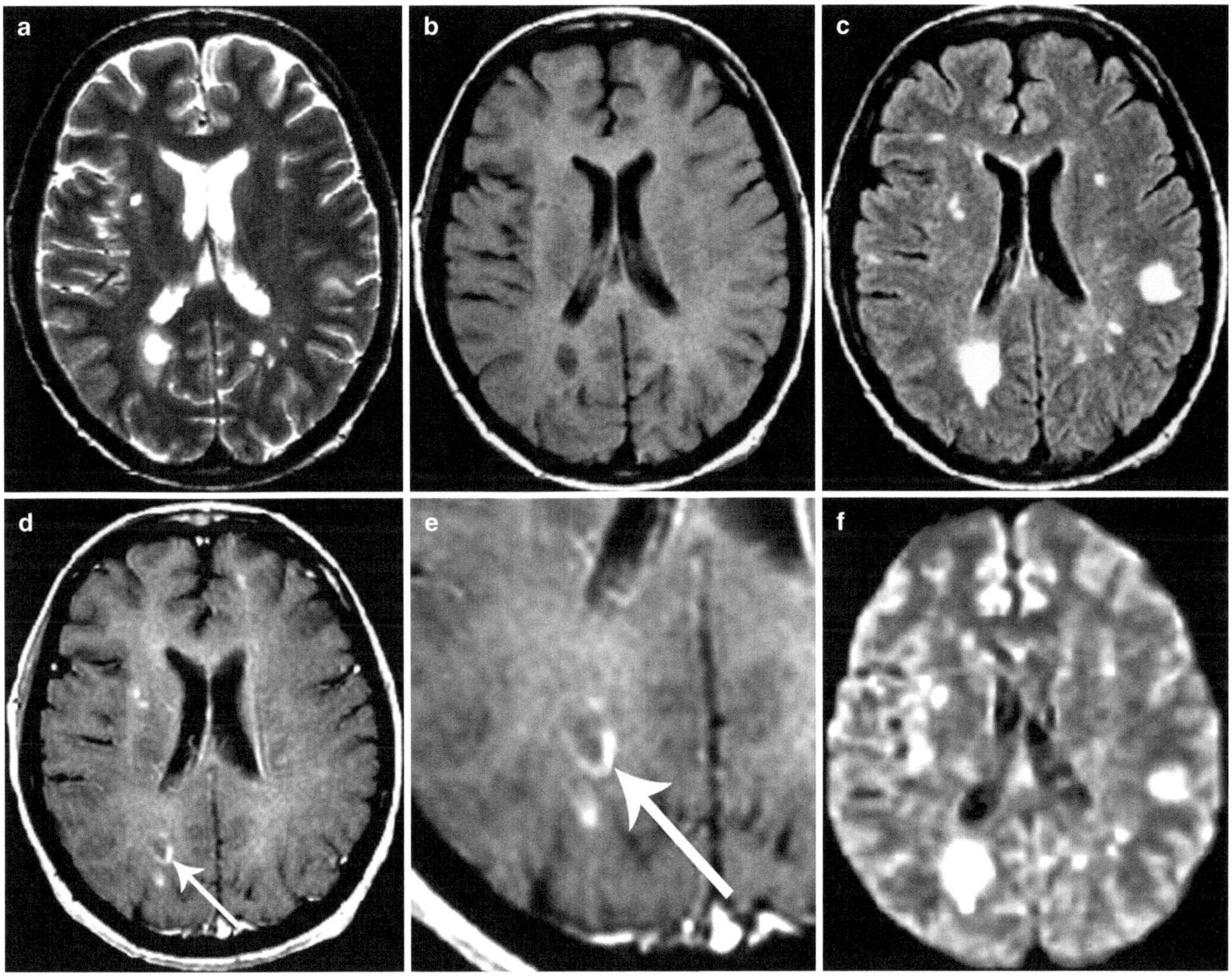

Fig. 41.2 Multiple sclerosis. On T2-weighted (**a**), T1-WI (**b**), T2-FLAIR (**c**), and T1-weighted MRI after intravenous contrast enhancement (**d**, **e**), there are multiple areas with an altered signal. Contrast enhancement in the form of a "half-ring" is observed along the edge of one of the portions (indicated by the *arrow*). All lesions are hyperintensive on T2-FLAIR (**c**). On DWI (**f**), the signal from demyelination foci is increased

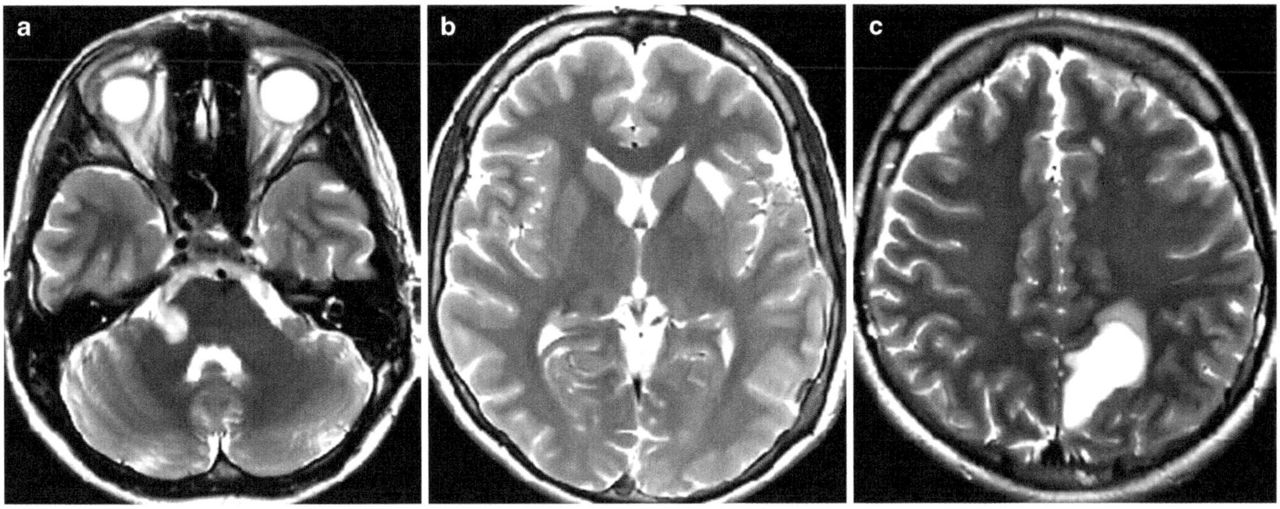

Fig. 41.3 Multiple sclerosis (pseudotumor form). On T2-weighted (**a**–**c**) and T1-weighted MRI with contrast enhancement (**d**), there are multiple demyelination foci. Contrast enhancement has open, peripheral character (**d**). On CBV and CBF perfusion maps (**e**, **f**), at the level of a major lesion in the right parietal region, there is a marked area with reduced perfusion

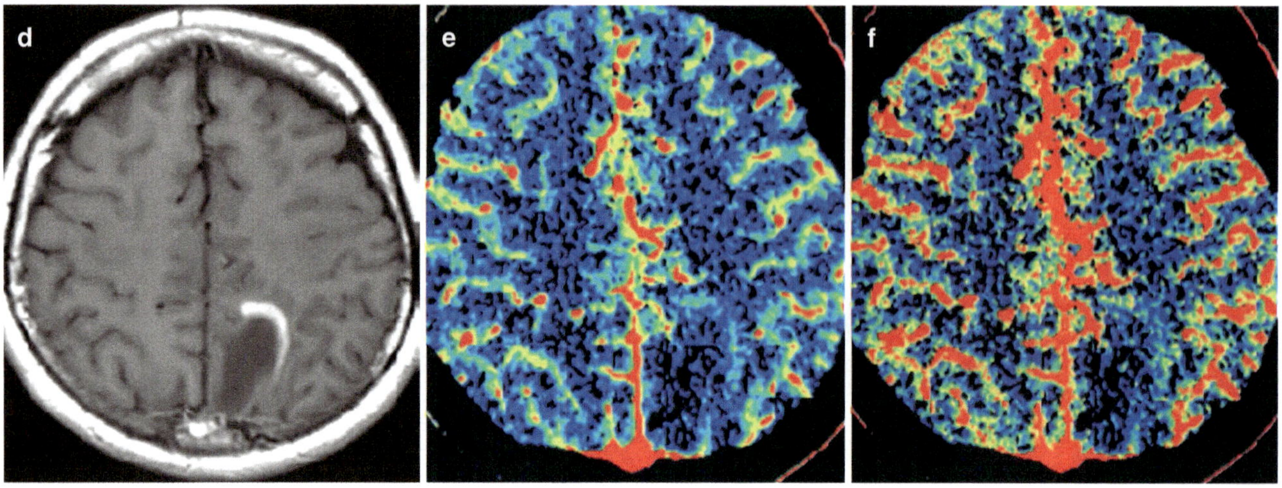

Fig. 41.3 (continued)

41.2 Acute Disseminated Encephalomyelitis (ADEM)

It is an inflammatory demyelinating disease that is more common in children but can occur in all age groups. Usually, it is clinically manifested in the form of a single-phase process limited by the central nervous system, developing in a few weeks after a nonspecific viral infection (measles, rubella, mumps, chicken pox, mononucleosis, Epstein-Barr virus, pertussis, mycoplasma, or Coxsackie B infection) or after vaccination (rabies, diphtheria, smallpox, tetanus, and typhoid). The disease can occur spontaneously on the background of good health.

MRI in ADEM visualizes a pattern identical to initial stages of the acute phase of MS. A number of patients diagnosed with ADEM subsequently experience a marked exacerbation, and the diagnosis is changed to MS. On T2-WI, there are multiple foci with a high homogeneous (due to the simultaneous occurrence) signal in the supratentorial white matter, brainstem, and cerebellum with frequent involvement of the deep gray matter. Lesions may be large, but a mass effect is usually minimal. MR follow-up usually identifies a marked reduction in the size of lesions (Figs. 41.4 and 41.5). In some cases, a full recovery after steroid therapy occurs. Exacerbations and new lesions can occur as a result of delays in discontinuation of therapy with corticosteroids.

In ADEM (similar to MS), in most cases, there is annular contrast enhancement. Accumulation of a contrast agent in the form of "half-rings" is less typical, since the demyelinating process is acute and monophasic; however, the lack of contrast enhancement of foci in ADEM does not contradict the diagnosis.

The use of new technologies, in particular, new study programs in MRI, allowed to objectify earlier assumptions about the relationship between a lesion with acute demyelination and cerebral veins—the hypothesis of perivenous inflammatory demyelination. The use of MRI with high magnetic field (1.5 T or greater) as well as 3D gradient echo pulse sequence or the SWI (SWAN) sequence "sensitive" to magnetic field inhomogeneities (susceptibility-weighted imaging) allows to visualize the venous structures passing through the entire acute demyelination plaque (Fig. 41.6).

Demyelinating processes, even in the active stage, are not characterized by an unusual increase in perfusion parameters; on the contrary, there is a decrease in CBV and CBF values. ADEM is no exception. An increase in MTT values is noted along the contour of large lesions due to mechanical effects on the brain tissue (Fig. 41.7). A marked reduction in the RP accumulation is noted with the

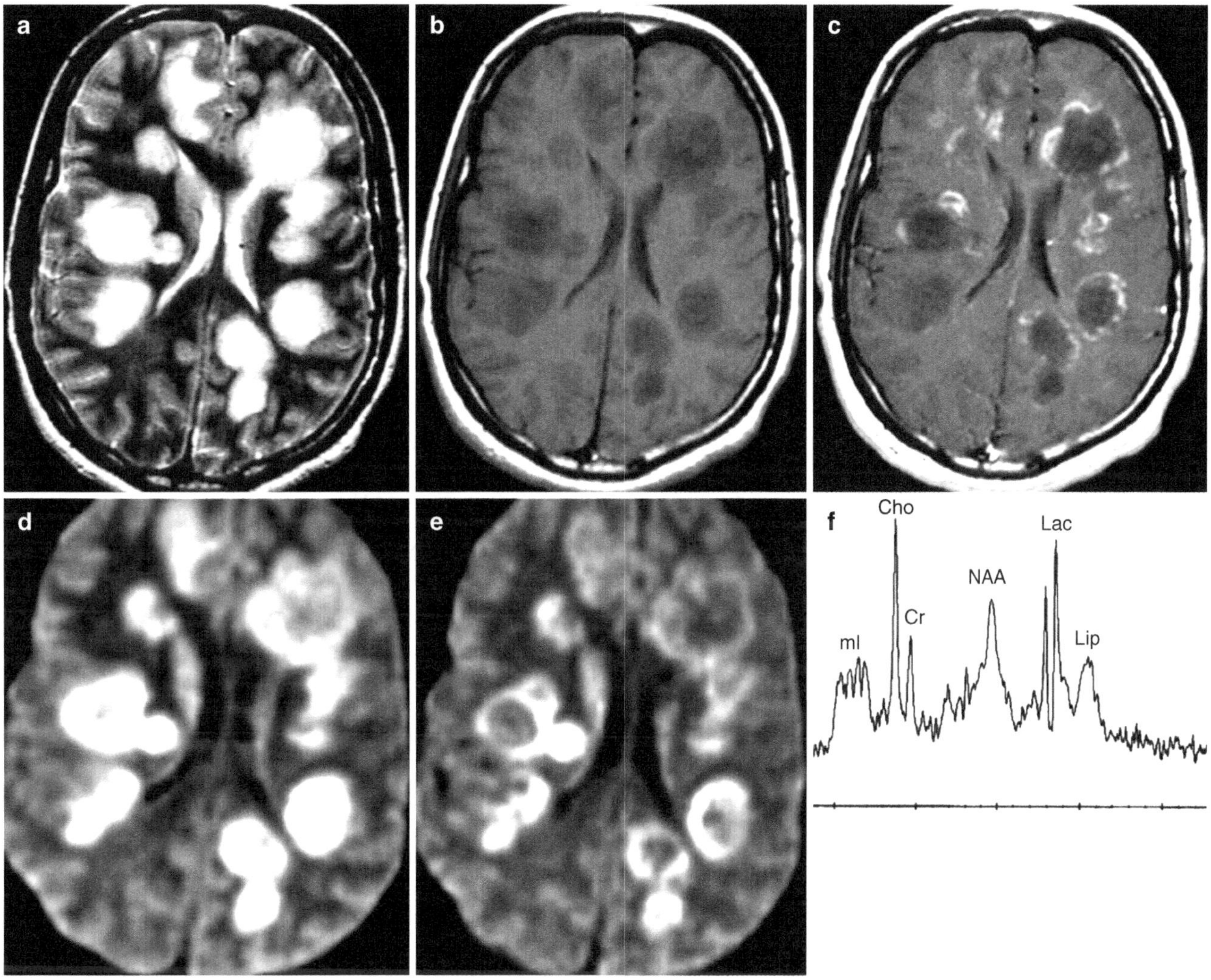

Fig. 41.4 Acute disseminated encephalomyelitis. MRI identifies multiple large foci of demyelination in the white matter of the cerebral hemispheres on both sides, with a hyperintense signal in T2-weighted images (**a**) and a hypointense signal in T1-weighted images (**b**). Accumulation of the intravenous contrast agent on the peripheral border of the lesions in the form of "rings" and "half-rings" (**c**). On DWI MRI with $b = 500$ (**d**) and $b = 1000$ (**e**), there is a decrease in the signal from the central areas of demyelination foci (areas of myelin destruction) and a high signal from the periphery of the foci. MR spectroscopy (**f**) shows a high double-humped Lac peak, a decrease in the NAA peak, and an increase in Cho peaks

use of ^{18}F–FDG. We performed several studies with ^{18}F-tyrosine in MS and ADEM patients at different stages of the disease and noted a moderate increase in its accumulation in the projection of demyelinating lesions but by several orders of magnitude lower than that in metastatic tumors (Fig. 41.8).

Thus, demyelinating diseases may mimic metastases only in case of multifocal manifestation. Accumulation of the contrast agent allows almost completely to eliminate metastases due to its heterogeneity and blurring. Additional study protocols—MR spectroscopy and perfusion protocols—leave no doubt as to the non-tumoral nature of lesions.

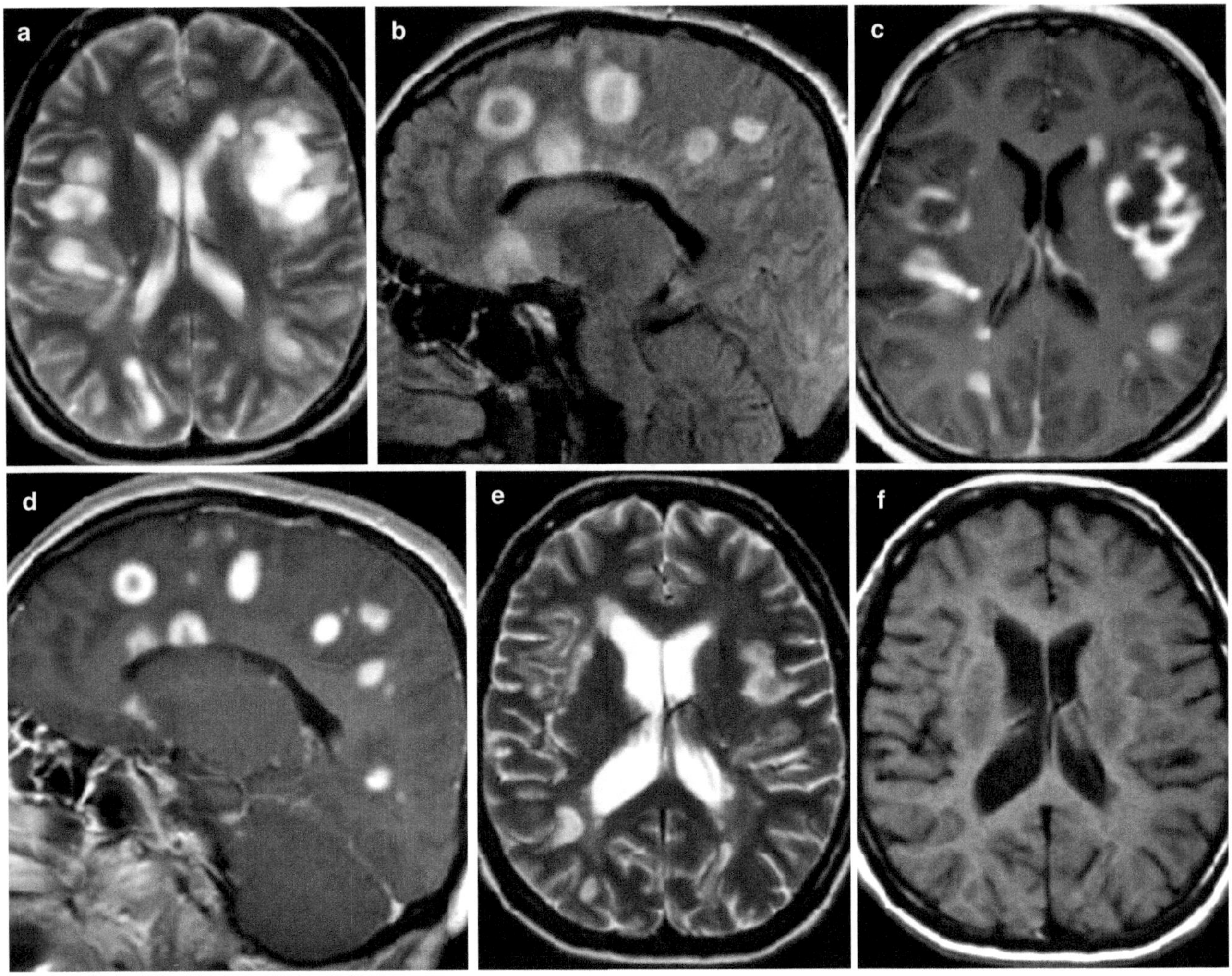

Fig. 41.5 Acute disseminated encephalomyelitis. Follow-up MRI studies. On T2-weighted (**a**) MRI in the axial projection and T2-FLAIR MRI (**b**) in the sagittal projection, there are multiple foci with an altered signal and different sizes and shapes, supratentorially in the white matter of the cerebral hemispheres and the corpus callosum. On T1-weighted MRI after intravenous contrast enhancement (**c**, **d**), the foci intensely and unevenly accumulate the contrast agent. One month after the first study (**e**, **f**), there is a decrease in the number and size of demyelination foci, regression of perifocal edema in the lesions, and a decrease in the volume of white matter with a compensatory expansion of the lateral ventricles

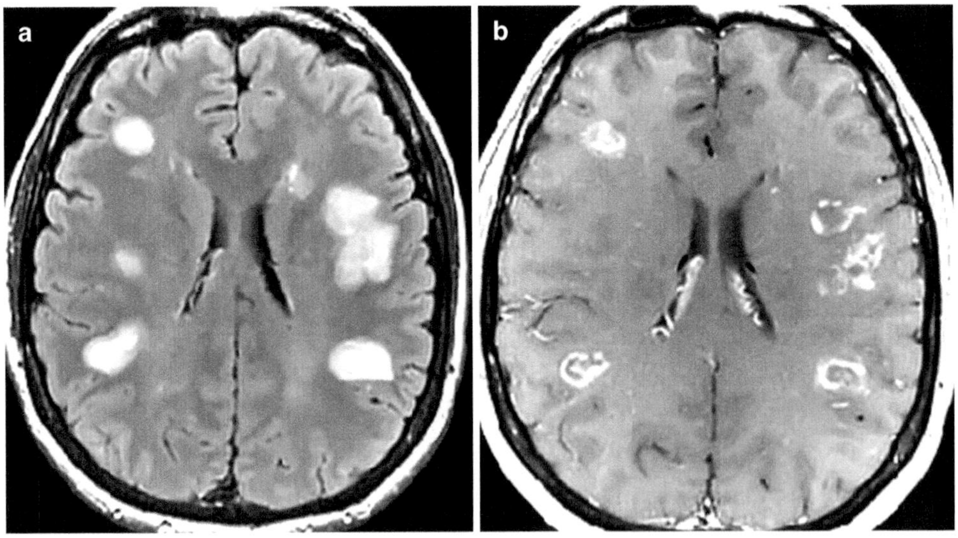

Fig. 41.6 Acute disseminated encephalomyelitis. T2-FLAIR MRI (**a**) shows the presence of multiple large lesions with abnormal changes in MR signal located in the subcortical region of both cerebral hemispheres. All lesions are characterized by the same type of peripheral contrast enhancement (**b**), followed by diffuse opacification of the entire plaque on delayed post-contrast images (**c**). 3D GRE sequence clearly demonstrates hypointense linear structures passing through the entire demyelination lesion—veins (**d**)—in individual plaques (the *arrows*)

Fig. 41.6 (continued)

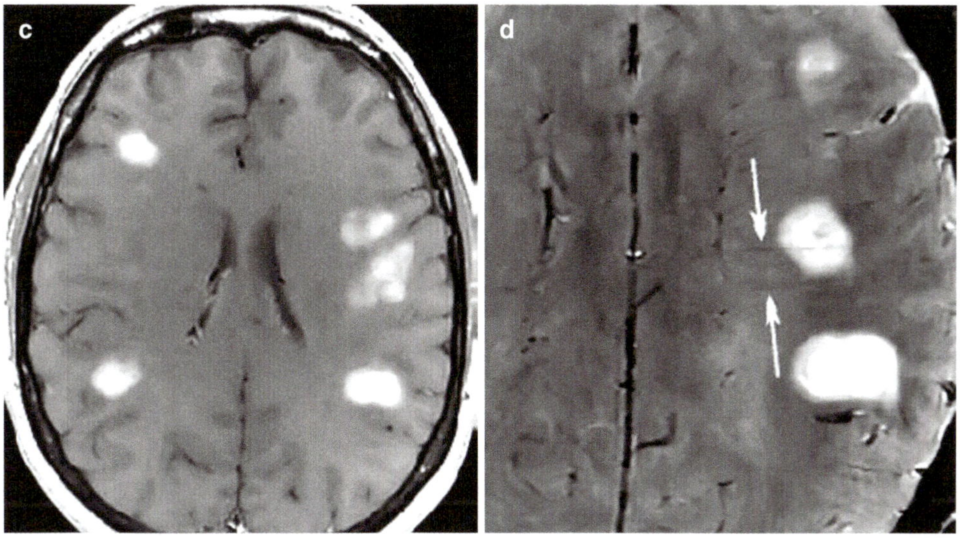

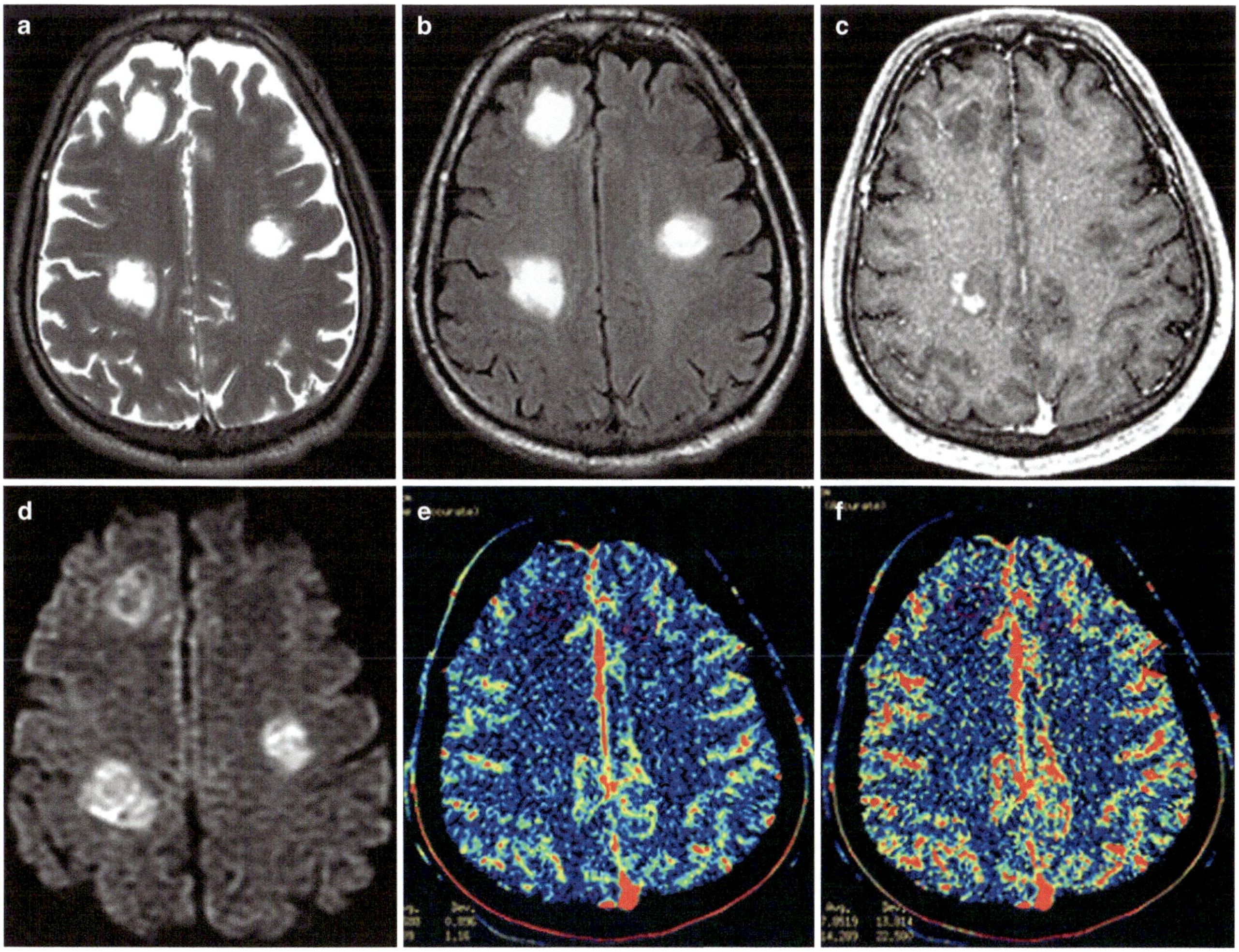

Fig. 41.7 Acute disseminated encephalomyelitis. In the tissue of the cerebral hemispheres, there are multiple areas with unclear and irregular contours with an increased signal in T2-weighted, T2-FLAIR, DWI MRI (**a**, **b**, **d**). On T1-weighted MRI (**c**) with contrast enhancement, low accumulation of the contrast agent is noted in one of the areas located in the right frontoparietal region; the rest of the lesions have no signs of accumulation of the contrast agent. On CT-perfusion maps of CBV (**e**) and CBF (**f**), perfusion values are low in these areas

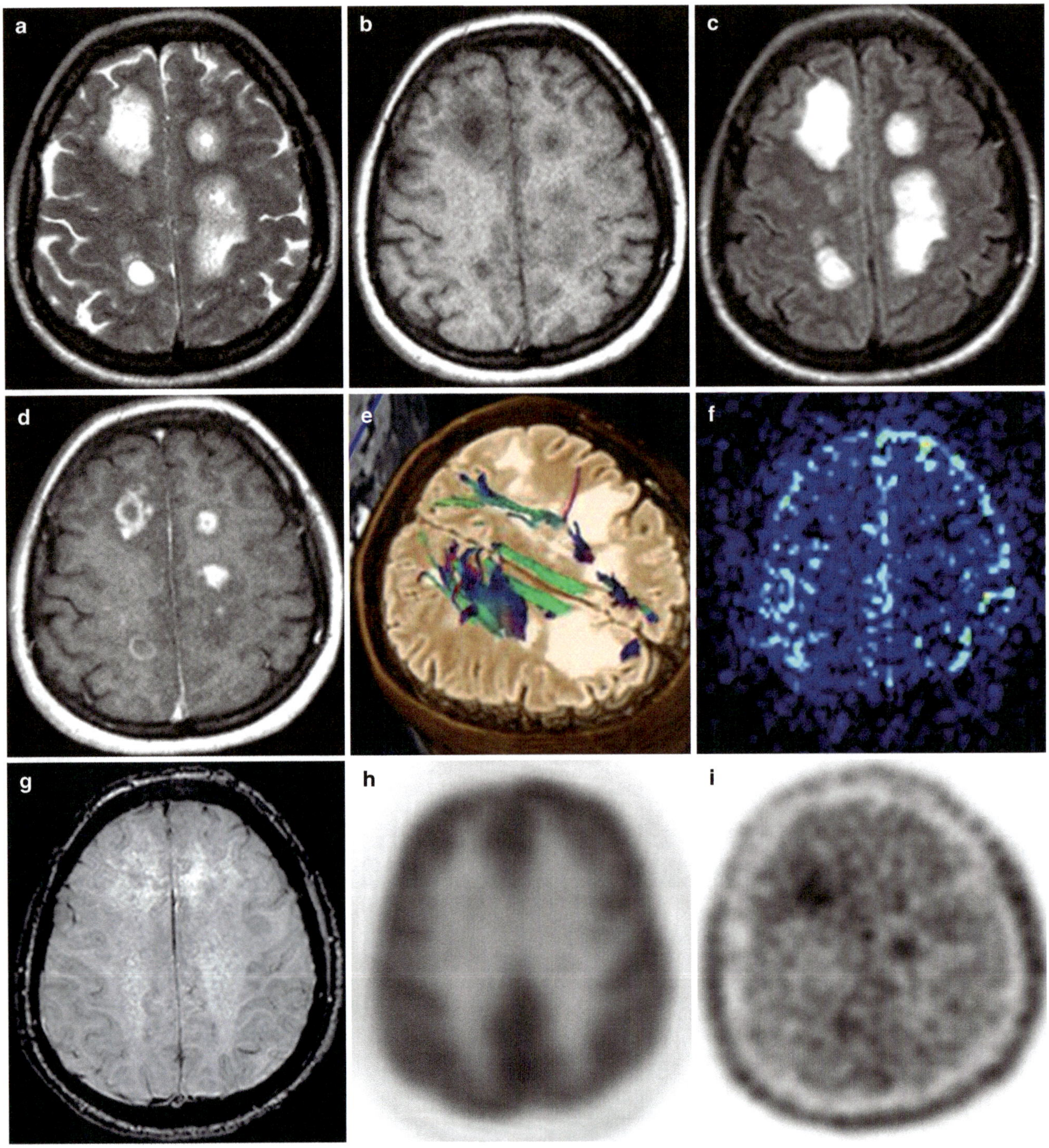

Fig. 41.8 Acute disseminated encephalomyelitis. In the tissue of the cerebral hemispheres, there are multiple areas with unclear and irregular contours with an increased signal in T2-weighted, T2-FLAIR MRI (**a**, **c**) and a decreased signal in T1-weighted MRI (**b**). On T1-weighted contrast-enhanced MRI (**d**), there are areas of intense and inhomogeneous accumulation of contrast agent. On MR tractography (**e**), individual fibers from conductive tracts are absent in the abnormal areas. On ASL MRI (**f**), there is decreased perfusion. In SWI (SWAN) images (**g**), low signal areas are not visualized. On PET with ^{18}F-FDG (**h**), no signs of abnormal radiopharmaceutical accumulation were identified; on PET with 18F-tyrosine (**i**), there are areas with increased radiopharmaceutical accumulation in some zones. On CT perfusion maps, no increase in CBV (**j**), CBF (**k**), and MTT (**l**) was observed

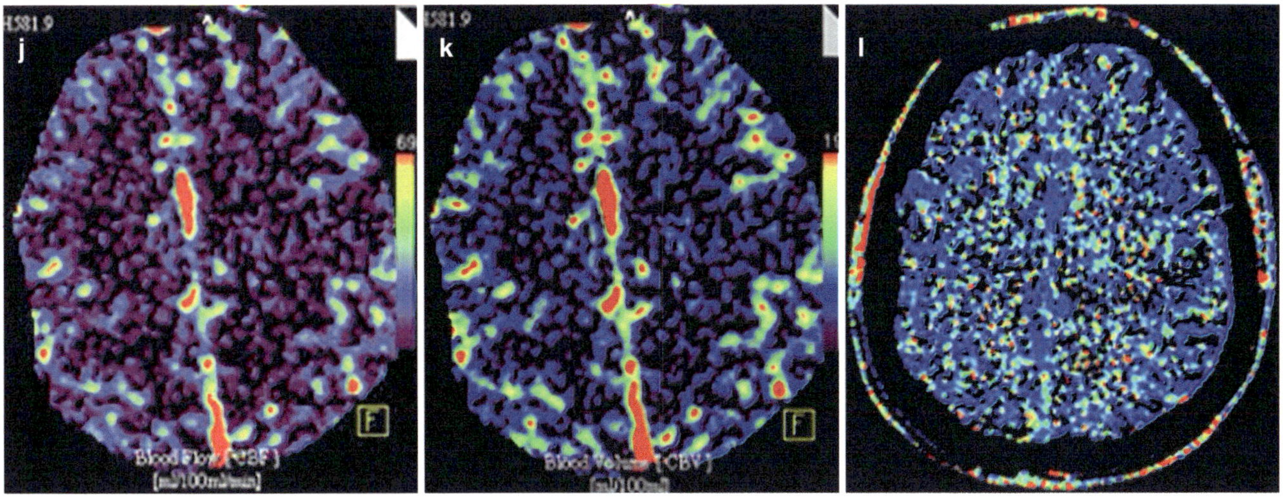

Fig. 41.8 (continued)

42 Traumatic Brain Injury

Acute hemorrhagic lesions from multiple contusions (up to 3 days) of the brain can be visualized by MRI with a certain degree of similarity of the tissue characteristics to those in metastatic lesions. A situation, when patients can be transported to the hospital in an unconscious state, cannot be excluded, since this can also occur as a result of strokes and hemorrhages into tumor lesions.

Such lesions in the acute stage contain mostly intracellular paramagnetic deoxyhemoglobin, which is formed upon dissociation of oxygen and hemoglobin. Since deoxyhemoglobin in undamaged hypoxic red cells does not cause a shortening of T1, hemorrhagic injuries have a normal or weakly hypointense signal in this sequence. The high concentration of red blood cells and fibrin in the clot is causing shortening of T2 and the emergence of very low signal areas in T2-weighted and T2*-weighted, T2-FLAIR images (Fig. 42.1). A few days later, the lesion of subacute contusion begins to "liquefy" with the development of a vasogenic edema that increases within the first week, which may be the cause of cerebral herniations. With the transformation of deoxyhemoglobin to the paramagnetic intracellular methemoglobin, the interaction between hydrogen atoms and the paramagnetic methemoglobin center is the cause of high signal intensity in T1-weighted images, which first manifests along the periphery of the contusion. Intracellular methemoglobin is characterized by a low signal in T2-weighted images.

After the rupture of the membranes of red blood cells and migration of methemoglobin into the extracellular space (a subacute phase), a change in the hemorrhagic contusion or hematoma occurs on the MRI scan—a high signal from extracellular methemoglobin in T1- and T2-weighted images. New vessels on the periphery of the lesion have no close endothelial connection, as it happens in the intact blood-brain barrier; therefore, accumulation of the contrast agent can be determined on the periphery of the lesion on CT and MRI, while blood vessels of the fragile granulation tissue predispose to repeated hemorrhages. At the same time, CT shows a decrease in the density of the contusion lesion and a mass effect due to the reduction in edema. The peripheral rim of hemosiderin and ferritin has a weekly intense signal in T1-weighted images and a significantly lower in T2-weighted images—the beginning of transition into the chronic phase of hematoma. The clot resorption starts from the periphery to the center, depending on the size of a hemorrhage. The duration of this process may vary from one to several weeks.

M. Dolgushin et al., *Brain Metastases*, DOI 10.1007/978-3-319-57760-9_42

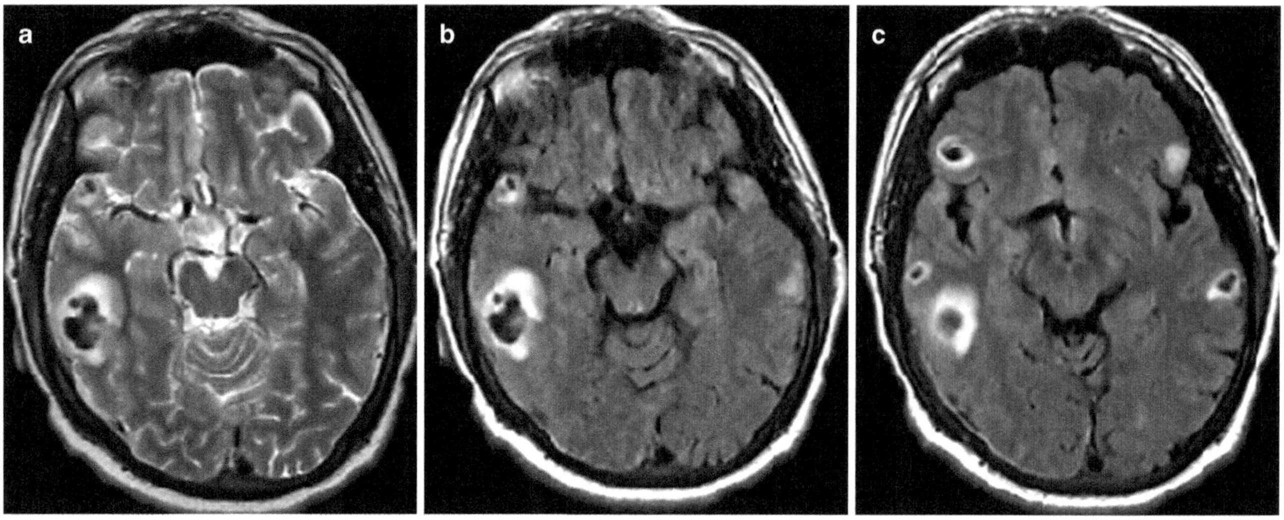

Fig. 42.1 Multiple brain contusion lesions. In both cerebral hemispheres on T2-weighted (**a**) and T2-FLAIR MRI (**b**, **c**), there are areas with a low signal in the center and an increased signal in the periphery

43 Fungal Infections (Mycoses) of CNS

Affecting the central nervous system, a fungal infection is regarded as an opportunistic granulomatous disease that can be acute and fulminant or chronic and slow. Fungi can invade the central nervous system and cause meningitis or parenchymal focal lesions in some patients suffering from systemic fungal infections.

MRI and CT manifestations of fungal infections are similar to those of tuberculosis (Lyons and Andriole 1986; Sze et al. 1998). CT and MRI can identify a space-occupying brain lesion, abscesses, infection foci in the eye sockets or sinuses, and hydrocephalus. The most common fungi are divided into opportunistic microorganisms that affect only immunocompromised patients (*Candida*, *Aspergillus*, *Mucor*) and microorganisms that also infect immunocompetent individuals. Cryptococcosis, histoplasmosis, and blastomycosis may arise both in previously healthy individuals and in patients with compromised immunity. *Candida*, *Aspergillus*, *Mucor*, *and Cryptococcus neoformans* live worldwide; the rest are endemic to certain geographical areas of the world. In addition, pathophysiology of fungal infections of the central nervous system depends on the fungus species. Fungi that reproduce as yeast (by division) enter the CNS via the hematogenous route (*Cryptococcus* and *Histoplasma*), enter the microvascular system of meninges, and penetrate the vascular wall, causing acute or chronic meningitis. Intracerebral lesions, such as granulomas or abscesses, are less common (Gaviani et al. 2005).

Fungi that reproduce in the infected tissue by hyphae (*Aspergillus*, *Mucor*) or pseudohyphae (*Candida*) tend to invade the parenchyma, not the meninges, since the blood supply of meninges is insufficient for them. Hyphae that form fungal colonies are able to penetrate and occlude large, medium, and small arteries, resulting in cerebral vascular accidents and cerebritis (Table 43.1).

CNS infection with *Candida* species often results in diffuse granulomatous intracerebral microabscesses, secondary to occlusion of small arterioles (Zimmenmann et al. 1987).

Cryptococcus neoformans is a fungus that most commonly affects the central nervous system in patients with AIDS. Clinically, fungal infection is observed in 6–7% of

Table 43.1 Pathogens of fungal meningitis

Pathogen	Opportunistic	Other affected structures	Characteristic changes in CSF
Cryptococcus neoformans	Sometimes in AIDS	Lungs, bones, joints	Viscous consistency, stained with ink, positive reaction to anti-cryptococcal antigen
Coccidioides immitis	No	Lungs, skin, bones	Positive reaction of complement binding
Candida	Yes	Mucous membranes, skin, esophagus, urinary tract, heart	Positive Gram stain
Aspergillus	Yes	Lungs, skin	*Neutrophilic pleocytosis*
Mucor	Yes (in diabetes mellitus)	Eye sockets, paranasal sinuses	
Histoplasma capsulatum	Occasionally	Lungs, skin, mucous membranes, heart, visceral peritoneum	
Blastomyces dermatitidis	No	Lungs, skin, bones, joints, visceral peritoneum	
*Actinomyces*1	No	Jaws, lungs, abdominal cavity, eye socket, sinus, skin.	
Nocardia[a]	Yes	Lungs, skin	

[a]Microorganisms that occupy an intermediate place between bacteria and fungi

M. Dolgushin et al., *Brain Metastases*, DOI 10.1007/978-3-319-57760-9_43

patients. Moreover, in 45% of HIV-infected patients with cryptococcosis, the clinical picture is manifested simultaneously with manifestations of the fungal infection (Davenport et al. 1992). The usual route of infection is inhalation. CNS cryptococcosis causes meningitis of the brain base. A common and often the only symptom of subacute fungal meningitis is headache. Clinical manifestations can also include neck stiffness, seizures, and signs of increased intracranial pressure.

Diagnosis is made based on staining, isolation of cryptococcal antigens, or fungal culture of cerebrospinal fluid.

MR manifestations of fungal meningitis are nonspecific. The CT picture is often negative. Signs identified by CT in the form of atrophy and open hydrocephalus are nonspecific. Contrast enhancement of meninges may be observed in patients with compromised immunity, but not always. MRI is more sensitive to fungal infections, than CT, but it often does not detect any abnormalities. Contrast-enhanced MRI can visualize opacification of meninges, which is usually not determined by MRI without contrast enhancement (Whiteman et al. 2002).

Virchow-Robin spaces are the place where fungi settle and begin to propagate. A fungal infection produces a large amount of mucus in these perforating vessels coming from the basal cisterns into the brain substance, which fills and dilates the perivascular spaces. This is most evident in the basal ganglia and the midbrain but is also sometimes detected in all brain tissues (Mathews et al. 1992). In such cases, the infectious agent is extrinsic relative to the brain tissue and does not cause any visible inflammatory response. Parenchymal/leptomeningeal nodules are presented in the cortex by small granulomas (Sze et al. 1987).

MR manifestations of *candidiasis* are nonspecific. On T2-weighted MRI, abscesses caused by *Candida* spp. appear as clearly delimited hypointense signal areas surrounded by a large high signal area representing an edema (Sze et al. 1998). Some call this manifestation a "target" (like in a shooting range). Rarely CNS candidiasis may cause meningitis and meningoencephalitis or form a granuloma (Fig. 43.1).

The most common signs on CT and MRI are an abnormal increase in contrast enhancement of the meninges on the surface of the cerebral hemispheres and basal cisterns, communicating hydrocephalus, and constriction of the fourth ventricle and a part of the third or lateral ventricles with formation of obstructive hydrocephalus. Less commonly observed is induration of the white or deep gray matter, which represents granulomas. Vascular occlusions are quite rare, but vasculitis can occur in Coccidioides.

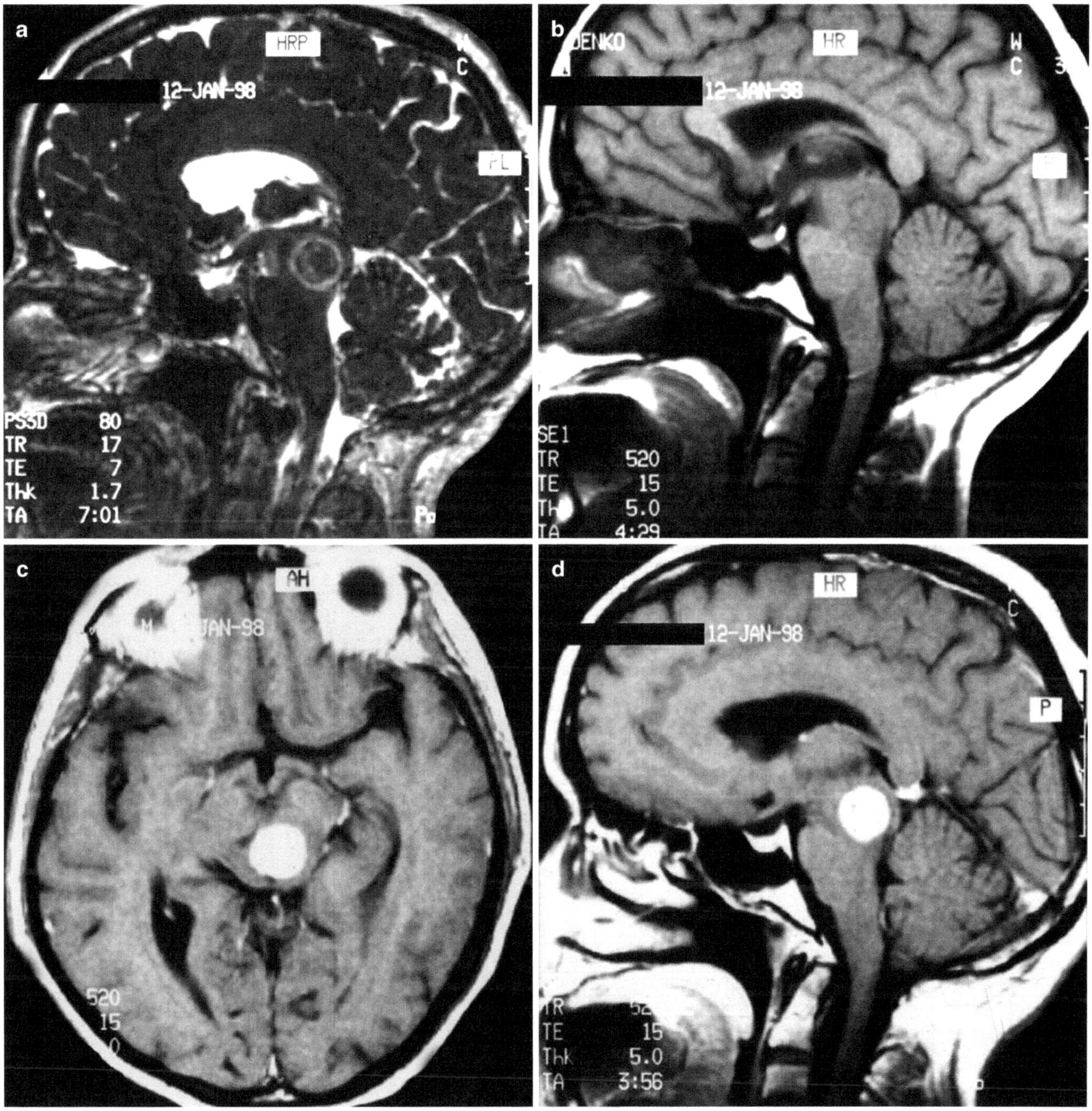

Fig. 43.1 Cryptococcosis. On MRI in the projection of the cerebral aqueduct, there is a round space-occupying lesion with an iso-hypointense signal in the MR-myelography sequence (**a**) with a well-determined thin CSF rim and isointense in T1-weighted MRI (**b**) and intensely, homogeneously accumulating the contrast agent (**c**, **d**). The quadrigeminal plate is deformed backwards. There is no pronounced edema of the brain tissue

Conclusion

As it has been repeatedly noted, the number of patients with metastatic brain lesions is growing, including due to improved quality of treatment of cancer patients—patients live longer and, as expected, this increases the long-term risk of distant metastases.

Metastatic brain involvement is an issue that really unites oncologists of any specialization, as this secondary brain damage can be observed in various malignant tumors. The decision on the tactics of treatment in this type of patients is very individual: drug therapy or radiosurgery can be used in case of small metastatic lesions, while surgery or symptomatic treatment is the option for solitary large lesions. Such decisions are always made on a collegiate basis by a joint discussion of neurosurgeons, radiologists, and chemotherapists. Patients with neuro-oncological diseases should be provided specialized medical care to a certain extent, and the designated vector of our professional aspirations has irrefutable and compelling reasons: real progress in the treatment of these patients, a significant reduction in the proportion of patients who were previously condemned for symptomatic treatment due to the feeling of hopelessness and despair. The breakthrough in modern technology of drug and radiation treatment of neuro-oncological patients allows to provide therapy with a complete "response" even in cases of multiple metastatic lesions. Undoubtedly, in case of the slightest suspicion of metastatic brain lesions or when searching the primary focus, the information about the disease dissemination and the history of cancer must be obtained as quickly as possible. Therefore, our ability to objectively and precisely identify metastases in the patient's body in general and in the brain in particular is an extremely important factor. How much we can rely on the modern diagnostic technology, including neuroimaging, depends on the justified choice of treatment tactics, possibly determining the fate of the patient: what should be done in a particular case—antitumor or symptomatic treatment?!

Undoubtedly, successful treatment cannot be imagined without a preliminary comprehensive investigation. This is also applicable to interim investigations to assess the effectiveness of the therapy.

In this monograph based on the results of the diagnosis and treatment of more than 3000 patients with metastatic brain lesions from malignant tumors with various origins and sites, the authors present to the professional audience their expertise and opinions on the essence of the issue of indication and identification of metastases in the brain in the context of current and future possibilities, as well as of what should be strived for in general.

The first part of the monograph is devoted to the main biological and pathophysiological processes associated with the occurrence and further growth of metastatic tumors in the brain, as well as conditions, causes, and mechanisms resulting in their characteristic clinical manifestation or characteristic sings that can be detected and recorded by means of modern radiology technologies. Despite the fact that the authors focus on visual characteristics of tumors, it is the complex of clinical data and diagnostic images obtained using radiation methods that allows to make a diagnostic conclusion.

The second part discusses current technical possibilities of CT, MRI, PET diagnostics, as well as their findings "synthesized" as relevant diagnostic images obtained in the study of metastases in the brain from primary tumors with various histogenesis and sites. The authors hope that images with CT and MR manifestations of various metastatic lesions and comments to them will help our colleagues in their professional activities. In addition, a number of patterns discovered of the authors in the interpretation of diagnostic images could also be useful. Among them are, for example:

- a decreased signal in T2-weighted images, more characteristic of colon cancer metastases in the brain;
- radiologic signs of a hemorrhage in the tumor stroma are typical for melanoma metastases;
- a cystic nature of metastatic lesions is more common in metastases of ovarian cancer and pancreatic cancer;
- the highest perfusion parameters (CBV, CBF) are typical for metastases of renal cancer and melanoma metastases, while low—for metastases of ovarian cancer;
- the use of perfusion protocols, as well as PET with ^{18}F-tyrosine allows to identify the tumor tissue on the background of a hemorrhage.

M. Dolgushin et al., *Brain Metastases,* DOI 10.1007/978-3-319-57760-9

Unfortunately, in the real-world practice MRI and CT studies without contrast enhancement are still performed in patients with suspected focal brain lesions, which is unacceptable. MR protocols such as DWI, MR spectroscopy, ASL, and some others did not allow us to identify any signs that show the "nature" of metastases, however, these protocols found their use in the differential diagnosis of metastases with other focal brain lesions. First of all, the difficulties in identification occur with the most common metastases of lung cancer and breast cancer, but eventually the solution will be probably found by investigating the receptor properties of tumors using radioisotope techniques (for example, PET). The search for a possible relationship between the site of metastatic lesions in the brain and the histogenesis of a primary tumor continues: preliminary data published by a number of researchers support the existence of such a relationship.

The attention should be paid to the issue of finding and identifying the primary tumor, manifested for the first time exclusively by intracranial metastases: in 17% of our cases of these patients, PET with ^{18}F-FDG did not reveal any abnormal accumulation of RP outside the brain. At the same time, the assessment of the total diagnostic information including CT, MRI, and PET findings gave a reason to consider extracranial cancer in 10% of cases (a false negative result), while the histological examination of biopsy and surgery material confirmed the secondary nature of brain lesions.

Undoubtedly, PET is currently the most sensitive and specific method for the diagnosis of unknown primary tumor in patients with metastatic brain lesions, although there is an increase in the role of a relatively simple-to-use "whole body" methods, such as DWI MRI. A comparison of the whole body PET cost, whose high cost is one of the main disadvantages, to the total cost of a standard set of diagnostic procedures (ultrasound, X-ray, endoscopic diagnosis, CT and MRI scans of the chest or abdomen, etc.) aimed at achieving the same goal (identification of the primary tumor) showed that a PET study is cheaper and, just as importantly, allows to solve diagnostic issues in a much shorter time. However, despite its clear advantages over the above complex of diagnostic measures, the PET method still has some significant limitations that do not allow to use it as a screening method. First of all, it is a technically demanding procedure; in addition, not all tumors have affinity for the most commonly used radiotracer—^{18}F-FDG. Nevertheless, subject to further development of radiochemistry, the method has great prospects.

The third part is devoted to the results of the use of diagnostic technologies in numerous cases of patients with metastatic tumors in the brain with a differentiated analysis by the location of the primary tumor. The statistical data on the incidence of certain cancers and the risk of metastasizing to the brain are provided. The use of the complex of methods in particular, including CT, MRI, and PET, allowed the authors to suggest the secondary nature of intracranial tumors in most cases. In case brain metastases were initially suspected, one-study whole body and brain DWI MRI or PET were used for the detection of the primary tumor and evaluation of the disease dissemination in general.

In the fourth part, we undertook a comparative analysis of the results of radiation diagnosis, based on a comparable number of cases of primary tumors and other focal brain lesions. This analysis was needed to find reliable criteria for the differential diagnosis of pathological conditions with such similar clinical and neuroimaging manifestations. In the context of secondary tumor lesions of the brain, solutions to differential diagnostic difficulties are presented by a large number of relevant illustrations and comments.

Primary brain tumors have their patterns of growth and development, rarely metastasize, and are an object of professional interest of neuro-oncologists and neurosurgeons. Accumulation of a contrast agent by an intracerebral tumor is not always a sign that it is malignant, however, the authors did not encounter a single case of metastatic lesions without abnormal accumulation of the contrast medium by secondary tumors of the brain. It has been shown that neither multiplicity nor solitarity of intracranial lesions, nor the size of tumor lesions, nor the presence of perifocal edema is specific symptom of metastases or glial tumors. The use of advanced MRI protocol can significantly improve the quality of diagnosis:

- on DWI MRI, the signal from the solid metastasis portion is higher than the signal from intracerebral tumors due to a denser structure of secondary tumors,
- intactness of the conductive tracts in the tumor structure established in MR tractography suggests a primary brain tumor,
- the presence of a choline peak in the spectrum is more typical for an intracerebral tumor,
- a small number of hypointense inclusions or their complete absence on SWI (SWAN) MRI is characteristic for metastatic, not primary malignant brain tumors,
- a sharp increase in the accumulation of ^{18}F-FDG by the tumor is more characteristic for lymphomas, than for gliomas or metastases (except for melanoma metastases);
- a significantly increased signal on DWI MRI is more characteristic for inflammatory changes (abscesses);
- a decrease in perfusion values (both in CT and MRI perfusion) is not characteristic of malignant tumors, at the same time allows to think about a demyelinating or inflammatory disease.

The authors pay particular attention to identification, verification, and differential diagnosis of treatment-induced changes in the brain tissue at the tumor lesion. The issue of identifying post-radiation changes (necrosis) after various radiotherapy regimens is relevant for almost half of cases of patients who received this treatment: modern possibilities of evaluating the effectiveness of antitumor treatment using radiation diagnostic technologies have found a worthy reflection in this monograph. DWI MRI and MR spectroscopy did not show any diagnostic value in differentiation of a residual tumor from post-radiation changes in the brain substance, in contrast, PET and perfusion methods allow to determine the presence of a residual tumor tissue in most cases. It must be said in fairness that the mixed nature of the changes in patients treated for intracranial malignant neoplasms (a combination of a residual tumor with necrotic tissue in the area of therapeutic intervention) occurs much more frequently, and this is due to the lack of any reasonable time frames to perform follow-up studies after the treatment, while a simplified interpretation of changes with time in the size of lesions is not an unambiguous reflection of a benefit or failure of the treatment.

Of course, it is extremely difficult to summarize and display all the cumulative experience of the authors. The scientific results of many years of work became instantly obsolete as new technological opportunities occurred, encouraging the authors to investigate them, while constantly emerging new analytical data delayed the publication of this book over and over again. The authors sincerely hope that their work will not be ignored by the professional community and will broaden the range of researchers of the diagnosis issues related to metastatic tumors in the brain and will hasten their effective solution.

The authors express their deep gratitude to the scientific personnel, doctors, nurses, and radiologic technologists of diagnostic departments at the research institutions of the Ministry of Health of the Russian Federation—N. N. Blokhin Russian Cancer Research Center and N. N. Burdenko National Scientific and Practical Center for Neurosurgery for their participation in the clinical work that underlies this monograph.

Bibliography

Aalders J, Syde R, Poppema S, et al. Prognostic factors and changing trends in the treatment of stage 1 endometrial cancer: a clinical and histopathological study of 182 patients. Int J Radiat Oncol Biol Phys. 1984;10:2083–8.

Abasheev-Konstantinovsky LA. Psychopathology in brain tumors, vol. 200. Moscow: M. Medicine; 1973.

Abdelmalik A, Alenezi S, Muzaffar R. The incremental added value of including the head in (18)F-FDG PET/CT imaging for cancer patients. Front Oncol. 2013;3:71.

Abrakov LV. Lung cancer metastases in the brain and their treatment. Vestn Khir. 1955;2:33–9.

Abrams H, Spiro R, Goldstein N. Metastases in carcinoma. Analysis of 1000 autopsied cases. Cancer. 1950;3:74–85.

Adamovich-Razumovskaya AI, Goryunova MT. Clinical and morphological properties of metastatic tumors of the central nervous system. Coll. of scientific works of Sverdlovsk Med. Inst. in the XX century. Sverdlovsk;1958. p. 172–201.

Adams J, Lodge J, Parker D. Liver transplantation for metastatic hemangiopericytoma associated with hypoglycemia. Transplantation. 1999;67:488–9.

Adams R, Victor M. Multiple sclerosis and allied demyelinative diseases. In: Adams R, Victor M, editors. Principles of neurology. 5th ed. New York: McGraw-Hill; 1993. p. 776–98.

Aitken J, Martinez Z, McDonald G, et al. Sensation of smell does not determine motional status with cystic fibrosis. Pediatr Pulmonol. 1997;24:52–6.

Akeson P, Larsson E, Kristoffersen D, et al. Brain metastases – comparison of gadodiamide injection-enhanced MR imaging at standard and high dose, contrast-enhanced CT and non-contrast-enhanced MR imaging. Acta Radiol. 1995;36(3):300–6.

Akimov MA, Gershanowitch ML. Clinical evaluation of the effectiveness of modern chemotherapy regimens of first, second and third lines for patients with disseminated melanoma. Vopr Oncol. 2001;47(4):428–35.

Alazraki N, Shumate M, Kooby D. A clinican's guide to nuclear oncology. Practicak molecular imaging and radionuclide therapies. Reston: The Society of Nuclear Medicine; 2007. p. 206.

Al-Dhahri S, Al-Amro A, Al-Shakwer W. Cerebellar mass as a primary presentation of papillary thyroid carcinoma: case report and literature review. Head Neck Oncol. 2009;29:1–23.

Alexander E, Moriarty T, Loeffler J. Radiosurgery for metastases. J Neuro-Oncol. 1996;27:279–85.

Allen J, Bruce J, Larry E et al. Pineal region tumors. In: Diagnostic pathology pediatric neoplasms. On-line: Levin_ch07_p193-207.pdf.

Alperovich PN. Differential diagnostic features of single and multiple metastases to the brain. J Neuropathol Psychiatry S S Korsakova. 1975;9:1333–9.

Alperovich PN. Metastatic brain cancer. Nevrol Psykhiatr Kiev. 1977;6:3–11.

Alsop D, Detre J, Golay X, et al. Recommended implementation of arterial spin-labeled perfusion MRI for clinical applications: a consensus of the ISMRM perfusion study group and the European consortium for ASL in dementia. Magn Reson Med. 2015;73(1):102–16.

Althuis M, Fergenbaum J, Garcia-Closas M. Etiology of hormone receptor-defined breast cancer: a systematic review of the literature. Cancer Epidemiol Biomark Prev. 2004;13(10):1558–68.

Altimari-Romero R, Montenegro P, Michaluart P, et al. Brain metastases from papillary thyroid carcinoma: a case report and review of the literature. Rev Hosp Clin. 1997;52:263–6.

Altundag K, Bondy M, Mirza N, et al. Clinicopathologic characteristics and prognostic factors in 420 metastatic breast cancer patients with central nervous system metastasis. Cancer. 2007;110:2640–7.

Amane S, Honig M, Milner T, et al. Sites of acetylcholine synthesis and release associated with microvessels in cerebral cortex: ultrastructural and neurochemical studies. J Cereb Blood Flow Metab. 1987;7:5330.

Ambrose J, Hounsfield G. Computed transverse axial tomography. Proceedings of the British Institute of Radiology. Br J Radiol. 1973;46:148–9.

Amer M, Al-Sarraf M, Baker L, et al. Malignant melanoma and central nervous system metastases: incidence, diagnosis, treatment and survival. Cancer. 1978;42:660–8.

Ammirati M, Cobbs C, Linskey M, et al. The role of retreatment in the management of recurrent/progressive brain metastases: a systemic review and evidence-based clinical practice guideline. J Neuro-Oncol. 2010;96:85–96.

Andre F, Slimane K, Bachelot T, et al. Breast cancer with synchronous metastases: trends in survival during a 14-year period. J Clin Oncol. 2004;22:3302–8.

Araujo L. A new brainwave in non-small cell lung cancer: driving targeted therapy to central nervous system metastases. Transl Cancer Res. 2013;2(1):51–3.

Arbelaez A, Castillo M, Armao D. Imaging features of intraventricular melanoma. Am J Neuroradiol. 1999;20:691–3.

Ariel IM. Incidence of metastases to lymph nodes from soft tissue sarcomas. Semin Surg Oncol. 1988;4(1):27–9.

Arslanoglu A, et al. MR imaging characteristics of polimyxoidastrocytomas. Am J Neuroradiol. 2003;24:1906–8.

Arutyunov AI, Kornienko VN. Total cerebral angiography. Moscow: M. Medicine; 1971. p. 167.

Asa S. Practical pituitary pathology: what does the pathologist need to know? Arch Pathol Lab Med. 2008;132:1231–40.

Atlas S, Grossman R, Gomori J, et al. MR imaging of intracranial metastatic melanoma. J Comput Assist Tomogr. 1987a;11:577–82.

Atlas S, Grossman R, et al. MR imaging of metastatic melanoma. Radiology. 1987b;3:577–82.

Attenberger U, Runge V, Jackson C, et al. Comparative evaluation of lesion enhancement using 1 M gadobutrol vs. 2 conventional gadolinium chelates, all at a dose of 0.1 mmol/kg, in a rat brain tumor model at 3 T. Investig Radiol. 2009;44:251–6.

Axel EM. Morbidity and mortality from breast cancer in Russia. Materials of the conference "Breast Cancer", Moscow, January 22–24, 2014. p. 34–38.

M. Dolgushin et al., *Brain Metastases*, DOI 10.1007/978-3-319-57760-9

Axel EM. Statistics of gynecologic malignant neoplasms. J Oncogynecol. 2012;1:18–23.

Axel EM. Status of oncological aid to the population in Russia and the CIS in 2007. Bull NN Blokhin Russ Cancer Res Center. 2009;20(3/annex 1):8–155.

Axel L. Tissue mean transit time from dynamic computed tomography by a simple deconvolution technique. Investig Radiol. 1983;18:94–9.

Babchin IS, Babchin IP, Kalkun VR. Metastatic brain cancer. Moscow: Meditsina; 1974. p. 192.

Babchin IS, Babchin IP, Kalkun VR. Metastatic brain cancer. L.; 1974. p. 192.

Badalament R, Kreutzer E, Gluck R, et al. Surgical treatment of brain metastases from renal cell carcinoma. Urology. 1990;36:112–7.

Baert A, Sartor K. Imaging of orbital and visual pathway pathology. Berlin: Springer; 2006. p. 429.

Baert A, Sartor K. In: Jackson A, Buckley DL, Parker GJM, editors. Dynamic contrast-enhanced magnetic resonance imaging in oncology. Berlin Heidelberg: Springer-Verlag; 2005. p. 313.

Baker A. Metastatic tumors of the nervous system. Arch Pathol Lab Med. 1942;34:495–537.

Baker G, Kernohan J, Kiefer E. Metastatic tumors of the brain. Surg Clin North Am. 1951;31:1143–5.

Balch C, Kirkwood J. Cutaneous melanoma. In: Cancer principles and practice of oncology. Philadelphia, PA: Lippincott Williams & Wilkins; 1997. p. 1947–94.

Baltaci S, Orhan D, Soyupek S, et al. Influence of tumor stage, size, grade, vascular involvement, histological cell type and histological pattern on multifocality of renal cell carcinoma. J Urol. 2000;164(1):36–9.

Barajas R, Cha S. Imaging diagnosis of brain metastasis. Prog Neurol Surg. 2012;25:55–73.

Barnholtz-Sloan J, Sloan A, Davis F, et al. Incidence proportions of brain metastases in patients diagnosed (1973 to 2001) in the Metropolitan Detroit Cancer Surveillance System. J Clin Oncol. 2004;22(14):2865–72.

Basser P, Pierpaoli C. A simplified method to measure the diffusion tensor from seven MR images. Magn Reson Med. 1998;39:928–34.

Basser P, Pierpaoli C. Microstructural and physiological features of tissues elucidated by quantitative-diffusion-tensor MRI. J Magn Reson B. 1996;111:209–19.

Behney C. Advanced carcinoma of the cervix with a report of 166 necropsies. Am J Obstet Gynecol. 1933;26:608–14.

Behranwala K, A'Hern R, Omar A-M, et al. Prognosis of lymph node metastasis in soft tissue sarcoma. Ann Surg Oncol. 2004;11(7):714–9.

Bektas H, Länger F, Piso P, et al. Neuroendocrine tumors of the stomach. Surgery therapy and prognosis. Chirurg. 2002;73(4):331–5.

Belohlavek O, Simonova G, Kantorova I, et al. Brain metastases after stereotactic radiosurgery using the Leksell gamma knife: can FDG PET help to differentiate radionecrosis from tumor progression? Eur J Nucl Med Mol Imaging. 2003;30:96–100.

Belov DM, Karahan VB, Bekyashev AH, et al. Surgical stage in the complex treatment of patients with cerebral metastases of breast cancer. Malignant Tumours. 2014;10(3):110–5.

Bendell J, Domchek S, Winer E. Central nervous system metastases in women who receive trastuzumab-based therapy by metastatic breast carcinoma. Cancer. 2003;97:2972–7.

Bergmann M, Edel G. Primary intracerebral non-Hodgkin's lymphoma. Pathology. 1991;12:246–53.

Bernaerts A, Vanhoenacker F, Parizel P, et al. Tuberculosis of the central nervous system: overview of neuroradiological findings. Eur Radiol. 2003;13:1876–90.

Bhatia R, Tandon P, Banerji A. Brain abscess: an analysis of 55 cases. Int Surg. 1973;58(8):565.

Bianchi M, Sun M, Jeldres C, et al. Distribution of metastatic sites in renal cell carcinoma: a population-based analysis. Ann Oncol. 2012;23(4):973–80.

Bindal AK, Bindal RK, Hess KR, Shiu A, Hassenbusch SJ, Shi WM, et al. Surgery versus radiosurgery in the treatment of brain metastasis. J Neurosurg. 1996;84(5):748–54.

Bisese J. MRI of cranial metastasis. Semin Ultrasound CT MRI. 1992;3:473–83.

Bishop J. Molecular themes in oncogenesis. Cell. 1991;64:235–48.

Biswas G, Bhagwat R, Khurana R, et al. Brain metastasis evidence based management. J Cancer Res Ther. 2006;2(1):513.

Blanco A, Teh S, Amato R. Role of radiation therapy in the management of renal cell cancer. Cancers. 2011;3:4010–23.

Bliznyukov OP, Cosmin LD, Olyushin VE, et al. Malignant tumors of the central nervous system may be available for an attack with specific antibodies. Vopr Onkol. 2001;47(1):49–51.

Bloch F, Hanson H, Packard M. Nuclear induction. Phys Rev. 1946;70:460–74.

Blouw B, et al. The hypoxic response of tumors is dependent on their microenvironment. Cancer Cell. 2003;4:133–46.

Boogerd W, Vos V, Hart A, et al. Brain metastases in breast cancer: natural history, prognostic factors and outcome. J Neuro-Oncol. 1993;15(2):165–74.

Bouffet E, Doumi N, Thiesse P, et al. Brain metastases in children with solid tumors. Cancer. 1997;79:403–10.

Boyle P, Leon M. Epidemiology of colorectal cancer. Br Med Bull. 2002;64:1–25.

Bradbury M. The concept of blood–brain barrier. Moscow: M. Medicine; 1983. p. 480.

Breckwoldt M, Bendszus M, Cerebral MR. imaging of malignant melanoma (article in German). Radiologe. 2015;55(2):113–9.

Brehar F, Gorgan R, Neacsu A. Brain metastases of neuroendocrine tumor with unknown primary location – case report. Rom Neurosurg. 2013;20(2):159–65.

Brennan J, Boyle J, Koch W, et al. Association between cigarette smoking and mutation of the p53 gene in head and neck squamous carcinoma. N Engl J Med. 1995;332:712–7.

Broadwell R, Sofroniew M. Serum proteins bypass the blood–brain fluid barriers for extracellular entry to the central nervous system. Exp Neurol. 1993;120(2):245–63.

Brovkina AF. Diseases of the orbit: Meditsinskoye Informatsionnoe Agentstvo LLC, M; 2008. p. 256.

Brovkina AF. Endocrine ophthalmopathy. Moscow: M. GEOTAR Media; 2004. p. 174.

Brovkina AF. Ophthalmooncology: a guide for physicians, vol. 420. Moscow: Meditsina M; 2002.

Brown K, Cheng Y, Haacke M, et al. Magnetic resonance imaging: physical principles and sequence design. 2nd ed. Hoboken: Wiley; 2014.

Bruce J, Stein B. Complications of surgery for pineal region tumors. In: Post K, Freidman E, McCormick PC, editors. Postoperative complications in intracranial neurosurgery. New York: Thieme; 1993. p. 74–86.

Brunschwig A, Pierce V. Necropsy findings in patients with carcinoma of the cervix. Am J Obstet Gynecol. 1948;56:1134–7.

Bruzzone M, Campora E, Chiara S, et al. Cerebral metastases secondary to ovarian cancer: still an unusual event. Gynecol Oncol. 1993;49:37–40.

Bryusova SS. Brain angiography. 1951.

Buetow M, Burton P, Smirniotopoulos J. Typical, atypical and misleading features in meningioma. Radiographics. 1991;11:1087–100.

Bulakbasi N, Kocaoglu M, Somuncu I. Assessment of diagnostic accuracy of perfusion MR imaging in primary and metastatic solitary malignant brain tumors. Am J Neuroradiol. 2005;26:2187–99.

Bullard D, Cox E. Central nervous system metastases in malignant melanoma. Neurosurgery. 1981;8:26–30.

Burt M, Wronski M, Arbit E, et al. Resection of brain metastases from non-small-cell lung carcinoma. Results of therapy. Memorial Sloan-Kettering Cancer Center Thoracic Surgical Staff. J Thorac Cardiovasc Surg. 1992;103:399–410.

Burt R, Bishop D, et al. Risk and surveillance of individuals with heritable factors for colorectal cancer. WHO Collaborating Centre for the Prevention of Colorectal Cancer. Bull World Health Organ. 1990;68(5):655–65.

Burtscher I, Holtas S. In vivo proton MR spectroscopy of untreated and treated brain abscesses. Am J Neuroradiol. 1999;20(6):1049–53.
Burtscher I, Holtas S. Proton MR spectroscopy in clinical routine. J Magn Reson Imaging. 2001;13(4):560–7.
Cairncross J, Kim J, Posner J. Radiation therapy for brain metastases. Ann Neurol. 1980;7:529–41.
Campos S, Davey P, Hird A, et al. Brain metastasis from an unknown primary, or primary brain tumour? A diagnostic dilemma. Curr Oncol. 2009;16:62–6.
Cappuzzo F, Mazzoni F, Maestri A, et al. Medical treatment of brain metastases from solid tumors. Forum (Genova). 2000;10(2):137–48.
Caricato M, Borzomati D, Ausania F, et al. Cerebellar metastasis from pancreatic adenocarcinoma. A case report. Pancreatology. 2006;6:306–8.
Carney D. Prophylactic cranial irradiation and small-cell lung cancer. N Engl J Med. 1999;341:524–6.
Caroli M, Di Cristofori A, Lucarella F, et al. Surgical brain metastases: management and outcome related to prognostic indexes: a critical review of a ten-year series. ISRN Surg. 2011;2011:207103.
Carswell R. Melanoma – pathological anatomy, part 9. London: Longman; 1838.
Cascino T, Byrne T, Deck M, Posner JB. Intra-arterial BCNU in the treatment of metastatic brain tumors. J Neuro-Oncol. 1983;1(3):211–8.
Casentino C, Poulton T, Esquerra J. Giant cranial hemangiopericytoma: MR and angiographic findings. Am J Neuroradiol. 1993;14:253–6.
Castaldo J, Bernat J, Meier F, et al. Intracranial metastases due to prostatic carcinoma. Cancer. 1983;52:1739–47.
Catane R, Kaufman J, West C, et al. Brain metastasis from prostatic carcinoma. Cancer. 1976;38(6):2583–7.
Cenic A, Nabavi D, Craen R, et al. A CT method to measure hemodynamics in brain tumors: validation and application of cerebral blood flow maps. Am J Neuroradiol. 2000;21:462–70.
Ceresoli G, Cappuzzo F, Gregorc V, et al. Gefitinib in patients with brain metastases from non-small-cell lung cancer: a prospective trial. Ann Oncol. 2004;7:1042–7.
Cha S, Lupo J, Chen M, et al. Differentiation of glioblastoma multiforme and single brain metastasis by peak height and percentage of signal intensity recovery derived from dynamic susceptibility-weighted contrast-enhanced perfusion MR imaging. Am J Neuroradiol. 2007;28:1078–84.
Chambers A, Groom A, MacDonald I. Dissemination and growth of cancer cells in metastatic sites. Nat Rev Cancer. 2002;2:563–72.
Chang S, Lai P, Chen W. Diffusion-weighted MRI features of brain abscess and cystic or necrotic brain tumors: comparison with conventional MRI. Clin Imaging. 2002;26(4):227–36.
Chao C, Martin R, Ross M, et al. Correlation between prognostic factors and increasing age in melanoma. Ann Surg Oncol. 2004;11:259–64.
Chao S, Suh J, Raja S, et al. The sensitivity and specificity of FDG PET in distinguishing recurrent brain tumor from radionecrosis in patients treated with stereotactic radiosurgery. Int J Cancer. 2001;96:191–7.
Chason J, Walker F, Landers J. Metastatic carcinoma in the central nervous system and dorsal root ganglia. A prospective autopsy studies. Cancer. 1963;16:781–7.
Chaudhry I, O'Donovan D, Brenchley P, et al. Vascular endothelial growth factor expression correlates with tumor grade and vascularity in gliomas. Histopathology. 2001;39:409–15.
Chen W. Clinical applications of PET in brain tumors. J Nucl Med. 2007;48(9):1468–81.
Chiang I, Hsieh T, Chiu M, et al. Distinction between pyogenic brain abscess and necrotic brain tumor using 3-tesla MR spectroscopy, diffusion and perfusion imaging. Br J Radiol. 2009;82(982):813–20.
Chiang I, Kuo Y-T, Lu C-Y, et al. Distinction between high-grade gliomas and solitary metastases using peritumoral 3-T magnetic resonance spectroscopy, diffusion, and perfusion imagings. Neuroradiology. 2004;46:619–27.
Chissov VI, Davydov MI. Onkologiya. National guideline. Moscow: GEOTAR-Media; 2008. p. 1038–44.
Chissov VI, Starinsky VV, Kovalev BV, et al. Status of cancer care for the population of the Russian Federation. Moscow; 2000. p. 24.
Cho S, Lee D, Hong S. Intracranial aspergillosis involving the internal auditory canal and inner ear in an immunocompetent patient. Am J Neuroradiol. 2007;28:38–140.
Christensen T, Spindler K, Palshof J, et al. Systematic review: brain metastases from colorectal cancer – incidence and patient characteristics. BMC Cancer. 2016;16:260.
Christiaans M, Kelder J, Tijssen C. Prediction of intracranial metastases in cancer patients with headache. Cancer. 2002;94:2063–8.
Chung J, Kim Y, Kim S, et al. Usefulness of 11C-methionine PET in the evaluation of brain lesions that are hypo- or isometabolic on 18F-FDG PET. Eur J Nucl Med Mol Imaging. 2002;29:176–82.
Chura J, Shukla K, Argenta P. Brain metastasis from cervical carcinoma. Int J Gynecol Cancer. 2007;17:141–6.
Chute C, Greenberg E, Baron J, et al. Presenting conditions of 1539 population-based lung cancer patients by cell type and stage in New Hampshire and Vermont. Cancer. 1985;56:2107–11.
Cifuentes N, Pickren J. Metastases from carcinoma of mammary gland: an autopsy study. Surg Oncol. 1979;11:193–205.
Clague J, Lin J, Cassidy A, et al. Family history and risk of renal cell carcinoma: results from a case–control study and systematic meta-analysis. Cancer Epidemiol Biomark Prev. 2009;18:801–7.
Coppic C, Porzsot F, Awa A, et al. Immunotherapy for advanced renal cancer. Cochrane Database Syst Rev. 2000;1:CD001425.
Coughlin S, Neaton J, Randall B, et al. Predictors of mortality from kidney cancer in 332 547 men screened for the Multiple Risk Factor Intervention Trial. Cancer. 1997;79:2171–7.
Cox JD, Barber-Derus S, Hartz AJ, et al. Is adenocarcinoma/large cell carcinoma the most radio curable type of cancer of the lung. Int J Radiat Oncol Biol Phys. 1986;12:1801–5.
Crispen P, Lohse C, Blute M. Multifocal renal cell carcinoma: clinicopathologic features and outcomes for tumors ≤4 cm. Adv Urol. 2008;2008:7.
Cubilla A, Fortner J, Fitzgerald P. Lymph node involvement in carcinoma the pancreas area. Cancer. 1978;41:880–7.
Cuddapah V, Sontheimer H. Ion channels and transporters in cancer. 2. Ion channels and the control of cancer cell migration. Am J Physiol Cell Physiol. 2011;301(3):541–9.
Da Silva A, Nagayama K, Schlesinger D, et al. Gamma knife surgery for brain metastases from gastrointestinal cancer. J Neurosurg. 2009;111(3):423–30.
Damek DM. Melanoma. In: Cancer neurology in clinical practice. Berlin: Springer; 2003. p. 339–53.
Dandy W. Rontgenography of the brain after the injection of air into the spinal canal. Ann Surg. 1919;70:397–403.
Davenport C, Dillon W, Sze G. Neuroradiology of the immunosuppressed state. Radiol Clin N Am. 1992;30:611–37.
Davey P. Brain metastases: treatment options to improve outcomes. CNS Drugs. 2002;16:325–38.
Davydov MI, Axel EM. Statistics of malignancies in Russia and the CIS in 2012. Moscow: IOP Science; 2014. p. 39–42.
Davydov MI, Axel EM. Statistics of malignancies in Russia and the CIS in 2012. Moscow: M. Publishing Group of Russian Cancer Research Center; 2014. p. 226.
Davydov MI, Axel EM. Statistics of malignancies in Russia and the CIS in 2008. Moscow: M. Publishing Group of Russian Cancer Research Center; 2010.
Davydov MI, Polotsky BE. Lung cancer: M Radix; 1994. p. 216.
Daykhes NA, Bykov VP, Ponomarev AB, et al. Clinical pathology of the larynx: guideline atlas for postgraduate training of specialists of scientific, medical and academic medical institutions. Moscow: Med. News Agency; 2009. p. 160.
de Bree R, Mehta D, Snow G, et al. Intracranial metastases in patients with squamous cell carcinoma of the head and neck. Otolaryngol Head Neck Surg. 2001;124(2):217–21.
de Groot P, Munden R. Lung cancer epidemiology, risk factors, and prevention. Radiol Clin N Am. 2012;50:863–76.

De Potter P, Shields J, Shields C. Secondary orbit tumors. In: MRI of the eye and orbit. Philadelphia: JB Lippincott; 1995. p. 225–68.
Decker K. Klinische neuroradiologie. Stuttgart: Thieme; 1960.
Dedov II, et al. Magnetic resonance imaging in the diagnosis of diseases of the pituitary-hypothalamic system and the adrenal glands. Moscow: M Medicine; 1997. p. 159.
Defesche H. Cerebral metastases from pulmonary and mammary carcinomas. Clin Neurol Neurosurg. 1982;84(1):45–50.
DeGrado T, Coleman R, Wang S, et al. Synthesis and evaluation of ^{18}F-labeled choline as an oncologic tracer for positron emission tomography: Initial findings in prostate cancer. Cancer Res. 2001;61:110–7.
Deibler A, Pollock J, Kraft R, et al. Arterial spin-labeling in routine clinical practice, part 1: technique and artifacts. Am J Neuroradiol. 2008;29(7):1228–34.
Delattre J, George K, Howard T, et al. Distribution of brain metastases. Arch Neurol. 1988;45(7):741–4.
Delektorskaya VV, Perevoshchikov AG, Golovkov DA, et al. Prognostic significance of the expression of matrix metalloproteinases in colon adenocarcinoma and metastases. Bull Exp Biol Med. 2007;143(4):434–7.
Denkins Y, Reiland J, Roy M, et al. Brain metastases in melanoma: roles of neurotrophins. Neuro-Oncology. 2004;6(2):154–65.
Derlon J, Bourdet C, Bustany P, et al. [11C]L-methionine uptake in gliomas. Neurosurgery. 1989;25(5):720–8.
Dev R, Gupta R, Poptani H, et al. Role of in vivo proton magnetic resonance spectroscopy in the diagnosis and management of brain abscess. Neurosurgery. 1998;42(1):37–42.
Diyora B, Nayak N, Kamble H. Brain metastasis from papillary carcinoma of thyroid gland. J Neurosci Rural Pract. 2010;1(1):55–7.
Doglietto F, Colosimo C, Lauriola L, et al. Intracranial melanocytic meningeal tumours and melanosis oculi: case report and literature review. BMC Cancer. 2012;12:220.
Dolgushin M, et al. Use of CT perfusion to discriminate between brain metastases from different primaries. Clin Imaging. 2015;39:9–14.
Dolgushin MB, et al. A CT perfusion method in the differential diagnosis of a secondary tumor lesions of the brain. J Med Imaging. 2007;4:100–6.
Dolgushin MB, Fadeeva LM, Zaitseva AY, et al. 3D-diffusion-weighted magnetic resonance imaging of the whole body in patients with metastatic brain lesions. J Med Imaging. 2008a;1:118–23.
Dolgushin MB, Pronin IN, Kornienko VN, et al. Perfusion CT in dynamic evaluation of the effectiveness of radiation therapy in secondary brain tumors. Bull NN Blokhin Russ Cancer Res Center. 2008b;19(4):36–46.
Dolgushin MB, Pronin IN, Turkin AM, et al. 3D SWI (SWAN) in the evaluation of the structure characteristics of glioblastoma brain metastases on a 3 Tl MR tomograph. J Med Imaging. 2012a;1:26–35.
Dolgushin MB, Pronin IN, Fadeeva LM, et al. The pulse sequence SWI (SWAN) (3T) and CT perfusion in a comprehensive assessment of structural features of brain metastases and malignant gliomas. Radial Diagn Ther. 2012b;3:51–7.
Dolgushin MB. Abstract of dissertation for the degree of Doctor of Medical Sciences, Moscow. 2012.
Douglas J, Margolin K. The treatment of brain metastases from malignant melanoma. Semin Oncol. 2002;29:518–24.
Durnov LA et al. Malignant tumors of the skin in children. M Sirius Complex. 2000.
Eastwood J, Provenzale J. Cerebral blood flow, blood volume, and vascular permeability of cerebral gliomas assessed with dynamic CT perfusion imaging. Neuroradiology. 2003;45(6):373.
Ebisu T, Tanaka C, Umeda M, et al. Discrimination of brain abscess from necrotic or cystic tumors by diffusion-weighted echo planar imaging. Magn Reson Imaging. 1996;14:1113–6.
Ecker A, Riemenschneider P. Angiografic localization of intracranial masses. Springfield: Thomas; 1955.
Ecker A. The normal cerebral angiogram. Springfield: Thomas; 1951.
Edelman R, Zlatkin M, Hesselink J. Clinical magnetic resonance imaging. Philadelphia: Saunders; 1996.
Egeblad M, Werb Z. New functions for the matrix metalloproteinases in cancer progression. Nat Rev Cancer. 2002;2:161–74.
Eichler A, Kuter I, Ryan P, et al. Survival in patients with brain metastases from breast cancer: the importance of HER-2 status. Cancer. 2008;112(11):2359–67.
El Kamar F, Jindal K, Grossbard M, et al. Pancreatic carcinoma with brain metastases: case report and literature review. Dig Liver Dis. 2004;36:355–60.
Emami B, Graham MV. Lung. In: Perez CA, Brady LW, editors. Principles and practice of radiation oncology. 3rd ed. Philadelphia: Lippincot – Raven; 1997. p. 1181–220.
Engeset A, Kristiansen K. Cerebral angiography. London: Butterworth; 1940.
Erdogan C, Hakyemez B, Yildirim N, et al. Brain abscess and cystic brain tumor: discrimination with dynamic susceptibility contrast perfusion-weighted MRI. J Comput Assist Tomogr. 2005;29(5):663–7.
Escott E. A variety of appearances of malignant melanoma in the head: a review. Radiographics. 2001;21:625–39.
Estrada C, Bready J, Berliner J, et al. Choline uptake by cerebral capillaryendothelial cells in culture. J Neurochem. 1990;54: 1467–73.
Ewend M, Brem S, Gilbert M et al. The treatment of single brain metastasis with surgery, BCNU-polymer wafers, and radiation therapy: Results of phase I-II trial. ASCO, 2001, abstract 226. 2001.
Fabi A, Felici A, Metro G, et al. Brain metastases from solid tumors: disease outcome according to type of treatment and therapeutic resources of the treating center. J Exp Clin Cancer Res. 2011;30(1):10.
Faivre J, Bouvier AM, Bonithon-Kopp C. Epidemiology and screening of colorectal cancer. Best Pract Res Clin Gastroenterol. 2002;16:187–99.
Fan G, Sun B, Wu Z, et al. In vivo single-voxel proton MR spectroscopy in the differentiation of high-grade gliomas and solitary metastases. Clin Radiol. 2004;59:77–85.
Faro S, Koenigsberg R, Turtz A, et al. Melanocytoma of the cavernous sinus: CT and MRI findings. Am J Neuroradiol. 1996;17:1087–90.
Farrokh D, Fransen P, et al. MR finding of a primary intramedullary malignant melanoma: case report and literature review. Am J Neuroradiol. 2001;22:1864–6.
Ferlay J, Soerjomataram I, Dikshit R, Eser S, Mathers C, Rebelo M, et al. Cancer incidence and mortality worldwide: sources, methods and major patterns in GLOBOCAN 2012. Int J Cancer. 2015;136(5):359–86.
Fertikh D, Krejza J, Cunqueiro A. Discrimination of capsular stage brain abscesses from necrotic or cystic neoplasms using diffusion-weighted magnetic resonance imaging. J Neurosurg. 2007;106:76–81.
Fidler I. Critical factors in the biology of human cancer metastasis: twenty-eighth GHA Clowes memorial award lecture. Cancer Res. 1990;50:6130–8.
Fidler I. Molecular biology of cancer: invasion and metastasis. In: DeVita V, Hellman S, Rosenberg S, editors. Cancer: principles and practice of oncology. Philadelphia: Lippincott-Raven; 1997. p. 135–52.
Finegold M. Clinic and diagnosis of metastatic brain cancer with a primary source in the lungs. Nevrol Psykhiatr Kiev. 1977;6:58–63.
Fink K, Fink J. Imaging of brain metastases. Surg Neurol Int. 2013;4(4):209–19.
Fisher B, Osborne CK, et al. Neoplasms of the breast. In: Holland JF, editor. Cancer medicine, vol. 2. 4th ed; 1997. p. 2349–429. Baltimore, Philadelphia, London, Paris, Bangkok, Buenos Aires, Hong Kong, Munich, Sydney, Tokyo, Wroclaw.

Fitzgerald D, Palmieri D, Hua E, et al. Reactive glia are recruited by highly proliferative brain metastases of breast cancer and promote tumor cell colonization. Clin Exp Metastasis. 2008;25:799–810.

Flowers A, Levin V. Management of brain metastases from breast carcinoma. Oncology (Huntington). 1993;7(3):21–6.

Folkert M, Timmerman R. Review of treatment options for oligometastatic non–small cell lung cancer. Clin Adv Hematol Oncol. 2015;13(3):186–93.

Friedrichs N, Hahne J, Pepper M, et al. Immunohistochemical quantification of lymph vessels, VEGF-C and VEGF receptor 3 in human sarcomas. Histopathology. 2006;49(1):87–8.

Gaddikeri S, Gaddikeri RS, Tailor T, et al. Dynamic contrast-enchanced MR imaging in head and neck cancer: techniques and clinical applications. Am J Neuroradiol. 2016;37(4):588–95.

Gaidar BV, et al. Therapeutic tactics in renal cancer with metastatic lesions of the central nervous system. Prakticheskaya Onkol. 2005;3:172–7.

Galperin MD. Angiography in diagnosis of tumors and cerebral vascular diseases. L. 1962.

Ganina KP, Naleskina LA, Polishchuk LZ, et al. Morphology, histochemistry and cytogenetics of pigmented human skin tumors. Kiev: Naukova Dumka; 1978. p. 182.

Ganina KP, Naleskina LA. Malignant melanoma of the skin and previous skin changes. Kiev: Naukova Dumka; 1991. p. 147.

Ganov DI, Varlamov SA, Lazarev AF. Prostate cancer metastases in young and middle-aged men. Russ J Oncol. 2014;5:28–30.

Ganusevich II. The role of matrix metalloproteinases (MMPs) in malignant tumors. Characteristics of MMP, regulation of their activity, prognostic significance. Onkologiya. 2010;12(1):10–6.

Gaspar L, Mehta M, Patchell R, et al. The role of whole brain radiation therapy in the management of newly diagnosed brain metastases: a systematic review and evidence-based clinical practice guideline. J Neuro-Oncol. 2010;96(1):17–32.

Gaspar L, Scott C, Rotman M, et al. Recursive partitioning analysis (RPA) of prognostic factors in three Radiation Therapy Oncology Group (RTOG) brain metastases trials. Int J Radiat Oncol Biol Phys. 1997;37(4):745–51.

Gasperini C, Paolillo A, Rovaris M, et al. A comparison of the sensitivity of MRI after double- and triple-dose Gd-DTPA for detecting enhancing lesions in multiple sclerosis. Magn Reson Imaging. 2000;18:761–3.

Gauthier S, Diksic M, Yamamoto L, et al. Positron emission tomography with C-choline in human subjects. Can J Neurol Sci. 1985;12:214.

Gaviani P, Mullins M, Braga T, et al. Improved detection of metastatic melanoma by T2*-weighted imaging. Am J Neuroradiol. 2006;27:605–8.

Gaviani P, Schwartz R, Hedley-Whyte E. Diffusion-weighted imaging of fungal cerebral infection. Am J Neuroradiol. 2005;26(5):1115–21.

Gavrilovic I, Posner J. Brain metastases: epidemiology and pathophysiology. J Neuro-Oncol. 2005;75:5–14.

Gebarski S, Blaivas M. Imaging of normal Leptomeningeal Melanin. Am J Neuroradiol. 1996;17(1):55–60.

Ghosh S, Prabhash K. Brain metastases in head and neck cancers. Otorhinolaryngol Clin Int J. 2011;3(2):3–6.

Ginsberg M, Chang J, Kelley R, et al. Increases in both cerebral glucose utilization and blood flow during execution of a somatosensory task. Ann Neurol. 1988;23:152–60.

Girard N, Zimmerman R. Infectious and inflammatory diseases of brain and spinal cord. In: Zimmerman R, Gibby W, Carmody R, editors. Neuroimaging: clinical and physical principles. Berlin Heidelberg: Springer; 2000. p. 909–50.

Gnepp D, Brandwein M, Henley J. Salivary and lacrimal glands. In: Gnepp DR, editor. Diagnostic surgical pathology of the head and neck. Philadelphia: WB Saunders; 2001. p. 325–430.

Go P, Klaassen Z, Meadows M, et al. Gastrointestinal cancer and brain metastasis: a rare and ominous sign. Cancer. 2011;117(16):3630–40.

Godley P, Stinchcombe T. Renal cell carcinoma. Curr Opin Oncol. 1999;11(3):213–7.

Goebell E, Paustenbach S, et al. Low-grade and anaplastic gliomas: differences in architecture evaluated with diffusion-tensor MR imaging. Radiology. 2006;239:217–22.

Gohji K, Hara I, Gotoh A, et al. Multifocal renal cell carcinoma in Japanese patients with tumors with maximal diameters of 50 mm or less. J Urol. 1998;159(4):1144–7.

Golan AV, Banov SM, Vetlova ER. Metastatic brain lesions: a change in the radiation treatment paradigm. Probl Onkol. 2015;61(4):530–45.

Golan AV, Banov SM, Vetlova ER. Stereotactic radiotherapy of large metastases in the brain. Results of a randomized study. Educational materials for the congress X-ray diagnostics and radiotherapy in. Oncology. 2015:42–3.

Golanov AV, Kotelnikova TM, Melikyan AG, Dolgushin MB. Experience using SPECT/CT in neurosurgical clinic. Issues Neurosurg. 2012;1:85–92.

Golbert ZV. Histogenesis, histology, classification of pigmented (melanocytic) skin tumors. In: Pigment tumors in humans. Moscow; 1975. p. 5–81.

Goritz C, Dias D, Tomilin N, et al. A pericyte origin of spinal cord scar tissue. Science. 2011;333(6039):238–42.

Goulart CR, Alecio Mattei T, Ramina R. Cerebral melanoma metastases: a critical review on diagnostic methods and therapeutic options. ISRN Surg. 2011;2011:9. Article ID 276908.

Graf A, Buchberger W, Langmayr H, et al. Site preference of metastatic tumours of the brain. Virchows Arch A. 1988;412:493–8.

Gramada FM, Indrei A, Iencean SM. Management of unknown origin cerebral metastases. Rom Neurosurg. 2011;XVIII(1):60–7.

Granov A, Tiutin L. Positron emission tomography. London: Springer; 2013. p. 384.

Granov A, Tiutin L. Positron emission tomography. Heidelberg: Springer; 2013. p. 384.

Granov AM, Tyutin LA. Positron emission tomography Guidelines for physicians. St Petersburg: Foliant; 2008. p. 365.

Grant F. Concerning intracranial malignant metastases: their frequency and the value of surgery in their treatment. Ann Surg. 1926;84:635–46.

Graus F, Elkon K, Cordon-Cardo C, et al. Sensory neuronopathy and small cell lung cancer. Antineuronal antibody that also reacts with the tumor. Am J Med. 1986;80:45–52.

Graus F, Walker R, Alien J. Brain metastases in children. J Pediatr. 1983;103:558–61.

Greenlee R, Hill-Harmon M, Murray T, et al. Cancer statistics, 2001. CA Cancer J Clin. 2001;51:15–36.

Griffith B, Jain R. Perfusion imaging in neuro-oncology basic techniques and clinical applications. J Pathol. 2015;53(3):497–511.

Grigorov SV, Plotnikova VE. Features of metastatic brain involvement in breast cancer depending on the state of ovarian cycle. Vrach-Aspirant. 2012;6(55):4–8.

Grigsby P, Siegel B, Dehdashti F. Lymph node staging by positron emission tomography in patients with carcinoma of the cervix. J Clin Oncol. 2001;19(17):3745–9.

Grossman S, Finkelstein D, Ruckdeschel D, et al. Randomized prospective comparison of intraventricular methotrexate and thiotepa in patients with previously untreated neoplastic meningitis. J Clin Oncol. 1993;11:561–9.

Grossman S, Krabak M. Leptomeningeal carcinomatosis. Cancer Treat Rev. 1999;25:103–19.

Guenot M, Wager M, Bataille B, et al. Metastases cerebrales des cancers testiculaires. A propos de deux cas et revue de la literature. Neurochirurgie. 1994;40:135–7.

Gulec S, Mountcasile T, Frey D, et al. Cytoreductive surgery in patients with advanced-stage carcinoid tumors. Am Surg. 2002;68:667–72.

Guo A, Cummings T, Dash R, et al. Lymphomas and high grade astrocytomas: comparison of water diffusibility and histologic characteristics. Radiology. 2002;224:177–83.

Gustavo A, Gustavo B, Ellen C, et al. Whole brain radiotherapy with radiosensitizer for brain metastases. J Exp Clin Cancer Res. 2009:28–31.

Haacke E, Ayaz M, Khan A, et al. Establishing a baseline phase behavior in magnetic resonance imaging to determine normal vs. abnormal iron content in the brain. J Magn Reson Imaging. 2007;26:256–64.

Haacke E, Cheng N, House M, et al. Imaging iron stores in the brain using magnetic resonance imaging. J Magn Reson Imaging. 2005;23(1):1–25.

Haacke E, Tang J, Neelavalli J, et al. Susceptibility mapping as a means to visualize veins and quantify oxygen saturation. J Magn Reson Imaging. 2010;32:663–76.

Hahn E. Spin echoes. Phys Rev. 1950;80:580–94.

Hakyemez B, Ergin N, Uysal S, et al. Diffusion-weighted MRI in the differentiation of brain abscesses and necrotic tumors. Tani Girisim Radyol. 2004;10(2):110–8.

Hamel E, Assumel-Lurdin C, Edvinsson L, et al. Neuronal versus endothelial origin of vasoactive acethylcholine in pial vessels. Brain Res. 1987;420:391–6.

Hara T, Inagaki K. Sensitive detection of mediastinal lymph node metastasis of lung cancer with ^{11}C-choline PET. J Nucl Med. 2000;41:1507–13.

Hara T, Kosaka N, Kishi H. Development of (18)F-fluoroethylcholine for cancer imaging with PET: synthesis, biochemistry, and prostate cancer imaging. J Nucl Med. 2002;43:187–99.

Hara T, Kosaka N, Shinoura N, et al. PET imaging of brain tumor with [methyl-11C] choline. J Nucl Med. 1997;38:842–7.

Harada Y, Nonomura N, Kondo M, et al. Clinical study of brain metastasis of renal cell carcinoma. Eur Urol. 1999;36:230–5.

Hardy J, Harvey V. Cerebral metastases in patients with ovarian cancer treated with chemotherapy. Gynecol Oncol. 1989;33:296–300.

Hardy J, Smith I, Cherryman G, et al. The value of computed tomographic (CT) scan surveillance in the detection and management of brain metastases in patients with small-cell lung cancer. Br J Cancer. 1990;62:684–6.

Hatiboglu M, Chang E, Suki D, et al. Outcomes and prognostic factors for patients with brainstem metastases undergoing stereotactic radiosurgery. Neurosurgery. 2011;69:796–806.

Hatzoglou V, Patel G, Morris M, et al. Brain metastases from prostate cancer: an 11-year analysis in the MRI era with emphasis on imaging characteristics, incidence, and prognosis. J Neuroimaging. 2014;24(2):161–6.

Hauward R, Hayward R. Malignant melanoma and the central nervous system. A guide for classification based on the clinical findings. J Neurol Neurosurg Psychiatry. 1976;39:526–30.

Hawk M, Shahlaie K, Kim K, et al. Neurocysticercosis: a review. Surg Neurol. 2005;63:123–32.

Helfre S, Pierga J. Cerebral metastases: radiotherapy and chemotherapy. Neurochirurgie. 1999;45(5):382–92.

Helmy A, Antoun N, Hutchinson P. Cerebral tuberculoma and magnetic resonance imaging. J R Soc Med. 2011;104(7):299–301.

Henderson J, Campbell R, Farrow G, et al. Orbital tumors. 3rd ed. New York: Raven; 1993. p. 361–75.

Henriksen E. The lymphatic dissemination in endometrial carcinoma. A study of 188 necropsies. Am J Obstet Gynecol. 1975;123:570–6.

Heon S, Yeap B, Britt G, et al. Development of central nervous system metastases in patients with advanced non-small cell lung cancer and somatic EGFR mutations treated with gefitinib or erlotinib. Clin Cancer Res. 2010;16:5873–82.

Hirsch F, Paulson O, Hansen H, et al. Intracranial metastases in small cell carcinoma of the lung: correlation of clinical and autopsy findings. Cancer. 1982;50:2433–7.

Ho SI, Chung D, Saw R, et al. Imaging in cutaneous melanoma. Nucl Med Commun. 2008;29:847.

Hochberg F, Pruitt A. Assumptions in the radiotherapy of glioblastoma. Neurology. 1980;30(9):907–11.

Holzaepfel J, Ezell H. Sites of metastasis of uterine carcinoma. Am J Obstet Gynecol. 1955;69:1027–38.

Hounsfild G. Computerized transverse axial scanning (tomography). Part I. Description of system. Br J Radiol. 1973;46:1016–22.

Hsu S, Chou M, Ko C, et al. Proton MR spectroscopy in patients with pyogenic brain abscess: MR spectroscopic imaging versus single-voxel spectroscopy. Eur J Radiol. 2013;82(8):1299–307.

Huisman T, Sorensen A. Perfusion-weighted magnetic resonance imaging of the brain: techniques and application in children. Eur Radiol. 2004;14:59–72.

Hurwitz H, Fehrenbacher I, Novotny W, et al. Bevacizumab plus irinotecan, fluorouracil and leucovorian for metastases colorectal cancer cells. Oncogene. 2005;24:2647–53.

Idris M, Sokrab T, Arbab A, et al. Tuberculoma of the brain: a series of 16 cases treated with anti-tuberculosis drugs. Int J Tuberc Lung Dis. 2007;11:91–5.

Idrisov MI. Brain lesions in lung cancer. Moscow: Diss cand med nauk; 1980. p. 212.

Ikeda S, Yamada T, Katsumata N. Cerebral metastasis in patients with uterine cervical cancer. Jpn J Clin Oncol. 1998;28(1):27–9.

Ikonopisov RL, Kirov SM, Raichev RD, et al. Pigmented tumors. Sofia 1977;192.

Raizer J, Abrey L, Rosen ST, editors. Brain metastases. New York: Springer-Science; 2007.

Isiklar I, Leeds N, Fuller G, et al. Intracranial metastatic melanoma: correlation between MR imaging characteristics and melanin content. AJR. 1995;165:1503–12.

Iwadate Y, Namba H, Yamaura A. Significance of surgical resection for the treatment of multiple brain metastases. Anticancer Res. 2000;20(1B):573–7.

Jänne P, Freidlin B, Saxman S, et al. Twenty-five years of clinical research for patients with limited-stage small cell lung carcinoma in North America. Cancer. 2002;95(7):1528–38.

Järnum H, Steffensen E, Knutsson L. Perfusion MRI of brain tumours: a comparative study of pseudo-continuous arterial spin labelling and dynamic susceptibility contrast imaging. Neuroradiology. 2010;52(4):307–17.

Jellison B, et al. Diffusion tensor imaging of cerebral matter: a pictorial review of physics. Fiber tract anatomy and tumor imaging patterns. Am J Neuroradiol. 2004;25:356–69.

Jemal A, Bray F, Center M, et al. Global cancer statistics. CA Cancer J Clin. 2011;61:69–90.

Jemal A, Siegel R, Ward E, et al. Cancer statistics. CA Cancer J Clin. 2007;57(1):43–66.

Jena A, Taneja S, Talwar V, et al. Magnetic resonance (MR) patterns of brain metastasis in lung cancer patients: correlation of imaging findings with symptom. J Thorac Oncol. 2008;3(2):140–4.

Jennings M, Gelman R, Hochberg F. Intracranial germ-cell tumors: natural history and pathogenesis. J Neurosurg. 1985;63:155–67.

Jereczek B, et al. Autopsy findings in small cell lung cancer. Neoplasma. 1996;43(2):133.

Ji S, Hua Y, Zhuang J, et al. Significance of COX-2, p53, proliferating cell nuclear antigen and nm23 expressions in gastric cancer and its behavior. Ai Zheng. 2002;21(6):619–24. (Chinese)

Johnson T, Smith J. Current therapy for cutaneous melanoma. J Am Acad Dermatol. 1995;32:689–707.

Jooma R, Kendall B. Diagnosis and management of pineal tumors. J Neurosurg. 1983;58(5):654–65.

Jyothirmayi R, Edison J, Nayar P, et al. Case report: brain metastases from papillary carcinoma thyroid. Br J Radiol. 1995;68:767–9.

Kaal E, Taphoorn M, Vecht CJ. Symptomatic management and imaging of brain metastases. J Neuro-Oncol. 2005a;75:15–20.

Kaal E, Niël C, Vecht C. Therapeutic management of brain metastasis. Lancet Neurol. 2005b;4(5):289–98.

Kabaria R, Klaassen Z, Terris M. Renal cell carcinoma: links and risks. Int J Nephrol Renovasc Dis. 2016;9:45–52.

Kadashev BA. Indications for various methods of treatment of pituitary adenomas. Author's abstract for the degree of Doctor of Medical Sciences, Moscow;1992.

Kahlenberg M, Sullivan J, Witmer D, et al. Molecular prognostics in colorectal cancer. Surg Oncol. 2003;12:173–86.

Kalkanis S, Kondziolka D, Gaspar L, et al. The role of surgical resection in the management of newly diagnosed brain metastases: a systematic review and evidence-based clinical practice guideline. J Neuro-Oncol. 2010;96(1):33–43.

Kalkun VR. On clinical manifestations of metastatic brain cancer. 1963;4:105–110.

Karami S, Schwartz K, Purdue M, et al. Family history of cancer and renal cell cancer risk in Caucasians and African Americans. Br J Cancer. 2010;102(11):1676–80.

Karp VN, Susin VM, Pronko AV et al. Some clinical aspects of metastatic melanoma in the brain. IIIrd Congress of Neurosurgeons of Russia: Congress of Materials (St. Petersburg, June 2002). St. Petersburg 2002. p. 110–111.

Kashiwagi S, Hatano M, Yokoyama T. Metastatic small cell carcinoma to the pineal body: case report. Neurosurgery. 1989;25:810–3.

Kastrup O, Wanke I, Maschke M. Neuroimaging of infections of the central nervous system. Semin Neurol. 2008;28(4):511–22.

Katz-Brull R, Degani H. Kinetics of choline transport and phosphorylationin human breast cancer cells NMR application of the zero trans method. Anticancer Res. 1996;16:1375–80.

Kaufmann S. Envisioning future strategies for vaccination against tuberculosis. Nat Rev Immunol. 2006;6:699–704.

Kebudi R, Ayan I, Görgün O, et al. Brain metastasis in pediatric extracranial solid tumors: survey and literature review. J Neuro-Oncol. 2005;71(1):43–8.

Kellinghaus C, Schilling M, Ludemann P. Neurosarcoidosis: clinical experience and diagnostic pitfalls. Eur Neurol. 2004;51:84–8.

Kety S, Schmidt C. The nitrous oxide method for the quantitative determination of cerebral blood flow in man: theory, procedure and normal values. J Clin Invest. 1948;27:476–83.

Khalimova HM. Clinic, diagnostics and some issues of prognosis in metastatic brain tumors. Autoref Cand Diss. 1982;16.

Khanevich MD, Manikhas GM, Luzin VV. Colorectal cancer. The choice of surgical tactics in colonic obstruction Spb., Agraf +; 2008. p. 136.

Khanjanasthiti P, Issaragrisil R. CT findings of brain metastases. J Med Assoc Thail. 1989;72(7):361–70.

Khanson K, Imyanitov E. Epidemiology and biology of prostate cancer. Pract Oncol. 2001;2:3–7.

Khmelev AV. Positron emission tomography. Physical and technical aspects: M Trovant; 2016. p. 336.

Khosla A, et al. Brain metastasis imaging: eMedscape; 2015.

Kim E, Chang J, Choi H, et al. Diagnostic yield of double-dose gadobutrol in the detection of brain metastasis: intraindividual comparison with double-dose gadopentetate dimeglumine. Am J Neuroradiol. 2010;31:1055–8.

Kim H, Im S, Keam B, et al. Clinical outcome of central nervous system metastases from breast cancer: differences in survival depending on systemic treatment. J Neuro-Oncol. 2012;106:303–13.

Kim LS, Huang S, Lu W, et al. Vascular endothelial growth factor expression promotes the growth of breast cancer brain metastases in nude mice. Clin Exp Metastasis. 2004;21:107–18.

Kim M. Intracranial involvement by metastatic advanced gastric carcinoma. Neuro-Oncol. 1999;43:59–62.

Kim Y, Kwon J, Lim S. A clinical analysis of brain metastasis in gynecologic cancer: a retrospective multi-institute analysis. J Korean Med Sci. 2015;30(1):66–73.

Kirkali Z, Tuz E, Mungan M. Recent advances in kidney cancer and metastatic disease. BJU Int. 2001;88:818–24.

Kitajima K, Murakami K, Yamasaki E, et al. Performance of integrated FDG-PET/contrast-enhanced CT in the diagnosis of recurrent uterine cancer: comparison with PET and enhanced CT. Eur J Nucl Med Mol Imaging. 2009;36(3):362–72.

Kleihues P, Cavenee W. Tumors of the nervous system; pathology and genetics: world health organization international classification of tumours. Lyon: IARC Press; 2000.

Kleinberg L. Brain metastases: a multidisciplinary approach. New York: Demos; 2009. p. 224.

Koh D, Collins D. Diffusion Weighted MRI in the body: application in oncology. AJR. 2007;188(6):1622–35.

Kolomainen D, Larkin J, Bardan M, et al. Epithelial ovarian cancer metastasizing to the brain: a late manifestation of the disease with an increasing incidence. J Clin Oncol. 2002;20:982–6.

Kondziolka D, Bernstein M, et al. Significance of hemorrhage into brain tumors: clinicopathological study. J Neurosurg. 1987;67:852–7.

Konig M. Brain perfusion CR in acute stroke: current status. Eur J Radiol. 2003;45(1):11–22.

Konovalov AN, et al. Surgical removal of giant meningeal hemangiopericytoma. In: Kobayashi S, editor. Neurosurgery of complex vascular lesions and tumors. NewYork: Thieme; 2005. p. 244–8.

Konovalov AN, Kornienko VN, Pronin IN, et al. Hematomas and occult vascular malformations of the brainstem. Med Imaging. 2001;2:13–8.

Konovalov AN, Kornienko VN, Pronin IN. Magnetic resonance imaging in neurosurgery. Moscow: Vidar; 1997a. p. 472.

Konovalov AN, Kornienko VN, Pronin IN. Magnetic resonance imaging in neurosurgery. Vidar: Moscow; 1997b.

Konovalov AN, Kornienko VN, Pronin IN. Magnetic resonance imaging in neurosurgery. Moscow: Vidar; 1997. p. 471.

Konovalov AN, Kornienko VN. Computed tomography in the neurosurgical clinic. Moscow: M Medicine; 1985. p. 293.

Konovalov AN, Kornienko VN. Computed tomography in the neurosurgical clinic, vol. 296. Moscow: M Medicine; 1985.

Konovalov AN, Pitskhelauri DI. Treatment of pineal tumors. Moscow; 2004. p. 278.

Konstas A, Goldmakher G, Lee T, et al. Theoretic basis and technical implementations of CT perfusion in acute ischemic stroke, part 2: technical implementations. Am J Neuroradiol. 2009;30:885–92.

Kopylov MB. Fundamentals of X-ray diagnosis brain disease. Moscow: M Medicine; 1968.

Kornienko VN, Ozerov VI. Pediatric neuroradiology. Moscow: M Medicine; 1993. p. 444.

Kornienko VN, Pronin IN. Diagnostic neuroradiology, vol. 1. Moscow: Andreeva TM; 2008a. p. 454.

Kornienko VN, Pronin IN, editors. Neuroimaging: selected articles (2000–2007). Moscow: Andreeva TM; 2008b. p. 256.

Kornienko VN, Pronin IN, et al. Neuroradiology. Current state and prospects of development. In: Konovalov AN, editor. Modern technologies and clinical research in neurosurgery, vol. 1. Moscow: Alexeeva TM; 2012. p. 113–58.

Kornienko VN, Pronin IN, Pyanykh OS, Fadeeva LM. A study of brain tissue perfusion by computed tomography. J Med Imaging. 2007;2:70–81.

Kornienko VN, Pronin IN. Contrast enhancement in neuroradiology. Moscow: Alexeeva TM; 2010. p. 256.

Kornienko VN, Pronin IN. Diagnostic neuroradiology, vol. 2. Moscow: Andreeva TM; 2009a. p. 462.

Kornienko VN, Pronin IN. Diagnostic neuroradiology, vol. 3. Moscow: Andreeva TM; 2009b. p. 463.

Kornienko V, Pronin I. Diagnostic neuroradiology. Berlin-Heidelberg: Springer-Verlag; 2009c. p. 1388.

Kornienko VN, Pronin IN. Diagnostic neuroradiology, vol. III. Moscow: Andreeva TM; 2009d. p. 182–346.

Kornienko VN, Pronin IN. Diagnostic neuroradiology. Moscow: Andreeva TM; 2006. p. 1327.

Kornienko VN, Pronin IN. Diagnostic neuroradiology. In: Tumors of the skull base, vol. 4. Alexeeva TM: Moscow; 2012. p. 502.

Kovacs K. Metastatic cancer of the pituitary gland. Oncology. 1973;27:533–42.

Kozhanov LG, Sdvizhkov AM, Mulyarets MV, et al. Clinical significance of echosonography in the diagnosis of laryngeal cancer. Bull Otorhinolaryngol. 2008;2:46–9.

Krasovsky AB. Tumors of the brain and meninges, vol. 2. Philadelphia: Lea & Febiger; 1958. p. 710.

Krayenbuhl H, Yasargil M, Huber P. Zerebrale angiographie fur klinik and praxis. Stuttgart: Georg Thieme Verlag; 1979.

Kristijansen P. The role of cranial irradiation in the management of patients with small cell lung cancer. Lung Cancer. 1989;5:264–74.

Kryuchkov AV, Yartsev VV. Diagnosis and surgical treatment of pulmonary bronchial cancer metastases in the brain. In: Current issues of neurosurgery. Moscow; 1974. p. 51–7.

Kuhn M, Hammer G, Swenson L, et al. MRI evaluation of "solitary" brain metastases with triple-dose gadoteridol: comparison with contrast-enhanced CT and conventional-dose gadopentetate dimeglumine MRI studies in the same patients. Comput Med Imaging Graph. 1994;18(5):391–9.

Kumar R, Halanaik D, Malhotra A. Clinical applications of positron emission tomography-computed tomography in oncology. Rev Indian J Cancer. 2010;47(2):100–19.

Kumar R, Jain R, Kaur A, et al. Brain stem tuberculosis in children. Br J Neurosurg. 2000;14:356–61.

Kuratsu J, Murakami M, Uemura S, et al. Brain and skull metastases of hepatic or pancreatic cancer – report of six cases. Neurol Med Chir (Tokyo). 1990;30:476–82.

Kurennaya SS. Tumors with brain metastases. Vrach Delo. 1986;3:99–101.

Kusters B, de Waal R, Wesseling P, et al. Differential effects of vascular endothelial growth factor isoforms in a mouse brain metastases model of human melanoma. Cancer Res. 2003;63:5408–13.

Kusuda Y, Miyake H, Terakawa T, et al. Treatment of brain metastases from renal cell carcinoma with sunitinib and radiotherapy: our experience and review of the literature. Int J Urol. 2011;18:326–9.

Kutuki S, Ito H, Shigematsu N, et al. Palliation of brain metastases: factors associated with survival. Nippon Igaku Hoshasen Gakkai Zasshi. 1996;56(6):426–31.

Kwee S, Ko J, Jiang C, et al. Solitary brain lesions enhancing at MR imaging: evaluation with fluorine 18 fluorocholine PET. Radiology. 2007;244:557–65.

Lagergren J, Lagergren P. Clinical review: oesophageal cancer. Br Int J Cancer. 2002;99(5):751–4.

Lagerwaard F, Levendag P, Nowak P, et al. Identification of prognostic factors in patients with brain metastases: a review of 1292 patients. Int J Radiat Oncol Biol Phys. 1999;43:795–803.

Lai P, Kun T, Shu S, et al. Pyogenic brain abscess: findings from in vivo 1.5-T and 11.7-T in vitro proton MRS. Am J Neuroradiol. 2005;26:279–88.

Laigle-Donadey F, Taillibert S, Mokhtari K, et al. Dural metastases. J Neuro-Oncol. 2005;75(1):57–61.

Lang E, Slater J. Metastatic brain tumors. Results of surgical and nonsurgical treatment. Surg Clin North Am. 1964;44:865–72.

Lang F, Sawaya R. Surgical management of cerebral metastases. Neurosurg Clin N Am. 1996;7(3):459–84.

Lang H, Lindner V, Martin M, et al. Prognostic value of multifocality on progression and survival in localized renal cell carcinoma. Eur Urol. 2004;45(6):749–53.

Langen K, Jarosch M, Muhlensiepen H, et al. Comparison of fluorotyrosines and methionine uptake in F98 rat gliomas. Nucl Med Biol. 2003;30:501–8.

Langer C, Mehta M. Current management of brain metastases, with a focus on systemic options. J Clin Oncol. 2005;23:6207–19.

Langleben D, Segall G. PET in differentiation of recurrent brain tumor from radiation injury. J Nucl Med. 2000;41:1861–7.

Langley R, Fidler I. The biology of brain metastasis. Clin Chem. 2013;59(1):180–9.

Lassman A, De Angelis L. Brain metastases. Neurol Clin. 2003;21(1):1–7.

Lassman A, DeAngelis L. Brain metastases. Neurol Clin N Am. 2003;21:1–23.

Lauterbour P. Image information by induced local interactions: examples employing NMR. Nature. 1973;242:190–1.

Law M, Cha S, Knopp E, et al. High-grade gliomas and solitary metastases: differentiation by using perfusion and proton spectroscopic MR imaging. Radiology. 2002;222:715–22.

Lawlor P, Gagnon B, Mancini I. Occurrence, causes and outcomes of delirium in patients with advanced cancer: prospective study. Arch Intern Med. 2000;160:786–94.

Le Bihan D, Breton E. Imagieri de diffusion in-vivo par resonance magnetique. C R Acad Sci (II). 1985;15:1109–12.

Le Bihan D, Turner R, Mooner C, et al. Imaging of diffusion and microvasculation with gradient sensitization: design, strategy and significance. J Magn Reson Imaging. 1991;1:7–28.

Le Bihan D, van Zijl P. From the diffusion coefficient to the diffusion tensor. NMR Biomed. 2002;15:431–4.

Le Chevalier T, Smith FP, Caille P, et al. Sites of primary malignancies in patients presenting with cerebral metastases. A review of 120 cases. Cancer. 1985;56:880–2.

Lee B, Vo K, Lim T. NMR Venography using susceptibility effect produced by deoxyhemoglobin. Magn Reson Med. 1992;28:25–38.

Lee K, Lee H, Yu H, et al. Prognostic significance of ps3, nm23, PCNA and c-erbB-2 in gastric cancer. Jpn J Clin Oncol. 2003;33(4):173–9.

Leenders W, Kusters B, Pikkemaat J. Vascular endothelial growth factor-A determines detectability of experimental melanoma brain metastasis in GD-DTPA-enhanced MRI. Int J Cancer. 2003;105:437–43.

Lemke J, Scheele J, Kapapa T, et al. Brain metastasis in pancreatic cancer. Int J Mol Sci. 2013;14(2):4163–73.

Leon S, Folkerth R, Black P. Microvessel density is a prognostic indicator for patients with astroglial brain tumors. Cancer. 2007;77:362–77.

Leone JP, Leone BA. Breast cancer brain metastases: the last frontier. Exp Hematol Oncol. 2015;4:33.

Lester J, Macbeth F, Coles B. Prophylactic cranial irradiation for preventing brain metastases in patients undergoing radical treatment for non-small-cell lung cancer: a Cochrane review. Int J Radiat Oncol Biol Phys. 2005;63(3):690–4.

Lev M, Nichols S. Computed tomographic angiography and computed tomographic perfusion imaging of hyperacute stroke. Top Magn Reson Imaging. 2000;11:283–7.

Levine P, Silberfarb P, Lipowski Z. Mental disorders in cancer patients: a study of 100 psychiatric referrals. Cancer. 1978;42:1385–91.

Li C, Shan S, Huang Q, et al. Initial stages of tumor cell-induced angiogenesis: evaluation via skin window chambers in rodent models. J Natl Cancer Inst. 2000;92:143–214.

Lieb W. Tumoren und tumorähnliche Läsionen der Orbita. HNO. 2010;58(7):661–71.

Likhterman LB. Clinical diagnosis of tumors of the cerebral hemispheres. Moscow: M Meditsina; 1979.

Lima P. Cerebral angiography. New York: Thieme-Stratton; 1950.

Lin N, Bellon J, Winer E. CNS metastases in breast cancer. J Clin Oncol. 2004;22(17):3608.

Lindblad P, Mellemgaard A, Schlehofer B, et al. International renal-cell cancer study. V. Reproductive factors, gynecologic operations and exogenous hormones. Int J Cancer. 1995;61:192–8.

Liotta L, Kohn E. Cancer's deadly signature. Nat Genet. 2003;33(1):10.

Liu H, Wang X, Zhou G, et al. Cancerous inhibitor of protein phosphatase 2A is overexpressed in cervical cancer and upregulated by human papillomavirus 16 E7 oncoprotein. Gynecol Oncol. 2011;122:430–6.

Ljungberg B, Campbell S, Choi H, et al. The epidemiology of renal cell carcinoma. Eur Urol. 2011;60:615–21.

Loevner L, Grossman R, Cohen J, et al. Microscopic disease in normal-appearing white matter on conventional MR images in patients with multiple sclerosis: assessment with magnetization transfer measurements. J Radiol. 1995;196:511–5.

Lonardo E, Cioffi M, Sancho P. Studying pancreatic cancer stem cell characteristics for developing new treatment strategies. J Vis Exp. 2015;(100):52801.

Lonnroth K, Castro K, Chakaya J, et al. Tuberculosis control and elimination 2010–50: cure, care, and social development. Lancet. 2010;375:1814–29.

Loshakov VA. Intracranial metastatic tumors. In: Konovalov AN, editors. Clinical neurology, part 1; vol 3, 2005. p. 402–408.

Loshakov VA. Intrakranial'nye metastaticheskie opukholi: klinicheskaya nevrologiya pod redaktsiei. Konovalova AN M. 2005;II(1):402–8. (russian)

Loudyi A, Samlowski W. Brain metastasis in renal cell carcinoma patients. Chapter 6. In: Hayat MA, editor. Tumors of the central nervous system, vol. 3. Dordrecht: Springer; 2011.

Lowther E, Whitlow C, Maldjian J. Clinical applications of ASL brain perfusion imaging, chapter 14. In: Saremi F, editor. Perfusion imaging in clinical practice. A multimodality approach to tissue perfusion analysis. New York: Wolters Klumer; 2015. p. 240–61.

Lu S, Ahn D, Johnson G, et al. Peritumoral diffusion tensor imaging of high-grade gliomas and metastatic brain tumors. Am J Neuroradiol. 2003;24(5):937–41.

Luna A, Vilanova J, da Cruz LC Jr, et al. Functional imaging in oncology clinical applications, vol 2. Berlin Heidelberg: Springer; 2014. p. 1478.

Lwu S, Goetz P, Monsalves E, et al. Stereotactic radiosurgery for the treatment of melanoma and renal cell carcinoma brain metastases. Oncol Rep. 2013;29(2):407–12.

Lynes W, Bostwick D, Freiha F, et al. Parenchymal brain metastases from adenocarcinoma of prostate. Urology. 1986;28:280–7.

Lyons R, Andriole V. Fungal infections of the CNS. Neurol Clin. 1986;4(1):159–70.

Mac GE. Surgical treatment of cerebral metastases from lung cancer. The effect on quality and duration of survival. Neurosurgery. 1971;35:416–20.

Mafee M, Dorodi S. Sarcoidosis of the eye, orbit and central nervous system: role of MR imaging. Radiol Clin N Am. 1999;37:73–87.

Mahajan A, Borden J, Tsai J-S. Carcinomatous meningitis: are surgery or gamma knife radiosurgery treatment risk factors? J Neurosurg. 2002;97(5):441–4.

Maiuri F, Iaconetta G, Gallicchio B, et al. Intraoperative sonography for spinal tumors: correlations with MR findings and surgery. J Neurosurg Sci. 2000;44:115–22.

Mandybur T. Intracranial hemorrhage caused by metastatic tumors. Neurology. 1977;27(7):650–5.

Mansfield P, Grannel P. NMR diffraction in solids. J Phys C Solid State Phys. 1973;6:422–6.

Mansfield P, Mandsley A. Medical imaging by NMR. Br J Radiol. 1973;50:188–94.

Mansfield P. Multi-planar image-formation using NMR spin echoes. J Phys C Solid State Phys. 1977;10:55–8.

Marin F, Kovacs K, Scheithauer B, et al. The pituitary gland in patients with breast carcinoma: a histological and immunocytochemical study of 125 cases. Mayo Clin Proc. 1992;67:949–56.

Markesbery W, Brooks W, Gupta G, et al. Treatment for patients with cerebral metastases. Arch Neurol. 1978;35:754–6.

Marshall M, Butler K, Pearson T, et al. Low incidence of asymptomatic brain metastases in patients with renal cell carcinoma. Urology. 1990;36:300–2.

Martinez-Manas R, Brell M, Rumia J, et al. Brain metastases in endometrial carcinoma. Gynecol Oncol. 1998;70:282–4.

Martínez-Mañas R, Brell M, Rumià J, et al. Brain metastases in endometrial carcinoma. Gynecol Oncol. 1998;70(2):282–4.

Martino L, Martino F, et al. Renal metastases from pancreatic adenocarcinoma. Arch Ital Urol Androl. 2004;76(1):37–9.

Martynov BV, Gaidar BV, Shchigolev YS, et al. Metastatic brain tumor. In: Practical neurosurgery: guidelines for physicians. St Petersburg: Gippokrat; 2002. p. 476–84.

Martynov YS, Idrisova MI. Brain involvement in lung cancer. J Neuropathol Psychiatry Korsakov. 1981;11:1601–6.

Martynyuk VV. Colon cancer (morbidity, mortality, risk factors, screening). In: Practical oncology: selected lectures. St. Petersburg; 2004. p. 151–61.

Maruyama I, Sadato N, Waki A, et al. Hyperacute changes in glucose metabolism of brain tumors after stereotaxic radiosurgery: a PET study. J Nucl Med. 1999;40:1085–90.

Mathews V, Alo P, Glass J, et al. AIDS-related CNS cryptococcosis: radiologic-pathologic correlation. Am J Neuroradiol. 1992;13:1477–86.

Matsko DE, Korshunova AG. Atlas of tumors of the central nervous system. In: SPb, editor, Russian Research Neurosurgical Institute n.a. prof. A.L. Polenov: St. Petersburg;1998. p. 277.

Matsumoto H, Yoshida Y. Brain metastasis from pancreatic cancer: a case report and literature review. Asian J Neurosurg. 2015;10(1): 35–9.

Matsumura T, Ohzato H, Yamamoto T, et al. A case of postoperative brain metastasis originated from pancreatic cancer which was successfully treated by resection and postoperative irradiation. Gan To Kagaku Ryoho Cancer Chemother. 2009;36:2433–5.

Matsuyama T, Tsukamoto N, Imachi M, et al. Bone metastasis from cervix cancer. Gynecol Oncol. 1989;32(1):72–5.

Maxwell M, Chir M, Phil D. Renal cell carcinoma: a rare source of cauda equina metastasis – case report. J Neurosurg. 1999;90(Spine 1):129–32.

Mayer R, Berkowitz R, Griffiths C. Central nervous system involvement by ovarian carcinoma: a complication of prolonged survival with metastatic disease. Cancer. 1978;41:776–83.

Mayor S. Cancer of unknown primary: a diagnostic and therapeutic dilemma. 2010. http://www.cancerworld.org/Articles/Issues/39/November-December-2010/e-Grand-Round/440/Cancer-of-unknown-primary-a-diagnostic-and-therapeutic-dilemma.html

Mayor S. Cancer of unknown primary: a diagnostic and therapeutic dilemma. 2015. http://www.cancerworld.org/Articles/Issues/39/November-December-2010/e-Grand-Round/440/Cancer-of-unknown-primary-a-diagnostic-and-therapeutic-dilemma.html

Mazzaferri E, Harmer K, Mallick U, et al. Practical management of thyroid cancer. A multidisciplinary approach. London: Springer; 2006. p. 440.

McCutcheon I, Eng D, Logothetis C. Brain metastasis from prostate carcinoma: ante-mortem recognition and outcome after treatment. Cancer. 1999;86:2301–11.

McDonald D, Choyke P. Imaging of angiogenesis: from microscope to clinic. Nat Med. 2003;9:713–25.

McWilliams R, et al. Melanoma-induced brain metastases. Expert Rev Anticancer Ther. 2008;8:743–55.

Mege D, Quassi M, Fuks D, et al. Patients with brain metastases from colorectal cancer are not condemned. Anticancer Res. 2013;33:5645–8.

Mehta M, Rodrigus P, Terhaard C, et al. Survival and neurologic outcomes in a randomized trial of motexafin gadolinium and whole-brain radiation therapy in brain metastases. J Clin Oncol. 2003;21:2529–36.

Mehta MP, Paleologos NA, Mikkelsen T, et al. The role of chemotherapy in the management of newly diagnosed brain metastases. J Neuro-Oncol. 2010;96(1):71–83.

Meier P, Zierler K. On the theory of the indicator-dilution measurement of blood flow and volume. J Appl Physiol. 1954;6:731–44.

Merseburger A, Merseburger A, Muller C, et al. A rare case of isolated prostate metastasis from primary pancreatic cancer. Urology. 2005;44(5):527–9.

Miles K, Charnsangavej C, Cuenod C. Multi-detector computed tomography in oncology CT perfusion imaging. London: Informa Helthcare; 2007.

Miller D, Grossman R, Reingold S, et al. The role of magnetic resonance techniques in understanding and managing multiple sclerosis. Brain. 1998;121:3–24.

Mintz A, Kestle J, Rathbone M, et al. A randomized trial to assess the efficacy of surgery in addition to radiotherapy in patients with a single cerebral metastasis. Cancer. 1996;8(7):1470–6.

Mintz A., Perry J, Cairncross G. Management of single brain metastases. Practice guideline report 9-1. 2004.

Mitomo M, Kawai R, Miura T, et al. Radiation necrosis of the brain and radiation-induced cerebrovasculopathy. Acta Radiol Suppl. 1986;369:227–30.

Mogila VV. The clinic, diagnosis and treatment of brain metastatic melanomas. Author's abstract of Cand. of Med. Sciences, Kiev; 1979. p. 21.

Moniz E. Arterial encephalography, its importance in the localization of cerebral tumors. Rev Neurol. 1927;2:72–89.

Moniz E. L'angiographie cerebrale. Paris: Masson; 1934.

Montero F, Ajuria E, Pereda G, et al. Cerebral metastasis, idiopathic pneumoperitoneum and obstructive jaundice as clinical manifestations of carcinoma of the pancreas. Rev Esp Oncol. 1983;30:399–409.

Mori Y, Kondziolka D, Flickinger J, et al. Stereotactic radiosurgery for cerebral metastatic melanoma: factors affecting local disease control and survival. Int J Radiat Oncol Biol Phys. 1998;42:581–9.

Moritani T, Hiwatashi A, Shrier D, et al. CNS vasculitis and vasculopathy: efficacy and usefulness of diffusion-weighted echoplanar MR imaging. Clin Imaging. 2004;28:261–70.

Motoyama S, Maruyama K, Sato Y. A case of recurrent malignant melanoma of esophagus responsive to combined chemotherapy, radiotherapy and cellular immunotherapy. Gan To Kadaku Ryoho Cancer Chemother. 2011;38(4):639–42.

Motzer R, Bacik J, Schwartz L, et al. Prognostic factors for survival in previously treated patients with metastatic renal cell carcinoma. J Clin Oncol. 2004;22(3):454–63.

Murase K. Dynamic contrast-enhanced perfusion CT: basic of mathematical tracer kinetic models and applications. Chapter 4. In: Saremi F, editor. Perfusion imaging in clinical practice. A multimodality approach to tissue perfusion analysis. New York: Wolters Klumer; 2015. p. 62–76.

Muscat J. The epidemiology of renal cell carcinoma. In: Bukowski RM, Novick AC, editors. Renal cell carcinoma: molecular biology, immunology, and clinical Management. Totowa: Human Press; 2000. p. 3–13.

Mut M. Surgical treatment of brain metastasis: a review. Clin Neurol Neurosurg. 2012;114(1):1–8.

Nakagami K, Nakagami K, Uchida T, et al. Increased choline kinase activity and elevated phosphocholine levels in human colon cancer. Jpn J Cancer Res. 1999;90:419–24.

Nakagawa H, Fujita T, Izumoto S, et al. Cis-diamminedichloroplatinum (CDDP) therapy for brain metastasis of lung cancer. I. Distribution within the central nervous system after intravenous and intracarotid infusion. J Neuro-Oncol. 1993;16(1):61–7.

Nakagawa H, Hagiwara Y, Yamada M, et al. Treatment of metastatic brain tumors from lung cancer: analysis of performance status between treatment methods. Neurol Surg. 1997;25(2):117–22.

Nakajima M, Irimura T, Nicolson G. Heparanases and tumor metastasis. J Cell Biochem. 1988;36:157–67.

Naskhletashvili DR. Primary and metastatic brain tumors. In: Davydova MI, Gorbunova VA, editors. Guideline "rational pharmacotherapy in oncology"; 2015. p. 552–9.

Naugler C, Xu Z. Pancreatic adenocarcinoma metastatic to the pineal gland. J Clin Neurosci. 2008;15(11):1284–6.

Navi B, Reichman J, Berlin D, et al. Intracerebral and subarachnoid hemorrhage in patients with cancer. Neurology. 2010;74(6):494–501.

NCCN (National Comprehensive Cancer Network) recommendations. 2015.

Nechipay EA, Dolgushin MB, Pronin IN, et al. DCE MRI in Differential Diagnosis of Primary and Secondary Brain Tumors. J Medical Imaging. 2015;4:18–30.

Nelson S, et al. Characterization of untreated gliomas: magnetic resonance spectroscopic imaging. Neuroimaging Clin N Am. 2002;12:599–613.

Nemeth A, Henson J, Mullins M, et al. Improved detection of skull metastasis with diffusion weighted MR imaging. Am J Neuroradiol. 2007;28(6):1088–92.

Nersesyants SI. On the issue of metastatic brain tumors and metastatic pathways.1951;3:25–30.

Nersesyants SI. Clinic and morphology of metastatic brain cancer: author's abstract of Cand. of Med. M Sciences. 1955.

Neubauer H, Platzer I, Mueller V, et al. Diffusion-weighted MRI of abscess formations in children and young adults. World J Pediatr. 2012;8(3):229–34.

Neumann H, Bausch B, McWhinney S, et al. Germ-line mutations in nonsyndromic pheochromatocytoma. N Engl J Med. 2002;346:1549–66.

Nicolson G, Menter D, Herrmann J, et al. Brain metastasis: role of trophic, autocrine, and paracrine factors in tumor invasion and colonization of the central nervous system. Curr Top Microbiol Immunol. 1996;213:89–115.

Nisce L, Hilaris B, Chu FC. A review of experience with irradiation of brain metastasis. Amer J Roentgenol. 1971;111(2):329–33.

Nieder C, Berberich W, Schnabel K. Tumor-related prognostic factors for remission of brain metastases after radiotherapy. Int J Radiat Oncol Biol Phys. 1997;39:25–30.

Nieder C, Grosu A, Mehta M. Brain metastases research 1990–2010: pattern of citation and systematic review of highly cited articles. Sci World J. 2012;2012:721598.

Nieder C, Marienhagen K, Thamm R, et al. Prediction of very short survival in patients with brain metastases from breast cancer. Clin Oncol. 2008;20:337–9.

Nieder C, Norum J, Stemland J, et al. Resource utilization in patients with brain metastases managed with best supportive care, radiotherapy and/or surgical resection: a markov analysis. Oncology. 2010;78(5–6):348–55.

Nieder C, Spanne O, Mehta M, et al. Presentation, patterns of care, and survival in patients with brain metastases: what has changed in the last 20 years? Cancer. 2011a;117(11):2505–12.

Nieder C, Spanne O, Nordoy T, et al. Treatment of brain metastases from renal cell cancer. Urol Oncol. 2011b;29(4):405–10.

Nugent JL, Bunn PA, Matthews MJ, et al. CNS metastases in small cell bronchogenic carcinoma: increasing frequency and changing pattern with lengthening survival. Cancer. 1979;44:1885–93.

Nussbaum E, Djalilian H, Cho K, et al. Brain metastases. Histology, multiplicity, surgery, and survival. Cancer. 1996;78(8):1781–8.

Ogava K, Yoshii Y, Aoki Y, et al. Treatment and prognosis of brain metastases from gynecological cancers. Neurol Med Chir (Tokyo). 2008;48(2):57–62.

Ogawa S, Horio Y, Yatabe Y, et al. Patterns of recurrence and outcome in patients with surgically resected small cell lung cancer. Int J Clin Oncol. 2012;17:218–24.

Ohtani T, Kurihara H, Ishiuchi S, et al. Brain tumour imaging with carbon-11-choline: comparison with FDG PET and gadolinium-enhanced MR imaging. Eur J Nucl Med. 2001;28:1664–70.

Oldberg E. Surgical considerations of carcinomatous metastases to the brain. JAMA. 1933;101:1458–61.

Olivecrona H, Tonnis W. Handbuch der Neurochirurgie. Bd.2. Roentgenologie von E. Stockholm: Lindgren; 1954.

Olsen K, Lewis J. Carcinoma ex pleomorphic adenoma: a clinicopathologic review. Head Neck. 2001;23:705–12.

Oneschuk D, Bruera E. Palliative management of brain metastases. Support Care Cancer. 1998;6(4):365–72.

Oppenheim H. Die h'lyasthenische Paraiyse (Bulbarpzu'alyse oline anatornischen Behind). Berlin: S. Karger; 1901.

Opstad K, Murphy M, Wilkins P, et al. Differentiation of metastases from high-grade gliomas using short echo time 1H spectroscopy. J Magn Reson Imaging. 2004;20:187–92.

Orrison W, Hart B. Intra-axial brain tumors. In: Neuroimaging. Philadelphia: WB Saunders Company; 2000. p. 583–611.

Ortega P, Malamud N, Shimkin MB. Metastasis to the pineal body. AMA Arch Pathol. 1951;52:518–28.

Osborn A. Brain diagnostic imaging. Salt Lake City: Amirsys; 2004. p. 936.

Osborn AG. Diagnostic neuroradiology. St. Louis: C.V. Mosby; 1994.

Osenbach R, Loftus C. Diagnosis and management of brain abscesses. Neurosurg Clin N Am. 1992;3:403–20.

Ostergaard L. Principles of cerebral perfusion imaging by bolus tracking. J Magn Reson Imaging. 2005;22(6):710–7.

Otegbayo J, Oluswasola O, Akere A, et al. Pancreatic carcinoma presenting as cutaneous nodules in a diabetic Nigerian male. West Afr J Med. 2005;24(2):180.

Ottaiano A, de Chiara A, Fazioli F, et al. Biological prognostic factors in adult soft tissue sarcomas. Anticancer Res. 2005;25:4519–26.

Owonikoko T, Zhang G, Deng X, et al. Poly (ADP) ribose polymerase enzyme inhibitor, veliparib, potentiates chemotherapy and radiation in vitro and in vivo in small cell lung cancer. Cancer Med. 2014;3(6):1579–94.

Ozawa Y, Omae M, Fujii M, et al. Management of brain metastasis with magnetic resonance imaging and stereotactic irradiation attenuated benefits of prophylactic cranial irradiation in patients with limited-stage small cell lung cancer. BMC Cancer. 2015;15:589.

Ozbayrak M, Ulus O, Berkman M, et al. Atypical pyogenic brain abscess evaluation by diffusion-weighted imaging: diagnosis with multimodality MR imaging. Jpn J Radiol. 2015;33(10):668–71.

Paches AI, Propp RM. Thyroid cancer. Moscow: M Medicine; 1995. p. 372.

Paches AI. Head and neck tumors. Moscow: M Medicine; 2000. p. 300.

Paches AI. Head and neck tumors. Moscow: M Medicine; 2000. p. 479.

Pacini F, Castagna M, Brilli L. Advances in the diagnosis and management of differentiated thyroid cancer. Thyroid disorders. Eur Endocrinol. 2008;4(2):100–2.

Pacini F, Ladenson P, Schlumberger M, et al. Radioiodine ablation of thyroid remnants after preparation with recombinant human thyrotropin in differentiated thyroid carcinoma: results of an international, randomized, controlled study. J Clin Endocrinol Metab. 2006;91:926–32.

Pack G, Ariel I. Tumors of the soft somatic tissues. New York: Hoeber-Harper; 1958.

Paek S, Audu P, Sperling M, et al. Reevaluation of surgery for the treatment of brain metastases: review of 208 patients with single or multiple brain metastases treated at one institution with modern neurosurgical techniques. Neurosurgery. 2005;56:1021–34.

Paget S. The distribution of secondary growths in cancer of the breast. Lancet. 1889;1:99–101.

Painter T, Chaljub G, Sethi R, et al. Intracranial and intraspinal meningeal melanocytosis. Am J Neuroradiol. 2000;21:1349–53.

Pal D, Bhattacharyya A, Husain M, et al. In vivo proton MR spectroscopy evaluation of pyogenic brain abscesses: a report of 194 cases. Am J Neuroradiol. 2010;31(2):360–6.

Papapolychroniadis C. Environmental and other risk factors for colorectal carcinogenesis. Tech Coloproctol. 2004;8(1):7–9.

Parashar B, Patro K, Smith M, et al. Role of radiation therapy for renal tumors. Semin Intervent Radiol. 2014;31(1):86–90.

Park K, Kim M, Park S, et al. Nervous system involvement by pancreatic cancer. J Neuro-Oncol. 2003;63:313–6.

Parker L, Wu S, Kim D, et al. Recurrence of papillary thyroid carcinoma presenting as a focal neurologic deficit. Arch Intern Med. 1986;146(10):1985–7.

Pasche B, Mulcahy M, Benson A. Molecular markers in prognosis of colorectal cancer and prediction of response to treatment. Best Pract Res Clin Gastroenterol. 2002;16:331–45.

Passik S, Ricketts P. Central nervous system tumors. In: Holland JC, editor. Psycho-oncology. New York: Oxford Press; 1998. p. 303–13.

Patanaphan V, Salaazar O. Colorectal cancer: metastatic patterns and prognosis. South Med J. 1993;86(1):38–41.

Patchell R, Tibbs P, Walsh J, et al. A randomized trial of surgery in the treatment of single metastases to the brain. N Engl J Med. 1990a;322:753–9.

Patchell R, Tibbs P, Walsh J, et al. A randomized trial of surgery in the treatment of single metastases to the brain. New Engl J Med. 1990b;322(8):494–500.

Patel N, Attwood K, Terrance M, et al. Comparative analysis of smoking as a risk factor among renal cell carcinoma histological subtypes. J Urol. 2015;194(3):640–6.

Patel T, Knisely J, Chiang V. Management of brain metastases surgery, radiation, or both? Hematol Oncol Clin N Am. 2012;26(4):933–47.

Patten R, Shuman W, Teefey S. Metastases from malignant melanoma to the axial skeleton: a CT study of frequency and appearance. AJR. 1990;155:109.

Paulino A, Nguyen T, Barker J, et al. Brain metastases in children with sarcoma, neuroblastoma and Willms' tumor. Int J Radiat Oncol Biol Phys. 2003;57:177–83.

Pectasides D, Pectasides M, Economopoulos T. Brain metastases from epithelial ovarian cancer: a review of the literature. Oncologist. 2006;11(3):252–60.

Peel R, Gnepp D. Diseases of the salivary glands. In: Surgical pathology of the head and neck. New York: Marcel Dekker; 1985. p. 533–645.

Pelletier E, Shim B, Goodman S, et al. Epidemiology and economic burden of brain metastases among patients with primary breast cancer: results from a US claims data analysis. Breast Cancer Res Treat. 2008;108(2):297–305.

Pemberton J. Malignant lesions of thyroid gland; a review of 774 cases. Surg Gynecol Obstet. 1939;69:417–30.

Peppiatt CM, Howarth C, Mobbs P, Attwell D. Bidirectional control of CNS capillary diameter by pericytes. Nature. 2006;443:700–4.

Pestalozzi B, Zahrieh D, Price K, et al. International Breast Cancer Study Group (IBCSG) Identifying breast cancer patients at risk for central nervous system (CNS) metastases in trials of the international breast cancer study group (IBCSG). Ann Oncol. 2006;17(6):935–44.

Peters S, Adjei A, Gridelli C, et al. Metastatic non-small-cell lung cancer (NSCLC): ESMO Clinical Practice Guidelines for diagnosis, treatment and follow-up. Ann Oncol. 2012;23(7):56–64.

Pfaffenroth E, Linchan W. Genetic basis for kidney cancer: opportunity for disease-specific approaches to therapy. Expert Opin Biol Ther. 2008;8(6):779–90.

Phuttharak W, Hesslink S, Wixon C. MR features of cerebral aspergillosis in an immunocompetent patient: correlation with histology and elemental analysis. Am J Neuroradiol. 2005;26:835–8.

Pieper D, Hess K, Sawaya R. Role of surgery in the treatment of brain metastases in patients with breast cancer. Ann Surg Oncol. 1997;4(6):481–90.

Piura E, Piura B. Brain metastases from endometrial carcinoma. ISRN Oncol. 2012;2012:13.

Pizzinni F, Smits M, Wesolowski R, et al. Arterial spin-labeled MR perfusion imaging techniques. Chapter 9. In: Saremi F, editor. Perfusion imaging in clinical practice a multimodality approach to tissue perfusion analysis. New York: Wolters Klumer; 2015. p. 149–81.

Pneumaticos SG, Savidou C, Korres DS, et al. Pancreatic cancer's initial presentation: Back pain due to osteoblastic bone metastasis. Eur J Cancer Care (Engl). 2009;19:137–40.

Poddubnaya IV. Achievements of modern chemotherapy. Sovrem Onkol. 2013;2(5):49.

Podoprigora AE, Pronin IN, Fadeeva LM, et al. Proton magnetic resonance spectroscopy in neuroradiology. J Med Imaging. 2001a;3:26–30.

Podoprigora AE, Klimchuk OV, Rodionov PV. Proton magnetic resonance spectroscopy: diagnosis of brain lesions of different etiology. In: Bersneva VP, Kondakova EN, editors. Polenovskie reading Scientific works of the conference of young neurosurgeons, vol. II. St Petersburg: Russian Research Neurosurgical Institute na prof AL Polenov; 2001b. p. 67.

Popovich M, Arthur R, Helmer E. CT of intracranial cryptococcosis. Am J Neuroradiol. 1990;11:139–42.

Posner J. Management of cerebral nervous system metastases. Semin Oncol. 1977;4(1):81–91.

Posner J. Neurologic complications of cancer, vol. 3–14. Philadelphia: F. A. Davis; 1995. p. 77–110.

Post M, Chan J, Hensley G, et al. Toxoplasma encephalitis in Haitian adults with HIV: a clinical-pathologic-CT correlation. AJR. 1983;140:861–8.

Post M, Floros J, Smith B, et al. Inhibition of lung maturation by monoclonal antibodies against fibroblast-pneumonocyte. Nature. 1984;308:284.

Potts D, Abbott G. National cancer institute study: evaluation of computed tomography in the diagnosis of intracranial neoplasm. III Metastatic tumors. Radiology. 1980;136:657–64.

Pronin IN, et al. The use of CT perfusion imaging in stereotactic biopsy of diffuse gliomas. In: Nevsky radiological forum. St Petersburg; 2005. p. 189.

Pronin IN, Kornienko VN, Fadeeva LM, et al. Diffusion-weighted images in the study of brain tumors and peritumoral edema. J Issues Neurosurgery. 2000;3:14–7.

Pronin IN, Kornienko VN, Podoprigora AE, et al. Comprehensive MR diagnosis of brain abscesses. J Issues Neurosurgery Burdenko. 2002;1:7–11.

Pronin IN, Turkin AM, Dolgushin MB, et al. Tissue contrast due to magnetic susceptibility: application in neuroradiology. J Med Imaging. 2011;2:4.

Provenzale J, McGraw P, Mhatre P, et al. Peritumoral brain regions in gliomas and meningiomas: investigation with isotropic diffusion weighted MR imaging and diffusion-tensor MR imaging. Radiology. 2004;232:451–60.

Pursell E, Toney H, Pound R. Resonance absorption by nuclear magnetic moments in a solid. Phys Rev. 1946;69:37–83.

Radinsky R, Aukerman S, Fidler I. The heterogeneous nature of metastatic neoplasms: relevance to biotherapy. In: Oldham RK, editor. Principles of cancer biotherapy. 3rd ed. Boston: Kluwer; 1998. p. 16–38.

Radley M, McDonald J, et al. Late solitary cerebral metastases from renal cell carcinoma: report of two cases. Surg J Neurol. 1993;39:230–4.

Ragayshene VN. Radiation therapy in the combination treatment of brain tumors. Autoref Dokt Diss Obninsk. 1985;37.

Raman R, Vaena D. Immunotherapy in metastatic renal cell carcinoma: a comprehensive review. Biomed Res Int. 2015;2015:8.

Ramazanova MS, Kislichko AG. Small cell lung cancer: the effectiveness of different treatment regimens, long-term results and prognosis. Kazan Med J. 2012;93(4):623–7.

Ramirez de Molina A, Rodriguez-Gonzalez A, Gutierrez R, et al. Overexpression of choline kinase is a frequent feature in human tumorderivedcell lines and in lung, prostate, and colorectal human cancers. Biochem Biophys Res Commun. 2002;296(3):580.

Reichenbach J. High resolution blood oxygenation level dependent MR venography (HRVG): a new technique. Neuroradiology. 2001;43:364–9.

Remler M, Marcussen W, Tiller-Borsich J. The late effects of radiation on the blood brain barrier. Int J Radiat Oncol Biol Phys. 1986;12:1965–9.

Rhodes A, Weistock M, Fitzpatrick T, et al. Risk factors for cutaneous melanoma. A practical method of recognizing predisposed individuals. JAMA. 1987;258(2):3146.

Richstone L, Scherr D, Reuter V, et al. Multifocal renal cortical tumors: frequency, associated clinicopathological features and impact on survival. J Urol. 2004;171(2, part 1):615–20.

Ries L, Melbert D, Krapcho M, et al. SEER cancer statistics review. 1975–2005. National Cancer Institute: Bethesda; 2008. Available from http://seer.cancer.gov/csr/1975-2005

Rigel D, Carucci J, et al. Malignant melanoma: prevention, early detection and treatment in the 21st century. CA Cancer J Clin. 2000;50:215–30.

Rink P. Magnetic resonance in medicine. Translation by prof. E.I. Fedin. Oxford: Blackwell; 2003.

Riquet M, Manac'h D, Dujon A, et al. Place of radical surgery in the treatment of non-small cell lung cancer. Apropos of 969 cases. Cancer Radiother. 1997;1(2):165–9.

Roberts T. Physiologic measurements by contrast-enhanced MR imaging: evaluate expectations and limitations. J Magn Reson Imaging. 1997;7:82–90.

Robertson E. Pneumoencephalography. Springfield: Charles C. Thomas; 1967.

Robinson B, Lewis R. Myocardial metastases from carcinoma of pancreas presenting as acute myocardial infarction. J R Soc Med. 1982;75(7):560–2.

Rodriguez-Galindo C, Pappo A, Kaste S, et al. Brain metastases in children with melanoma. Cancer. 1997;79:2440–5.

Rohren E, Provenzale J, Barboriak D, et al. Screening for cerebral metastases with FDG-PET in patients undergoing whole body of non-central nervous system malignancy. Radiology. 2003; 226(1):181–7.

Romodanov AP, Zozulya YA, Sosov YD. Metastatic brain tumor. Kyiv; 1973. p. 192.

Romodanov AP, Zozulya YA, Sosov YD. Metastatic brain tumor. Kyiv; 1973.

Rootman J, Robertson W. Tumors. In: Rootman J, editor. Diseases of the orbit. Philadelphia: JB Lippincott; 1988. p. 231.

Roser F, Rosahl S, Samii M. Single cerebral metastasis 3 and 19 years after primary renal cell carcinoma: case report and review of the literature. J Neurol Neurosurg Psychiatry. 2002;72(2):257–8.

Rosner D, Nemoto T, Lane W. Chemotherapy induces regression of brain metastases in breast carcinoma. Cancer. 1986;58(4):832–9.

Rossi S, Trinidad C, Luna A. Lung cancer: PET, perfusion CT, functional MR imaging. In: Luna A, et al., editors. Functional imaging in oncology: clinical applications, vol. 2. Berlin: Springer; 2014. p. 723–49.

Rowley H, Scialfa G, Gao P, et al. Contrast-enhanced MR imaging of brain lesions: a large-scale intraindividual crossover comparison of gadobenate dimeglumine versus gadodiamide. Am J Neuroradiol. 2008;29:1684–91.

Rubino G, King W, Quinn B, et al. Primary pineal melanoma: case report. Neurosurgery. 1993;33(3):511–5.

Rudà R, Borgognone M, Benech F, Vasario E, Soffietti R. Brain metastases from unknown primary tumor. J Neurol. 2001;248:394–8.

Rudas MS, Nasnikova IY, Matyakin GG. Positron emission tomography in clinical practice. Moscow: Teaching aid; 2007. p. 46.

Ruhlmann J, Oehr P, Biersack H. PET in oncology. Basics and clinical application. Berlin Heidelberg: Springer; 1999. p. 203.

Russell D, Rubinstein L. Pathology of tumors of the nervous system. 5th ed. Baltimore: Williams and Wilkins; 1989. p. 470.

Russell D. Who puts the tubercle in tuberculosis? Nat Rev Microbiol. 2007;5:39–47.

Ryabukha DO. Clinical and diagnostic features of cerebral metastases. Author Diss Cand Med Nauk, Rostov-on-Don. 2010;24.

Said A, Raufman J-P, Xie G. The role of matrix metalloproteinases in colorectal cancer. Cancers. 2014;6:366–75.

Saitoh H. Distant metastasis of renal adenocarcinoma. Cancer. 1981;48:1487–91.

Salvati M, Cervoni L, Celli P. Solitary brain metastases from thyroid carcinoma: study of 6 cases. Tumori. 1995;81:142–3.

Salvati M, D'Elia A, Frati A, et al. Sarcoma metastatic to the brain: a series of 35 cases and considerations from 27 years of experience. J Neuro-Oncol. 2010;98(3):373–7.

Salvati M, Frati A, Rocchi G, et al. Single brain metastasis from thyroid cancer: report of twelve cases and review of the literature. J Neuro-Oncol. 2001;51(1):33–40.

Sancho-Chust J, Ferreres J, et al. Pulmonary tumor embolism as an initial manifestation of pancreatic adenocarcinoma. Respir Care. 2009;54(12):1732–5.

Santy K, Nan P, Chantana Y, et al. The diagnosis of brain tuberculoma by (1)H-magnetic resonance spectroscopy. Eur J Pediatr. 2011;170(3):379–87.

Saparadin A, Bronstein M, Saparadin S. Prevalence of patient misperseptions regarding melanoma. Dermatology. 2012;66(4):AB147.

Saremi F. Perfusion imaging in clinical practice. A multimodality approach to tissue perfusion analysis. New York: Wolters Klumer; 2015. p. 592.

Sawaya R, Ribalta R, Fuller G. Brain metastases: histopathological evaluation and diagnostic pitfalls, Chapter 4. In: Sawaya R, editor. Intracranial metastases current management strategies: Blackwell; 2004.

Schackert G, Sobottka S, Steinmetz A, et al. Current treatment strategies in brain metastases. Onkologie. 2000;23:98–104.

Schellinger P, Meinck H, Thron A. Diagnostic accuracy of MRI compared to CCT in patients with brain metastases. J Neuro-Oncol. 1999;44(3):275–81.

Schneider G, Siveke J, Eckel F, et al. Pancreatic cancer: basic and clinical aspects. Gastroenterology. 2005;128:1606–25.

Schouten L, Rutten J, Huveneers H, et al. Incidence of brain metastases in a cohort of patients with carcinoma of the breast, colon, kidney, lung and melanoma. Cancer. 2002;94:2698–705.

Schroth G, Gawehn J, Thron A, et al. Early diagnosis of herpes simplex encephalitis by MRI. Neurology. 1987;37:179–83.

Schuster J, Rostomily R, Hahn C, et al. Two cases of esophageal carcinoma metastatic to the pineal region with a review of the literature. Surg Neurol. 1998;49:100–3.

Scott B, Kesari S. Leptomeningeal metastases in breast cancer. Am J Cancer Res. 2013;3(2):117–26.

Scott BJ, Oberheim-Bush NA, Kesari S. Leptomeningeal metastasis in breast cancer – a systematic review. Oncotarget. 2016;7(4): 3740–7.

Semiglazov VF, Semiglazov VV, Kletse AE. Non-invasive and invasive breast cancer. St. Petersburg; 2006. p. 349.

Sen M, Demiral AS, Cetingoz R, et al. Prognostic factors in lung cancer with brain metastasis. Radiother Oncol. 1998;46:33–8.

Setoodeh R, Hakam A, Shan Y. Cerebral metastasis of cervical cancer, report of two cases and review of the literature. Int J Clin Exp Pathol. 2012;5(7):710–4.

Seyedin S, Geffen D. All About cancer of unknown primary March 17, 2014. http://www.oncolink.org/cancers/miscellaneous-other-diseases/carcinoma-of-unknown-primary/all-about-cancer-of-unknown-primary.

Shakur S, Bit-Ivan E, Watkin W. Multifocal and multicentric glioblastoma with leptomeningeal gliomatosis: a case report and review of the literature. Case Rep Med. 2013;2013:132679.

Shangaĭ V, Gavrik I. Metastasis of pancreatic cancer to the brain. (Article in Russian). Vrach Delo. 1984;11:77–9.

Shaw E, Scott C, Souhami L, et al. Single dose radiosurgical treatment of recurrent previously irradiated primary brain tumors and brain metastases: final report of RTOG protocol 90–05. Int J Radiat Oncol Biol Phys. 2000;47(2):291–8.

Sheehan J, Kondziolka D, Flickinger J. Radiosurgery for patients with recurrent small cell lung carcinoma metastatic to the brain: outcomes and prognostic factors. J Neurosurg. 2005;102(Suppl): 247–54.

Sheehy J, Crockard H. Multiple meningiomas: a long-term review. J Neurosurg. 1983;59:1–5.

Shetty P, Moiyadi A, Pantvaidya G, et al. Cystic metastasis versus brain abscess: role of MR imaging in accurate diagnosis and implications on treatment. J Can Res Ther. 2010;6:356–8.

Shinoura N, Nishijima M, Hara T, et al. Brain tumors: detection with C-11 choline PET. Radiology. 1997;202(2):497–503.

Shiroishi M, Castellazzi G, Boxerman J, et al. Principles of T2*-weighted dynamic susceptibility contrast MRI technique in brain tumor imaging. J Magn Reson Imaging. 2015;41:296–313.

Shlifer IG. Radiology. V I. Head. Gosmedizdat: Kiev; 1941.

Shus AV. Optimization of diagnostic and treatment tactics in multifocal renal cancer. Intern Med J. 2003;9(3):95–7.

Shweiki D, Itin A, Soffer D, et al. Vascular endothelial growth factor induced by hypoxia may mediate hypoxia-initiated angiogenesis. Nature. 1992;359:843–5.

Siegel R, Miller K, Jemal A. Cancer statistics. CA Cancer J Clin. 2016;66(1):7–30.

Sierra A, Price J, Garcia-Ramirez M. Astrocyte-derived cytokines contribute to the metastatic brain specificity of breast cancer cells. Lab Investig. 1997;77(4):357–68.

Sierra T, Nguyen L, Mascitelli J, et al. Brain metastasis from uterine serous carcinoma: a case report and review of literature. Gynecol Oncol Rep. 2015;11:34–7.

Skvortsova TY, Brodskaya ZL, Gurchin AF. Possibilities of positron emission tomography c 11S-methionine in the recognition pseudoprogression of cerebral gliomas after combination treatment. J Issues Neurosurgery. 2014;78(4):50–8.

Slack B, Richardson U, Nitsch R, et al. Dioctanoylglycerol stimulates accumulation of [methyl-14C]choline and its incorporation into acetylcholine and phosphatidylcholine in a human cholinergic neuroblastoma cell line. Brain Res. 1972;585:169–76.

Slotman B, Faivre-Finn C, Kramer G, et al. Prophylactic cranial irradiation in extensive small-cell lung cancer. N Engl J Med. 2007;357(7):664–72.

Smedby K, Brandt L, Backlund M, et al. Brain metastases admissions in Sweden between 1987 and 2006. Br J Cancer. 2009;101(11):1919–24.

Smirnov LI. Tumors of the brain and spinal cord. Moscow: Medgiz; 1962.

Snee M, Rodger A. Brain metastases from carcinoma of breast: a review of 90 cases. Clin Radiol. 1985;33:365–7.

Soffietti R, Ruda R, Mutani R. Management of brain metastases. J Neurol. 2002;249:1357–69.

Soga J. Endocrinocarcinomas (carcinoids and their variants) of the duodenum. An evaluation of 927 cases. J Exp Clin Cancer Res. 2003;22:349–63.

Som P, Brandwein M. Salivary glands: anatomy and pathology. In: Som PM, Curtin HD, editors. Head and neck imaging. St Louis: Mosby; 2003. p. 2067–76.

Som P, Shugar J, Sacher M, et al. Benign and malignant parotid pleomorphic adenomas: CT and MR studies. J Comput Assist Tomogr. 1988;12:65–9.

Song Z, Lin B, Shao L, et al. Brain metastases from esophageal cancer: clinical review of 26 cases. World Neurosurg. 2014;81:131–5.

Sorensen A, Reimer P. Cerebral MR perfusion imaging: principles and current applications. New York: Thieme; 2000.

Spencer H. Pathology of the lung cancer, vol. 799. 3rd ed. New York: Pergamon Press; 1977.

Sperduto P, Berkey B, Gaspar L, et al. A new prognostic index and comparison to three other indices for patients with brain metastases: an analysis of 1960 patients in the RTOG database. Int J Radiat Oncol Biol Phys. 2008;70:510–4.

Sperduto P, Kased N, Roberge D, et al. Summary report on the graded prognostic assessment: an accurate and facile diagnosis-specific tool to estimate survival for patients with brain metastases. J Clin Oncol. 2012a;30(4):419–25.

Sperduto P, Kased N, Roberge D, et al. Effect of tumor subtype on survival and the graded prognostic assessment for patients with breast cancer and brain metastases. Int J Radiat Oncol Biol Phys. 2012b;82:2111–7.

Stark A, Tscheslog H, Buhl R, et al. Surgical treatment for brain metastases: prognostic factors and survival in 177 patients. Neurosurg Rev. 2005;28:115–9.

Stark A. Neurosurgical treatment for brain metastases: clinical features, operative strategies, recurrence and survival. In: Tumors of central nervous system, vol. 12. Dordrecht: Springer; 2011. p. 301–11.

Starkey J, Moritani T, Kirby P. MRI of CNS fungal infections: review of aspergillosis to histoplasmosis and everything in between. Clin Neuroradiol. 2014;24:217–30.

Steblov EM, Mandelbeym NV. Changes in the cellular composition of cerebrospinal fluid in metastatic brain tumors. J Nevropatol Psikhiatr. 1962;4:529–36.
Steeg P. Targeting metastasis. Nat Rev Cancer. 2016;16:201–18.
Stehlin J, Clark R. Melanoma of the extremities: experiences with conventional treatment and perfusion in 339 cases. Am J Surg. 1965;110(3):366–83.
Stehlin J, Hilis W, Rifino C. Disseminated melanoma. Arch Surg. 1965;94:495–501.
Steliarova-Foucher E, Parkin D. Cancer registration in Europe. In: Razum O, Spallek J, Reeske A, Arnold M, editors. Migration-sensitive cancer registration in Europe. Challenges and potentials. Frankfurt: Peter Lang Verlag; 2011.
Stelzer K. Epidemiology and prognosis of brain metastases. Surg Neurol Int. 2013;4(4):192–202.
Stortebecker T. Metastatic tumors of the brain from a neurosurgical point of view: a follow-up study of 158 cases. Neurosurgery. 1954;11:84–111.
Strauss L, Conti P. The application of PET in clinical oncology. J Nucl Med. 1991;32:623–47.
Sundaresan N, Galicich J. Surgical treatment of brain metastases: clinical and computerized tomography evaluation of the results of treatment. Cancer. 1985;55:1382–138.
Sundelof M, Ye W, Dickman P, et al. Improved survival in both histologic types of oesophageal cancer in Sweden. Int J Cancer Med J. 2010;26(341):6280.
Sutton M, Watkins H, Green L, et al. Intracranial metastases as the first manifestation of prostate cancer. Urology. 1996;48:789–93.
Sze G, Brant-Zawadzki M, Norman D, et al. The neuroradiology of AIDS. Semin Roentgenol. 1987;12:42–53.
Sze G, Johnson C, Kawamura Y, et al. Comparison of single- and triple-dose contrast material in the MR screening of brain metastases. Am J Neuroradiol. 1998;19:821–8.
Sze G, Johnson E, Heier L. Detection of brain metastases: comparison of contrast-enhanced MR with unenhanced MR and enhanced CT. Am J Neuroradiol. 1990;11:785–91.
Sze G, Zimmermann R. The MRI of infections and inflammatory diseases. Radiol Clin N Am. 1988;26:839–59.
Takahara T, Imai Y, Yamashita T, et al. Diffusion weighted whole body imaging with background body signal suppression (DWIBS): technical improvement using free breathing, STIR and high resolution 3D display. Radiat Med. 2004;22:275–82.
Takakura K, Sano K, Hojo S, et al. Metastatic tumors of the central nervous system. Tokyo: Igaku-Shoin; 1982. p. 5–35.
Takamori H, Kanemitsu K, et al. Metastatic gastric tumor secondary to pancreatic adenocarcinoma. J Gastroenterol. 2005;40(2):209–12.
Tan H, Chen L, Guan Y, et al. Comparison of MRI, F-18 FDG, and ^{11}C-choline PET/CT for their potentials in differentiating brain tumor recurrence from brain tumor necrosis following radiotherapy. Clin Nucl Med. 2011;36(11):978–81.
Tan W, Ho K, Eu K. Brain metastases in colorectal cancers. World J Surg. 2009;33:817–21.
Tasdemiroglu E, Patchell R. Cerebral metastases in childhood malignancies. Acta Neurochir. 1997;139:182–7.
Tatagiba M, Boker D, Brandis A, et al. Meningeal melanocytoma of the C8 nerve root: case report. Neurosurgery. 1992;31:945–7.
Tatsuno S, Hata Y, Tada S. Double-dose Gd-DTPA: detectability of intraparenchymal brain metastasis (in Japanese). Nippon Igaku Hoshasen Gakkai Zasshi. 1996;56:855–9.
Taylor G, Nathanson I. Lymph node metastases. New York: Oxford University Press; 1942.
Temple D, Ledesma E, Mittelman A. Cerebral metastases. From adenocarcinoma of the colon and rectum. NY State J Med. 1982;82:1812–4.
Tevaarwerk A, et al. Survival in patients with metastatic recurrent breast cancer after adjuvant chemotherapy: little evidence of improvement over the past 30 years. Cancer. 2013;119:1140–8.
Thackray A, Lucas R. Tumors of the major salivary glands. In: Atlas of tumor pathology. Washington: Armed Forces Institute of Pathology; 1983. p. 107–11.
Tien R, Chu P, Hesselink J, et al. Intracranial cryptococcosis in immunocompromised patients: CT and MR findings in 29 cases. Am J Neuroradiol. 1991;12:283–9.
Tikhtman A, Patchell R. Brain metastasis. In: Morantz R, Walsh J, editors. Brain tumors. New York: Marcel Dekker; 1995. p. 553–6.
Tiraspolskaya MM. Some findings on the morphological diversity of melanomas. Arch Pathol. 1975;37(8):75–7.
Tiwari A, Kumar N, Bajpai R, et al. Bone metastasis from ovarian cancer. J Cancer Res Ther. 2007;3:34–6.
Tofts P, Brix G, Buckley D, et al. Estimating kinetic parameters from dynamic contrast-enhanced T(1)-weighted MRI of a diffusible tracer: standardized quantities and symbols. Magn Reson Imaging. 1999;10(3):223–32.
Tofts P, Kermode A. Measurement of the blood–brain barrier permeability and leakage space using dynamic MR imaging. 1. Fundamental concepts. Magn Reson Med. 1991;17:357–67.
Tofts P. Quantitative MRI of the brain. Chichester: Wiley; 2004. p. 633.
Tokumaru A, O'Uchi T, Eguchi T, et al. Prominent meningeal enhancement adjacent to meningioma on Gd-DTPA enhanced MR images: histopathologic correlation. Radiology. 1990;175:431–3.
Tomiak A, Chu Q, Kocha W, et al. Effect of brain metastasis presentation on survival of small cell lung cancer. ASCO, 2001, abstract 1277. 2001.
Tomita N, Kodaira T, Tachibana H, et al. Helical tomotherapy for brain metastases: dosimetric evaluation of treatment plans and early clinical results. Technol Cancer Res Treat. 2008;7(6):417–24.
Toro J, et al. Incidence patterns of soft tissue sarcomas, regardless of primary site, in the surveillance, epidemiology and end results program, 1978–2001: an analysis of 26,758 cases. Int J Cancer. 2006;119(12):2922–30.
Tourdias T, Rodrigo S, Oppenheim C, et al. Pulsed arterial spin labeling applications in brain tumors: practical review. J Neuroradiol. 2008;35:79–89.
Trachtenberg AKH. Lung cancer. Moscow: M Medicine; 1987. p. 304.
Tremont-Lukats I, Bobustuc G, Lagos G, et al. Brain metastasis from prostate carcinoma. Cancer. 2003;98:363–8.
Tsuda K, Tsurushima H, Takano S, et al. Brain metastasis from papillary thyroid carcinomas. Mol Clin Oncol. 2013;1(5):817–9.
Turiaf J, Battesti J, Basset F, et al. Metastatic pleurisy in pancreatic cancer with the presence of considerable quantities of amylase in the pleural effusion and a major paraneoplastic peripheral neurologic syndrome. Ann Med Interne. 1969;120(6):449–58.
Turkin AM, Belov TV. Using three-dimensional reconstruction in neuroradiology. In: Neuroimaging: selected articles (2000–2007). Moscow: Andreeva TM; 2000. p. 256.
Ushakov VS, Ivanov SV. Laryngeal cancer: modern possibilities and prospects. Pract Oncol. 2003;4(1):56–0.
Vaalavirta L, Rasulova N, Partanen K, et al. [18F]-estradiol PET/CT imaging in breast cancer patients. J Diag Imag Ther. 2014;1(1):59–72.
Valdina EA. Thyroid disorders. Guidelines. 3rd ed. St. Petersburg: Peter; 2006. p. 368.
van der Ree TC, Dippel D, Avezaat C. Leptomeningeal metastasis after surgical resection of brain metastases. J Neurol Neurosurg Psychiatry. 1999;66:225–7.
van Eck J, Go K, Ebels E. Metastatic tumors of the brain. Psychiatr Neurol Neurochir. 1965;68:443–62.
Vannucci R, Baten M. Cerebral metastatic disease in childhood. Neurology. 1974;24:981–5.
Vanpouille C, Le Jeune N, Kryza D, et al. Influence of multidrug resistance on (18)F-FCH cellular uptake in a glioblastoma model. Eur J Nucl Med Mol Imaging. 2009;36(8):1256–64.
Vansteenkiste J, Stroobants S. FDG-PET scan in potentially operable non-small cell lung cancer: do anatomical PET-CT fusion images improve the localization of regional lymph node metastases? Eur J Nucl Med. 1998;25:1495–501.

Vecht C, Haaxma-Reiche H, Noordijk E, et al. Treatment of single brain metastasis: radiotherapy alone or combined with neurosurgery? Ann Neurol. 1993;33(6):583–90.
Vecht C. Clinical management of brain metastasis. J Neurol. 1998;245(3):127–31.
Verlato G, Di L, Rossi G, et al. Epidemiology of gastric cancer and screening programs. In: de Manzoni G, Roviello F, Siquini W, editors. Surgery in the multimodal management of gastric cancer. Mailand: Springer; 2012. p. 300.
Verma R, Singh P, Kumar A, et al. Cranial aspergilloma masquerading as meningioma. BMJ Case Rep. 2013; doi:10.1136/bcr-2012-008118.
Vikhert AM, Galil-Ogly GA, Poroshin KK. The atlas of diagnostic skin biopsies. Moscow: M Medicine; 1973. p. 173.
Villà S, Weber D, Moretones C, et al. Validation of the new graded prognostic assessment scale for brain metastases: a multicenter prospective study. Radiat Oncol. 2011;6:23.
Vlodavsky I, Friedmann Y. Molecular properties and involvement of heparanase in cancer metastasis and angiogenesis. J Clin Invest. 2001;108(3):341–7.
Vogel I, Soeth E, Roder C, et al. Multivariable analysis reveals RT-PCR-detected tumor cells in the blood and/or bone marrow of patients with colorectal carcinoma as an independent prognostic factor. Ann Oncol. 2000;11(4):43.
Vogel I, Soeth E, Ruder C, et al. Disseminated tumor cells in the blood and or bone marrow of patients with colorectal carcinoma are an independent prognostic factor. Ann Oncol. 2000;1. Abstr. 183
Vogl TJ, Friebe CE, Balzer T, et al. Diagnosis of cerebral metastasis with standard dose gadobutrol vs. a high dose protocol: intraindividual evaluation of a phase II high dose study (in German). Radiologe. 1995;35:508–16.
Vokes E, Weichselbaum R, Lippman S, et al. Head and neck cancer. N Engl J Med. 1993;328(3):184–95.
Vuong D, Rades D, Vo S, et al. Extracranial metastatic patterns on occurrence of brain metastases. J Neuro-Oncol. 2011;105(1):83–90.
Wafflart E, Gibaud H, Lerat F, et al. Muscular metastases of cancer of the pancreas. J Chir. 1996;133(4):167–70.
Walker A, Robins M, Weinfeld F. Epidemiology of brain tumors: the national survey of intracranial neoplasms. Neurology. 1985;35:219–26.
Wang S, Kim S, Chawla S, et al. Differentiation between glioblastomas, solitary brain metastases, and primary cerebral lymphomas using diffusion tensor and dynamic susceptibility contrast-enhanced MR imaging. Am J Neuroradiol. 2011;32:507–14.
Wang Z, Fernández-Seara M, Alsop D, et al. Assessment of functional development in normal infant brain using arterial spin labeled perfusion MRI. NeuroImage. 2008;39(3):973–8.
Warren S, Meyer R. Lymph node metastasis of sarcoma. Am J Pathol. 1938;XIV:605–19.
Webb WR, Muller NL, Naidich D. High-resolution CT of the lung. Philadelphia: Lippincott Williams & Wilking; 2001. p. 259–355.
Weidner N. Intratumoral microvessels density as a prognostic in cancer. Am J Pathol. 1995;147:9–19.
Weidner N. Tumoural vascularity as a prognostic factor in cancer patients: the evidence continues to grow. J Pathol. 1998;184(2):119–22.
Weinberg J, Suki D, Hanbali F, et al. Metastasis of esophageal carcinoma to the brain. Cancer. 2003;98:1925–33.
Weisberg L. Computerized tomographic findings in intracranial metastatic malignant melanoma. Comput Radiol. 1985;9(6):365–72.
Weissman D. Glucocorticoid treatment for brain metastases and epidural spinal cord compression: a review. J Clin Oncol. 1988;6:543–51.
Werner M, Burger P, Heinz E, et al. Intracranial atherosclerosis following radiotherapy. Neurology. 1988;38(7):1158–60.
Wester H, Herz M, Weber W, et al. Synthesis and radiopharmacology of O-(2-[18F]fluoroethyl)-L-tyrosine for tumor imaging. J Nucl Med. 1999;40:205–12.
Wetzel S, Cha S, Johnson G, et al. Relative cerebral blood volume measurements in intracranial mass lesions: interobserver and intraobserver reproducibility study. Radiology. 2002;224:797–803.
Whiteman M, Bowen B, Post M, Bell M. Intracranial infection. In: Atlas W, editor. MRI of the brain and spine. Philadelphia: Lippincott Williams & Wilkins; 2002. p. 1099–175.
Wikman H, Lamszus K, Detels N, et al. Relevance of PTEN loss in brain metastasis formation in breast cancer patients. Breast Cancer Res. 2012;14(2):R49.
Willis R. The spread of tumors in the human body. 2nd ed. London: Butterworth; 1952.
Wintermark M, et al. Admission perfusion CT: prognostic value in patients with severe head trauma. Radiology. 2004;232: 211–20.
Wolf R, Detre J. Clinical neuroimaging using arterial spin-labeled perfusion magnetic resonance imaging. Neurotherapeutics. 2007;4:346–59.
Worni M, Guller U, White R, et al. Modest improvement in overall survival for patients with metastatic pancreatic cancer: a trend analysis using the surveillance, epidemiology, and end results registry from 1988 to 2008. Pancreas. 2008;42:1157–63.
Wronski M, Arbit E, Bilsky M, et al. Resection of brain metastases (BMET) from breast cancer (BRC): retrospective review of 70 patients (Meeting abstract). Proc An Meet ASCO 1996;15:A165.
Wroński M, Arbit E, Russo P, et al. Surgical resection of brain metastases from renal cell carcinoma in 50 patients. Urology. 1996;47(2):187–93.
Wyss MT, Spaeth N, Biollaz G, et al. Uptake of ^{18}F-Fluorocholine, ^{18}F-FET, and ^{18}F-FDG in C6 gliomas and correlation with ^{131}I-SIP(L19), a marker of angiogenesis. J Nucl Med. 2007;48(4):608–14.
Yakhno NN, Shtulman DR. Diseases of the nervous system: Guidelines for physicians in 2 volumes. V. 2. Moscow: M Medicine; 2001. p. 480.
Yamada K, Miura M, Miyayama H, et al. Brain metastases from asymptomatic adenocarcinoma of the pancreas: an autopsy case report. Surg Neurol. 2002;58(5):332–6.
Yamada K, Murakami M, Kuroda Y. Treatment results of brain metastasis from breast cancer: course of the disease and radiation therapy. Nippon Igaku Hoshasen Gakkai Zasshi. 1997;57(1):34–40.
Yamaguchi N, Yamashima T, Yamashita J. A histological and flow cytometric study of dog brain endothelial cell injuries in delayed radiation necrosis. J Neurosurg. 1991;74:625–32.
Yamaguchi S, Nagasawa H, Suzuki T, et al. Sarcomas of the oral and maxillofacial region: a review of 32 cases in 25 years. Clin Oral Investig. 2004;8(2):52–5.
Yamasaki F, Kurisu K, Satoh K, et al. Apparent diffusion coefficient of human brain tumors at MR imaging. Radiology. 2005; 235:985–91.
Yanagawa T, Saito K, Takagishi K. Risk factors for lymphatic metastasis of malignant bone and soft-tissue tumors: a retrospective cohort study of 242 patients. Medicine. 2014;93(27):1–5.
Yancik R, Ries L. Cancer in older persons: an international issue in an aging world. Semin Oncol. 2004;31(2):128–36.
Yano S, Shinohara H, Herbst R, et al. Expression of vascular endothelial growth factor is necessary but not sufficient for production and growth of brain metastasis. Cancer Res. 2000;60:4959–67.
Yap C, Schiepers C, Fishbein M, et al. FDG-PET imaging in lung cancer: how sensitive is it for bronchioloalveolar carcinoma? Eur J Nucl Med Mol Imaging. 2002;29(9):1166–73.
Yawn B, Wollin P, Schroeder C. Temporal and gender-related trends in brain metastases from breast and lung cancer. Minn Med. 2003;86:32–7.
York J, Stringer J, Ajani J, et al. Gastric cancer and metastasis to the brain. Ann Surg Oncol. 1999;6:771–6.
Yoshida K, Gage F. Cooperative regulation of nerve growth factor synthesis and secretion in fibroblasts and astrocytes by fibroblast growth factor and other cytokines. Brain Res. 1992;569: 14–25.
Yoshida S. Brain metastasis in patients with esophageal carcinoma. Surg Neurol. 2007;67:288–90.

Yuh W, Engelken J, Muhonen M, et al. Experience with high-dose gadolinium MR imaging in the evaluation of brain metastases. Am J Neuroradiol. 1992;13:335–45.

Yurin AG. Epidemiology, new in classification of kidney cancer. Arch Pathol. 2007;69(1):49–54.

Zaitsev A, Kurzhupov M, Potapova E, Kirsanova. On the treatment of metastatic brain lesions. Sci Pract Res J Pract Med. 2015;2(2):8–14.

Zakaria R, Das K, Radon M, et al. Diffusion-weighted MRI characteristics of the cerebral metastasis to brain boundary predicts patient outcomes. BMC Med Imag. 2014;14:26.

Zakharova NE, Kornienko VN, Potapov AA, et al. Neuroimaging of structural and hemodynamic abnormalities in brain injury. Moscow; 2013. p. 156.

Zakharova NE, Pronin IN, Potapov AA, et al. Quantitative and qualitative assessment of the brain conductive pathways using diffusion tensor magnetic resonance imaging in normal and diffuse axonal injuries. J Radiat Diagn Ther. 2012;3(3):92–108.

Zayats RG, Rachkovskaya IV, Karpov IA. Fundamentals of general and medical parasitology. Rostov-on-Don: Fenix; 2002. p. 224.

Zedeler K, Keiding N, Kamby C. Differential influence of prognostic factors on the occurrence of metastases at various anatomical sites in human breast cancer. Stat Med. 1992;11(3):281–94.

Zhang M, Olsson Y. Hematogenous metastases of the human brain - Characteristics of peritumoral brain changes: a review. J Neuro-Oncol. 1997;35(1):81–9.

Zhuravlev KV, Barchuk AS, Wagner RI, et al. Prophylactic lymphadenectomy in melanomas of lower extremities. Issues Oncol. 1994;45(1):59–64.

Zimm S, Wampler G, Stablein D. Intracerebral metastases in solid-tumor patients: natural history and results of treatment. Cancer. 1981;48(2):384–94.

Zimmenmann R, Bilaniuk L, Sze G. Intracranial infection. In: Brant-Zawadzki M, Norton D, editors. MRI of the central nervous system. New York: Raven; 1987. p. 235–57.

Index

M. Dolgushin et al., *Brain Metastases*, https://doi.org/10.1007/978-3-319-57760-9

D